Cancer and Immunotherapy

Cancer and Immunotherapy

Editor: Meaghan Crockett

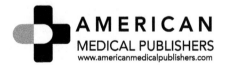

AMERICAN
MEDICAL PUBLISHERS
www.americanmedicalpublishers.com

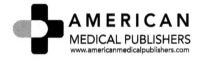

Cataloging-in-Publication Data

Cancer and immunotherapy / edited by Meaghan Crockett.
   p. cm.
Includes bibliographical references and index.
ISBN 978-1-63927-950-0
1. Cancer. 2. Cancer--Immunotherapy. 3. Immunotherapy.
4. Cancer--Treatment. I. Crockett, Meaghan.
RC271.I45 C36 2023
616.994 061--dc23

American Medical Publishers,
41 Flatbush Avenue,
1st Floor, New York,
NY 11217, USA

ISBN 978-1-63927-950-0 (Hardback)

Contents

Permissions

List of Contributors

Index

Preface

Immunotherapy refers to a treatment that utilizes immune system of the body to fight disease. This therapy has the capability to transform and boost the manner in which the immune system works, in order to find and attack cancer cells in the body. Various types of immunotherapy are utilized for treatment of cancer, such as immune system modulators, immune checkpoint inhibitors, treatment vaccines, T-cell transfer therapy and monoclonal antibodies. It can be administered in different ways, including intravesical, intravenous, topical and oral methods. Immunotherapy is a biological therapy, as it uses substances to treat cancer that are created from living organisms. However, it can have side effects, which can occur when the immune system has received the boost to fight against the cancer cells and it also attacks the healthy tissues and cells in the human body. This book unravels the recent studies on cancer and immunotherapy. The readers would gain knowledge that would broaden their perspective in this area of medicine.

This book is the end result of constructive efforts and intensive research done by experts in this field. The aim of this book is to enlighten the readers with recent information in this area of research. The information provided in this profound book would serve as a valuable reference to students and researchers in this field.

At the end, I would like to thank all the authors for devoting their precious time and providing their valuable contribution to this book. I would also like to express my gratitude to my fellow colleagues who encouraged me throughout the process.

Editor

Tryptophan Metabolism in Inflammaging: From Biomarker to Therapeutic Target

Freek J. H. Sorgdrager [1,2,3,4], *Petrus J. W. Naudé* [3,5], *Ido P. Kema* [4], *Ellen A. Nollen* [1] *and Peter P. De Deyn* [2,3,6*]

[1] European Research Institute for the Biology of Ageing, University Medical Center Groningen, University of Groningen, Groningen, Netherlands, [2] Laboratory of Neurochemistry and Behavior, Department of Biomedical Sciences, Institute Born-Bunge, University of Antwerp, Antwerp, Belgium, [3] Department of Neurology and Alzheimer Center, University Medical Center Groningen, University of Groningen, Groningen, Netherlands, [4] Department of Laboratory Medicine, University Medical Center Groningen, University of Groningen, Groningen, Netherlands, [5] Department of Molecular Neurobiology, Groningen Institute for Evolutionary Life Sciences (GELIFES), University of Groningen, Groningen, Netherlands, [6] Department of Neurology, Memory Clinic of Hospital Network Antwerp (ZNA) Middelheim and Hoge Beuken, Antwerp, Belgium

Correspondence:
Peter P. De Deyn
p.p.de.deyn@umcg.nl

Inflammation aims to restore tissue homeostasis after injury or infection. Age-related decline of tissue homeostasis causes a physiological low-grade chronic inflammatory phenotype known as inflammaging that is involved in many age-related diseases. Activation of tryptophan (Trp) metabolism along the kynurenine (Kyn) pathway prevents hyperinflammation and induces long-term immune tolerance. Systemic Trp and Kyn levels change upon aging and in age-related diseases. Moreover, modulation of Trp metabolism can either aggravate or prevent inflammaging-related diseases. In this review, we discuss how age-related Kyn/Trp activation is necessary to control inflammaging and alters the functioning of other metabolic faiths of Trp including Kyn metabolites, microbiota-derived indoles and nicotinamide adenine dinucleotide (NAD^+). We explore the potential of the Kyn/Trp ratio as a biomarker of inflammaging and discuss how intervening in Trp metabolism might extend health- and lifespan.

Keywords: tryptophan, aging, inflammation, kynurenine, inflammaging, tryptophan 2,3-dioxygenase (TDO), indoleamine 2,3 dioxygenases (IDO)

INFLAMMAGING: CHRONIC INFLAMMATION THAT DRIVES THE AGING PROCESS

Inflammation is initiated by the innate immune system in response to mechanical, infectious, or metabolic tissue stress and aims to restore homeostasis by eliminating damaged cells (1). Aging is characterized by progressive decline of tissue homeostasis resulting from damaged cellular components and aberrant functioning of damage-response mechanisms (2).

Age-related changes of the innate immune system are common and include shifts in the composition of immune cell populations, altered secretory phenotypes and impaired signaling transduction (3). These changes are paralleled by the development of a chronic inflammatory state referred to as *inflammaging*. This is characterized by an imbalance between pro- and anti-inflammatory responses and fluctuations of inflammatory cytokines, such as interleukin-6 (IL-6), high-sensitive C reactive protein (hsCRP), IL-10 and tissue growth factor beta (TGF-β) (4, 5). The rate of inflammaging, quantified by measuring these markers, is strongly associated with age-related disability, disease and mortality (6). It is theorized that inflammaging is driven by endogenous ligands released upon age-related tissue damage and can be aggravated by food excess and attenuated by caloric restriction, suggesting relevant cross-talk between metabolic and immune functioning (7).

Understanding how inflammaging is controlled could aid in the development of diagnostic and therapeutic tools for many age-related diseases associated with inflammation such as cancer, atherosclerosis, diabetes mellitus, and Alzheimer's disease. Tryptophan (Trp) metabolism is associated with aging and produces metabolites that control inflammation, regulate energy homeostasis and modulate behavior (8). We discuss how activation of Trp metabolism could be involved in the control of inflammaging and how this can alter the Trp metabolite milieu. We hypothesize on how this could impact health- and lifespan and how interfering with Trp metabolism could be used in the treatment of neurodegenerative diseases.

ACTIVATION OF TRYPTOPHAN METABOLISM REGULATES INFLAMMATION

Inflammation Activates Tryptophan Metabolism

The essential amino acid Trp fuels the synthesis of kynurenine (Kyn), serotonin (5-HT) and indoles (9, 10). The Kyn pathway of Trp is the most active pathway of Trp metabolism and produces metabolites including kynurenic acid and nicotinamide adenine dinucleotide (NAD$^+$). The Kyn pathway is initiated by the enzymes tryptophan 2,3-dioxygenase (TDO) and indoleamine 2,3-dioxygenase (IDO and IDO2). In this review, we focus on the role of IDO1, which we refer to as IDO. Expression of TDO and IDO (and other enzymes in the Kyn pathway) is species-, cell type-, and context-specific (11–13).

While IDO plays a minor role in Trp metabolism under normal circumstances, IDO-dependent Trp metabolism is strongly activated in response to interferons and other cytokines that are released upon inflammation (14). Interferon gamma (IFN-γ) is considered the most potent IDO-activating cytokine and induces expression in a variety of cell types after it binds to the IDO promotor-region. The effect of IFN-γ on IDO activation is best-characterized in macrophages and dendritic cells (DCs) but is also evident in connective (e.g., fibroblast) and epithelial tissue (e.g., pulmonary, renal, gastro-intestinal, and vascular) (15–19).

Other inflammatory signals that activate IDO include lipid mediators such as prostaglandin E2 (PGE2) and pathogen particles such as lipopolysaccharides (LPS) (20). In addition, while the regulation of IDO is often transcriptional, specific mediators of inflammation induce post-transcriptional and post-translational modifications that either promote ubiquitination and proteasomal degradation of IDO or sustain its activity through phosphorylation (21, 22).

Inflammation-related IDO activity is often measured by the Kyn/Trp ratio in blood in diseases characterized by excessive or chronic inflammation including infections, auto-immune disorders, cardiovascular disease, and cancer (23).

Activation of Tryptophan Metabolism Has Anti-inflammatory and Immunosuppressive Effects

Trp metabolism controls hyperinflammation and induces long term immune tolerance. These effects pivot on the ability of IDO to alter the local and systemic Kyn/Trp balance (**Figure 1A**). This balance directly affects metabolic and immune signaling pathways that drive an anti-inflammatory response in IDO-competent cells (e.g., antigen-presenting cells and epithelial cells). In addition, it changes the function of neighboring cells (e.g., T cells) by creating a local (and sometimes systemic) environment high in Kyn and low in Trp. Several molecular pathways mediate immune and non-immune responses to changes in intracellular Trp and Kyn levels (**Figure 1B**).

Trp Depletion in the Metabolic Regulation of Inflammation and Tolerance

Trp levels influence nutrient sensing systems such as the general control non-derepressable 2 (GCN2) stress kinase and mechanistic target of rapamycin complex 1 (mTORC1). The kinase GCN2 is activated during amino acid depletion (or imbalance) and causes phosphorylation of eukaryotic initiation factor (eIF)2α that has cell-type specific effects on translation. mTORC1 is active during amino acid sufficiency and governs anabolic metabolism and energy expenditure. GCN2 and mTORC1 are implicated in the metabolic control of inflammation by immune and non-immune cells (24).

Trp depletion activates GCN2 in IDO-expressing dendritic cells and macrophages causing them to produce anti-inflammatory cytokines including interleukin-10 (IL-10) and TGF-β instead of immunogenic cytokines (25, 26). Additionally, Trp depletion can alter the secretory phenotype of neighboring IDO-incompetent dendritic cells, cause GCN2-dependent differentiation and recruitment of regulatory T cells (T$_{reg}$) (27, 28) and prevent T cell activation and proliferation (25). These concepts seem to be involved in providing tolerance to apoptotic cells in the spleen (26, 29). However, the role of IDO/GCN2-signaling is not limited to immune cells. In an antibody-induced model for glomerulonephritis in mice, which is lethal in mice lacking *IDO* expression, IDO/GCN2 signaling limited inflammatory tissue damage by inducing autophagy in renal epithelial cells (15). Taken together, these studies indicate that IDO can prevent inflammation and promote tolerance in a context-specific manner by regulating GCN2 activity in immune and non-immune cells.

mTORC1 is a central regulator of cellular function. Cells of the innate immune system largely depend on mTORC1 to enable the metabolic transition that is required for their activation (30). mTORC1 orchestrates the cellular immune behavior in response to extracellular and intracellular factors such as inflammatory stimuli, glucose availability and amino acid sufficiency. *In vitro* studies showed that IFN-γ inhibited mTORC1 by depleting cellular Trp levels in IDO-expressing cells (31) causing suppression of mTORC1 co-localization to the lysosome and altering the metabolic functioning of human primary macrophages (32). The relevance of IDO/mTORC1

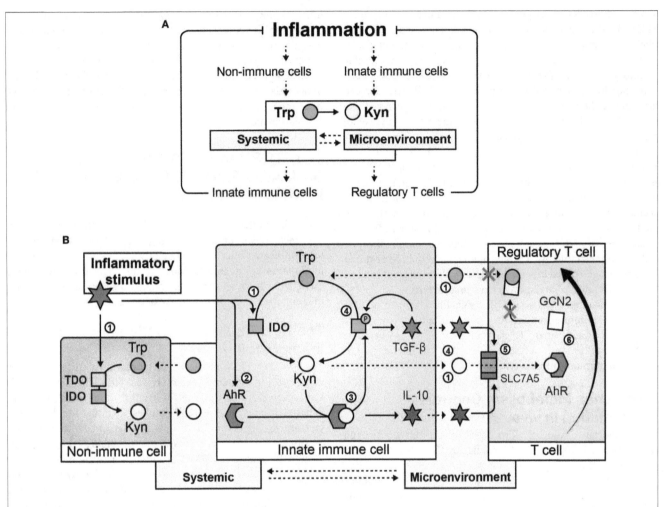

FIGURE 1 | Mechanisms involved the regulation of inflammation by Trp metabolism. Inflammation activates Trp metabolism and causes systemic and intra- and extra-cellular changes in the Kyn/Trp ratio that suppress the inflammatory response **(A)**. The molecular steps involved in the immunomodulatory effect of activation of Trp metabolism **(B)**: An inflammatory stimulus activates IDO (and in specific instances TDO) in immune and non-immune cells causing reduced Trp systemic and local Trp levels and increased intra- and extracellular Kyn content (1); inflammation induces increased expression of AhR (2) that is activated by its ligand Kyn and results in the secretion of anti-inflammatory cytokines such as IL-10 (3); AhR ligand-activation causes phosphorylation of IDO and results in sustained IDO activity and the secretion of TGF-β, which is involved in a feedback loop by inducing IDO phosphorylation (4); inflammatory cytokines such as TGF-β and IL-10 induce the amino acid transporter SLC7A5 on the plasma membrane of naïve T-cells causing transport of Kyn into the T cell (5); activation of GCN2 by Trp depletion and AhR ligand-activation by Kyn cause the differentiation of naïve T cells toward regulatory T cells (6). Solid arrows indicate regulatory (transcriptional or translational) and enzymatic effects, dashed arrows indicate active or passive cross-cellular and cross-compartmental transport of Trp and Kyn. Trp, Tryptophan; Kyn, Kynurenine, IDO, indoleamine 2,3-dioxygenase; TDO, tryptophan 2,3-dioxygenase; AhR, aryl hydrocarbon receptor; TGF-β, tissue growth factor beta; IL-10, interleukin 10; SLC7A5, solute carrier family 7 member 5; GCN2, general control non-derepressable 2 stress kinase.

signaling in controlling inflammation *in vivo* is yet to be established.

Future studies are needed to determine how the cellular Trp content is regulated in response to exogenous and endogenous inflammatory stimuli and how Trp levels affect GCN2 and mTORC1 signaling to determine the metabolic control of inflammation *in vivo*.

Kyn Activates the Aryl Hydrocarbon Receptor

Activated Trp metabolism results in increased Kyn production. The role of Kyn in the regulation of inflammation is largely mediated through its function as a ligand of the aryl hydrocarbon receptor (AhR), a transcription factor that controls local and

systemic immune responses. Recent studies are suggesting that Kyn/AhR signaling is involved in the generation of T_{reg} cells and the modulation of the immune phenotype of DCs.

T_{reg} cells are derived from naïve T cells and are involved in maintenance of immunological tolerance but also aid macrophages during the resolution of inflammation by stimulating them to secrete anti-inflammatory cytokines (33) and aging is associated with increased T_{reg} populations in immune and non-immune tissue (34). Kyn supplementation can activate AhR in naïve T cells in the presence of specific inflammatory cytokines and directly drive T_{reg} differentiation (35). Although Kyn passes relatively easily across the cell membrane of most cell types, recent data suggest that Kyn-dependent AhR activation in

T cells requires Kyn transport across the amino acid transporter SLC7A5, which is expressed upon T cell activation (36). DCs play an essential role in creating the microenvironment that is required for T_{reg} differentiation. To do so, DCs take on a specific secretory phenotype that is also driven by Kyn-dependent AhR activation by Nguyen et al. (37). Interestingly, AhR activation can also induce the expression of *IDO,* suggesting a Kyn/AhR/IDO feedback loop that is possibly involved in the maintenance of an immunosuppressive phenotype in DCs (38).

IDO function in DCs seems to be sustained by phosphorylation caused either by a chaperone of AhR that is released upon Kyn binding (39) or through autocrine TGF-β and NF-κB dependent signaling (22). In the latter study, IDO seemed to act through a non-catalytic mechanism. In both studies, IDO phosphorylation sustained the immunomodulatory phenotype of DCs necessary for long-term tolerance to inflammatory stimuli. As this type of tolerance could be required to dampen age-related inflammation, it would be of great interest to study IDO phosphorylation in aged immune tissue.

To conclude, IDO/Kyn/AhR signaling can modulate the innate immune system to create an anti-inflammatory microenvironment that is favorable for the generation of T_{reg} cells and critical for the maintenance of long-term immunosuppression.

Tryptophan Metabolism Controls Inflammation *in vivo*

The important role of Trp metabolism in controlling inflammation is highlighted by studies in IDO deficient mice. These mice show no apparent inflammatory phenotype or auto-immune disorders (within controlled, pathogen-free laboratory facilities). Yet, when confronted with an inflammatory stimulus they develop severe inflammatory diseases. These include pulmonary infections in response to stem cell transplantation (40), antibody-induced renal inflammation (15), auto-immunity in response to chronic exposure to apoptotic cells (29), severe colitis in response to 2,4,6-trinitrobenzene sulfonic acid (17), aggravation of hepatic inflammation in response to a high-fat diet (41) and aggravation of hypercholesterolemia-related atherosclerosis (42). Of note, IDO-deficiency protected from inflammation in a mouse model of chronic gastric inflammation by modulating B cell immunity and suppressing cytotoxicity of natural killer cells (43). The fact that IDO seems to control inflammation in response to so many non-infectious stimuli including metabolic stress, underlines its function as a general regulator of inflammation and suggests that it could be involved in the regulation of inflammaging.

Other Tryptophan Metabolites Involved in Inflammation

Other Trp metabolites are also involved in the control of inflammation and tissue damage. Examples of this include serotonin, implicated in intestinal inflammation (44); kynurenic acid, which exerts anti-inflammatory changes in adipose tissue (45); 3-hydroxyanthranilic acid and cinnabarinic acid (two other Kyn metabolites) that are, respectively, connected to vascular

inflammation (46) and autoimmune encephalomyelitis (47); NAD$^+$, which prevents renal kidney injury (48, 49) and regulates macrophage immune responses (50); and indoles, crucially involved in gastro-intestinal and neuronal inflammation (51).

Although a discussion of the specific roles of these metabolites in age-related inflammation is outside the scope of this review, it is important to consider the broad role of Trp metabolism in inflammation.

TRYPTOPHAN METABOLISM AS A BIOMARKER AND THERAPEUTIC TARGET IN INFLAMMAGING

There is limited evidence of a direct, mechanistic, role of Trp metabolism in inflammaging. Yet, observational studies have indicated that Trp metabolism could be a biomarker for inflammaging. In addition, Trp metabolism could provide therapeutic targets to treat age-related diseases associated with inflammation and possibly even extend lifespan.

The Kyn/Trp Ratio as a Biomarker for Inflammaging

The Kyn/Trp ratio, measured in blood, is robustly associated with aging in humans (**Table S1**) (52–60). The fact that this association is already evident in healthy young adults (61) and persists throughout life (56), implies that the age-dependent increase in the Kyn/Trp ratio is not secondary to the onset of disease but rather represents a physiological age-related change. In addition, markers of immune activation are, already in young adults, strongly associated with the Kyn/Trp ratio (62). Taken together, these observational data suggests that the Kyn/Trp ratio could provide a valuable marker for the rate of (physiological) inflammaging.

As inflammaging is involved in the onset of age-related diseases, a marker for inflammaging should also predict the onset of age-related diseases. This is the case for the Kyn/Trp ratio. For example, an increased Kyn/Trp ratio was found to be associated with increased frailty (63), reduced cognitive performance (64), increased risk of cardiovascular disease (65, 66) and mortality (56, 66) in aged individuals. Other Kyn metabolites, including the 3-hydroxyanthranilic acid/anthranilic acid ratio and kynurenic acid, have also been associated with inflammation and poor outcome in the context of (age-related) diseases of the brain (67, 68).

The Kyn/Trp ratio—and potentially other Kyn pathway metabolites—could thus be valuable readouts of the rate of physiological inflammaging in healthy individuals and predict the onset of age-related diseases associated with chronic inflammation. In addition, the Kyn/Trp ratio meets the criteria for a biological age biomarker (as opposed to chronological age) (69). As a single biomarker is seldomly able to predict complex biological processes, the use of the Kyn/Trp ratio in the prediction of inflammaging and biological aging should be validated in concordance with other potential biomarkers of aging preferably in combination with immune markers for sustained inflammation [e.g., GlycA (70)]. These studies should

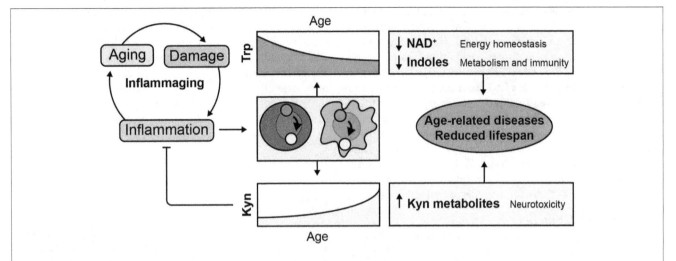

FIGURE 2 | Implications of inflammaging-dependent shunt of Trp metabolism. Age-related decline of tissue homeostasis causes a physiological low-grade chronic inflammatory phenotype known as inflammaging. We hypothesize that Trp is metabolized toward the Kyn pathway in order to control age-related inflammation. Consequent disturbances of Trp and Kyn metabolites could be involved in age-related diseases and reduced lifespan.

ideally address intraindividual variability of such markers by making use of longitudinal study designs.

Consequences of Kyn/Trp Shunt in Inflammaging

An inflammaging-related shunt of Trp metabolism toward extrahepatic Kyn production could impact the functioning of Trp metabolites in a range of organs during aging (**Figure 2**).

Indoles in Gastro-Intestinal and Metabolic Functioning

The microbiome is increasingly recognized to play an important role in aging and age-related disease (71). Indoles are microbiota-derived Trp metabolites that are implicated in immune regulation and affect gastro-intestinal functioning (51). A recent paper showed that dietary-induced obesity increased intestinal IDO activity shifting Trp metabolism toward the production of Kyn and away from microbiota-derived metabolites (72). Inhibition of IDO in the gut improved insulin sensitivity and resulted in reduced chronic inflammation. In addition, age-related changes to the microbiome were associated with increased expression of enzymes involved in microbial Trp metabolism (73). These data highlights the importance of microbiota-dependent Trp metabolism and suggest that activation of intestinal IDO and age-related changes in microbiome composition can deplete the body of health-promoting indoles while affecting the systemic Kyn/Trp balance. In addition, it provides relevant evidence that links metabolic inflammation (metaflammation) to gastro-intestinal Trp metabolism and metabolic health. In this context, it is interesting to note that Trp metabolites and indoles are emerging as modulators of adipose tissue homeostasis and obesity (45, 74, 75). Age-related gastro-intestinal metaflammation could thus cause metabolic disturbances through altering microbiome and host Trp metabolism.

De novo NAD+ Synthesis in Age-Related Tissue Decline

The liver metabolizes the majority of Trp in a TDO-dependent manner producing NAD+ or acetoacetyl-CoA (9). NAD+ is a coenzyme and cosubstrate for several important regulatory proteins involved in cellular metabolism and damage such as sirtuins and Poly(ADP-ribose) polymerases (PARPs). NAD+ can be generated *de novo* from Trp or through salvage pathways. While *in vitro* the contribution of *de novo* NAD+ synthesis is limited, *in vivo* NAD+ is actively synthesized *de novo* from Trp, especially in the liver and the kidney (76).

Declining cellular NAD+ content is a cross-species phenotype of aging that is associated with a range of age-related diseases (77). Boosting *de novo* synthesis of NAD+ from Trp in the liver—by blocking acetoacetyl-CoA production—improved hepatic function and inflammation in mice on a high fat diet through modulation of mitochondrial function (78). Similarly, increasing *de novo* synthesis of NAD+ was protective in mouse models of renal damage (49, 78) and restored age-related functional decline of macrophages (50). These recent studies underline the relevance of *de novo* NAD+ synthesis in modulating health and lifespan by regulating mitochondrial function in metabolically active tissue such as immune cells and the liver. Inflammaging could shunt Trp metabolism toward extrahepatic tissue and possibly contribute to age-related hepatic NAD+ deficits, providing new evidence for theories that link age-related inflammation and metabolic dysfunction (7).

Peripheral Trp Metabolism as a Target for Neurodegenerative Diseases

TDO2 and *IDO* expression in the brain is low and restricted to specific brain regions. Trp metabolism in the brain is therefore largely dependent on transport of Trp and Kyn across the blood-brain barrier. Modulating peripheral Trp metabolism can thus alter the functioning of Trp and Trp metabolites in the brain

(13). In mouse models of Alzheimer's disease and Huntington's disease peripheral inhibition of the Kyn pathway prevented neurodegeneration and memory-deficits (79, 80). Similarly, inhibition of TDO was neuroprotective in fly and worm models of Alzheimer's and Parkinson's disease (81–83). Although the mechanisms that underlie these findings are largely unknown and are difficult to study due to cell type-specific expression of Kyn pathway enzymes in the brain, they could involve a direct effect on protein aggregation, altered immune responses, changed mitochondrial function, or variations in levels of kynurenic acid–a modulator of neurotransmission (13). In addition, the long-term activation of AhR potentially contributes to vascular aging, which is a known risk factor for neurodegenerative diseases (84).

Trp in the Regulation of Lifespan

Evidence from studies in *Caenorhabditis elegans* and rodents suggests that targeting Trp metabolism could extend lifespan. For example, we showed that knockdown of *tdo-2* in *C. elegans* increased lifespan with ~15% (83). This effect was dependent on *daf-16*, the *C. elegans* homolog of the forkhead box protein O (FOXO) family of transcription factors. Accordingly, TDO inhibition and Trp feeding extended lifespan in other studies in a daf-16-dependent manner (85, 86).

In rats Trp content in liver, kidney and brains decreases with age while Kyn content in these organs increases (87). A study across 26 mammalian species showed that the Kyn/Trp ratio in the liver of healthy adult animals was associated with species-specific maximum lifespan (88); species that showed a higher Kyn/Trp ratio were shorter lived.

As TDO inhibitors are readily available and TDO knockout mice are viable, these models could be used to study the effects of TDO inhibition on lifespan. However, caution should be warranted as inhibition of Trp metabolism could aggravate immune responses upon inflammatory stimuli (not present in a laboratory context) and may lead to an exacerbated inflammatory environment during inflammaging, which could have dire consequences on health. In addition, failure of recent clinical trials with IDO inhibitors in cancer have underlined that a more thorough understanding of the physiological functions of the Kyn pathway is needed to successfully target the Kyn pathway in disease (10).

CONCLUSION

Trp metabolism regulates inflammation, energy homeostasis, and brain functioning. Age-related chronic inflammation—inflammaging—shunts Trp metabolism toward its immunomodulatory catabolite Kyn. Alterations of other Trp metabolites, as a consequence of this adaptive anti-inflammatory mechanism, could drive aging and underlie pathophysiology of age-related diseases. Future studies should address the value of Trp metabolism as a biomarker for (un)healthy aging and as drug target for inflammaging-related disease.

AUTHOR CONTRIBUTIONS

FS managed the literature searches and wrote the first draft of the manuscript. PN, IK, EN, and PD critically reviewed the manuscript.

REFERENCES

1. Medzhitov R. Origin and physiological roles of inflammation. *Nature.* (2008) 454:428–35. doi: 10.1038/nature07201
2. López-Otín C, Blasco MA, Partridge L, Serrano M, Kroemer G. The hallmarks of aging. *Cell.* (2013) 153:1194–217. doi: 10.1016/j.cell.2013.05.039
3. Shaw AC, Goldstein DR, Montgomery RR. Age-dependent dysregulation of innate immunity. *Nat Rev Immunol.* (2013) 13:875–87. doi: 10.1038/nri3547
4. Franceschi C, Bonafè M, Valensin S, Olivieri F, De Luca M, Ottaviani E, et al. Inflamm-aging. An evolutionary perspective on immunosenescence. *Ann N Y Acad Sci.* (2000) 908:244–54. doi: 10.1111/j.1749-6632.2000.tb06651.x
5. Franceschi C, Garagnani P, Vitale G, Capri M, Salvioli S. Inflammaging and 'Garb-aging.' *Trends Endocrinol Metab.* (2017) 28:199–212. doi: 10.1016/j.tem.2016.09.005
6. Fulop T, Witkowski JM, Olivieri F, Larbi A. The integration of inflammaging in age-related diseases. *Semin Immunol.* (2018) 40:17–35. doi: 10.1016/j.smim.2018.09.003
7. Franceschi C, Garagnani P, Parini P, Giuliani C, Santoro A. Inflammaging: a new immune–metabolic viewpoint for age-related diseases. *Nat Rev Endocrinol.* (2018) 14:576–90. doi: 10.1038/s41574-018-0059-4
8. Cervenka I, Agudelo LZ, Ruas JL. Kynurenines: tryptophan's metabolites in exercise, inflammation, and mental health. *Science.* (2017) 357:eaaf9794. doi: 10.1126/science.aaf9794
9. Bender DA. Biochemistry of tryptophan in health and disease. *Mol Aspects Med.* (1983) 6:101–97. doi: 10.1016/0098-2997(83)90005-5
10. Platten M, Nollen EAA, Röhrig UF, Fallarino F, Opitz CA. Tryptophan metabolism as a common therapeutic target in cancer, neurodegeneration and beyond. *Nat Rev Drug Discov.* (2019) 18:379–401. doi: 10.1038/s41573-019-0016-5
11. Badawy AA-B. Kynurenine pathway of tryptophan metabolism: regulatory and functional aspects. *Int J Tryptophan Res.* (2017) 10:1178646917691938. doi: 10.1177/1178646917691938
12. Murakami Y, Saito K. Species and cell types difference in tryptophan metabolism. *Int J Tryptophan Res.* (2013) 6(Suppl 1):47–54. doi: 10.4137/IJTR.S11558
13. Schwarcz R, Bruno JP, Muchowski PJ, Wu HQ. Kynurenines in the mammalian brain: when physiology meets pathology. *Nat Rev Neurosci.* (2012) 13:465–77. doi: 10.1038/nrn3257
14. Yeung AWS, Terentis AC, King NJC, Thomas SR. Role of indoleamine 2,3-dioxygenase in health and disease. *Clin Sci.* (2015) 129:601–72. doi: 10.1042/CS20140392
15. Chaudhary K, Shinde R, Liu H, Gnana-Prakasam JP, Veeranan-Karmegam R, Huang L, et al. Amino acid metabolism inhibits antibody-driven kidney injury by inducing autophagy. *J Immunol.* (2015) 194:5713–24. doi: 10.4049/jimmunol.1500277
16. Curran T-A, Jalili RB, Farrokhi A, Ghahary A. IDO expressing fibroblasts promote the expansion of antigen specific regulatory T cells. *Immunobiology.* (2014) 219:17–24. doi: 10.1016/j.imbio.2013.06.008

17. Takamatsu M, Hirata A, Ohtaki H, Hoshi M, Hatano Y, Tomita H, et al. IDO1 plays an immunosuppressive role in 2,4,6-trinitrobenzene sulfate-induced colitis in mice. *J Immunol.* (2013) 191:3057–64. doi: 10.4049/jimmunol.1203306

18. Wang Y, Liu H, McKenzie G, Witting PK, Stasch JP, Hahn M, et al. Kynurenine is an endothelium-derived relaxing factor produced during inflammation. *Nat Med.* (2010) 16:279–85. doi: 10.1038/nm.2092

19. Yoshida R, Imanishi J, Oku T, Kishida T, Hayaishi O. Induction of pulmonary indoleamine 2,3-dioxygenase by interferon. *Proc Natl Acad Sci USA.* (1981) 78:129–32. doi: 10.1073/pnas.78.1.129

20. Baumgartner R, Forteza MJ, Ketelhuth DFJ. The interplay between cytokines and the Kynurenine pathway in inflammation and atherosclerosis. *Cytokine.* (2017) 122:154148. doi: 10.1016/j.cyto.2017.09.004

21. Orabona C, Pallotta MT, Volpi C, Fallarino F, Vacca C, Bianchi R, et al. SOCS3 drives proteasomal degradation of indoleamine 2,3-dioxygenase (IDO) and antagonizes IDO-dependent tolerogenesis. *Proc Natl Acad Sci USA.* (2008) 105:20828–33. doi: 10.1073/pnas.0810278105

22. Pallotta MT, Orabona C, Volpi C, Vacca C, Belladonna ML, Bianchi R, et al. Indoleamine 2,3-dioxygenase is a signaling protein in long-term tolerance by dendritic cells. *Nat Immunol.* (2011) 12:870–8. doi: 10.1038/ni.2077

23. Schröcksnadel K, Wirleitner B, Winkler C, Fuchs D. Monitoring tryptophan metabolism in chronic immune activation. *Clin Chim Acta.* (2006) 364:82–90. doi: 10.1016/j.cca.2005.06.013

24. Munn DH, Mellor AL. Indoleamine 2,3 dioxygenase and metabolic control of immune responses. *Trends Immunol.* (2013) 34:137–43. doi: 10.1016/j.it.2012.10.001

25. Munn DH, Sharma MD, Baban B, Harding HP, Zhang Y, Ron D, et al. GCN2 kinase in T cells mediates proliferative arrest and anergy induction in response to indoleamine 2,3-dioxygenase. *Immunity.* (2005) 22:633–42. doi: 10.1016/j.immuni.2005.03.013

26. Ravishankar B, Liu H, Shinde R, Chaudhary K, Xiao W, Bradley J, et al. The amino acid sensor GCN2 inhibits inflammatory responses to apoptotic cells promoting tolerance and suppressing systemic autoimmunity. *Proc Natl Acad Sci USA.* (2015) 112:10774–9. doi: 10.1073/pnas.1504276112

27. Fallarino F, Grohmann U, You S, McGrath BC, Cavener DR, Vacca C, et al. The combined effects of tryptophan starvation and tryptophan catabolites down-regulate T cell receptor ζ-chain and induce a regulatory phenotype in naive T cells. *J Immunol.* (2006) 176:6752–61. doi: 10.4049/jimmunol.176.11.6752

28. McGaha TL, Huang L, Lemos H, Metz R, Mautino M, Prendergast GC, et al. Amino acid catabolism: a pivotal regulator of innate and adaptive immunity. *Immunol Rev.* (2012) 249:135–57. doi: 10.1111/j.1600-065X.2012.01149.x

29. Ravishankar B, Liu H, Shinde R, Chandler P, Baban B, Tanaka M, et al. Tolerance to apoptotic cells is regulated by indoleamine 2,3-dioxygenase. *Proc Natl Acad Sci USA.* (2012) 109:3909–14. doi: 10.1073/pnas.1117736109

30. Weichhart T, Hengstschläger M, Linke M. Regulation of innate immune cell function by mTOR. *Nat Rev Immunol.* (2015) 15:599–614. doi: 10.1038/nri3901

31. Metz R, Rust S, DuHadaway JB, Mautino MR, Munn DH, Vahanian NN, et al. IDO inhibits a tryptophan sufficiency signal that stimulates mTOR: a novel IDO effector pathway targeted by D-1-methyl-tryptophan. *Oncoimmunology.* (2012) 1:1460–8. doi: 10.4161/onci.21716

32. Su X, Yu Y, Zhong Y, Giannopoulou EG, Hu X, Liu H, et al. Interferon-γ regulates cellular metabolism and mRNA translation to potentiate macrophage activation. *Nat Immunol.* (2015) 16:838–49. doi: 10.1038/ni.3205

33. Proto JD, Doran AC, Gusarova G, Yurdagul A, Sozen E, Subramanian M, et al. Regulatory T cells promote macrophage efferocytosis during inflammation resolution. *Immunity.* (2018) 49:666–77.e6. doi: 10.1016/j.immuni.2018.07.015

34. Jagger A, Shimojima Y, Goronzy JJ, Weyand CM. Regulatory T cells and the immune aging process: a mini-review. *Gerontology.* (2014) 60:130–7. doi: 10.1159/000355303

35. Mezrich JD, Fechner JH, Zhang X, Johnson BP, Burlingham WJ, Bradfield CA. An interaction between Kynurenine and the aryl hydrocarbon receptor can generate regulatory T cells. *J Immunol.* (2010) 185:3190–8. doi: 10.4049/jimmunol.0903670

36. Sinclair LV, Neyens D, Ramsay G, Taylor PM, Cantrell DA. Single cell analysis of kynurenine and system L amino acid transport in T cells. *Nat Commun.* (2018) 9:1981. doi: 10.1038/s41467-018-04366-7

37. Nguyen NT, Kimura A, Nakahama T, Chinen I, Masuda K, Nohara K, et al. Aryl hydrocarbon receptor negatively regulates dendritic cell immunogenicity via a kynurenine-dependent mechanism. *Proc Natl Acad Sci USA.* (2010) 107:19961–6. doi: 10.1073/pnas.1014465107

38. Vogel CFA, Goth SR, Dong B, Pessah IN, Matsumura F. Aryl hydrocarbon receptor signaling mediates expression of indoleamine 2,3-dioxygenase. *Biochem Biophys Res Commun.* (2008) 375:331–5. doi: 10.1016/j.bbrc.2008.07.156

39. Bessede A, Gargaro M, Pallotta MT, Matino D, Servillo G, Brunacci C, et al. Aryl hydrocarbon receptor control of a disease tolerance defence pathway. *Nature.* (2014) 511:184–90. doi: 10.1038/nature13323

40. Lee S-M, Park HY, Suh Y-S, Yoon EH, Kim J, Jang WH, et al. Inhibition of acute lethal pulmonary inflammation by the IDO-AhR pathway. *Proc Natl Acad Sci USA.* (2017) 114:E5881–90. doi: 10.1073/pnas.1615280114

41. Nagano J, Shimizu M, Hara T, Shirakami Y, Kochi T, Nakamura N, et al. Effects of indoleamine 2,3-dioxygenase deficiency on high-fat diet-induced hepatic inflammation. *PLoS ONE.* 8:e73404. doi: 10.1371/journal.pone.0073404

42. Cole JE, Astola N, Cribbs AP, Goddard ME, Park I, Green P, et al. Indoleamine 2,3-dioxygenase-1 is protective in atherosclerosis and its metabolites provide new opportunities for drug development. *Proc Natl Acad Sci USA.* (2015) 112:13033–8. doi: 10.1073/pnas.1517820112

43. El-Zaatari M, Bass AJ, Bowlby R, Zhang M, Syu L-J, Yang Y, et al. Indoleamine 2,3-dioxygenase 1, increased in human gastric pre-neoplasia, promotes inflammation and metaplasia in mice and is associated with type II hypersensitivity/autoimmunity. *Gastroenterology.* (2018) 154:140–53.e17. doi: 10.1053/j.gastro.2017.09.002

44. Spohn SN, Mawe GM. Non-conventional features of peripheral serotonin signalling - the gut and beyond. *Nat Rev Gastroenterol Hepatol.* (2017) 14:412–20. doi: 10.1038/nrgastro.2017.51

45. Agudelo LZ, Ferreira DMS, Cervenka I, Bryzgalova G, Dadvar S, Jannig PR, et al. Kynurenic acid and Gpr35 regulate adipose tissue energy homeostasis and inflammation. *Cell Metab.* (2018) 27:378–92.e5. doi: 10.1016/j.cmet.2018.01.004

46. Song P, Ramprasath T, Wang H, Zou MH. Abnormal kynurenine pathway of tryptophan catabolism in cardiovascular diseases. *Cell Mol Life Sci.* (2017) 74:2899–916. doi: 10.1007/s00018-017-2504-2

47. Fazio F, Zappulla C, Notartomaso S, Busceti C, Bessede A, Scarselli P, et al. Cinnabarinic acid, an endogenous agonist of type-4 metabotropic glutamate receptor, suppresses experimental autoimmune encephalomyelitis in mice. *Neuropharmacology.* (2014) 81:237–43. doi: 10.1016/j.neuropharm.2014.02.011

48. Gomes AP, Price NL, Ling AJY, Moslehi JJ, Montgomery MK, Rajman L, et al. Declining NAD(+) induces a pseudohypoxic state disrupting nuclear-mitochondrial communication during aging. *Cell.* (2013) 155:1624–38. doi: 10.1016/j.cell.2013.11.037

49. Poyan Mehr A, Tran MT, Ralto KM, Leaf DE, Washco V, Messmer J, et al. De novo NAD+ biosynthetic impairment in acute kidney injury in humans. *Nat Med.* (2018) 24:1351–9. doi: 10.1038/s41591-018-0138-z

50. Minhas PS, Liu L, Moon PK, Joshi AU, Dove C, Mhatre S, et al. Macrophage de novo NAD+ synthesis specifies immune function in aging and inflammation. *Nat Immunol.* (2018) 20:50–63. doi: 10.1038/s41590-018-0255-3

51. Roager HM, Licht TR. Microbial tryptophan catabolites in health and disease. *Nat Commun.* (2018) 9:3294. doi: 10.1038/s41467-018-05470-4

52. Capuron L, Schroecksnadel S, Féart C, Aubert A, Higueret D, Barberger-Gateau P, et al. Chronic low-grade inflammation in elderly persons is associated with altered tryptophan and tyrosine metabolism: role in neuropsychiatric symptoms. *Biol Psychiatry.* (2011) 70:175–82. doi: 10.1016/j.biopsych.2010.12.006

53. Collino S, Montoliu I, Martin F-PJ, Scherer M, Mari D, Salvioli S, et al. Metabolic signatures of extreme longevity in northern Italian centenarians reveal a complex remodeling of lipids, amino acids, and gut microbiota metabolism. *PLoS ONE.* (2013) 8:e56564. doi: 10.1371/journal.pone.0056564

54. Frick B, Schroecksnadel K, Neurauter G, Leblhuber F, Fuchs D. Increasing production of homocysteine and neopterin and degradation of tryptophan with older age. *Clin Biochem.* (2004) 37:684–7. doi: 10.1016/j.clinbiochem.2004.02.007

55. Niinisalo P, Raitala A, Pertovaara M, Oja SS, Lehtimäki T, Kähönen M, et al. Indoleamine 2,3-dioxygenase activity associates with cardiovascular

risk factors: the Health 2000 study. *Scand J Clin Lab Invest.* (2008) 68:767–70. doi: 10.1080/00365510802245685

56. Pertovaara M, Raitala A, Lehtimäki T, Karhunen PJ, Oja SS, Jylhä M, et al. Indoleamine 2,3-dioxygenase activity in nonagenarians is markedly increased and predicts mortality. *Mech Ageing Dev.* (2006) 127:497–9. doi: 10.1016/j.mad.2006.01.020

57. Ramos-Chávez LA, Roldán-Roldán G, García-Juárez B, González-Esquivel D, Pérez de la Cruz G, Pineda B, et al. Low serum tryptophan levels as an indicator of global cognitive performance in nondemented women over 50 years of age. *Oxid Med Cell Longev.* (2018) 2018:8604718. doi: 10.1155/2018/8604718

58. Rist MJ, Roth A, Frommherz L, Weinert CH, Krüger R, Merz B, et al. Metabolite patterns predicting sex and age in participants of the Karlsruhe Metabolomics and Nutrition (KarMeN) study. *PLoS ONE.* (2017) 12:1–21. doi: 10.1371/journal.pone.0183228

59. Theofylaktopoulou D, Midttun Ø, Ulvik A, Ueland PM, Tell GS, Vollset SE, et al. A community-based study on determinants of circulating markers of cellular immune activation and kynurenines: the Hordaland Health Study. *Clin Exp Immunol.* (2013) 173:121–30. doi: 10.1111/cei.12092

60. Yu Z, Zhai G, Singmann P, He Y, Xu T, Prehn C, et al. Human serum metabolic profiles are age dependent. *Aging Cell.* (2012) 11:960–7. doi: 10.1111/j.1474-9726.2012.00865.x

61. Pertovaara M, Raitala A, Juonala M, Lehtimäki T, Huhtala H, Oja SS, et al. Indoleamine 2,3-dioxygenase enzyme activity correlates with risk factors for atherosclerosis: the Cardiovascular Risk in Young Finns Study. *Clin Exp Immunol.* (2007) 148:106–11. doi: 10.1111/j.1365-2249.2007.03325.x

62. Deac OM, Mills JL, Gardiner CM, Shane B, Quinn L, Midttun Ø, et al. Serum immune system biomarkers neopterin and interleukin-10 are strongly related to tryptophan metabolism in healthy young adults. *J Nutr.* (2016) 146:1801–6. doi: 10.3945/jn.116.230698

63. Valdiglesias V, Marcos-Pérez D, Lorenzi M, Onder G, Gostner JM, Strasser B, et al. Immunological alterations in frail older adults: a cross sectional study. *Exp Gerontol.* (2018) 112:119–26. doi: 10.1016/j.exger.2018.09.010

64. Solvang SEH, Nordrehaug JE, Tell GS, Nygård O, McCann A, Ueland PM, et al. The kynurenine pathway and cognitive performance in community-dwelling older adults. The Hordaland health study. *Brain Behav Immun.* (2019) 75:155–62. doi: 10.1016/j.bbi.2018.10.003

65. Sulo G, Vollset SE, Nygård O, Midttun Ø, Ueland PM, Eussen SJPM, et al. Neopterin and kynurenine–tryptophan ratio as predictors of coronary events in older adults, the Hordaland Health Study. *Int J Cardiol.* (2013) 168:1435–40. doi: 10.1016/j.ijcard.2012.12.090

66. Zuo H, Ueland PM, Ulvik A, Eussen SJPM, Vollset SE, Nygård O, et al. Plasma biomarkers of inflammation, the Kynurenine pathway, and risks of all-cause, cancer, and cardiovascular disease mortality: the Hordaland health study. *Am J Epidemiol.* (2016) 183:249–58. doi: 10.1093/aje/kwv242

67. Darlington LG, Mackay GM, Forrest CM, Stoy N, George C, Stone TW. Altered kynurenine metabolism correlates with infarct volume in stroke. *Eur J Neurosci.* (2007). doi: 10.1111/j.1460-9568.2007.05838.x

68. Darlington LG, Forrest CM, Mackay GM, Smith RA, Smith AJ, Stoy N, et al. On the biological importance of the 3-hydroxyanthranilic acid: anthranilic acid ratio. *Int J Tryptophan Res.* (2010) 3:51–9. doi: 10.4137/IJTR.S4282

69. Moreno-Villanueva M, Bernhard J, Blasco M, Zondag G, Hoeijmakers JHJ, Toussaint O, et al. MARK-AGE biomarkers of ageing. *Mech Ageing Dev.* (2015) 151:2–12. doi: 10.1016/j.mad.2015.03.006

70. Connelly MA, Otvos JD, Shalaurova I, Playford MP, Mehta NN. GlycA, a novel biomarker of systemic inflammation and cardiovascular disease risk. *J Transl Med.* 15:219. doi: 10.1186/s12967-017-1321-6

71. Heintz C, Mair W. You are what you host: microbiome modulation of the aging process. *Cell.* (2014) 156:408–11. doi: 10.1016/j.cell.2014.01.025

72. Laurans L, Venteclef N, Haddad Y, Chajadine M, Alzaid F, Metghalchi S, et al. Genetic deficiency of indoleamine 2,3-dioxygenase promotes gut microbiota-mediated metabolic health. *Nat Med.* (2018) 24:1113–20. doi: 10.1038/s41591-018-0060-4

73. Rampelli S, Candela M, Turroni S, Collino EB, Franceschi C, O'Toole PW, et al. Functional metagenomic profiling of intestinal microbiome in extreme ageing. *Aging.* (2013) 5:902–12. doi: 10.18632/aging.100623

74. Crane JD, Palanivel R, Mottillo EP, Bujak AL, Wang H, Ford RJ, et al. Inhibiting peripheral serotonin synthesis reduces obesity and metabolic dysfunction by promoting brown adipose tissue thermogenesis. *Nat Med.* (2015) 21:166–72. doi: 10.1038/nm.3766

75. Oh C-M, Namkung J, Go Y, Shong KE, Kim K, Kim H, et al. Regulation of systemic energy homeostasis by serotonin in adipose tissues. *Nat Commun.* (2015) 6:6794. doi: 10.1038/ncomms7794

76. Liu L, Su X, Quinn WJ, Hui S, Krukenberg K, Frederick DW, et al. Quantitative analysis of NAD synthesis-breakdown fluxes. *Cell Metab.* (2018) 27:1067–80.e5. doi: 10.1016/j.cmet.2018.03.018

77. Fang EF, Lautrup S, Hou Y, Demarest TG, Croteau DL, Mattson MP, et al. NAD+ in aging: molecular mechanisms and translational implications. *Trends Mol Med.* (2017) 23:899–916. doi: 10.1016/j.molmed.2017.08.001

78. Katsyuba E, Mottis A, Zietak M, De Franco F, van der Velpen V, Gariani K, et al. *De novo* NAD+ synthesis enhances mitochondrial function and improves health. *Nature.* (2018) 563:354–9. doi: 10.1038/s41586-018-0645-6

79. Woodling NS, Colas D, Wang Q, Minhas P, Panchal M, Liang X, et al. Cyclooxygenase inhibition targets neurons to prevent early behavioural decline in Alzheimer's disease model mice. *Brain.* (2016) 139:2063–81. doi: 10.1093/brain/aww117

80. Zwilling D, Huang SY, Sathyasaikumar KV, Notarangelo FM, Guidetti P, Wu HQ, et al. Kynurenine 3-monooxygenase inhibition in blood ameliorates neurodegeneration. *Cell.* (2011) 145:863–74. doi: 10.1016/j.cell.2011.05.020

81. Breda C, Sathyasaikumar KV, Sograte Idrissi S, Notarangelo FM, Estranero JG, Moore GGL, et al. Tryptophan-2,3-dioxygenase (TDO) inhibition ameliorates neurodegeneration by modulation of kynurenine pathway metabolites. *Proc Natl Acad Sci USA.* (2016) 113:5435–40. doi: 10.1073/pnas.1604453113

82. Campesan S, Green EW, Breda C, Sathyasaikumar KV, Muchowski PJ, Schwarcz R, et al. The kynurenine pathway modulates neurodegeneration in a Drosophila model of Huntington's disease. *Curr Biol.* (2011) 21:961–6. doi: 10.1016/j.cub.2011.04.028

83. van der Goot AT, Zhu W, Vazquez-Manrique RP, Seinstra RI, Dettmer K, Michels H, et al. Delaying aging and the aging-associated decline in protein homeostasis by inhibition of tryptophan degradation. *Proc Natl Acad Sci USA.* (2012) 109:14912–7. doi: 10.1073/pnas.1203083109

84. Eckers A, Jakob S, Heiss C, Haarmann-Stemmann T, Goy C, Brinkmann V, et al. The aryl hydrocarbon receptor promotes aging phenotypes across species. *Sci Rep.* (2016) 6:19618. doi: 10.1038/srep19618

85. Edwards C, Canfield J, Copes N, Brito A, Rehan M, Lipps D, et al. Mechanisms of amino acid-mediated lifespan extension in *Caenorhabditis elegans*. *BMC Genet.* (2015) 16:18. doi: 10.1186/s12863-015-0167-2

86. Sutphin GL, Backer G, Sheehan S, Bean S, Corban C, Liu T, et al. *Caenorhabditis elegans* orthologs of human genes differentially expressed with age are enriched for determinants of longevity. *Aging Cell.* (2017) 16:672–82. doi: 10.1111/acel.12595

87. Braidy N, Guillemin GJ, Mansour H, Chan-Ling T, Grant R. Changes in kynurenine pathway metabolism in the brain, liver and kidney of aged female Wistar rats. *FEBS J.* (2011) 278:4425–34. doi: 10.1111/j.1742-4658.2011.08366.x

88. Ma S, Yim SH, Lee S-G, Kim EB, Lee S-R, Chang K-T, et al. Organization of the mammalian metabolome according to organ function, lineage specialization, and longevity. *Cell Metab.* (2015) 22:332–43. doi: 10.1016/j.cmet.2015.07.005

2

Hypoxia Inducible Factor 1α Inhibits the Expression of Immunosuppressive Tryptophan-2,3-Dioxygenase in Glioblastoma

Soumya R. Mohapatra[1], Ahmed Sadik[1,2], Lars-Oliver Tykocinski[3], Jørn Dietze[4],
Gernot Poschet[5], Ines Heiland[4] and Christiane A. Opitz[1,6*]

[1] DKTK Brain Cancer Metabolism Group, German Cancer Research Center (DKFZ), Heidelberg, Germany, [2] Faculty of Bioscience, Heidelberg University, Heidelberg, Germany, [3] Division of Rheumatology, Department of Medicine V, University Hospital of Heidelberg, Heidelberg, Germany, [4] Department of Arctic and Marine Biology, UiT The Arctic University of Norway, Tromsø, Norway, [5] Centre for Organismal Studies (COS), University of Heidelberg, Heidelberg, Germany, [6] Neurology Clinic and National Center for Tumor Diseases, University Hospital of Heidelberg, Heidelberg, Germany

*Correspondence:
Christiane A. Opitz
c.opitz@dkfz.de

Abnormal circulation in solid tumors results in hypoxia, which modulates both tumor intrinsic malignant properties as well as anti-tumor immune responses. Given the importance of hypoxia in glioblastoma (GBM) biology and particularly in shaping anti-tumor immunity, we analyzed which immunomodulatory genes are differentially regulated in response to hypoxia in GBM cells. Gene expression analyses identified the immunosuppressive enzyme tryptophan-2,3-dioxygenase (TDO2) as the second most downregulated gene in GBM cells cultured under hypoxic conditions. TDO2 catalyses the oxidation of tryptophan to N-formyl kynurenine, which is the first and rate-limiting step of Trp degradation along the kynurenine pathway (KP). In multiple GBM cell lines hypoxia reduced TDO2 expression both at mRNA and protein levels. The downregulation of TDO2 through hypoxia was reversible as re-oxygenation rescued TDO2 expression. Computational modeling of tryptophan metabolism predicted reduced flux through the KP and lower intracellular concentrations of kynurenine and its downstream metabolite 3-hydroxyanthranilic acid under hypoxia. Metabolic measurements confirmed the predicted changes, thus demonstrating the ability of the mathematical model to infer intracellular tryptophan metabolite concentrations. Moreover, we identified hypoxia inducible factor 1α (HIF1α) to regulate TDO2 expression under hypoxic conditions, as the HIF1α-stabilizing agents dimethyloxalylglycine (DMOG) and cobalt chloride reduced TDO2 expression. Knockdown of HIF1α restored the expression of TDO2 upon cobalt chloride treatment, confirming that HIF1α controls TDO2 expression. To investigate the immunoregulatory effects of this novel mechanism of TDO2 regulation, we co-cultured isolated T cells with TDO2-expressing GBM cells under normoxic and hypoxic conditions. Under normoxia TDO2-expressing GBM cells suppressed T cell proliferation, while hypoxia restored the proliferation of the T cells, likely due to the reduction in kynurenine levels produced by the GBM cells. Taken together, our data suggest that the regulation of TDO2 expression by HIF1α may be involved in modulating anti-tumor immunity in GBM.

Keywords: hypoxia, HIF1α, tryptophan, TDO2, immunosuppression

INTRODUCTION

More than 60 years ago, Thomlinson and Gray postulated the occurrence of hypoxic regions in solid tumors (1). Initial interest in studying hypoxia in tumors was due to the realization that hypoxic cells are more resistant to radiotherapy (2) resulting in adverse clinical outcomes for the patients. Measurements of intra-tumoral oxygen levels revealed a highly heterogeneous hypoxic landscape within a tumor. The oxygen concentration in moderately hypoxic regions was determined to be $\sim$1% oxygen (O_2), while in severely hypoxic tumor regions it fell below 1% O_2 (3).

Cells under hypoxic conditions are known to shut down non-essential processes by chromatin modifications and a global downregulation of gene expression (4), while simultaneously genes needed for cell survival under oxygen limitation are upregulated through hypoxia inducible transcription factors (HIFs) (5). The most well-known HIF family member HIF1α is degraded under normoxic conditions by the action of prolyl-hydroxylase (PHD) enzymes. However, under hypoxic conditions PHD function is inhibited, thus stabilizing HIF1α and activating the expression of its target genes (6). Furthermore, HIF1α can also inhibit the expression of genes during hypoxia (7).

Similar to other solid tumors, the most aggressive primary brain tumor, glioblastoma multiforme (GBM), is prone to severe hypoxia. GBM are characterized by the presence of necrotic foci and surrounding severely hypoxic pseudopalisades consisting of outwardly migrating GBM cells trying to escape the core hypoxic regions (8). Measurements of O_2 levels in tumors from 14 GBM patients revealed a median O_2 level of 0.7% (9). Bio-availability of oxygen to a tumor cell in a solid tumor depends on a number of factors such as the distance of the tumor cell from the nearest blood vessel and diminished blood supply due to the abnormal vasculature found in tumors (10, 11). Irrespective of the factors causing hypoxic stress, hypoxia has been shown to drive established hallmarks of cancer progression in GBM such as inhibition of cell death (12), induction of angiogenesis (13), activation of endothelial to mesenchymal transition (14), modulation of cellular metabolism (15), and tumor immune escape (16).

Of note, hypoxic regions of solid tumors often harbor a large number of immunosuppressive cells, which inhibit anti-tumor immune responses (17). Tumor hypoxia in GBM has been shown to exert immune suppression by activation of regulatory T cells (Tregs) (18). HIF1α-mediated gene regulation is involved in promoting hypoxic suppression of anti-tumor immunity (19, 20). For instance, HIF1α induces the expression of the inhibitory immune checkpoint regulator programmed death-ligand 1 (PD-L1), which facilitates the suppression of anti-tumor immune effects (21, 22). Furthermore, hypoxia also obstructs anti-tumor immunity by reduction of tumor cell MHC presentation and the tumor cell expression of chemokines essential for immune cell infiltration (23).

In light of the important role played by hypoxia in GBM biology and particularly in modulating anti-tumor immune responses, we analyzed GBM cells for genes involved in the regulation of anti-tumor immunity that are differentially regulated upon hypoxia. We find that hypoxia significantly reduces the expression of the immunosuppressive enzyme tryptophan-2,3-dioxygenase (TDO2). TDO2 catalyses the first step of tryptophan (Trp) catabolism along the kynurenine pathway (KP) and is known to play an important role in GBM as it promotes tumor cell motility and suppresses anti-tumor immune responses via production of Trp metabolities that activate the aryl hydrocarbon receptor (AHR) (24).

MATERIALS AND METHODS

Cell Culture

Human GBM cell lines A172, U-87 MG, and LN-18 were obtained from ATCC. Cells were cultivated in DMEM (Gibco) containing 10% FBS (Gibco), 2 mM Glutamine (Gibco), 1 mM Sodium Pyruvate (Gibco), 100 μg/ml Streptomycin, and 100 U/ml Penicillin (Gibco). Cells were authenticated by Multiplex Cell Authentication service (Multiplexion GmbH) and were routinely monitored using the Venor® GeM Classic mycoplasma detection kit (Minerva Biolabs). Twenty-four hours after cell seeding a medium change was done following which, various treatments were carried out. Unless stated otherwise, cells were normally cultivated at normoxic conditions i.e., 18.6% O_2 concentration (conc.) (25) in a SANYO MCO-18AIC incubator with 5% CO_2 and at 37°C.

Long Term Hypoxic Exposure

A172, U-87 MG, and LN-18 cells in T25 flasks containing 5 ml medium, were subjected to either normoxic or hypoxic conditions for 3, 5, 8, and 10 days. For hypoxic conditions (i.e., 1% O_2) cells were placed in the Labotect incubator C42. For each time point, cells were seeded in duplicates; one of the flasks was incubated in normoxic conditions and served as a control for the other flask incubated under hypoxic conditions. At the indicated time points, 1 ml culture supernatant from each treatment was harvested and used for metabolic measurements. Subsequently, the cells were harvested by trypsinization in 1.5 ml PBS. The cell count of the harvested cells was measured using 10 μl of cell suspension and Trypan Blue dye (Gibco) in a 1:1 ratio with an automated Cell Counter (Countess, Invitrogen). The remaining cells were further processed for either RNA, protein or intracellular metabolite extraction.

Treatment With Hypoxia Mimetics

HIF1α protein stabilization was attained by using the hypoxia mimetic compounds dimethyloxalylglycine (DMOG) and cobalt chloride ($CoCl_2$). DMOG was obtained from Frontier Scientific Inc. and reconstituted in 100% ethanol (Sigma). Cells were treated such that the final DMOG concentrations of 0.5, 1, 2, and 3 mM were obtained according to the treatment specifications. EtOH was used as carrier control. A second hypoxia mimetic agent, cobalt chloride ($CoCl_2$) was obtained from Sigma and reconstituted in ddH_2O. Cells were treated for 24 h such that a final treatment concentration of 100, 150, 200, 250, and 300 μM of $CoCl_2$ was obtained.

RNA Isolation and Quantitative (q)RT-PCR

Total RNA was isolated using the RNAeasy Mini Kit (Qiagen). cDNA was reverse transcribed from 1 μg total RNA using the High Capacity cDNA reverse transcriptase kit (Applied Biosystems). cDNA amplification was performed using the SYBR Select Master Mix (Thermo Fisher Scientific) during the (q)RT-PCR on a StepOnePlus real-time PCR system (Applied Biosystems). For all (q)RT-PCR measurements 18s RNA was used as a housekeeping gene for normalization. (q)RT-PCR primers for a gene were designed using Primer Blast (NCBI), such that on the genomic DNA at least one intron separated the forward and reverse primers.

Primer sequences used:

TDO2	Forward	5′-CAAATCCTCTGGGAGTTGGA-3′
	Reverse	5′-GTCCAAGGCTGTCATCGTCT-3′
18s RNA	Forward	5′-GATGGGCGGCGGAAAATAG-3′
	Reverse	5′-GCGTGGATTCTGCATAATGGT-3′
NDRG1	Forward	5′-TCAAGATGGCGGACTGTG-3′
	Reverse	5′-GAAGGCCTCAGCGAGCTT-3′

Protein Isolation and Western Blots

Total protein was harvested using ice-cold RIPA lysis buffer (1% IGEPAL/NP40, 12 mM sodium-deoxycholate, 3.5 mM sodium dodecyl sulfate (SDS) supplemented with a protease and phosphatase inhibitor (Roche/Sigma-Aldrich). The Bradford protein assay (Biorad) was employed for total protein content measurement and subsequent normalization between samples across one experiment. Protein samples were separated using a 10% SDS-PAGE gel and transferred onto an activated 0.45 μm PVDF membrane (Sigma-Aldrich), subsequently the membrane was blocked with 5% BSA for 30 min and incubated with primary antibodies overnight. The primary antibodies were used in 1:1000 dilution for mouse anti-human TDO2 (#TA504730, Origene), rabbit anti-human NDRG1 (#HPA006881, Sigma), and rabbit anti-human Tubulin (#ab108629, Abcam plc.). Membranes were subsequently incubated for 1 h with 1:5000 diluted HRP-conjugated secondary antibodies (anti-rabbit ab.: #GENA9340-1M, anti-mouse ab.: #GENXA931, both from GE Healthcare). Either Pierce® ECL Western Blotting Substrate or SuperSignal® West Femto Maximum Sensitivity Substrate (both Thermo Scientific) were used to generate the signals, which were captured either on an autoradiography film (Amersham Hyperfilm, GE Healthcare) or on the ChemiDoc XRS+ (Bio-Rad Laboratories) using Image Lab Software 5.2.1.

siRNA-Mediated HIF1α Knockdown

siRNA stocks (20 μM) were prepared by reconstituting ON-TARGETplus Human SMARTPOOL siRNA reagent targeting HIF1α (Dharmacon) in sterile PBS in accordance to the manufacturer's recommended ratio. ON-TARGETplus Non-targeting Pool siRNA (Dharmacon) was used as a control. siRNA transfection mix was prepared using siRNA stocks and Lipofectamine RNAiMAX (Thermo Fisher Scientific) according to the manufacturer's protocol. Cells were treated with the transfection mix for 24 h, which was followed by a fresh medium change and incubation with cobalt chloride for 24 h before harvest.

High Performance Liquid Chromatography (HPLC)

For Trp and Kyn measurements (**Figures 2A,B**) in cell culture supernatants, 72% trichloroacetic acid (Sigma-Aldrich) was added in a ratio of 162.8 μl per 1 ml of supernatant for protein precipitation. Samples were then centrifuged at full speed for 12 min, following which the supernatants were analyzed in a Dionex Ultimate® 3000 uHPLC (Thermo Scientific, Waltham, MA, USA) by chromatographic separation. An Accucore™ aQ column (Thermo Scientific™) with 2.6 μm particle size with a gradient mobile phase consisting of 0.1% trifluoroacetic acid (TFA) in water (A) and 0.1% TFA in acetonitrile (B) was utilized for separation of Trp and Kyn, which were detected at UV emission spectra of 280 and 365 nm, respectively. The Chromeleon™ 7.2 Chromatography Data System (Thermo Scientific™ Dionex™) was used for data analysis.

For intracellular analyses of Trp and Trp-derived compounds (**Figure 2C**), the samples were rapidly frozen in liquid nitrogen following trypsinization and pelleting of harvested cells. Subsequently, metabolites were extracted with 0.1 ml 6% perchloric acid per million of cells in an ultrasonic ice-bath for 10 min. For analyses of extracellular content, supernatants were mixed with an equal volume of 12% perchloric acid and incubated on ice for 10 min. Prior analysis, samples were centrifuged for 10 min at 4°C and 16.400 g to precipitate proteins and to remove remaining cell debris. Metabolites were separated by reversed phase chromatography on an Acquity HSS T3 column (100 × 2.1 mm, 1.7 μm, Waters) connected to an Acquity H-class UPLC system (Waters). The column was heated to 37°C and equilibrated with 5 column volumes of 100% solvent A (20 mM sodium acetate, 3 mM zinc acetate, pH 6) at a flow rate of 0.55 ml min^{-1}. Clear separation of Trp and Trp-derived compounds was achieved by increasing the concentration of solvent B (Acetonitrile) in solvent A as follows: 4 min 0% B, 10 min 5% B, 13 min 15% B, 15 min 25% B, and return to 0% B in 3 min. Trp, 3HAA, KynA and tryptamine were detected by fluorescence (Acquity FLR detector, Waters, excitation: 254 nm, emission: 401 nm). Kyn and OH-Kyn were determined by simultaneous recording of absorption at 365 nm (Acquity PDA detector, Waters). For quantification, ultrapure standards were used (Sigma). Data acquisition and processing was performed with the Empower3 software suite (Waters).

Microarray Analysis

RNA was harvested after 5 days from the control and hypoxic cells, using the RNAeasy Mini Kit (Qiagen). Labeled ss-cDNA was generated from 100 ng total RNA using the Affymetrix WT PLUS Reagent Kit, as per the manufacturer's instructions. Subsequently, 5.5 μg of fragmented and labeled ss-cDNA were hybridized for 17 h at 45°C on Affymetrix Human Gene 2.0 ST chip following the manufacturer's instructions. The Affymetrix GeneChip® Scanner 3000 was used for scanning the hybridized chips according to the GeneChip® Expression Wash, Stain and Scan Manual for Cartridge Arrays (P/N 702731). The Raw CEL files were imported from disk followed by RMA normalization and summarization using the *oligo* package and were annotated at the probeset level using NetAffx (26). Differential gene expression was conducted by fitting a linear model and estimating a moderated *t*-statistic followed by eBayes adjustment as described in the *limma* package (27, 28). All analyses were run in R, version 3.4.4 (https://cran.r-project.org/) and Bioconductor version 3.6 (https://bioconductor.org/). All graphical representations were generated using *ggplot2*, *ggpubr*, and *RcolorBrewer*. All datasets have been made publicly available in the Gene Expression Omnibus (GEO) repository under accession number GSE138535.

Modeling of Trp Metabolism

To simulate Trp metabolism in A172 cells, we employed the previously published comprehensive kinetic model of Trp metabolism (29). Microarray data previously generated for A172 cells exposed to normoxia or hypoxia for 5 days, were integrated into the Trp model using SBMLmod as described previously (30). No transporters and no external metabolites were used. Instead the concentration of cellular Trp was set to the measured intracellular concentration, assuming a cell volume of 10 pL. Steady-state concentrations and fluxes were calculated using the steady state task of COPASI 4.26 (31).

Proliferation Measurements in T Cell Co-cultures

The functional characterization of PBMC from healthy donors was approved by the Ethics Committee of the University of Heidelberg. PBMC isolation was carried by density-gradient centrifugation and T cells were enriched using the MojoSort Human CD4 T cell isolation kit (Biolegend) according to the manufacturer's instructions. T cells were cultured in 96 well plates either alone or in a co-culture with A172 cells in RPMI1640 (Thermo Fisher Scientific) containing 10% FCS in the presence of 5 μg/ml phytohaemagglutinin (PHA) (Sigma) and 1 U/μl rhIL-2 (Novartis). All cultures were performed in duplicate sets, one set under normoxia and the second under hypoxia. A glove box (Coylab) and an incubator (Heracell 150i, Thermo Fisher Scientific) with oxygen level regulation were used for ensuring continued hypoxia conditions during all steps of culturing. PKH26 (Sigma-Aldrich) was used to label T cells prior to culture. After 6 days of culturing, PKH26 mean fluorescence intensity (MFI) was measured by flow cytometry (BD FACSCanto II (BD Biosciences). The degree of reduction in PKH26 fluorescence intensity reflected the number of cell divisions undergone by the cells. Suppression of T cell proliferation by hypoxia was measured by calculating the ratio between the PKH26 MFI of T cell co-cultured with A172 cells and the PKH26 MFI of T cells cultured alone, for both normoxia and hypoxia culture conditions.

Statistical Analysis

GraphPad Prism v5.04 (GraphPad Software Inc.) was used for performing statistical analysis. For single comparisons between two datasets, two-tailed unpaired Student's *t*-test was utilized. Rank sum analysis by the Mann–Whitney *U*-test was carried out wherever necessary. For multiple comparisons, one-way ANOVA with Tukey's multiple comparisons test was employed. Data was collected from at least three independent experiments. All data are plotted as mean ± SEM, unless stated otherwise. Differences with a $p \leq 0.05$ were considered to be statistically significant (ns: not significant i.e., $p > 0.05$; *$p \leq 0.05$; **$p \leq 0.01$; ***$p \leq 0.001$; ****$p \leq 0.0001$).

RESULTS

TDO2 Expression Is Suppressed Under Hypoxia

To investigate if hypoxia differentially regulates genes that play a role in anti-tumor immune responses in GBM cells, we performed microarray analysis of A172 GBM cells exposed to 5 days of hypoxia (1% O_2) as compared to cells cultured in normoxia (18.6% O_2) (GSE138535). Analysis of the microarray data revealed tryptophan-2,3-dioxygenase (TDO2) to be the second most downregulated gene under hypoxia (**Figure 1A**, **Supplementary Table 1**). TDO2 is an immunosuppressive enzyme, whose metabolic products have been shown to modulate anti-tumor immune responses by inhibition of T cell proliferation as well as induction of apoptosis in T cells (32, 33). Apart from TDO2, other immune-regulatory genes, such as TLR3 and CCL2 were also strongly downregulated under hypoxia (**Supplementary Table 1**). However, in the present study we focussed our attention on TDO2, the strongest differentially regulated gene candidate among the genes with known effects on immune responses. TDO2 integrates molecular O_2 into Trp to generate formyl-kynurenine, which is further converted to kynurenine (34). Therefore, reduced O_2 concentrations under hypoxia would be expected to affect the enzymatic activity of TDO2, however our microarray data revealed that also the expression of TDO2 may be reduced upon hypoxia in GBM cells.

To validate the results of the microarray, we next performed qRT-PCR measurements. To test for the presence of hypoxia we assayed N-myc downstream regulated 1 (NDRG1), a gene known to be upregulated under hypoxia in GBM (35, 36), as a surrogate hypoxia marker that was also significantly upregulated by hypoxia in the microarray (**Supplementary Table 1**). Analysis of mRNA transcript levels in A172 cells exposed to hypoxic conditions for different durations, confirmed the presence of hypoxia as NDRG1 was significantly upregulated (**Figure 1B**, left). Further, the qRT-PCR measurements confirmed the result of the microarray analysis, as a significant reduction in TDO2 mRNA levels was observed at all-time points upon hypoxic exposure (**Figure 1B**, right). Downregulation of TDO2 mRNA in response to hypoxia was not limited to A172 cells, but was also observed in U-87 MG and LN-18 GBM cells (**Figures 1C,D**). Western blot analysis of all three GBM cell lines exposed to either normoxia or hypoxia revealed that TDO2 protein expression was reduced under hypoxia, while expression of the hypoxia surrogate marker NDRG1 was increased (**Figure 1E**). To investigate whether the hypoxic

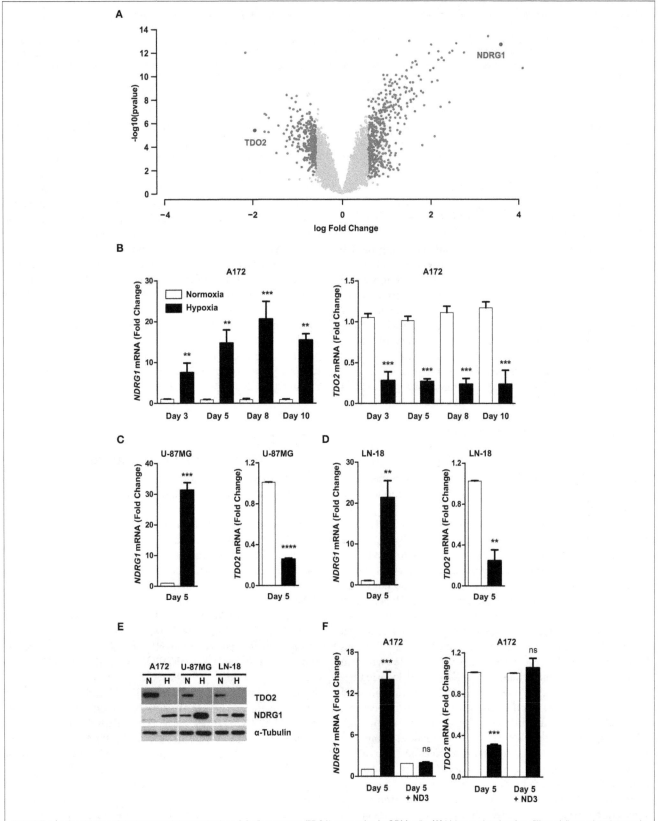

FIGURE 1 | Hypoxia reversibly downregulates tryptophan-2,3-dioxygenase (TDO2) expression in GBM cells. **(A)** Volcano plot showing differentially regulated genes in A172 cells upon exposure to 5 days of hypoxia compared to 5 days normoxic controls. **(B)** qRT-PCR analysis of NDRG1 (left) and TDO2 (right) mRNA expression in A172 cells after 3, 5, 8, or 10 days of exposure to either normoxia (white) or hypoxia (back). **(C)** qRT-PCR analysis of NDRG1 (left) and TDO2 (right) mRNA expression

(Continued)

FIGURE 1 | in U-87MG cells after 5 days of either normoxia (white) or hypoxia (black) exposure. **(D)** qRT-PCR analysis of NDRG1 (left) and TDO2 (right) mRNA expression in LN-18 cells after 5 days of either normoxia or hypoxia. **(E)** Western blot analysis of TDO2 and NDRG1 protein expression in A172, U-87MG, and LN-18 cells subsequent to 5 days normoxia or hypoxia. α-Tubulin protein expression was used as a loading control. **(F)** NDRG1 (left) and TDO2 (right) mRNA expression in A172 cells analyzed by qRT-PCR after exposure to hypoxia for 5 days followed by re-oxygenation for 3 days under normoxic conditions (ND3). Data from at least three independent experiments are expressed as mean ± S.E.M. Statistical significance was assumed at $p < 0.05$ (**$p < 0.01$, ***$p < 0.001$, ****$p \leq 0.0001$). n.s., not significant.

---

downregulation of TDO2 expression can be restored by re-oxygenation, we subjected A172 cells to 3 days of normoxia after 5 days of hypoxia. Re-oxygenation completely restored the expression of TDO2 (**Figure 1F**), indicating that the observed hypoxic downregulation of TDO2 is reversible.

Hypoxia-Mediated TDO2 Downregulation Reduces Flux Through the KP

TDO2 catalyses the first step of Trp degradation along the KP (37). However, after establishing the regulatory effects of hypoxia on TDO2 expression, we aimed to investigate effects of reduced oxygen on Trp degradation and KP metabolite production, which likely results from both the hypoxia-mediated reduction in TDO2 expression and possibly also reduced TDO2 catalytic activity due to O_2 limitation. Analysis of supernatants harvested from the long-term hypoxia experiments with A172 cells (shown in **Figure 1B**), revealed that cells growing under hypoxic conditions produced less Kyn than the cells cultured under normoxia (**Figure 2A**). This reduction in Kyn production corresponded to the high amount of Trp that remained present in the supernatants of the hypoxic cells (**Figure 2B**). Taken together, these results indicate that hypoxia downregulates Trp catabolism.

We next hypothesized that the reduced amount of Kyn produced by TDO2 upon hypoxia should affect the metabolic flux of the entire KP. We therefore performed computational modeling of Trp metabolism to predict the steady state fluxes and metabolite concentrations in the KP. To this end, gene expression data from A172 GBM cells cultivated under either hypoxia or normoxia (see **Figure 1A**) was integrated into the previously mentioned mathematical model of Trp metabolism (29). In line with our hypothesis, the model predicted a significantly decreased Trp catabolic flux mainly caused by the reduced enzymatic flux through TDO2, while the flux through DOPA decarboxylase (DDC) remained unperturbed (**Figure 2C**). Further, reduced metabolic flux was also predicted for downstream enzymes that degrade Kyn, such as the kynurenine aminotransferases (KATs) and kynurenine-3-monooxygenase (KMO), which generate kynurenic acid (KynA) and 3-hydroxy-anthranilic acid (3HAA), respectively (**Figure 2C**). This reduced metabolic flux under hypoxia through major enzymes of the KP resulted in reduced simulated intracellular concentrations not only of Kyn but also of its downstream metabolite 3HAA (**Figure 2C**, gray plots). In contrast, the simulated production of Trp metabolites not directly dependent on TDO2 activity such as tryptamine were predicted to remain unaffected under hypoxia (**Figure 2C**, gray plots).

To validate the predictions of the mathematical model of Trp metabolism, we analyzed the changes in intracellular concentrations of Trp metabolites in the A172 GBM cells after 5 days of exposure to hypoxia. In line with the simulations, the intracellular concentrations of the KP metabolites Kyn and 3HAA were significantly reduced under hypoxia (**Figure 2C**, black plots). Although intracellular KynA concentrations were reduced, this decrease failed to attain significance (**Figure 2C**, black plots). Furthermore, confirming the predictions, the intracellular tryptamine concentrations remained unchanged under hypoxia. In the cell supernatants no changes in 3HAA and KynA levels were observed under hypoxia and tryptamine was undetectable (**Supplementary Figure 1**). However, in line with our simulations and previous observations, Trp levels in the supernatants increased significantly under hypoxic conditions consistent with the significant decrease in Kyn production (**Supplementary Figure 1**). Taken together, these results confirm our computational predictions and show that hypoxic downregulation of TDO2 expression reduces flux through the KP.

TDO2 Expression Is Reduced Upon Stabilization of HIF1α by Chemical Hypoxia Mimetics

Hypoxia mediates most of its effects through the master regulator HIF1α, however a HIF1α independent global downregulation of gene expression by hypoxia has also been described (4). Therefore, we next investigated if HIF1α plays a role in the hypoxia-mediated downregulation of TDO2. For this, we stabilized HIF1α protein under normoxic conditions by the use of chemical hypoxia mimetics such as dimethyloxalylglycine (DMOG) or cobalt chloride ($CoCl_2$). Microarray analysis of A172 cells incubated for 24 h in the presence of 3 mM DMOG (GSE138535), revealed that TDO2 gene expression was strongly downregulated upon HIF1α stabilization (**Figure 3A**, **Supplementary Table 2**). qRT-PCR analysis of A172 cells exposed to a range of DMOG concentrations, confirmed the microarray data, as elevated NDRG1 mRNA levels upon DMOG exposure (**Figure 3B**, left) corresponded to a decrease in TDO2 mRNA expression at tested DMOG concentrations (**Figure 3B**, right). Analysis of the mRNA expression of A172 cells exposed to a second hypoxia mimetic, cobalt chloride ($CoCl_2$), also significantly reduced TDO2 mRNA expression at concentrations of 250 μM $CoCl_2$ and above (**Figure 3C**, right). Correspondingly, mRNA levels of the surrogate hypoxia marker NDRG1 were elevated upon exposure to 200 μM $CoCl_2$ and above (**Figure 3C**, left). In summary, these results indicate that TDO2 expression is regulated by HIF1α.

Hypoxia Inducible Factor 1α Inhibits the Expression of Immunosuppressive Tryptophan-2,3-Dioxygenase...

15

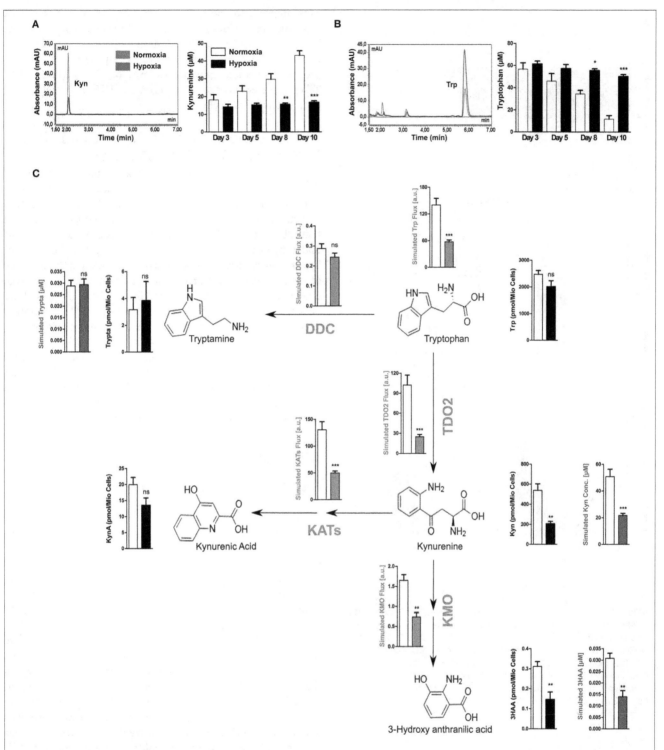

FIGURE 2 | Reduced TDO2 expression leads to reduced Trp flux through the KP. **(A)** uHPLC chromatogram (left) showing Kyn measured in supernatants of A172 cells exposed to 5 days of either normoxia (blue) or hypoxia (red). Quantification of Kyn measurements (right) in supernatants of A172 cells cultured either under normoxia (white) or hypoxia (black) for 3, 5, or 10 days. **(B)** uHPLC chromatogram (left) showing Trp measured in supernatants of A172 cells exposed to 5 days of either normoxia (blue) or hypoxia (red). Quantification of Trp (right) in A172 cell supernatants cultured either under normoxia (white) or hypoxia (black) for 3, 5, 8, or 10 days. **(C)** Scheme depicting the most prominent changes in the flux through the Trp degradation pathway upon exposure to hypoxia (blue plots). Microarray data from A172 GBM cells upon 5 days of hypoxia exposure was integrated into a computational model of Trp metabolism to calculate the fluxes through different enzymes and the general flux through the entire pathway (blue plots) as well as to predict the intracellular metabolite concentrations (gray plots). These intracellular predictions were validated by measurements of the intracellular concentrations (black plots). Data from at least three independent experiments are expressed as mean ± S.E.M. Statistical significance is assumed at $p < 0.05$ (*$p < 0.05$, **$p < 0.01$, ***$p < 0.001$). n.s., not significant.

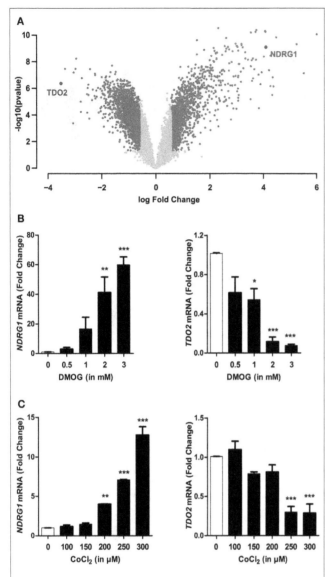

FIGURE 3 | HIF1α stabilization recapitulates hypoxia-mediated reduction in TDO2 expression. **(A)** Volcano plot showing differentially regulated genes in A172 cells exposed to 3 mM DMOG for 24 h compared to DMSO controls. **(B)** qRT-PCR analysis of NDRG1 (left) and TDO2 (right) mRNA expression in A172 cells exposed to 0.5, 1, 2, and 3 mM DMOG for 24 h. **(C)** qRT-PCR analysis of NDRG1 (left) and TDO2 (right) mRNA expression in A172 cells after treatment with 100, 150, 200, 250, and 300 μM of a second HIF1α stabilizing agent, CoCl$_2$, for 24 h. Data from at least three independent experiments are expressed as mean ± S.E.M. Statistical significance is assumed at $p < 0.05$ (*$p < 0.05$, **$p < 0.01$, ***$p < 0.001$).

siRNA-Mediated Silencing of HIF1α Restores TDO2 Expression

We next investigated whether the absence of HIF1α can abrogate the observed reduction in TDO2 expression. siRNA-mediated silencing of HIF1α resulted in a significant reduction in HIF1α mRNA (**Figure 4A**). The reduction of HIF1α was functionally relevant as it prevented the mRNA induction of the surrogate hypoxia marker NDRG1 upon exposure to CoCl$_2$ (**Figure 4B**).

Most importantly, however, the suppression of TDO2 mRNA expression upon CoCl$_2$ exposure was abrogated in the absence of HIF1α (**Figure 4C**). Finally, Western blot analysis of A172 cells under the above conditions revealed a complete rescue of TDO2 protein expression upon knockdown of HIF1α (**Figure 4D**). Taken together, these results confirm that HIF1α controls TDO2 expression in GBM cells.

Hypoxia Impairs the Ability of Tumor Cells to Suppress T Cell Proliferation

TDO2 expression in tumor cells enables them to effectively downregulate the proliferation and thus the anti-tumor activity of infiltrating T cells through production of KP metabolites (32) and the depletion of Trp (38, 39). As our results demonstrate that TDO2 expression is significantly reduced in GBM cells under hypoxic conditions, we next investigated the effect of hypoxia on the proliferation of activated T cells in the presence of A172 GBM cells cultured under either normoxia or hypoxia. Under normoxic conditions, the GBM cells in the co-culture system were clearly capable of suppressing T cell proliferation as compared to the normoxic T cell mono-cultures (**Figure 5A**). However, under hypoxic conditions the previously observed T cell suppression by GBM cells was reduced (**Figure 5B**). Quantification of T cell proliferation expressed as PKH26 mean fluorescent intensity (MFI) revealed that exposure to hypoxia significantly reduced the T cell suppressive capacity of A172 GBM cells in the co-culture system (**Figure 5C**).

DISCUSSION

Over the past decades, the role of hypoxia in shaping the tumor microenvironment and its contribution to tumor cell intrinsic properties as well as anti-tumor immunity has been well-documented (17). Hypoxia is a frequently occurring feature in most solid tumors including GBM, where it not only drives tumor malignancy but also determines tumor morphology (8).

Here, we set out to investigate the role of hypoxia in controlling GBM-derived factors that impact anti-tumor immune responses. Gene expression analysis identified TDO2 as the immunomodulatory factor most strongly regulated in response to hypoxia. TDO2 is a heme containing dioxygenase enzyme, which catalyses the first step of the KP, namely the conversion of Trp to formyl-kynurenine (32). Trp is the least abundant essential amino acid in humans, which in addition to its role in protein synthesis also functions as the precursor for diverse neurotransmitters, hormones and vitamins including serotonin, tryptamine, melatonin, and nicotinamide (40, 41). Trp catabolism along the KP is a well-known modulator of immune responses. Initially identified as an immunosuppressive mechanism preventing the rejection of allogeneic fetuses (42), Trp catabolism has also been implicated in neuropsychiatric disorders (43, 44), auto-immune and inflammatory diseases (45, 46).

Moreover, human cancers often express high levels of indoleamine-2,3-dioxygenase 1 (IDO1) and/or TDO2, the initial Trp-catabolic enzymes of the KP (37). TDO2, for instance is

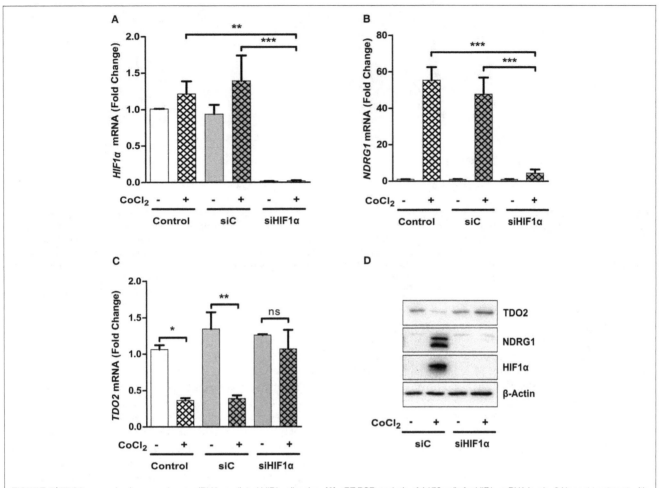

FIGURE 4 | TDO2 expression is rescued upon siRNA-mediated HIF1α silencing. **(A)** qRT-PCR analysis of A172 cells for HIF1α mRNA levels, 24 h post treatment with CoCl$_2$ and 48 h post treatments with either non-targeting siC or siRNA targeting HIF1α. **(B)** qRT-PCR analysis of A172 cells as in **(A)**. showing NDRG1 mRNA levels post HIF1α silencing and CoCl$_2$ treatment. **(C)** TDO2 mRNA levels analyzed by qRT-PCR in A172 cells treated as in **(A,B)**. **(D)** Western blot analysis of TDO2 and NDRG1 in A172 cells subsequent to siRNA-mediated HIF1α silencing and CoCl$_2$ treatment. β-Actin was used as loading control. Data from at least three independent experiments are expressed as mean ± S.E.M. Statistical significance is assumed at $p < 0.05$ (*$p < 0.05$, **$p < 0.01$, ***$p < 0.001$). n.s., not significant.

expressed in diverse tumor entities including breast cancer, bladder cancer, hepatocellular carcinoma, melanoma, non-small cell lung cancer, ovarian carcinoma, renal cell carcinoma, and GBM, where it promotes tumor cell motility and suppresses T cell proliferation and function (24, 47, 48). As Trp catabolism along the KP plays an important tumor-promoting role, this has resulted in interest toward targeting the enzymes of this pathway for cancer therapy (49).

Abnormal or inadequate vasculature in GBM results in formation of regions that have restricted nutrient and oxygen supply (50). Malignant cells in these nutrient-deprived hypoxic regions adapt to survive by profound metabolic reprogramming. In human GBM cells, numerous genes involved in global cellular metabolism are downregulated in response to hypoxia (15). This enables the cells to conserve nutrients in order to redirect them toward essential life-sustaining processes. Hypoxic regions in GBM, due to their nutrient-restricted microenvironment, tend to have a limited supply of Trp, which would dictate that cells

conserve Trp under hypoxia. Here, we show that indeed upon hypoxic exposure GBM cells reversibly downregulate TDO2 expression (**Figures 1A–E**), which is restored upon availability of oxygen (**Figure 1F**). This reversibility may enable tumor cells to effectively regulate Trp catabolism as necessary under cyclic hypoxia, which has been described to frequently occur during tumor progression and metastasis (51). In line with the downregulation of TDO2, the amount of downstream Kyn produced under hypoxia was reduced significantly (**Figure 2A**), corresponding to higher levels of Trp remaining in the extracellular space (**Figure 2B**).

In humans, Trp can be degraded by a number of enzymes along different metabolic pathways, however a majority of the available free Trp has been reported to be degraded via the KP (37). Therefore, we hypothesized that hypoxic control of TDO2 expression, might influence global Trp flux in a tumor cell. We employed a previously described computational model (29) to integrate gene expression data in order to predict

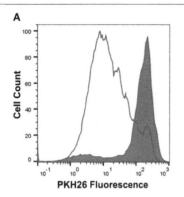
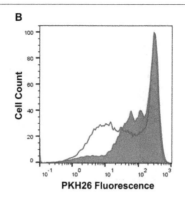
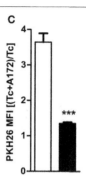

FIGURE 5 | Ability of GBM cells to suppress T cell proliferation is reduced under hypoxia. **(A)** PKH26-labeled CD4+ T cells were stimulated and cultured for 6 days either alone or in co-culture with A172 GBM cells. Histogram from a representative experiment where cultures were placed under normoxia (line histogram represents T cells cultured alone, while filled histogram represents T cells co-cultured with A172 cells). **(B)** Experimental setup as described in **(A)**, except that the cells were cultured under hypoxia. **(C)** Plot showing the change in the ratio between the PKH26 mean fluorescence intensity (MFI) of T cells co-cultured with A172 GBM cells vs. those cultured alone, either under normoxia (white) or hypoxia (black). Data from at least three independent experiments are expressed as mean ± S.E.M. Statistical significance is assumed at $p < 0.05$ (***$p < 0.001$).

changes in Trp metabolism under hypoxia. Our predictions revealed that indeed under hypoxia, the global Trp flux was significantly reduced (**Figure 2C**, blue plots). This reduction upon hypoxia can be attributed to the reduction in metabolic flux through TDO2 and consequently other downstream enzymes in the KP (**Figure 2C**, blue plots). In line, the computational model predicted that intracellular concentrations of Kyn and its downstream metabolite 3HAA were significantly reduced under hypoxia (**Figure 2C**, gray plots). In contrast, the flux through enzymes outside the KP, such as DDC, which degrades Trp to the neuromodulator tryptamine, remained virtually unperturbed (**Figure 2C**, blue plots). These predictions substantiate our hypothesis, that under hypoxia tumor cells downregulate TDO2 expression in order to conserve Trp.

To validate the computational predictions, we next measured intracellular metabolite concentrations of A172 GBM cells cultured under the same conditions as for the microarray analysis. The measured intracellular concentrations of Kyn and other Trp metabolites reflected the exact pattern of the predicted concentrations (**Figure 2C**, black plots), demonstrating that prediction of Trp metabolite concentrations accurately reflects their relative changes. The measurements showed that under hypoxic conditions the intracellular pool of Trp remains largely unchanged due to a significant reduction in the flux through TDO2. The latter was reflected by a reduced production of Kyn and downstream metabolites, while the concentration of other Trp metabolites such as tryptamine was unaltered (**Figure 2C**). Previously, we have shown that tumor cells in a nutrient-deficient but normoxic microenvironment upregulate the expression of tryptophanyl-tRNA synthetase to better utilize the available Trp pool for protein synthesis (52). Taken together, our current results establish the presence of a second adaptation to limited Trp availability under nutrient stress, where tumor cells conserve Trp by downregulation of TDO2 under hypoxic conditions.

Reduced Kyn levels in response to hypoxia have previously been attributed in tumor cells and fibroblasts to reduced expression and activity of IDO1 (53–55), which catalyzes the same reaction as TDO2. The presence of chemokines or chemokine-producing immune cells can however increase the expression of IDO1 under hypoxia (54, 56). Other studies have also reported the upregulation of IDO1 expression upon hypoxic exposure or HIF1α stabilization in neural and immune cells (57–59). Taken together, these studies indicate that the regulation of IDO1 under hypoxic conditions is highly cell type specific and also depends upon microenvironmental factors such as immune cell infiltration. Elbers and colleagues also previously described hypoxia-mediated downregulation of Trp metabolism, which they attributed to reduced TDO2 enzymatic activity under hypoxia (60). The authors used recombinant TDO2 protein in an overexpression system to arrive at the aforementioned conclusions. However, our results provide evidence for the existence of a transcriptional mechanism regulating TDO2-mediated Trp degradation under hypoxia.

Most biological effects of TDO2 including its immunosuppressive actions can be attributed either to the depletion of Trp, which activates nutrient sensing mechanisms such as GCN2 (61) or to the accumulation of downstream KP metabolites. The KP metabolite 3HAA modulates immune functions by enhancing the differentiation of Tregs, reducing T cell proliferation and inducing T cell death (62–64). 3HAA can also interfere with the anti-tumor activity of macrophages by inhibiting their NO production (64). Moreover, 3HAA can be converted further along the KP to quinolinic acid (QA) (65), which can serve as a precursor for NAD+ biosynthesis (66–68). In line with immunosuppressive effects of 3HAA, its metabolic product QA can also modulate immune cell function by suppressing T cell proliferation and increasing Tregs (64).

AHR activation accounts for many of the effects of Trp degradation (24, 69–72). KP metabolites including Kyn, kynurenic acid, xanthurenic acid, and cinnabarinic acid are potent AHR activators (24, 69–72). Moreover, engagement of nuclear coactivator 7 by 3HAA has been reported to enhance activation of the AHR in dendritic cells (73). AHR activation results in AHR binding to HIF1β (ARNT), which also is a binding partner for HIF1α upon its hypoxia-mediated stabilization. Sharing a common binding partner increases the likelihood of competition between the two transcription factors for ARNT binding in scenarios where both AHR activation and HIF1α stabilization take place. In line, reports indicate that HIF1α stabilization adversely affects the activity and downstream gene regulation subsequent to AHR activation in an ARNT-dependent fashion (74). Thus, hypoxia could counteract TDO2 effects mediated via AHR. Furthermore, in GBM, signaling through HIF1α and AHR can crossregulate each other at several points of contact, coordinating metabolic regulation of anti-tumor immunity as well as tumor growth (75).

In this light, we investigated if HIF1α can also interfere upstream of AHR by regulating TDO2 expression or whether the observed hypoxia-mediated TDO2 downregulation is a general HIF1α- independent hypoxia effect. We used the hypoxia mimetic DMOG to stabilize HIF1α in A172 GBM cells under normoxic conditions. Microarray results and qRT-PCR measurements identified TDO2 to be the most downregulated gene upon HIF1α stabilization by DMOG (**Figures 3A,B**). Further, use of a second HIF1α stabilizing agent, $CoCl_2$, also resulted in a significant reduction in TDO2 expression (**Figure 3C**). siRNA-mediated knockdown of HIF1α rescued TDO2 expression (**Figures 4A–D**). Taken together, these results suggest that HIF1α employs a two-pronged strategy to regulate AHR activity, first by direct competitive binding of ARNT (74) and second by downregulating TDO2 expression, thus reducing the concentration of AHR-activating Trp-metabolites.

Although lower oxygen levels are essential for immune cell maturation, extreme pathological hypoxia especially in a tumor acts as an effective immunosuppressive strategy, helping tumors escape immune surveillance (20). TDO2 also helps tumor immune evasion by activating the AHR through its downstream metabolites (24). In light of the existence of these two distinct modi operandi of tumors to suppress anti-tumor immunity, we next ascertained their role in tumor immune suppression under hypoxic conditions. Our data revealed a significant reduction in the immune suppressive abilities of GBM cells in hypoxic co-cultures with T cells (**Figures 5A–C**).

In the present study, we report a HIF1α-dependent regulatory mechanism in GBM cells through which hypoxia can reversibly regulate the expression of the Trp-degrading enzyme TDO2 and thus the production of known immunosuppressive onco-metabolites. Our results further suggest that GBM cells in their quest to give anti-tumor immunity a slip, employ the immunosuppressive effects of both TDO2 and hypoxia in a well-coordinated fashion. In microenvironments with ample oxygen and nutrient availability, tumor cells can employ the TDO2-Kyn-AHR axis to suppress the immune system. While in a nutrient-

deficient hypoxic microenvironment, where hypoxia itself keeps the immune system in check, tumor cells in a HIF1α-dependent fashion can downregulate TDO2 expression so as to conserve Trp. This novel mechanism may present new insights for better clinical management of anti-tumor immune suppression by both TDO2 expression as well as by hypoxia.

AUTHOR CONTRIBUTIONS

SM and CO designed the study and wrote the manuscript. SM, L-OT, GP, and CO developed the methodology. SM, L-OT, and GP acquired the data. SM, AS, L-OT, JD, GP, IH, and CO analyzed and interpreted the data. All the authors read, reviewed, and revised the manuscript.

FUNDING

This work was supported by grants from the BMBF e: Med initiative (GlioPATH, 01ZX1402) and by the Deutsche Forschungsgemeinschaft (DFG, German Research Foundation)–Project-ID 404521405, SFB 1389–UNITE Glioblastoma, Work Package C04 to CO. SM was supported by a Helmholtz International Graduate School for Cancer Research Fellowship. AS was supported by a DAAD Ph.D. scholarship. JD and IH are supported by the Norwegian Research Foundation (250395/F20).

ACKNOWLEDGMENTS

We thank the Microarray Unit of the DKFZ Genomics and Proteomics Core Facility for their excellent services. SM thanks Naba Kishore Mohapatra for the guidance and support. We thank Pauline Pfander, Mirja Tamara Prentzell, Philipp Secker, and Verena Panitz for critically reading the manuscript.

SUPPLEMENTARY MATERIAL

Supplementary Table 1 | Top differentially regulated genes in A172 GBM cells post exposure to 5 days of hypoxia.

Supplementary Table 2 | Top differentially regulated genes in A172 GBM cells 24 h post-exposure to 3 mM DMOG.

Supplementary Figure 1 | Metabolic measurements of supernatants from A172 GBM cells cultured for 5 days either under normoxia (white) or hypoxia (black). **(A)** Trpyptophan (Trp), **(B)** Kynurenine (Kyn), **(C)** 3-hydroxyanthranilic acid (3HAA), **(D)** Kynurenic acid (KynA), **(E)** Tryptamine (Trypta). Data from at least three independent experiments are expressed as mean ± S.E.M. Statistical significance is assumed at $p < 0.05$ (***$p < 0.001$, ****$p \leq 0.0001$). n.s., not significant and n.d., not detected.

REFERENCES

1. Thomlinson RH, Gray LH. The histological structure of some human lung cancers and the possible implications for radiotherapy. *Br J Cancer.* (1955) 9:539–49. doi: 10.1038/bjc.1955.55

2. Gray LH, Conger AD, Ebert M, Hornsey S, Scott OCA. The concentration of oxygen dissolved in tissues at the time of irradiation as a factor in radiotherapy. *Br J Radiol.* (1953) 26:638–48. doi: 10.1259/0007-1285-26-312-638

3. Vaupel P, Mayer A. Hypoxia in cancer: significance and impact on clinical outcome. *Cancer Metastasis Rev.* (2007) 26:225–39. doi: 10.1007/s10555-007-9055-1

4. Johnson AB, Denko N, Barton MC. Hypoxia induces a novel signature of chromatin modifications and global repression of transcription. *Mutat Res.* (2008) 640:174–9. doi: 10.1016/j.mrfmmm.2008.01.001

5. Semenza GL. HIF-1 mediates metabolic responses to intratumoral hypoxia and oncogenic mutations. *J Clin Invest.* (2013) 123:3664. doi: 10.1172/JCI67230

6. Chua YL, Dufour E, Dassa EP, Rustin P, Jacobs HT, Taylor CT, et al. Stabilization of hypoxia-inducible factor-1α protein in hypoxia occurs independently of mitochondrial reactive oxygen species production. *J Biol Chem.* (2010) 285:31277–84. doi: 10.1074/jbc.M110.158485

7. MacLauchlan SC, Calabro NE, Huang Y, Krishna M, Bancroft T, Sharma T, et al. HIF-1alpha represses the expression of the angiogenesis inhibitor thrombospondin-2. *Matrix Biol.* (2018) 65:45–58. doi: 10.1016/j.matbio.2017.07.002

8. Rong Y, Durden DL, Van Meir EG, Brat DJ. "Pseudopalisading" necrosis in glioblastoma: a familiar morphologic feature that links vascular pathology, hypoxia, and angiogenesis. *J Neuropathol Exp Neurol.* (2006) 65:529–39. doi: 10.1097/00005072-200606000-00001

9. Brown JM, Wilson WR. Exploiting tumour hypoxia in cancer treatment. *Nat Rev Cancer.* (2004) 4:437–47. doi: 10.1038/nrc1367

10. Petrova V, Annicchiarico-petruzzelli M, Melino G, Amelio I. The hypoxic tumour microenvironment. *Oncogenesis.* (2018) 7:10. doi: 10.1038/s41389-017-0011-9

11. Challapalli A, Carroll L, Aboagye EO. Molecular mechanisms of hypoxia in cancer. *Clin Transl Imaging.* (2017) 5:225–53. doi: 10.1007/s40336-017-0231-1

12. Hu YL, DeLay M, Jahangiri A, Molinaro AM, Rose SD, Carbonell WS, et al. Hypoxia-induced autophagy promotes tumor cell survival and adaptation to antiangiogenic treatment in glioblastoma. *Cancer Res.* (2012) 72:1773–83. doi: 10.1158/0008-5472.CAN-11-3831

13. Murat A, Migliavacca E, Hussain SF, Heimberger AB, Desbaillets I, Hamou MF, et al. Modulation of angiogenic and inflammatory response in glioblastoma by hypoxia. *PLoS ONE.* (2009) 4:e5947. doi: 10.1371/journal.pone.0005947

14. Monteiro A, Hill R, Pilkington G, Madureira P. The role of hypoxia in glioblastoma invasion. *Cells.* (2017) 6:45. doi: 10.3390/cells6040045

15. Kucharzewska P, Christianson HC, Belting M. Global profiling of metabolic adaptation to hypoxic stress in human glioblastoma cells. *PLoS ONE.* (2015) 10:e116740. doi: 10.1371/journal.pone.0116740

16. Tost J, Daunay A, Poras I, Moreau P, Donadi EA, Carosella ED, et al. Hypoxia inducible factor-1 mediates the expression of the immune checkpoint HLA-G in glioma cells through hypoxia response element located in exon 2. *Oncotarget.* (2016) 7:63690–707. doi: 10.18632/oncotarget.11628

17. Noman MZ, Hasmim M, Messai Y, Terry S, Kieda C, Janji B, et al. Hypoxia: a key player in antitumor immune response. A Review in the theme: cellular responses to hypoxia. *Am J Physiol Cell Physiol.* (2015) 309:C569–79. doi: 10.1152/ajpcell.00207.2015

18. Wei J, Wu A, Kong LY, Wang Y, Fuller G, Fokt I, et al. Hypoxia potentiates glioma-mediated immunosuppression. *PLoS ONE.* (2011) 6:e16195. doi: 10.1371/journal.pone.0016195

19. Vuillefroy de Silly R, Dietrich PY, Walker PR. Hypoxia and antitumor CD8+ T cells: an incompatible alliance? *Oncoimmunology.* (2016) 5:1–8. doi: 10.1080/2162402X.2016.1232236

20. Taylor CT, Colgan SP. Regulation of immunity and inflammation by hypoxia in immunological niches. *Nat Rev Immunol.* (2017) 17:774–85. doi: 10.1038/nri.2017.103

21. Barsoum IB, Smallwood CA, Siemens DR, Graham CH. A mechanism of hypoxia-mediated escape from adaptive immunity in cancer cells. *Cancer Res.* (2014) 74:665–74. doi: 10.1158/0008-5472.CAN-13-0992

22. Noman MZ, Chouaib S. Targeting hypoxia at the forefront of anticancer immune responses. *Oncoimmunology.* (2014) 3:1–3. doi: 10.4161/21624011.2014.954463

23. Murthy A, Gerber SA, Koch CJ, Lord EM. Intratumoral hypoxia reduces IFN-γ-mediated immunity and MHC class I induction in a preclinical tumor model. *Immuno Horizons.* (2019) 3:149–60. doi: 10.4049/immunohorizons.1900017

24. Opitz CA, Litzenburger UM, Sahm F, Ott M, Tritschler I, Trump S, et al. An endogenous tumour-promoting ligand of the human aryl hydrocarbon receptor. *Nature.* (2011) 478:197–203. doi: 10.1038/nature10491

25. Wenger R, Kurtcuoglu V, Scholz C, Marti H, Hoogewijs D. Frequently asked questions in hypoxia research. *Hypoxia.* (2015) 3:35–43. doi: 10.2147/hp.s92198

26. Carvalho BS, Irizarry RA. A framework for oligonucleotide microarray preprocessing. *Bioinformatics.* (2010) 26:2363–7. doi: 10.1093/bioinformatics/btq431

27. You N, Wang X. An empirical Bayes method for robust variance estimation in detecting DEGs using microarray data. *J Bioinform Comput Biol.* (2017) 15:1–14. doi: 10.1142/S0219720017500202

28. Ritchie ME, Phipson B, Wu D, Hu Y, Law CW, Shi W, et al. Limma powers differential expression analyses for RNA-sequencing and microarray studies. *Nucleic Acids Res.* (2015) 43:e47. doi: 10.1093/nar/gkv007

29. Stavrum AK, Heiland I, Schuster S, Puntervoll P, Ziegler M. Model of tryptophan metabolism, readily scalable using tissue-specific gene expression data. *J Biol Chem.* (2013) 288:34555–66. doi: 10.1074/jbc.M113.474908

30. Schäuble S, Stavrum AK, Bockwoldt M, Puntervoll P, Heiland I. SBMLmod: a Python-based web application and web service for efficient data integration and model simulation. *BMC Bioinformatics.* (2017) 18:314. doi: 10.1186/s12859-017-1722-9

31. Hoops S, Gauges R, Lee C, Pahle J, Simus N, Singhal M, et al. COPASI - a COmplex PAthway SImulator. *Bioinformatics.* (2006) 22:3067–74. doi: 10.1093/bioinformatics/btl485

32. Baren N Van, Eynde BJ Van Den. Tryptophan-degrading enzymes in tumoral immune resistance. *Front Immunol.* (2015) 6:34. doi: 10.3389/fimmu.2015.00034

33. Fallarino F, Grohmann U, Vacca C, Bianchi R, Orabona C, Spreca A, et al. T cell apoptosis by tryptophan catabolism. *Cell Death Differ.* (2002) 9:1069–77. doi: 10.1038/sj.cdd.4401073

34. Lewis-Ballester A, Forouhar F, Kim SM, Lew S, Wang Y, Karkashon S, et al. Molecular basis for catalysis and substrate-mediated cellular stabilization of human tryptophan 2,3-dioxygenase. *Sci Rep.* (2016) 6:35169. doi: 10.1038/srep35169

35. Weiler M, Blaes J, Pusch S, Sahm F, Czabanka M, Luger S, et al. mTOR target NDRG1 confers MGMT-dependent resistance to alkylating chemotherapy. *Proc Natl Acad Sci USA.* (2014) 111:409–14. doi: 10.1073/pnas.1314469111

36. Said HM, Safari R, Al-Kafaji G, Ernestus RI, Löhr M, Katzer A, et al. Time- and oxygen-dependent expression and regulation of NDRG1 in human brain cancer cells. *Oncol Rep.* (2017) 37:3625–34. doi: 10.3892/or.2017.5620

37. Platten M, Nollen EAA, Röhrig UF, Fallarino F, Opitz CA. Tryptophan metabolism as a common therapeutic target in cancer, neurodegeneration and beyond. *Nat Rev Drug Discov.* (2019) 18:379–401. doi: 10.1038/s41573-019-0016-5

38. Munn DH, Shafizadeh E, Attwood JT, Bondarev I, Pashine A, Mellor AL. Inhibition of T cell proliferation by macrophage tryptophan catabolism. *J Exp Med.* (1999) 189:1363–72. doi: 10.1084/jem.189.9.1363

39. Fallarino F, Grohmann U, You S, McGrath BC, Cavener DR, Vacca C, et al. The combined effects of tryptophan starvation and tryptophan catabolites down-regulate T cell receptor ζ-chain and induce a regulatory phenotype in naive T cells. *J Immunol.* (2006) 176:6752–61. doi: 10.4049/jimmunol.176.11.6752

40. Richard DM, Dawes MA, Mathias CW, Acheson A, Hill-kapturczak N, Dougherty DM. L -tryptophan : basic metabolic functions, behavioral research and therapeutic indications. *Int J Tryptophan Res.* (2009) 2:45–60. doi: 10.4137/IJTR.S2129

41. Gostner JM, Geisler S, Stonig M, Mair L, Sperner-Unterweger B, Fuchs D. Tryptophan metabolism and related pathways in psychoneuroimmunology:

the impact of nutrition and lifestyle. *Neuropsychobiology*. (2019) doi: 10.1159/000496293

42. Munn DH. Prevention of allogeneic fetal rejection by tryptophan catabolism. *Science*. (1998) 281:1191–3. doi: 10.1126/science.281.5380.1191

43. Teraishi T, Hori H, Sasayama D, Matsuo J, Ogawa S, Ota M, et al. 13 C-tryptophan breath test detects increased catabolic turnover of tryptophan along the kynurenine pathway in patients with major depressive disorder. *Sci Rep*. (2015) 5:4–12. doi: 10.1038/srep15994

44. Jenkins TA, Nguyen JCD, Polglaze KE, Bertrand PP. Influence of tryptophan and serotonin on mood and cognition with a possible role of the gut-brain axis. *Nutrients*. (2016) 8:1–15. doi: 10.3390/nu8010056

45. Muller AJ, Sharma MD, Chandler PR, Duhadaway JB, Everhart ME, Johnson BA, et al. Chronic inflammation that facilitates tumor progression creates local immune suppression by inducing indoleamine 2,3 dioxygenase. *Proc Natl Acad Sci USA*. (2008) 105:17073–8. doi: 10.1073/pnas.0806173105

46. Opitz CA, Wick W, Steinman L, Platten M. Tryptophan degradation in autoimmune diseases. *Cell Mol life Sci*. (2007) 64:2542–63. doi: 10.1007/s00018-007-7140-9

47. Pilotte L, Larrieu P, Stroobant V, Plaen E De, Uyttenhove C, Wouters J, et al. Reversal of tumoral immune resistance by inhibition of tryptophab 2,3-dioxygenase. *Proc Natl Acad Sci USA*. (2012) 109:2497–502. doi: 10.1073/pnas.1113873109

48. Guastella AR, Michelhaugh SK, Klinger NV, Kupsky WJ, Polin LA, Muzik O, et al. Tryptophan PET imaging of the kynurenine pathway in patient-derived xenograft models of glioblastoma. *Mol Imaging*. (2016) 15:1–11. doi: 10.1177/1536012116644881

49. Prendergast GC, Malachowski WJ, Mondal A, Scherle P, Muller AJ. Indoleamine 2,3-dioxygenase and its therapeutic inhibition in cancer. *Int Rev Cell Mol Biol*. (2018) 336:175–203. doi: 10.1016/bs.ircmb.2017.07.004

50. Dimberg A. The glioblastoma vasculature as a target for cancer therapy. *Biochem Soc Trans*. (2014) 42:1647–52. doi: 10.1042/BST20140278

51. Saxena K, Jolly MK. Acute vs. chronic vs. cyclic hypoxia: their differential dynamics, molecular mechanisms, and effects on tumor progression. *Biomolecules*. (2019) 9:339. doi: 10.3390/biom9080339

52. Adam I, Dewi DL, Mooiweer J, Sadik A, Mohapatra SR, Berdel B, et al. Upregulation of tryptophanyl-tRNA synthethase adapts human cancer cells to nutritional stress caused by tryptophan degradation. *Oncoimmunology*. (2018) 7:1–14. doi: 10.1080/2162402X.2018.1486353

53. Schmidt SK, Ebel S, Keil E, Woite C, Ernst JF, Benzin AE, et al. Regulation of IDO activity by oxygen supply: inhibitory effects on antimicrobial and immunoregulatory functions. *PLoS ONE*. (2013) 8:e63301. doi: 10.1371/journal.pone.0063301

54. Liu J, Zhang H, Jia L, Sun H. Effects of Treg cells and IDO on human epithelialovarian cancer cells under hypoxic conditions. *Mol Med Rep*. (2015) 11:1708–14. doi: 10.3892/mmr.2014.2893

55. Mennan C, Garcia J, McCarthy H, Owen S, Perry J, Wright K, et al. Human articular chondrocytes retain their phenotype in sustained hypoxia while normoxia promotes their immunomodulatory potential. *Cartilage*. (2018) 10:467–79. doi: 10.1177/1947603518769714

56. Wobma HM, Kanai M, Ma SP, Shih Y, Li HW, Duran-Struuck R, et al. Dual IFN-γ/hypoxia priming enhances immunosuppression of mesenchymal stromal cells through regulatory proteins and metabolic mechanisms. *J Immunol Regen Med*. (2018) 1:45–56. doi: 10.1016/j.regen.2018.01.001

57. Song X, Zhang Y, Zhang L, Song W, Shi L. Hypoxia enhances indoleamine 2,3-dioxygenase production in dendritic cells. *Oncotarget*. (2018) 9:11572–80. doi: 10.18632/oncotarget.24098

58. Lam CS, Li JJ, Tipoe GL, Youdim MBH, Fung ML. Monoamine oxidase A upregulated by chronic intermittent hypoxia activates indoleamine 2,3-dioxygenase and neurodegeneration. *PLoS ONE*. (2017) 12:e0177940. doi: 10.1371/journal.pone.0177940

59. Keränen MAI, Raissadati A, Nykänen AI, Dashkevich A, Tuuminen R, Krebs R, et al. Hypoxia-inducible factor controls immunoregulatory properties of myeloid cells in mouse cardiac allografts – an experimental study. *Transpl Int*. (2019) 32:95–106. doi: 10.1111/tri.13310

60. Elbers F, Woite C, Antoni V, Stein S, Funakoshi H, Nakamura T, et al. Negative impact of hypoxia on tryptophan 2,3-dioxygenase function. *Mediators Inflamm*. (2016) 2016:1–11. doi: 10.1155/2016/1638916

61. Munn DH, Sharma MD, Baban B, Harding HP, Zhang Y, Ron D, et al. GCN2 kinase in T cells mediates proliferative arrest and anergy induction in response to indoleamine 2, 3-dioxygenase. *Immunity*. (2005) 22:633–42. doi: 10.1016/j.immuni.2005.03.013

62. Hornyák L, Dobos N, Koncz G, Karányi Z, Páll D, Szabó Z, et al. The role of indoleamine-2,3-dioxygenase in cancer development, diagnostics, and therapy. *Front Immunol*. (2018) 9:151. doi: 10.3389/fimmu.2018.00151

63. Sordillo PP, Sordillo LA, Helson L. The kynurenine pathway: a primary resistance mechanism in patients with glioblastoma. *Anticancer Res*. (2017) 37:2159–71. doi: 10.21873/anticanres.11551

64. Heng B, Lim CK, Lovejoy DB, Bessede A, Gluch L, Guillemin GJ. Understanding the role of the kynurenine pathway in human breast cancer immunobiology. *Oncotarget*. (2016) 7:6506–20. doi: 10.18632/oncotarget.6467

65. Adams S, Braidy N, Bessesde A, Brew BJ, Grant R, Teo C, et al. The kynurenine pathway in brain tumor pathogenesis. *Cancer Res*. (2012) 72:5649–57. doi: 10.1158/0008-5472.CAN-12-0549

66. Sundaram G, Brew BJ, Jones SP, Adams S, Lim CK, Guillemin GJ. Quinolinic acid toxicity on oligodendroglial cells: Relevance for multiple sclerosis and therapeutic strategies. *J Neuroinflammation*. (2014) 11:204. doi: 10.1186/s12974-014-0204-5

67. Sahm F, Oezen I, Opitz CA, Radlwimmer B, Von Deimling A, Ahrendt T, et al. The endogenous tryptophan metabolite and NAD+ precursor quinolinic acid confers resistance of gliomas to oxidative stress. *Cancer Res*. (2013) 73:3225–34. doi: 10.1158/0008-5472.CAN-12-3831

68. Katsyuba E, Mottis A, Zietak M, De Franco F, van der Velpen V, Gariani K, et al. De novo NAD + synthesis enhances mitochondrial function and improves health. *Nature*. (2018) 563:354–9. doi: 10.1038/s41586-018-0645-6

69. Mezrich JD, Fechner JH, Zhang X, Johnson BP, Burlingham WJ, Bradfield CA. An interaction between kynurenine and the aryl hydrocarbon receptor can generate regulatory T cells. *J Immunol*. (2010) 185:3190–8. doi: 10.4049/jimmunol.0903670

70. Novikov O, Wang Z, Stanford EA, Parks AJ, Ramirez-Cardenas A, Landesman E, et al. An aryl hydrocarbon receptor-mediated amplification loop that enforces cell migration in ER - /PR - /Her2 - human breast cancer cells. *Mol Pharmacol*. (2016) 90:674–88. doi: 10.1124/mol.116.105361

71. Bessede A, Gargaro M, Pallotta MT, Matino D, Servillo G, Brunacci C, et al. Aryl hydrocarbon receptor control of a disease tolerance defence pathway. *Nature*. (2014) 511:184–90. doi: 10.1038/nature13323

72. Lowe MM, Mold JE, Kanwar B, Huang Y, Louie A, Pollastri MP, et al. Identification of cinnabarinic acid as a novel endogenous aryl hydrocarbon receptor ligand that drives IL-22 production. *PLoS ONE*. (2014) 9:e87877. doi: 10.1371/journal.pone.0087877

73. Gargaro M, Vacca C, Massari S, Scalisi G, Manni G, Mondanelli G, et al. Engagement of nuclear coactivator 7 by 3-hydroxyanthranilic acid enhances activation of aryl hydrocarbon receptor in immunoregulatory dendritic cells. *Front Immunol*. (2019) 10:1973. doi: 10.3389/fimmu.2019.01973

74. Vorrink SU, Severson PL, Kulak M V, Futscher BW, Domann FE. Hypoxia perturbs aryl hydrocarbon receptor signaling and CYP1A1 expression induced by PCB 126 in human skin and liver-derived cell lines. *Toxicol Appl Pharmacol*. (2014) 274:408–16. doi: 10.1016/j.taap.2013.12.002

75. Gabriely G, Wheeler MA, Takenaka MC, Quintana FJ. Role of AHR and HIF-1α in glioblastoma metabolism. *Trends Endocrinol Metab*. (2017) 28:428–36. doi: 10.1016/j.tem.2017.02.009

3

Tryptophan Co-Metabolism at the Host-Pathogen Interface

Claudio Costantini[1], Marina M. Bellet[1], Giorgia Renga[1], Claudia Stincardini[1],
Monica Borghi[1], Marilena Pariano[1], Barbara Cellini[1], Nancy Keller[2], Luigina Romani[1] and
Teresa Zelante[1]*

[1] Department of Experimental Medicine, University of Perugia, Perugia, Italy, [2] Department of Medical Microbiology and
Immunology, Department of Bacteriology, University of Wisconsin-Madison, Madison, WI, United States

Keywords: tryptophan, co-metabolism, xenobiotic receptor, microbiota, kynurenine, 3-IAld

*Correspondence:
Teresa Zelante
teresa.zelante@unipg.it

HOST-MICROBE TRYPTOPHAN CO-METABOLISM

Microbes have evolved to exploit humans as a rich source of nutrients to support survival and replication. Although mammals and microbes may differ in their requirement for tryptophan (Trp), being an essential amino acid in the former and produced, with some exceptions, by bacteria and fungi, common catabolic enzymes are shared by both host and pathogens. Indoleamine 2,3-dioxygenases (IDOs) catabolize Trp to kynurenines and are widely distributed from bacteria to metazoans. The evolutionary conservation of the kynurenine pathway may be linked to the importance of the *de novo* synthesis of nicotinamide adenine dinucleotide (NAD+), to which it ultimately leads, although additional functions of kynurenines are increasingly being recognized. Indeed, it is now clearly established that mammalian IDOs regulate infection and drive immune tolerance by means of Trp deprivation and the generation of active metabolites, including kynurenines. An additional level of complexity can be envisaged when microbes utilize Trp *via* alternative pathways upon colonization of the host in a relationship that can be either commensalism or pathogenic. In these situations, the host and microbes are found to share common substrates but the presence of dissimilar metabolic pathways may result in the generation of metabolites, such as indoles or tryptamine that can cross-regulate each others metabolism. Here, we discuss the potential relevance of Co-Trp metabolism or alternative secondary pathways of Trp degradation in modulating host immune response and eventually the xenobiotic receptors (XRs), while regulating microbe fitness. These concepts are expected to open a novel scenario in which a comprehensive assessment of the metabolic status is crucial to correctly evaluate pathological colonization and drive the most appropriate therapeutic strategy.

CO-METABOLISM DICTATES PATHOGEN VIRULENCE

Trp is one of the 20 amino acids used for building proteins with the unique characteristic of bearing an indole, a bicyclic ring formed by a benzene and a pyrrole group, linked to the α-carbon by a –CH2-group (1). The presence of the indole group not only dictates the biochemical properties of Trp, a highly hydrophobic amino acid that guarantees the stabilization of protein and peptide structures, but also makes Trp a reservoir of indole-based bioactive molecules with fundamental implications in organism physiopathology (1, 2). The relevance of Trp and its catabolic pathways acquires a novel dimension when they are envisioned in the context of a relationship between host and microbes. Indeed, the different entities involved in the relationship share the same Trp substrate, which is fundamental for all the parties at play, but is catabolized along peculiar patterns. Therefore, multiple levels of interactions can be foreseen, starting from the competition of the Trp substrate to the generation of bioactive molecules *via* shared or exclusive catabolic pathways with cross-regulatory properties, and each will be discussed upon in the following sections.

First, the requirement for Trp differs between the organisms. Indeed, while Trp is an essential amino acid in mammals, microorganisms, and higher plants possess the ability to synthesize Trp from chorismate, a common precursor of aromatic amino acids produced by the shikimate pathway from phosphoenol pyruvate and erythrose-4-phosphate (3). This dependence of mammals from external sources of Trp creates a first level of interaction in the host/microbe interface. Indeed, mammals might obtain Trp not only from the diet, but also from commensal microorganisms that possess the shikimate pathway and may represent a source of Trp. On the contrary, pathogens may co-opt host mechanisms of Trp degradation as a strategy to evade the host immune response (4). For instance, in a murine model, the gut pathogen *Clostridium difficile* induced IDO1 expression to deplete the Trp pool and increase kynurenine production in the cecal tissue by IDO1-expressing CD11c$^+$ myeloid cells, among other stromal cells. As a consequence, neutrophil accumulation and pathogen clearance were limited (4, 5). Other pathogens however, depend on the host for Trp availability, including common intracellular pathogens, and it is the host that depletes the Trp pool to limit the virulence of the pathogens (4, 6). For instance, the parasite *Toxoplasma gondii* is Trp-auxotroph and IDO activity suppresses its growth, as first demonstrated by Pfefferkorn and co-workers in cultured human fibroblasts treated with IFNγ (7). Thus, Trp itself appears as a double-edged sword in the host-microbe interaction: on the one hand, it may ensure a positive symbioses between the host and Trp synthesizing microbes; on the other hand, it may be used as a weapon to deprive the host or, vice versa, Trp-auxotroph pathogens of Trp, resulting in increased or reduced virulence, respectively.

Second, Trp may be catabolized via shared catabolic pathways. In mammals, Trp is metabolized along four different pathways leading to the formation of (i) serotonin and melatonin, (ii) tryptamine, (iii) indolepyruvic acid, and (iv) kynurenine (8). The kynurenine pathway accounts for nearly 95% of all Trp degradation (8), and the rate-limiting step is catalyzed by one of three enzymes, namely indoleamine 2,3-dioxygenase 1 (IDO1), IDO2, and tryptophan 2,3-dioxygenase (TDO), with distinct localization, affinity, and regulation (8). The evolution of IDOs and TDO has been the subject of intense research. TDO is widely present in metazoan and many bacterial species, but not in fungi, and is characterized by a high efficiency for Trp degradation throughout the evolution (9). On the contrary, IDO is found in mammals, lower vertebrates, invertebrates, fungi, and bacterial species, but only mammalian IDO1 and fungal IDOs show high efficiency for Trp degradation (9). Irrespective of the ancestral role of IDOs and TDO and their evolution, it is evident that microorganisms are endowed with the ability to catabolize Trp along the kynurenine pathway, as partially demonstrated by experiments in germ-free mice that show a decrease in the kynurenine pathway (10). In this scenario, two opposite outcomes are possible. Indeed, not only the distinct dioxygenases might compete for the same substrate to produce kynurenine for self-advantage, but they can also compensate each other in physiological or pathological conditions characterized by kynurenine deficiency,

again identifying Trp and its catabolism as a double-edged sword in host-microbe interaction. Unfortunately, studies on the kynurenine pathway in microbes and how it intersects with host metabolism are still very scarce, and it is not possible to draw any conclusions in support of one or the other possibility.

As a third level of interaction, Trp may be catalyzed via distinct catabolic pathways by the host and microbes, resulting in the generation of metabolites that can cross-regulate each other metabolism. In recent years, we have identified and characterized the "postbiotic" molecule indole-3-aldehyde (3-IAld) derived from the microbial degradation of Trp and produced by probiotics such as lactobacilli (11). 3-IAld proved critical in the maintenance and restoration of intestinal epithelial integrity. Indeed, by binding the aryl hydrocarbon receptor (AhR) and activating the expression of IL-22, 3-IAld promotes the repair of the intestinal epithelial lining and the reduction of inflammatory markers (11). Another interesting example is represented by indole, produced by bacteria and some plants from Trp *via* the enzymes tryptophanase and indole-3-glycerol phosphate lyases, respectively (12). Interestingly, indole negatively regulates the virulence of various pathogens, such as the gastrointestinal tract pathogens enterohemorrhagic *Escherichia coli* (EHEC) (13, 14) and *Citrobacter rodentium* (14). For instance, mice infected with *C. rodentium* and manipulated to contain different concentrations of indole in the gastrointestinal tract showed an inverse correlation between colonization/mortality and amounts of indole (14). In addition, indole can enhance the competitiveness of commensal microorganisms, for instance by promoting the growth of *E. coli* in mixed-cultures with *Pseudomonas aeruginosa* via inhibition of quorum sensing (15). However, microorganisms may also adopt specialized ways to use Trp and catabolic intermediates as pathogenic molecules. For instance, *A. fumigatus* can incorporate Trp and/or anthranilate *via* non-ribosomal peptide synthetases to generate toxic molecules (16), such as the Trp-derived iron (III)-complex hexadehydroastechrome that increased the virulence of *A. fumigatus* and the mortality in a neutropenic murine pulmonary model upon overexpression (17).

Overall, these examples illustrate how Trp and catabolic molecules play a fundamental role in regulating the interaction between the host and the microbes, which can occur at multiple levels and with opposite outcomes. Indeed, Trp and its metabolites may serve to establish a symbiotic relationship or otherwise be used to weaken the partner by depleting essential molecules or creating toxic substances.

TRYPTOPHAN DEGRADATION BY MICROBES: TOXICITY VS. IMMUNOMODULATION

Indole: The Interkingdom Molecule

The enzyme tryptophanase (TnA) is responsible of Trp degradation and release of indole and indole-derivatives. Importantly, TnA is widely expressed in Gram-negative as well as in Gram-positive bacteria (14, 18). The indole ring is found in humans as the nucleus of human hormones as serotonin or melatonin, but is also found in plants in auxins, which may affect plant orientation by promoting cell division to one side of the plant in response to sunlight and gravity. Indole is also synthesized in the bowel by microbes, regulating the biofilm as quorum sensing molecule or the intestinal physiology. Thus, the indole ring being diffused in different ecosystems, is considered a type of "*archetypical hormone*" able to regulate the relation between the host and microbes in plants but also in the animal kingdom. The mechanisms of action in the host by indole and indole derivatives are not well-characterized yet, although a very large part of research has focused the mechanistic function on their capacity to bid the XRs (11, 19, 20). Interestingly, animals can't synthesize indole, while many bacteria and also fungi produce indole and indole-derivatives with some pathogens such as *A. fumigatus* synthesizing toxic indole alkaloids (21). In addition, indole and indole-derivatives are detected in the human blood as well as in peripheral tissues in physiological conditions. Frequently, indoles can be measured in urine but traces are also present in lymph nodes (22–24). A good example of co-metabolism with the host among the indole-derivatives is the indoxyl sulfate, typically representing a uremic toxin, derived from indole in the liver via the actions of cytochrome P450 enzymes (25).

The Indole Pyruvate (IPyA) Route: A Direct Effect on Immunity

The indole-3-pyruvic acid (IPyA) route is key to converting aromatic amino acids to aroma compounds via transamination of Trp (26). IPyA secondary metabolites are indol-3-acetaldehyde (3-IAAld), indole-3-acetic-acid (IAA), and indole-3-carboxaldehyde (3-IAld)—all known as being AhR ligands (11) (**Figure 1**). AhR is part of the XRs family. XRs have evolved as cellular sensors for ligands (endogenous and exogenous) able to transcribe for genes encoding for drug-metabolizing enzymes.

XRs are also extremely involved in regulating general physiology since they can also transcribe for genes involved in immune regulation, cell metabolism, energy homeostasis (**Figure 1**). Families of XRs may bind a very large family of unrelated ligands by direct or indirect binding (27, 28). XRs may include the pregnane X receptor (PXR), the AhR, the constitutive androstane receptor (CAR), and the peroxisome proliferator-activated receptors (PPARs) (**Figure 1**). More recently, XRs family has been deeply investigated for their ability to directly communicate with the gut microbiota (11, 29, 30).

XRs respond to different metabolites produced by the host as well as by the microbiota. Thus, metabolism and co-metabolism are strictly related to XR activation pathway (30). Therefore, the acute or chronic symptoms of dysbacteriosis generally reflect the XR role in regulating the host physiology as energy metabolism, glucose homeostasis, immune-regulation.

Indeed, it was demonstrated that certain bacterial tryptophan-derived metabolites activate PXR particularly expressed in intestinal epithelial cells. The downstream signaling of intestinal PXR affects murine intestinal permeability, gut inflammation, and in peripheral tissue bile acid metabolism and drug resistance. Thus, in case of dysbiosis, where there is a severe lack of PXR ligands homeostasis is seriously compromised. Restoration of PXR signaling by using gnotobiotic mice or by administering PXR ligands, may result in abolishing pro-inflammatory signs and loss of barrier dysfunction in the context of intestinal inflammation (31).

In addition, we have demonstrated in mice that the indole-derivative 3-IAld is an AhR ligand that promotes IL-22 production. 3-IAld restored antifungal resistance and increased IL-22 production, ameliorated colitis via gut NKp46$^+$ cells and via the XR AhR. These results suggest that the activity of 3-IAld could be exploited to

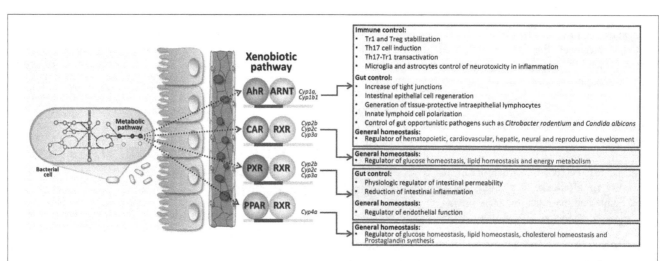

FIGURE 1 | Intricate microbiota-derived metabolic pathways may affect host XR activation and general host physiology. AhR, Aryl hydrocarbon receptor; ARNT, Aryl Hydrocarbon Receptor Nuclear Translocator; CAR, Constitutive Androstane Receptor; RXR, Retinoid X Receptor; PXR, Pregnane X Receptor; PPAR, Peroxisome Proliferator-Activated Receptors.

guarantee homeostasis and microbial cooperation at mucosal surfaces in conditions of immune dysregulation (11, 32). More recently, 3-IAld has been proved also changing together with a tryptophan-rich diet, the program of intraepithelial CD4$^+$ T cells into immunoregulatory T cells in mice (20).

Kynurenines: Immunomodulatory Functions

As in mammalians, Trp may also be degraded in to kynurenines by microbes. For example, *Pseudomonas aeruginosa*, a Gram-negative bacteria frequently involved in healthcare-associated pneumonia, catabolizes tryptophan through the kynurenine pathway. Thus, bacterial metabolites may interfere with the host's immune response during *in vivo* infection and acute lung injury (33). Another important evidence of co-metabolism, was demonstrated for the opportunistic fungus *Candida albicans* (34). Trp metabolites produced by the fungus *Candida*, in particular 5-hydroxytryptophan metabolites, are also able to modulate Th17 response, similarly to kynurenines as shown for mammalians (34). The opportunistic fungal pathogen *A. fumigatus* also has three *ido* genes (*idoA,B,C*) in its genome (35–37). Enzymatic studies suggest that Idos of *A. oryzae*, participate in Trp degradation (38). Furthermore, previous studies on *A. fumigatus* grown on Trp showed upregulation of these *ido* genes (36). However, the relative contributions of individual Idos and adaptation to the host's environment, as well as the impact of kynurenines released by the fungus during lung infection *in vivo*, remain unclear.

CONCLUSIONS

The scientific proof for a contribution of the XRs in the control of barrier function and immune regulation would serve as a basis toward improvement of non-toxic probes and ligands as drugs (30). This is also put forward by the fact that several of those microbial metabolites are found in human blood at levels comparable to host metabolites (3-IAld 0.01–0.1 μM; IAA 0.1–1 μM), suggesting that systemic responses may be easily activated by targeted XR-based therapy. These systems are thought to provide an additional level of interchange between the microbes and the host at the edge of their co-metabolism (**Figure 1**).

AUTHOR CONTRIBUTIONS

CC and TZ wrote the manuscript. MMB, GR, CS, MB, MP, BC, NK, and LR edited the manuscript and provided valuable discussions and criticisms.

FUNDING

This work was supported by the Specific Targeted Research Project FunMeta (ERC-2011-AdG-293714).

ACKNOWLEDGMENTS

The authors wish to thank C. Massi Benedetti for digital art and image editing.

REFERENCES

1. Palego L, Betti L, Rossi A, Giannaccini G. Tryptophan biochemistry: structural, nutritional, metabolic, and medical aspects in humans. *J Amino Acids.* (2016) 2016:8952520. doi: 10.1155/2016/8952520
2. Platten M, Nollen EAA, Rohrig UF, Fallarino F, Opitz CA. Tryptophan metabolism as a common therapeutic target in cancer, neurodegeneration and beyond. *Nat Rev Drug Discov.* (2019) 18:379–401. doi: 10.1038/s41573-019-0016-5
3. Parthasarathy A, Cross PJ, Dobson RCJ, Adams LE, Savka MA, Hudson AO. A three-ring circus: metabolism of the three proteogenic aromatic amino acids and their role in the health of plants and animals. *Front Mol Biosci.* (2018) 5:29. doi: 10.3389/fmolb.2018.00029
4. Ren W, Rajendran R, Zhao Y, Tan B, Wu G, Bazer FW, et al. Amino acids as mediators of metabolic cross talk between host and pathogen. *Front Immunol.* (2018) 9:319. doi: 10.3389/fimmu.2018.00319
5. El-Zaatari M, Chang YM, Zhang M, Franz M, Shreiner A, McDermott AJ, et al. Tryptophan catabolism restricts IFN-gamma-expressing neutrophils and *Clostridium difficile* immunopathology. *J Immunol.* (2014) 193:807–16. doi: 10.4049/jimmunol.1302913
6. Zhang YJ, Rubin EJ. Feast or famine: the host-pathogen battle over amino acids. *Cell Microbiol.* (2013) 15:1079–87. doi: 10.1111/cmi.12140
7. Pfefferkorn ER, Eckel M, Rebhun S. Interferon-gamma suppresses the growth of *Toxoplasma gondii* in human fibroblasts through starvation for tryptophan. *Mol Biochem Parasitol.* (1986) 20:215–24. doi: 10.1016/0166-6851(86)90101-5
8. Badawy AA. Kynurenine pathway of tryptophan metabolism: regulatory and functional aspects. *Int J Tryptophan Res.* (2017) 10:1178646917691938. doi: 10.1177/1178646917691938

9. Yuasa HJ, Ball HJ. Efficient tryptophan-catabolizing activity is consistently conserved through evolution of TDO enzymes, but not IDO enzymes. *J Exp Zool B Mol Dev Evol.* (2015) 324:128–40. doi: 10.1002/jez.b.22608
10. Gao J, Xu K, Liu H, Liu G, Bai M, Peng C, et al. Impact of the gut microbiota on intestinal immunity mediated by tryptophan metabolism. *Front Cell Infect Microbiol.* (2018) 8:13. doi: 10.3389/fcimb.2018.00013
11. Zelante T, Iannitti RG, Cunha C, De Luca A, Giovannini G, Pieraccini G, et al. Tryptophan catabolites from microbiota engage aryl hydrocarbon receptor and balance mucosal reactivity via interleukin-22. *Immunity.* (2013) 39:372–85. doi: 10.1016/j.immuni.2013.08.003
12. Lee JH, Wood TK, Lee J. Roles of indole as an interspecies and interkingdom signaling molecule. *Trends Microbiol.* (2015) 23:707–18. doi: 10.1016/j.tim.2015.08.001
13. Bansal T, Englert D, Lee J, Hegde M, Wood TK, Jayaraman A. Differential effects of epinephrine, norepinephrine, and indole on *Escherichia coli* O157:H7 chemotaxis, colonization, and gene expression. *Infect Immun.* (2007) 75:4597–607. doi: 10.1128/IAI.00630-07
14. Kumar A, Sperandio V. Indole signaling at the host-microbiota-pathogen interface. *MBio.* (2019) 10:e01031-19. doi: 10.1128/mBio.01031-19
15. Chu W, Zere TR, Weber MM, Wood TK, Whiteley M, Hidalgo-Romano B, et al. Indole production promotes *Escherichia coli* mixed-culture growth with *Pseudomonas aeruginosa* by inhibiting quorum signaling. *Appl Environ Microbiol.* (2012) 78:411–9. doi: 10.1128/AEM.06396-11
16. Choera T, Zelante T, Romani L, Keller NP. A multifaceted role of tryptophan metabolism and indoleamine 2,3-dioxygenase activity in *Aspergillus fumigatus*-host interactions. *Front Immunol.* (2017) 8:1996. doi: 10.3389/fimmu.2017.01996
17. Yin WB, Baccile JA, Bok JW, Chen Y, Keller NP, Schroeder FC. A nonribosomal peptide synthetase-derived iron(III) complex from the

pathogenic fungus *Aspergillus fumigatus. J Am Chem Soc.* (2013) 135:2064–7. doi: 10.1021/ja311145n

18. Berstad A, Raa J, Valeur J. Indole - the scent of a healthy 'inner soil'. *Microb Ecol Health Dis.* (2015) 26:27997. doi: 10.3402/mehd.v26.27997

19. Bessede A, Gargaro M, Pallotta MT, Matino D, Servillo G, Brunacci C, et al. Aryl hydrocarbon receptor control of a disease tolerance defence pathway. *Nature.* (2014) 511:184–90. doi: 10.1038/nature13323

20. Cervantes-Barragan L, Chai JN, Tianero MD, Di Luccia B, Ahern PP, Merriman J, et al. *Lactobacillus reuteri* induces gut intraepithelial CD4(+)CD8αα(+) T cells. *Science.* (2017) 357:806–10. doi: 10.1126/science.aah5825

21. Panaccione DG, Arnold SL. Ergot alkaloids contribute to virulence in an insect model of invasive aspergillosis. *Sci Rep.* (2017) 7:8930. doi: 10.1038/s41598-017-09107-2

22. Pavlova T, Vidova V, Bienertova-Vasku J, Janku P, Almasi M, Klanova J, et al. Urinary intermediates of tryptophan as indicators of the gut microbial metabolism. *Anal Chim Acta.* (2017) 987:72–80. doi: 10.1016/j.aca.2017.08.022

23. Williams BB, Van Benschoten AH, Cimermancic P, Donia MS, Zimmermann M, Taketani M, et al. Discovery and characterization of gut microbiota decarboxylases that can produce the neurotransmitter tryptamine. *Cell Host Microbe.* (2014) 16:495–503. doi: 10.1016/j.chom.2014. 09.001

24. Stoll ML, Kumar R, Lefkowitz EJ, Cron RQ, Morrow CD, Barnes S. Fecal metabolomics in pediatric spondyloarthritis implicate decreased metabolic diversity and altered tryptophan metabolism as pathogenic factors. *Genes Immun.* (2016) 17:400–5. doi: 10.1038/gene.2016.38

25. Gao H, Liu S. Role of uremic toxin indoxyl sulfate in the progression of cardiovascular disease. *Life Sci.* (2017) 185:23–9. doi: 10.1016/j.lfs.2017. 07.027

26. Rijnen L, Bonneau S, Yvon M. Genetic characterization of the major lactococcal aromatic aminotransferase and its involvement in conversion of amino acids to aroma compounds. *Appl Environ Microbiol.* (1999) 65:4873–80. doi: 10.1128/AEM.65.11.4873-4880.1999

27. Weems JM, Yost GS. 3-Methylindole metabolites induce lung CYP1A1 and CYP2F1 enzymes by AhR and non-AhR mechanisms, respectively. *Chem Res Toxicol.* (2010) 23:696–704. doi: 10.1021/tx9004506

28. Dolciami D, Gargaro M, Cerra B, Scalisi G, Bagnoli L, Servillo G, et al. Binding mode and structure-activity relationships of ITE as an aryl hydrocarbon receptor (AhR) agonist. *ChemMedChem.* (2018) 13:270–9. doi: 10.1002/cmdc.201700669

29. Gaitanis G, Magiatis P, Stathopoulou K, Bassukas ID, Alexopoulos EC, Velegraki A, et al. AhR ligands, malassezin, and indolo[3,2-b]carbazole are selectively produced by *Malassezia furfur* strains isolated from seborrheic dermatitis. *J Invest Dermatol.* (2008) 128:1620–5. doi: 10.1038/sj.jid.5701252

30. Ranhotra HS, Flannigan KL, Brave M, Mukherjee S, Lukin DJ, Hirota SA, et al. Xenobiotic receptor-mediated regulation of intestinal barrier function and innate immunity. *Nucl Receptor Res.* (2016) 3:101199. doi: 10.11131/2016/101199

31. Venkatesh M, Mukherjee S, Wang H, Li H, Sun K, Benechet AP, et al. Symbiotic bacterial metabolites regulate gastrointestinal barrier function via the xenobiotic sensor PXR and Toll-like receptor 4. *Immunity.* (2014) 41:296–310. doi: 10.1016/j.immuni.2014.06.014

32. Romani L, Zelante T, De Luca A, Iannitti RG, Moretti S, Bartoli A, et al. Microbiota control of a tryptophan-AhR pathway in disease tolerance to fungi. *Eur J Immunol.* (2014) 44:3192–200. doi: 10.1002/eji.201344406

33. Bortolotti P, Hennart B, Thieffry C, Jausions G, Faure E, Grandjean T, et al. Tryptophan catabolism in *Pseudomonas aeruginosa* and potential for inter-kingdom relationship. *BMC Microbiol.* (2016) 16:137. doi: 10.1186/s12866-016-0756-x

34. Cheng SC, van de Veerdonk F, Smeekens S, Joosten LA, van der Meer JW, Kullberg BJ, et al. Candida albicans dampens host defense by downregulating IL-17 production. *J Immunol.* (2010) 185:2450–7. doi: 10.4049/jimmunol.1000756

35. Yuasa HJ, Ball HJ. Indoleamine 2,3-dioxygenases with very low catalytic activity are well conserved across kingdoms: IDOs of basidiomycota. *Fung Genet Biol.* (2013) 56:98–106. doi: 10.1016/j.fgb.2013.03.003

36. Wang PM, Choera T, Wiemann P, Pisithkul T, Amador-Noguez D, Keller NP. TrpE feedback mutants reveal roadblocks and conduits toward increasing secondary metabolism in *Aspergillus fumigatus. Fung Genet Biol.* (2016) 89:102–13. doi: 10.1016/j.fgb.2015.12.002

37. Dindo M, Costanzi E, Pieroni M, Costantini C, Annunziato G, Bruno A, et al. Biochemical characterization of *Aspergillus fumigatus* AroH, a putative aromatic amino acid aminotransferase. *Front Mol Biosci.* (2018) 5:104. doi: 10.3389/fmolb.2018.00104

38. Yuasa HJ, Ball HJ. Molecular evolution and characterization of fungal indoleamine 2,3-dioxygenases. *J Mol Evol.* (2011) 72:160–8. doi: 10.1007/s00239-010-9412-5

4

Host and Microbial Tryptophan Metabolic Profiling in Multiple Sclerosis

Lorenzo Gaetani[1], Francesca Boscaro[2], Giuseppe Pieraccini[2], Paolo Calabresi[3], Luigina Romani[4], Massimiliano Di Filippo[1†] and Teresa Zelante[4*†]

[1] Section of Neurology, Department of Medicine, University of Perugia, Perugia, Italy, [2] Mass Spectrometry Centre (CISM), Department of Health Sciences, University of Florence, Florence, Italy, [3] Section of Neurology, Department of Neuroscience, Agostino Gemelli Hospital, Catholic University of the Sacred Heart, Rome, Italy, [4] Department of Experimental Medicine, University of Perugia, Perugia, Italy

*Correspondence:
Teresa Zelante
teresa.zelante@unipg.it

†These authors have contributed equally to this work

Multiple sclerosis (MS) is an autoimmune disease of the central nervous system (CNS) that is associated with demyelination and neuronal loss. Over recent years, the immunological and neuronal effects of tryptophan (Trp) metabolites have been largely investigated, leading to the hypothesis that these compounds and the related enzymes are possibly involved in the pathophysiology of MS. Specifically, the kynurenine pathway of Trp metabolism is responsible for the synthesis of intermediate products with potential immunological and neuronal effects. More recently, Trp metabolites, originating also from the host microbiome, have been identified in MS, and it has been shown that they are differently regulated in MS patients. Here, we sought to discuss whether, in MS patients, a specific urinary signature of host/microbiome Trp metabolism can be potentially identified so as to select novel biomarkers and guide toward the identification of specific metabolic pathways as drug targets in MS.

Keywords: tryptophan, urine, signature, metabolite, multiple sclerosis, kynurenine, indole-3-propionic acid, microbiota

INTRODUCTION

The levels of the essential amino acid Tryptophan (Trp) and the function of Trp derivatives have long been a subject of research interest in autoimmunity. Mammals utilize Trp for different reasons, such as protein synthesis, the release of immunomodulant catabolites, and the synthesis of the aminergic neurotransmitter serotonin, the neurohormone melatonin, several neuroactive kynuramine metabolites of melatonin, and trace amine tryptamine. Indeed, Trp is metabolized by the mammalian host cells via four different pathways, of which the most relevant is the kynurenine pathway. The other two pathways provide the transamination and decarboxylation of Trp. The hydroxylation in serotonin occurs for only 1% of dietary Trp. Interestingly, the metabolic products of the kynurenine pathway are known to have several effects on vascular system, immune system, immunotolerance, and infections.

From the time when Trp and Trp derivatives were administered in multiple sclerosis (MS) to treat autoimmunity empirically (1), many advances have been made on the knowledge of Trp metabolic functions (2). It is almost universally agreed that the catabolism of Trp has different physiological implications, such as having antimicrobial and immunomodulant properties. For all of these reasons, Trp metabolites have been largely investigated in MS (3).

From a pathophysiological point of view, MS is characterized, from its earliest stages, by the coexistence of acute focal inflammation, glial cell hyperactivation, and progressive neuro-axonal loss (4). In the relapsing-remitting phenotype of the disease, inflammatory mechanisms are prominent and are largely responsible for the clinical manifestations of the disease, which are usually transient and recurrent (4). On the contrary, the progressive phenotype of the disease, which often follows the relapsing-remitting phase, is thought to be largely sustained by neurodegenerative mechanisms, probably as the ultimate consequence of previous recurrent episodes of brain and spinal cord inflammation (5). Additionally, the development of meningeal lymphocytic infiltrates and B-cell follicle-like structures in progressive MS patients may enhance neurodegenerative phenomena (6). MS can be extremely variable between individuals, with huge differences in the frequency of episodes of focal inflammation, in the possibility of the transition from the relapsing-remitting to the progressive phenotype, in the rate of progression, and in disability outcomes (7). Among the numerous factors potentially underlying this variability, a link between environment, microbial commensals, and host immunity has been suggested (8).

The earlier findings that Trp metabolized by indoleamine-2,3-dioxygenase (IDO) along the kynurenine pathway, plays a role in the pathophysiology of neuroinflammatory and neurodegenerative disorders, led several groups of researchers to study the changes in the levels of kynurenines in plasma, urine and cerebrospinal fluid in MS patients or in mice with experimental autoimmune encephalitis (EAE), the animal model of MS (9–13).

Systemic activation of Trp metabolism may have critical effects in MS. For instance, it has been demonstrated that Trp degradation is increased in the brain during the acute phase of EAE (14). Experimental results obtained by the use of the pharmacological inhibitor of IDO (1-methyl-Trp) also support a role for this pathway in MS. Indeed, the treatment of mice with 1-methyl-Trp resulted in EAE exacerbation (14). This latter evidence might suggest a protective role of IDO metabolites in EAE, although some downstream products of the kynurenine pathway, such as quinolinic acid, may also promote neurotoxicity.

Recently, metabolomics provided new insights into the research field of MS immunopathology, showing significant promise for unraveling the sources of disease heterogeneity, for understanding the interaction between the environment and immunity, and for monitoring disease progression and response to treatment in MS patients. For instance, untargeted metabolomics has been used recently in plasma samples of EAE mice to find a signature of 44 metabolites corresponding to six major pathways that were considerably altered, including bile acid biosynthesis, taurine metabolism, tryptophan and histidine metabolism, and linoleic acid and D-arginine metabolic pathways (9). Interestingly, the signature also included various metabolites categorized under the xenobiotics class, which are normally not synthesized in the body but can be metabolized by the microbiome as equolsulphate, homostachydrine, hippurate, and a Trp-derivative, indoleacrylate, which is also excreted in urine.

Besides, another Trp-derivative metabolite produced by the microbiota, indole-3-propionic acid, was found to be elevated in the plasma of EAE mice (9).

From a clinical perspective, one of the most important outcomes in MS is the risk of developing a progressive disease course (15). Indeed, while the relapsing-remitting phase can be effectively managed with immunomodulatory drugs, few treatments are available for progressive MS, and the progression of neurological disability is difficult to manage (16). In this context, Lim et al. recently wrote a paper targeted at deciphering a metabolic signature in serum to predict the transition from relapsing-remitting to progressive MS and to find a metabolic biomarker. Accordingly, they examined the role of the kynurenine pathway in MS progression and found that this pathway has a strong association with MS subtypes, correlating with disease severity scores (17).

Metabolomics has also been done on urine samples, which are readily available for analysis, and this has been used as a potential source of biomarkers in MS (18). Nuclear magnetic resonance (NMR) spectroscopy of urine allowed for the identification of metabolites that differentiated EAE-mice from healthy and MS drug-treated EAE mice (19). More recently, the metabolic profile in urine of mice bearing chronic EAE was performed with an untargeted combined metabolomics approach using gas chromatography- and liquid chromatography-mass spectrometry (GC-MS and LC-MS) (20). The authors identified eight metabolites characterizing EAE mice that are commonly found in plasma and urine and are potential biomarkers (20). Interestingly, the amino acid metabolism was primarily affected during EAE, as supported by urine analysis (20).

It is worth noting that in the diagnostic and/or therapeutic work-up of MS patients, standard urine analysis is usually performed, which makes urine sampling feasible for other investigations also. Additionally, urine is a metabolite-rich fluid that reflects the body's homeostasis and gut microbiome changes. Thus, a combined metabolomics analysis in urine, where both changes in host inflammatory/metabolic responses and in gut microbiome during MS may be highlighted, might help identifying novel biomarkers. This may provide a model to characterize pathogenic aspects of MS and to develop therapeutic approaches. We have therefore decided to perform an observational study aimed at investigating a broad panel of Trp metabolites, of both human and microbial origin, in urine samples from relapsing-remitting MS (RRMS) patients, in order to specifically investigate the possible relationship of Trp metabolites with the earliest inflammatory phase of the disease. We have compared the findings in RRMS patients to a control group of healthy individuals, and we have specifically looked for differences between MS patients and controls and for possible associations with disease characteristics.

MATERIALS AND METHODS

Patients

Urine samples were obtained from 47 consecutive patients with RRMS and 43 healthy controls, i.e., individuals without MS or autoimmune or inflammatory diseases. Patients and healthy controls were prospectively and consecutively recruited over a 1-year period at the Section of Neurology, Department of Medicine, University of Perugia (Italy). For MS patients, inclusion criteria were: (i) a diagnosis of RRMS according to the 2010 revision of the McDonald criteria (21); (ii) no recent history of infectious disorders (i.e., <30 days before the inclusion in the study); (iii) age >18 years. The study was approved by the local Ethics Committee (# 2925/16), and patients gave informed consent for the collection of samples and subsequent analysis. The main demographic and clinical characteristics of patients were collected by experienced neurologists. For each patient, the disability level at the time of urine sampling was quantified by scoring on the Expanded Disability Status Scale (EDSS) (22). Urine samples were collected at the same time of the day (between 09:00 and 12:00) in order to avoid any potential confounding effect of diurnal rhythm. Urine samples were subsequently analyzed by laboratory technicians who were blinded to clinical data.

Urine Analysis

Urine Trp metabolites were assessed by means of high-performance liquid chromatography-tandem mass spectrometry (HPLC-MS/MS). We used a targeted approach where a set of host or microbial metabolites derived from Trp were measured in urine. Details of HPLC-MS/MS analysis are reported in the **Supplementary Methods**. The following Trp metabolites and ratios were determined: (i) Trp; (ii) kynurenine; (iii) anthranilate; (iv) kynurenine/Trp (K/T) ratio; (v) kynurenine/anthranilate (K/A) ratio; (vi) 3-hydroxykynurenine; (vii) 3-hydroxyanthranilate; (viii) serotonin; (ix) tryptamine; (x) indole-3-acetic acid; (xi) indole-3-acetamide; (xii) indole-3-lactic acid; (xiii) indole-3-propionic acid.

Statistical Analysis

Continuous variables are reported as mean ± standard deviation (SD) if normally distributed or as median, interquartile range (IQR), if non-normally distributed. Logarithmic transformation was applied to Trp metabolite values in order to reach normality, as verified with the Shapiro-Wilk test. Differences of (log) Trp metabolite values between groups were tested with the Student's t-test, while their association with continuous variables was tested with Pearson's correlation coefficient test. General linear models were performed for multivariable analysis. All tests were two-sided, and the significance threshold was set to $p < 0.05$. IBM SPSS Statistics software version 22 was used for statistical analysis.

RESULTS

The Trp Metabolic Urinary Signature of RRMS Patients

The main demographic and clinical characteristics of RRMS patients and controls are reported in **Table 1**. A total of 35 patients (74.5%) were under disease modifying drugs at the time of urine sampling. In the entire cohort of MS patients and controls, females had significantly lower urinary tryptophan ($p = 0.001$), kynurenine ($p = 0.01$), anthranilate ($p = 0.01$), and serotonin ($p = 0.01$) concentrations ($p = 0.04$) than males (data

TABLE 1 | Main patient and control characteristics.

		RRMS	HC	*p*-value
N[a]		47	43	ND
Age (years)[b]		31.8 ± 9.7	32.7 ± 10.6	NS
F/M		40/7	27/16	$p = 0.02$
Disease duration (years)[b]		7.5 ± 8.3	ND	ND
Ongoing therapy[a]	None	11 (23.4%)	ND	ND
	Interferons	15 (31.9%)		
	Glatiramer acetate	10 (21.3%)		
	Dimethylfumarate	6 (12.8%)		
	Fingolimod	3 (6.4%)		
	Natalizumab	1 (2.1%)		
	Alemtuzumab	1 (2.1%)		
EDSS[b]		1.6 ± 0.5	ND	ND
Recent relapse (<30 days)[a]		9 (19.1%)	ND	ND

[a]Data are shown as number (percentage).
[b]Data are shown as mean ± standard deviation.
EDSS, Expanded Disability Status Scale; HC, healthy controls; ND, not determinable; NS, not significant; RRMS, relapsing-remitting multiple sclerosis.

not shown). After adjusting for gender, RRMS patients had a significantly lower urine concentration of kynurenine (1.4 μM, IQR: 0.5–3 μM vs. 4 μM, IQR: 1.9–6.8 μ, $p = 0.01$) and a lower K/T ratio (19, IQR: 15.5–27.5 vs. 29.8, IQR: 13.5–43, $p = 0.04$) than healthy controls (**Figure 1**). In contrast, no significant difference between patients and control subjects was found in the other Trp analyzed metabolites (see Materials and Methods). Within the RRMS cohort, Trp metabolites were not correlated with age and disease duration. In contrast, we found significant correlations between EDSS scores and urine concentrations of the following metabolites: (i) tryptophan ($r = 0.5$, $p = 0.001$), (ii) K/T ($r = -0.3$, $p = 0.03$), and (iii) indole-3-propionic acid ($r = 0.5$, $p < 0.001$; **Figure 1**). In a multivariate model taking into account age and gender, the correlations were confirmed for tryptophan ($\beta = 0.1$, $p < 0.04$), K/T ($\beta = -0.02$, $p = 0.003$), and indole-3-propionic acid ($\beta = 4.4$, $p = 0.001$). Finally, in RRMS patients, we found no difference in treated compared to untreated individuals, nor were there significant variations depending on the type of ongoing treatment.

In our cohort of RRMS patients, we found that urinary Trp metabolites were differently expressed in patients who had had a recent relapse (i.e., within 30 days before urine sampling). Specifically, the urine K/A ratio was significantly lower in patients with a recent relapse than in clinically stable patients (2.3 μM, IQR: 1.2–4.3 μM vs. 6.6 μM, IQR: 2.5–13.7 μM, $p = 0.03$), with a significantly higher urinary anthranilate concentration in relapsing vs. stable patients (1.1 μM, IQR: 0.5–1.8 μM vs. 0.2 μM, IQR: 0.1–0.3 μM, $p = 0.02$) (data not shown). Finally, relapsing patients had significantly higher urine indole-3-propionic acid concentrations than stable patients (0.05 μM, IQR: 0–0.1 μM vs. 0.01 μM, IQR: 0–0.04 μM, $p = 0.04$; **Figure 1**).

DISCUSSION

The pathophysiology of MS is extremely complex since it relies on the interplay between several players, such as the peripheral immune system, central nervous system resident

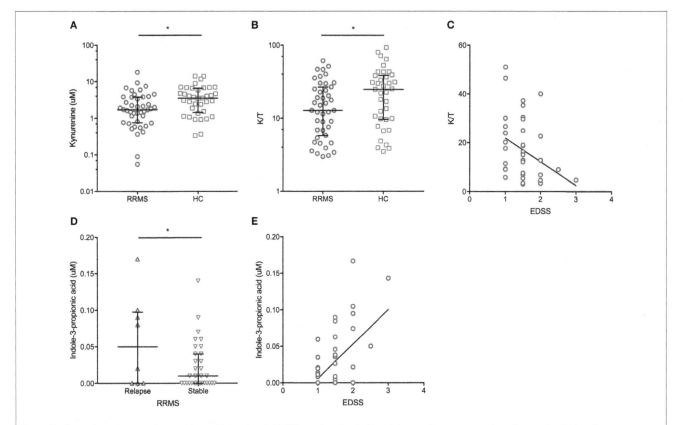

FIGURE 1 | In patients with relapsing-remitting multiple sclerosis (RRMS), we found a significantly lower urinary concentration of kynurenine **(A)** (median and interquartile range are reported) and kynurenine/tryptophan (K/T) ratio **(B)** (median and interquartile range are reported) than in healthy controls (HC). Additionally, a significant negative correlation between urinary K/T and the Expanded Disability Status Scale (EDSS) score at urine sampling was found **(C)**. In RRMS patients in proximity (i.e., <30 days) to a clinical relapse, significantly higher urinary indole-3-propionic acid concentrations were found than in clinically stable RRMS patients **(D)** (median and interquartile range are reported). Moreover, urinary indole-3-propionic acid concentrations were positively correlated with the EDSS score at urine sampling **(E)**. $^*p < 0.05$.

immune cells and glial cells, and neurons (23). MS is supposed to have a multifactorial etiology, and different environmental and genetic risk factors may play a role in determining the risk of developing the disease and in driving different phenotypic disease characteristics (24). Interestingly, Trp metabolism can be influenced both by the individual genetic background and interaction with environmental factors, such as diet. A great deal of interest is now being taken in determining how microbial commensals can modulate the host immune system, since this could lead to the potential discovery of new therapeutic targets.

In this study, we found some intriguing preliminary clues that a dysbalanced human Trp metabolism may have an association with MS, a finding that is supported by the evidence that this specific metabolism plays a central role in the control of immune activation (25). Specifically, we found that in the earliest and most inflammatory phenotype of MS, i.e., RRMS, there is a specific urinary Trp metabolite signature, which is characterized by a lower concentration of kynurenine and a lower K/T ratio than in healthy controls. Additionally, K/T was negatively and independently correlated with the degree of disability at the time of urine sampling. Taken together, these findings seem to suggest that in the earliest stages of MS, a reduced Trp

metabolism toward kynurenine can be found, and the lower the synthesis of kynurenine, the worse the degree of clinical impairment due to MS. Of interest, the synthesis of kynurenine via the IDO1 enzyme has been hypothesized to enhance the conversion of naïve T CD4+ cells into regulatory T cells (26), and kynurenine has shown immunoregulatory properties via the activation of the Aryl hydrocarbon Receptor (AhR) (27). Thereafter, reduced synthesis of kynurenine and a subsequent lower urinary kynurenine and K/T ratio may play a role in the pathophysiology of MS, where dysfunctional regulatory T cells favor autoimmune processes in the central nervous system (28).

From a biological point of view, once Trp is converted into kynurenine, the kynurenine pathway of Trp degradation is activated, which leads to the synthesis of a variety of compounds with both neurotoxic and neuroprotective properties that can influence MS pathology and, consequently, the degree of neurological impairment (29). Among the human urinary kynurenine downstream metabolites that we have measured in our study (i.e., 3-hydroxykynurenine and 3-hydroxyanthranilate), we did not find any significant association with the degree of disability apart from the above-mentioned negative correlation between K/T and EDSS. However, when interpreting this latter result, it should be noted that most of our patients had a low disability score. Therefore, the correlation between urinary Trp metabolites and the degree of neurological impairment deserves further confirmation on larger and more heterogeneous cohorts of MS patients, also including patients with progressive MS and with a longer disease duration.

Our findings are different from those reported for serum by Lim et al., who described higher serum K/T in MS patients than in controls (17). It is possible that this opposite result relies on the use of different biological samples (i.e., urine vs. serum), potentially reflecting different phases of Trp metabolism and/or different activities of the involved enzymes at different body sites. In this context, in order to understand the relationship between Trp metabolite concentrations in different biofluids, studies examining urine, blood, and cerebrospinal fluid in the same subjects at the same time are highly desirable.

Another possible explanation for the discrepancy between our findings and those coming from the literature might be the different characteristics of the enrolled patients. For instance, in the cohorts investigated by Lim et al., progressive MS patients were also included, and none of the patients was under disease-modifying drugs. Moreover, in the same paper, no information was provided on recent disease activity, although it can be assumed that enrolled patients had no history of recent relapses since, in the previous 3 months, they had not undergone steroid therapy (17).

The latter point could be extremely important in influencing Trp metabolite concentrations in body fluids, since we found that their urinary concentrations change in proximity to a clinical relapse, with a decrease in K/A and an increase in indole-3-propionic acid.

The decrease in K/A might either reflect a reduction in urinary kynurenine, a compound with immunoregulatory properties as discussed above, or an increase in anthranilate, or both. Of interest, anthranilate has been shown to increase in the blood in a wide range of human diseases, probably with a sort of "cleaning up" effect after an acute injury (30). Indeed, anthranilate has been associated with an antagonism to other neurotoxic kynurenines, such as quinolinic acid, as well as with a reduction in oxidative stress and in inflammatory responses (30–32). Thereafter, the decrease in urinary K/A in proximity of MS clinical relapses could reflect both a decrease in urinary kynurenine, which could enhance inflammatory responses, and an increase in urinary anthranilate, probably as a consequence of compensatory mechanisms following acute inflammation.

Also, the association between indole-3-propionic acid and MS disease activity is particularly interesting, since this molecule is one of the Trp-derived metabolites produced by the microbiota, called post-biotics (33, 34), that have been deeply investigated in recent years because of their presence in peripheral tissues and their ability to bind xenobiotic receptors. Indole-3-propionic acid is now known to contribute to changes in body weight gain on a tryptophan-rich diet (35). It may destroy indoxyl sulfate-induced expression of fibrosis and inflammation in kidney proximal tubular cells (36). More interestingly, it is also considered an antioxidant and has been reported to be neuroprotective (37). More recently, the mechanism by which the indole-3-propionic acid interacts with the mammalian host epithelial barrier has been described: the xenobiotic receptor pregnane X receptor (PXR) is, in fact, able to recognize this metabolite and reduce gut inflammation (38, 39). Interestingly, high blood levels of indole-3-propionic acid have also been found by other research groups in mice with EAE (9).

Since indole-3-propionic acid has been shown to have an antioxidant effect (40), its urinary increase may reflect an additional compensatory mechanism, driven by microbial commensals, trying to counteract the negative effects of acute inflammation. On the other hand, it is not possible to rule out a deleterious effect of indole-3-propionic acid, given the positive correlation that we have found between this Trp derivative and the degree of disability. Further studies investigating the possible immune and neuronal effects of indole-3-propionic acid are therefore needed to understand its pathophysiological role in MS.

In conclusion, although our findings are preliminary and deserve further confirmation on larger and unselected cohorts, they seem to suggest that a misbalanced human Trp metabolism is associated with MS, probably reflecting disease activity and severity. More interestingly, we found some clues that commensal microbials may interact with the host, especially in proximity to MS relapses, by synthesizing compounds such as indole-3-propionic acid.

FUTURE PERSPECTIVES

The study of Trp metabolites in MS is providing the scientific community with fascinating clues on the interaction between the microbiota and the human immune system in the context of autoimmune diseases. Our study, performed on urinary Trp metabolites, showed some preliminary and very interesting results, such as reduced urinary K/T in RRMS and its negative correlation with disability measures. In this sense, an altered Trp metabolism could either precede or follow autoimmune pathophysiological processes taking place in MS and could have an association with acute episodes of inflammatory activity during a chronic disease such as MS. More generally, it will be fundamental to understand if Trp metabolites are associated with a pathogenic effect and/or if they reflect the bystander activation of compensatory mechanisms to the ongoing MS-related autoimmunity. This step is required in order to proceed further in the Trp metabolism research field in search of novel potential therapeutic targets. In the near future, the study of Trp metabolism with the help of artificial intelligence and machine learning may become extremely effective in assisting medical doctors and biologists to address and solve complex diagnostic, prognostic, and therapeutic tasks. Indeed, probabilistic graphical models may be used to decipher or predict how the host and the microbiota share a common metabolic nutrient such as Trp and how this shared catabolism may be affected during immunopathology. Additionally, further studies on larger cohorts of MS patients are required in order to better investigate the correlations between Trp metabolites in different biofluids and more specific disease characteristics, such as neuroradiological and cerebrospinal fluid findings.

AUTHOR CONTRIBUTIONS

LG collected the samples, critically read, analyzed, and discussed the literature, and conceived the outline of the manuscript. LG, MD, and TZ wrote the manuscript. GP and FB performed mass spectrometry on urine samples. PC and LR edited the manuscript and provided valuable discussion and criticism.

FUNDING

This research came from the Italian Grant Programma per Giovani Ricercatori—Rita Levi Montalcini 2013 (Project No. PGR13XNIDJ) to TZ, the Specific Targeted Research Project FunMeta (ERC-2011-AdG-293714) to LR, and the Italian Fondazione Cassa di Risparmio di Perugia (Project No. 2018.0412.021) to TZ.

REFERENCES

1. Hyyppä MT, Jolma T, Riekkinen P, Rinne UK. Effects of L-tryptophan treatment on central indoleamine metabolism and short-lasting neurologic disturbances in multiple sclerosis. *J Neural Transm.* (1975) 37:297–304. doi: 10.1007/BF01258656

2. Fujigaki H, Yamamoto Y, Saito K. L-Tryptophan-kynurenine pathway enzymes are therapeutic target for neuropsychiatric diseases: focus on cell type differences. *Neuropharmacology.* (2017) 112(Pt B):264–74. doi: 10.1016/j.neuropharm.2016.01.011

3. Rothhammer V, Borucki DM, Tjon EC, Takenaka MC, Chao CC, Ardura-Fabregat A, et al. Microglial control of astrocytes in response to microbial metabolites. *Nature.* (2018) 557:724–8. doi: 10.1038/s41586-018-0119-x

4. Steinman L. Immunology of relapse and remission in multiple sclerosis. *Annu Rev Immunol.* (2014) 32: 257–81. doi: 10.1146/annurev-immunol-032713-120227

5. Correale J, Gaitán MI, Ysrraelit MC, Fiol MP. Progressive multiple sclerosis: from pathogenic mechanisms to treatment. *Brain.* (2017) 140:527–46. doi: 10.1093/brain/aww258

6. Magliozzi R, Howell O, Vora A, Serafini B, Nicholas R, Puopolo M, et al. Meningeal B-cell follicles in secondary progressive multiple sclerosis associate with early onset of disease and severe cortical pathology. *Brain.* (2007) 130(Pt 4): 1089–104. doi: 10.1093/brain/awm038

7. Filippi M, Bar-Or A, Piehl F, Preziosa P, Solari A, Vukusic S, et al. Multiple sclerosis. *Nat Rev Dis Primers.* (2018) 4:43. doi: 10.1038/s41572-018-0050-3

8. Kim D, Zeng MY, Núñez G. The interplay between host immune cells and gut microbiota in chronic inflammatory diseases. *Exp Mol Med.* (2017) 49:e339. doi: 10.1038/emm.2017.24

9. Mangalam A, Poisson L, Nemutlu E, Datta I, Denic A, Dzeja P, et al. Profile of circulatory metabolites in a relapsing-remitting animal model of multiple sclerosis using global metabolomics. *J Clin Cell Immunol.* (2013) 4. doi: 10.4172/2155-9899.1000150

10. Watzlawik JO, Wootla B, Rodriguez M. Tryptophan catabolites and their impact on multiple sclerosis progression. *Curr Pharm Des.* (2016) 22:1049–59. doi: 10.2174/1381612822666151215095940

11. Rothhammer V, Mascanfroni ID, Bunse L, Takenaka MC, Kenison JE, Mayo L, et al. Type I interferons and microbial metabolites of tryptophan modulate astrocyte activity and central nervous system inflammation via the aryl hydrocarbon receptor. *Nat Med.* (2016) 22:586–97. doi: 10.1038/nm.4106

12. Rogers GN, D'Souza BL. Receptor binding properties of human and animal H1 influenza virus isolates. *Virology.* (1989) 173:317–22. doi: 10.1016/0042-6822(89)90249-3

13. Monaco F, Fumero S, Mondino A, Mutani R. Plasma and cerebrospinal fluid tryptophan in multiple sclerosis and degenerative diseases. *J Neurol Neurosurg Psychiatry.* (1979) 42:640–1. doi: 10.1136/jnnp.42.7.640

14. Kwidzinski E, Bunse J, Aktas O, Richter D, Mutlu L, Zipp F, et al. Indolamine 2,3-dioxygenase is expressed in the CNS and down-regulates autoimmune inflammation. *FASEB J.* (2005) 19:1347–9. doi: 10.1096/fj.04-3228fje

15. Fambiatos A, Jokubaitis V, Horakova D, Kubala Havrdova E, Trojano M, Prat A, et al. Risk of secondary progressive multiple sclerosis: a longitudinal study. *Mult Scler.* (2019) 26:79–90. doi: 10.1177/1352458519868990

16. Feinstein A, Freeman J, Lo AC. Treatment of progressive multiple sclerosis: what works, what does not, and what is needed. *Lancet Neurol.* (2015) 14:194–207. doi: 10.1016/S1474-4422(14)70231-5

17. Lim CK, Bilgin A, Lovejoy DB, Tan V, Bustamante S, Taylor BV, et al. Kynurenine pathway metabolomics predicts and provides mechanistic insight into multiple sclerosis progression. *Sci Rep.* (2017) 7:41473. doi: 10.1038/srep41473

18. Dobson R. Urine: an under-studied source of biomarkers in multiple sclerosis? *Mult Scler Relat Disord.* (2012) 1:76–80. doi: 10.1016/j.msard.2012.01.002

19. Gebregiworgis T, Massilamany C, Gangaplara A, Thulasingam S, Kolli V, Werth MT, et al. Potential of urinary metabolites for diagnosing multiple sclerosis. *ACS Chem Biol.* (2013) 8:684–90. doi: 10.1021/cb300673e

20. Singh J, Cerghet M, Poisson LM, Datta I, Labuzek K, Suhail H, et al. Urinary and plasma metabolomics identify the distinct metabolic profile of disease state in chronic mouse model of multiple sclerosis. *J Neuroimmune Pharmacol.* (2019) 14:241–50. doi: 10.1007/s11481-018-9815-4

21. Polman CH, Reingold SC, Banwell B, Clanet M, Cohen JA, Filippi M, et al. Diagnostic criteria for multiple sclerosis: 2010 revisions to the McDonald criteria. *Ann Neurol.* (2011) 69:292–302. doi: 10.1002/ana.22366

22. Kurtzke JF. Rating neurologic impairment in multiple sclerosis: an expanded disability status scale. (EDSS). *Neurology.* (1983) 33:1444–52. doi: 10.1212/WNL.33.11.1444

23. Dendrou CA, Fugger L, Friese MA. Immunopathology of multiple sclerosis. *Nat Rev Immunol.* (2015) 15:545–58. doi: 10.1038/nri3871

24. Waubant E, Lucas R, Mowry E, Graves J, Olsson T, Alfredsson L, et al. Environmental and genetic risk factors for MS: an integrated review. *Ann Clin Transl Neurol.* (2019) 6:1905–22. doi: 10.1002/acn3.50862

25. Grohmann U, Bronte V. Control of immune response by amino acid metabolism. *Immunol Rev.* (2010) 236:243–64. doi: 10.1111/j.1600-065X.2010.00915.x

26. Puccetti P, Grohmann U. IDO and regulatory T cells: a role for reverse signalling and non-canonical NF-κB activation. *Nat Rev Immunol.* (2007) 7:817–23. doi: 10.1038/nri2163

27. Gutiérrez-Vázquez C, Quintana FJ. Regulation of the immune response by the Aryl hydrocarbon receptor. *Immunity.* (2018) 48:19–33. doi: 10.1016/j.immuni.2017.12.012

28. Astier AL, Hafler DA. Abnormal Tr1 differentiation in multiple sclerosis. *J Neuroimmunol.* (2007) 191:70–8. doi: 10.1016/j.jneuroim.2007.09.018

29. Lovelace MD, Varney B, Sundaram G, Franco NF, Ng ML, Pai S, et al. Current evidence for a role of the kynurenine pathway of tryptophan metabolism in multiple sclerosis. *Front Immunol.* (2016) 7:246. doi: 10.3389/fimmu.2016.00246

30. Darlington LG, Forrest CM, Mackay GM, Smith RA, Smith AJ, Stoy N, et al. On the biological importance of the 3-hydroxyanthranilic acid: anthranilic acid ratio. *Int J Tryptophan Res.* (2010) 3:51–9. doi: 10.4137/IJTR.S4282

31. Darlington LG, Mackay GM, Forrest CM, Stoy N, George C, Stone TW. Altered kynurenine metabolism correlates with infarct volume in stroke. *Eur J Neurosci.* (2007) 26:2211–21. doi: 10.1111/j.1460-9568.2007.05838.x

32. Forrest CM, Mackay GM, Oxford L, Stoy N, Stone TW, Darlington LG. Kynurenine pathway metabolism in patients with osteoporosis after 2 years of drug treatment. *Clin Exp Pharmacol Physiol.* (2006) 33:1078–87. doi: 10.1111/j.1440-1681.2006.04490.x

33. Tsilingiri K, Rescigno M. Postbiotics: what else? *Benef Microbes.* (2013) 4:101–7. doi: 10.3920/BM2012.0046

34. Oleskin AV, Shenderov BA. Probiotics and psychobiotics: the role of microbial neurochemicals. *Probiotics Antimicrob Proteins.* (2019) 11:1071–85. doi: 10.1007/s12602-019-09583-0

35. Konopelski P, Konop M, Gawrys-Kopczynska M, Podsadni P, Szczepanska A, Ufnal M. Indole-3-propionic acid, a tryptophan-derived bacterial metabolite, reduces weight gain in rats. *Nutrients.* (2019) 11:E591. doi: 10.3390/nu11030591

36. Yisireyili M, Takeshita K, Saito S, Murohara T, Niwa T. Indole-3-propionic acid suppresses indoxyl sulfate-induced expression of fibrotic and inflammatory genes in proximal tubular cells. *Nagoya J Med Sci.* (2017) 79:477–86. doi: 10.18999/nagjms.79.4.477

37. Chyan YJ, Poeggeler B, Omar RA, Chain DG, Frangione B, Ghiso J, et al. Potent neuroprotective properties against the Alzheimer beta-amyloid by an endogenous melatonin-related indole structure, indole-3-propionic acid. *J Biol Chem.* (1999) 274:21937–42. doi: 10.1074/jbc.274.31.21937

38. Venkatesh M, Mukherjee S, Wang H, Li H, Sun K, Benechet AP, et al. Symbiotic bacterial metabolites regulate gastrointestinal barrier function via the xenobiotic sensor PXR and Toll-like receptor 4. *Immunity.* (2014) 41:296–310. doi: 10.1016/j.immuni.2014.06.014

39. Pulakazhi Venu VK, Saifeddine M, Mihara K, Tsai YC, Nieves K, Alston L, et al. The pregnane X receptor and its microbiota-derived ligand indole 3-propionic acid regulate endothelium-dependent vasodilation. *Am J Physiol Endocrinol Metab.* (2019) 317:E350–61. doi: 10.1152/ajpendo.00572.2018

40. Karbownik M, Reiter RJ, Garcia JJ, Cabrera J, Burkhardt S, Osuna C, et al. Indole-3-propionic acid, a melatonin-related molecule, protects hepatic microsomal membranes from iron-induced oxidative damage: relevance to cancer reduction. *J Cell Biochem.* (2001) 81:507–13. doi: 10.1002/1097-4644(20010601)81:3<507::AID-JCB1064>3.0.CO;2-M

5

Quinolinate as a Marker for Kynurenine Metabolite Formation and the Unresolved Question of NAD$^+$ Synthesis During Inflammation and Infection

John R. Moffett[1]*, Peethambaran Arun[1], Narayanan Puthillathu[1], Ranjini Vengilote[1], John A. Ives[2], Abdulla A-B Badawy[3] and Aryan M. Namboodiri[1]

[1] Departments of Anatomy, Physiology and Genetics and Neuroscience Program, Uniformed Services University Medical School, Bethesda, MD, United States, [2] The Center for Brain, Mind, and Healing, Samueli Institute, Alexandria, VA, United States, [3] Independent Consultant, Cardiff, United Kingdom

*Correspondence:
John R. Moffett
jmoffett@usuhs.edu

Quinolinate (Quin) is a classic example of a biochemical double-edged sword, acting as both essential metabolite and potent neurotoxin. Quin is an important metabolite in the kynurenine pathway of tryptophan catabolism leading to the *de novo* synthesis of nicotinamide adenine dinucleotide (NAD$^+$). As a precursor for NAD$^+$, Quin can direct a portion of tryptophan catabolism toward replenishing cellular NAD$^+$ levels in response to inflammation and infection. Intracellular Quin levels increase dramatically in response to immune stimulation [e.g., lipopolysaccharide (LPS) or pokeweed mitogen (PWM)] in macrophages, microglia, dendritic cells, and other cells of the immune system. NAD$^+$ serves numerous functions including energy production, the poly ADP ribose polymerization (PARP) reaction involved in DNA repair, and the activity of various enzymes such as the NAD$^+$-dependent deacetylases known as sirtuins. We used highly specific antibodies to protein-coupled Quin to delineate cells that accumulate Quin as a key aspect of the response to immune stimulation and infection. Here, we describe Quin staining in the brain, spleen, and liver after LPS administration to the brain or systemic PWM administration. Quin expression was strong in immune cells in the periphery after both treatments, whereas very limited Quin expression was observed in the brain even after direct LPS injection. Immunoreactive cells exhibited diverse morphology ranging from foam cells to cells with membrane extensions related to cell motility. We also examined protein expression changes in the spleen after kynurenine administration. Acute (8 h) and prolonged (48 h) kynurenine administration led to significant changes in protein expression in the spleen, including multiple changes involved with cytoskeletal rearrangements associated with cell motility. Kynurenine administration resulted in several expression level changes in proteins associated with heat shock protein 90 (HSP90), a chaperone for the aryl-hydrocarbon receptor (AHR), which is the primary kynurenine metabolite receptor. We propose that cells with high levels of Quin are those that are currently releasing kynurenine pathway metabolites as well as accumulating Quin for sustained NAD^+ synthesis from tryptophan. Further, we propose that the kynurenine pathway may be linked to the regulation of cell motility in immune and cancer cells.

Keywords: quinolinic acid, indoleamine 2,3-dioxygenase, kynurenine pathway, PARP, cell motility, foam cells, HSP90, ERM proteins

INTRODUCTION

Considering the breadth of studies linking the tryptophan catabolite quinolinate (Quin) to neurotoxicity and neurological disorders, it is perhaps ironic that the earliest studies on Quin tied it to a critical biological function as a precursor for nicotinamide adenine dinucleotide (NAD^+) synthesis (1, 2). The irony lies in the rarity of subsequent studies investigating the role of Quin in the biosynthetic pathway from tryptophan to NAD^+ in different cell types, under various physiological and pathological circumstances. Many studies into Quin over the last several decades have focused on its connections to neurological disorders [reviewed in (3–9)]. More recently, attention has also turned to the immunomodulatory and immunosuppressive effects of kynurenine metabolites (10, 11). To this day, the extent and criticality of the contribution of tryptophan catabolism to NAD^+ synthesis in cells of the immune system during health and disease remain mostly unexplored (12). Yet, it is becoming increasingly clear that NAD^+ requirements in certain cell types can be elevated during inflammation, injury, and infection, and that this is critical for proper immune cell responsiveness (13–16). As such, the contribution of the kynurenine pathway to sustaining NAD^+ levels in the immune system during various challenges may turn out to be substantial in certain cell types.

One possible reason for the paucity of studies into NAD^+ synthesis from tryptophan in health and disease is that modern diets provide the majority of the requisite precursors for NAD^+ synthesis in the form of vitamin B3 (niacin; including both nicotinic acid and nicotinamide). However, when the diet does not provide sufficient niacin or the immune system is challenged, tryptophan catabolism is required to maintain sufficient NAD^+ synthesis. The pathway of tryptophan metabolism to NAD^+ is known as the *kynurenine pathway* because one of the early metabolites in this catabolic pathway is kynurenine (**Figure 1**). Two physiologically distinct, rate-limiting enzymes initiate tryptophan catabolism to NAD^+; tryptophan 2,3-dioxygenase (TDO) and indoleamine 2,3-dioxoygenase (IDO) [reviewed in (17)]. TDO is expressed extensively in hepatocytes, as well as in many other cell types throughout the body. IDO is expressed extensively in cells of the immune system, but is also found in many other cell types. The enzyme quinolinate phosphoribosyltransferase (QPRT) catalyzes the formation of nicotinic acid mononucleotide from Quin and 5-phosphoribosyl-1-pyrophosphate, fueling NAD^+ synthesis. Because NAD^+ is a cofactor in numerous redox and other important cellular reactions, some of which become substantially increased during inflammation and infection, the synthesis of NAD^+ may be enhanced when the immune system responds to challenges.

Despite these facts, the importance of Quin in the synthesis of NAD^+ during the immune system's responses to infections, cancer, or injury remains much more poorly understood than its neurotoxic effects.

The dramatic increase in tryptophan catabolism via IDO during immune system responses is evolutionarily conserved (18–21), indicating its pro-survival value. Yet, the precise nature of the benefits that the kynurenine pathway confers on fitness is a matter of ongoing debate (7, 9, 16, 22, 23). Known functions of the kynurenine pathway include the production of immune-regulatory metabolites, especially immunosuppressive ones, as well as NAD^+ synthesis. Both of these functions intersect during an immune response where immunosuppression and increased NAD^+ availability are necessary for a successful resolution of infection or injury. The surge in IDO expression during infection or after experimental immune stimulation is accompanied by an increase in kynurenine metabolites, including Quin, in blood and in tissues. Further, Quin levels increase in specific cell populations as shown by Quin immunohistochemistry. Specialized fixation and antibody purification methods permit the visualization of Quin in cells with very high sensitivity and specificity (24–27). These methods allow detailed visualization of cells that synthesize Quin and have demonstrated that specific cells of the immune system accumulate high intracellular concentrations of Quin. In the current study, we investigated this phenomenon by stimulating the immune system with either lipopolysaccharide (LPS) or pokeweed mitogen (PWM). We delivered LPS to the hippocampus of rats and administered PWM intraperitoneally (IP) to gerbils. We then used specialized immunohistochemistry to follow the course of Quin buildup in cells in the brain, spleen, and liver.

MATERIALS AND METHODS

The digital images presented here were generated from archival slides prepared previously and include material from both published (25–29) and unpublished studies. The methods used for the production, purification, and characterization of the polyclonal Quin antibodies have been described previously (26). The carbodiimide-based immunohistochemical methods have also been described (30). The Quin immunohistochemistry methods developed by us have been validated independently by another laboratory, using the same protocols (31). Imaging was done using an Olympus BX-51 microscope and Olympus DP-71 digital camera. Images were acquired using Image Pro Plus software (ver. 7.1; Media Cybernetics). Chemicals were from Sigma (St. Louis, MO). Horseradish peroxidase

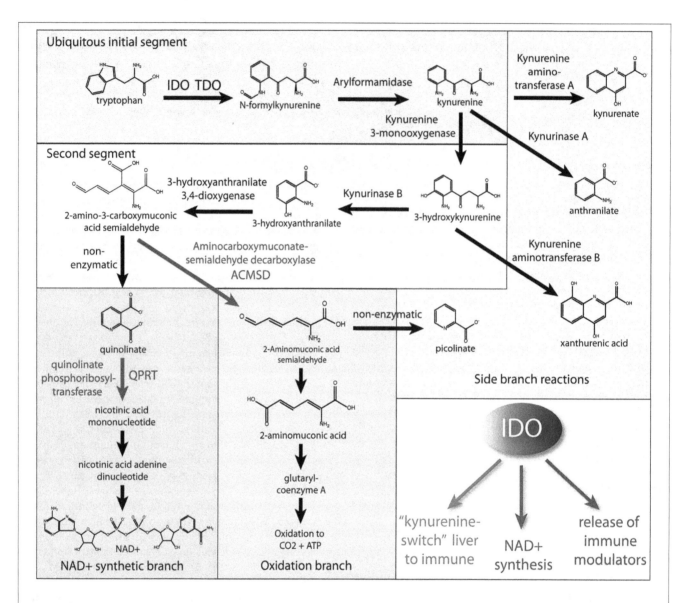

FIGURE 1 | Simplified diagram of the kynurenine pathway of tryptophan catabolism. Most cell types can initiate the kynurenine pathway via either TDO or IDO to produce kynurenine (initial segment of tryptophan metabolism). Hepatocytes have the full complement of enzymes to either produce NAD$^+$ or fully oxidize tryptophan to CO_2. Numerous cell types, including many of the immune system, express the enzymes through the NAD$^+$ synthetic branch. However, in order for Quin to build up in some immune cells during an immune response, the activities of the enzymes aminocarboxymuconate semialdehyde decarboxylase (ACMSD) and quinolinate phosphoribosyltransferase (QPRT) must be restricted to slow further metabolism to either NAD$^+$ or oxidation to CO_2. The fate of stockpiled Quin in those immune cells remains uncertain, but it is likely that both NAD$^+$ synthesis and oxidation to yield energy are employed by various cells of the immune system during an immune response. Also, these cells may be releasing upstream metabolites. As such, upregulation of QPRT activity (red arrow) would be the rate-limiting factor for further metabolism to NAD$^+$ when needed, and we propose this branch is predominantly utilized in cells of the immune system following IDO activation. In contrast, the activity of ACMSD would control the oxidative branch throughput for energy derivation. The three primary functions of IDO activation are (1) the extra-hepatic production of kynurenine, which is released for uptake by cells of the immune system thus diverting tryptophan metabolism to the immune system, (2) the production of NAD$^+$ in cells of the immune system for the PARP reaction to DNA damage and other critical functions in immune cells, and (3) the production and release of immune modulating metabolites to regulate the immune response, especially T cell responsiveness. NMNAT, nicotinamide mononucleotide adenylyltransferase; NADSYN1, NAD synthetase 1.

(HRP)-coupled goat anti-rabbit secondary antibodies were purchased from Kirkegaard and Perry (Gaithersburg, MD). Avidin–biotin complex kits (Vectastain Elite), normal goat serum (NGS), biotinylated GSL I-B$_4$, and HRP-labeled streptavidin were from Vector (Burlingame, CA). Polyclonal antibodies to GFAP (AB1980) were from Chemicon (Temecula, CA).

Immune Stimulation Models

Here, we compare the Quin-immunoreactivity (Quin-IR) response in two models of immune stimulation including (1) IP PWM injection in gerbils where we examined the Quin-IR response at 24 h and (2) LPS injection into the hippocampus of rats, examined at multiple time points. LPS and PWM act on immune cells via different receptor systems. For example, in Kupffer cells (hepatic macrophages), LPS activates TRL4 receptors, whereas PWM activates the complement system via cleavage of C3 (32). Both agents induce strong IDO activity in the immune system. Using these two models, we compared the Quin-IR response during peripheral immune stimulation vs. central nervous system immune stimulation.

We also examined the effects of L-kynurenine administration on protein expression in the spleen of mice. This model engaged the kynurenine pathway by bypassing the rate-limiting enzymes, IDO and TDO, providing a view into the effects of increased kynurenine pathway throughput on protein expression in the spleen in the absence of immune stimulation. All experimental protocols were approved by the Uniformed Services University of the Health Sciences (USUHS) animal care and use committee.

Intracerebral Injections of LPS

For these animals, under halothane anesthesia, a 30-gauge stainless steel cannula was inserted into the dorsal hippocampus (from bregma: AP = −4.2, Midline = +1.8, DV = −2.9), and 2 μl of sterile saline containing 4 μg of LPS from *Salmonella arbortus equi* was injected over a 10-min period. The cannula was withdrawn 30 min later, the incision closed, and the animals allowed to recover in a heated cage. Animals were perfused, as described below, from 1 to 30 days after LPS injection, with 2 to 3 animals per time point.

Intraperitoneal Injection of PWM

Methods for gerbils given IP injections of PWM have been previously described (28). Animals were anesthetized and perfused via carbodiimide fixation (described below) 24 h after PWM administration.

Animal Perfusions

The animals were anesthetized with pentobarbital and perfused transcardially with 400 ml of an aqueous solution of 6% 1-ethyl-3 (3-dimethylaminopropyl) carbodiimide hydrochloride, 6% DMSO, and 1 mM N-hydroxysuccinimide warmed to 37°C (26, 30). This fixative is required for Quin immunohistochemistry. The brains, spleens, and livers were removed to a solution of 4% paraformaldehyde in 100 mM phosphate buffer at pH 8 for 24 h. The tissues were then passed through a series of 10, 20, and 30% sucrose solutions in PBS.

Immunohistochemistry

The immunohistochemical methods have been described in detail previously (26, 27, 30). Briefly, tissues were cryo-sectioned at a thickness of 20 microns and were collected serially in groups of 5, and placed in 24-well tissue culture plates in the same solution. Endogenous peroxidase was blocked with a 50:50 mixture of methanol and water containing 1% H_2O_2 for 30 min with agitation. Tissue sections were incubated overnight with the Quin antibodies, diluted 1:10,000, using constant rotary agitation. The antibodies were visualized by the avidin–biotin complex method with HRP as the enzyme marker (Vectastain Elite, Vector Labs). The sections were

incubated with the biotinylated secondary antibody and avidin–biotin–peroxidase complex solutions for 90 min each, and then developed with diaminobenzidine and urea peroxide as chromogen and substrate (Sigmafast DAB tablets, Sigma) for 10–15 min. Lectin histochemistry with *Griffonia simplicifolia*-B4 lectin (GSL-IB4) and double staining with Quin was done as described earlier (27).

2D-DIGE PROTEOMICS AND LC-MS/MS

We used two-dimensional, differential image gel electrophoresis (2D-DIGE) to investigate the effects of kynurenine on protein expression in the spleen in the absence of inflammation, infection, or injury, and therefore in the absence of increased IDO activity. We administered high-dose L-kynurenine to normal mice and used fluorescent 2D proteomics to look for changes in protein expression in the spleen. Male C57 mice weighing between 20 and 25 g were used for these studies (Charles River Labs, Wilmington, MA). Animals were housed in the USUHS animal facility on a 12/12 h light–dark cycle, with *ad libitum* access to food and water. We compared a single high-dose IP injection of kynurenine to administration of kynurenine in drinking water for 48 h. In group 1, three experimental animals were given a single IP injection of 300 mg/kg of L-kynurenine diluted in sterile saline, whereas three control animals were given a single IP injection of sterile saline 8 h before sacrifice. In group 2, three mice were given free access to drinking water containing 5 mM kynurenine for 48 h before sacrifice, and three control animals were given access to plain tap water.

2D Gels

Eight hours after kynurenine injections or after 48 h of prolonged administration in drinking water, mice were anesthetized with pentobarbital (300 mg/kg) and killed by decapitation. Spleens were removed and frozen immediately on dry ice. The 2D-DIGE proteomics and mass spectroscopy were done at the Windber Research Institute (Windber, PA) as previously described (33). Spleen tissues were homogenized in an ice-cold lysis solution (2 M thiourea, 6 M urea, 4% CHAPS, 1% NP-40, 5 mM magnesium acetate, and 30 mM Tris–HCl at pH 8.5). Gels were run using the 2D-DIGE method (Amersham Biosciences). Experimental and control animals were paired randomly, and the experimental and control protein samples were labeled separately with a red or green fluorescent dye. A control mixture of the two samples was made with equal amounts of protein from each of the paired animals, and this was labeled with a yellow fluorescent dye. All three labeled protein samples from each pair of animals were mixed, and each mixture was subjected to 2-D gel electrophoresis (34). Gels were loaded with 50-μg samples, and the first dimension was run with an immobilized pH gradient from pH 3 to 10 (Immobiline dry strips). The second dimension was run on a 12% SDS-PAGE gel.

MALDI and LC/MS/MS

Gel image analysis was done using the DeCyder software package. Statistical analysis was done using the DeCyder biological variation analysis module (Amersham) and Student's *t*-test was used to determine differential expression (35). The destaining, digestion, extraction, and MALDI (matrix-assisted laser desorption/ionization) sample preparation were carried out robotically in an enclosed unit according to the manufacturer's instructions (Amersham). MALDI peptide mass fingerprinting was carried out on an Ettan Pro MALDI-ToF mass spectrometer (Amersham Biosciences) operating in reflectron mode. Sensitivity of the system allowed identification of 40 fmol of protein. The mass spectra were internally calibrated using trypsin autodigestion peaks at m/z 842.542 and 2211.109 to give a mass accuracy of better than 100 ppm. Protein identification by peptide mass fingerprinting was performed using the MASCOT search engine and the NCBInr protein database.

RESULTS

Intraperitoneal Injection of PWM in Gerbils

Our original short communication on PWM administration in the gerbil showed several images of the Quin-IR changes in the spleen and brain (28). Here, we provide a more detailed view of the observed changes. PWM is a potent immune stimulant that induces a large increase in Quin production (36). Further, PWM is one of the more potent inducers of INF-γ release (37). IP injection of PWM in gerbils elicited a very strong peripheral kynurenine pathway response in the spleen and liver, but no detectable increase in Quin-IR in brain parenchyma.

Quin-IR in Gerbil Brain

Quin-IR was absent from brain parenchyma in the gerbil 24 h after peripheral immune stimulation with PWM (**Figure 2A**). Careful examination of many brain tissue sections from three gerbils given PWM demonstrated that Quin-IR cells from the periphery were excluded from brain parenchyma. However, Quin-IR cells were observed within the vasculature of the brain (**Figure 2F**). Quin-IR cells were adherent to the vessel surface in arteries and veins of all diameters, including capillaries. Quin-IR cells were also present in the meninges (**Figure 2D**). A modest but consistent Quin-IR reaction was observed in the choroid plexus where Quin-IR cells were common in the PWM-treated group (**Figures 2B,C,E**). Some of the Quin-IR cells in the choroid plexus appeared to be foam cells, which are macrophages that are filled with lipid-laden vesicles [reviewed in (38)].

Quin-IR in Gerbil Spleen

Moderate splenomegaly was observed in gerbils 24 h after IP administration of 500 μg of PWM. Measurements of the longest dimensions in width and height showed that cross-sectional dimensions of spleen slices were increased 25% in width and 48% in height 24 h after PWM administration (see **Supplementary Figure 1**). A robust increase in Quin-IR was present in the red pulp and in the central region of the periarteriolar lymphoid sheaths (PALS) in gerbils given PWM (**Figure 3**). In the saline-injected control group, Quin-IR in the spleen was generally very low, and was present in large, irregularly shaped cells in the white pulp (PALS and follicles in **Figures 3A,C,E**). Twenty-four hours after PWM administration, Quin-IR increased dramatically in the red pulp and in the PALS

region of the white pulp (**Figures 3B,D,F**). Quin-IR in the cells in the B-cell-rich follicles also increased, but to a lesser degree than in the PALS and red pulp. These results show that in gerbils, as with other species, many cells of the immune system are capable of accumulating significant concentrations of Quin in their cytoplasm in response to potent immune stimulants.

Quin-IR in Gerbil Liver

Quin-IR in the liver of gerbils in the control group given saline was very low (**Figures 4A,C**). The vast majority of cells were unstained. Occasional cells at the margin of sinuses were lightly stained. Twenty-four hours after PWM challenge, Quin-IR in the liver was dramatically increased in cells with the morphology of activated Kupffer cells (**Figures 4B,D–F**), whereas most hepatocytes appeared very lightly stained as compared with controls (arrows in **Figures 4C,D**). Additionally, based on location and morphology, some of the Quin-IR cells appeared to be hepatic dendritic cells. At high magnification, many of the strongly stained Kupffer cells contained numerous visible inclusions that could be phagosomes or phagolysosomes (**Figures 4D–F**). Kupffer cells are resident hepatic macrophages (39), and it has been shown that they respond to IFN-γ by activation of IDO and production of kynurenine (40). These investigators reported that activated Kupffer cells inhibited T cell proliferation and induced apoptosis of allogeneic T cells. Our results show that Kupffer cells are capable of catabolizing tryptophan to the level of Quin, which can then be used for NAD$^+$ synthesis during an immune response.

LPS INJECTION INTO RAT HIPPOCAMPUS

Quin-IR in Rat Spleen

Even though we injected LPS only into the hippocampus of rats, a substantial increase in Quin staining was observed in the spleen that persisted for several days following the LPS challenge (**Figure 5**). In the control spleen from rats, Quin-IR was relatively modest, with very light staining of B-cell follicles, and strong staining of some cells in the T cell PALS (**Figure 5A**). However, most cells in the PALS were unstained. In the red pulp, which contains macrophages and erythrocytes, scattered macrophages were moderately to strongly stained for Quin in control spleens. In contrast, in the spleen of rats 1 day after injection of 4 μg of LPS into the hippocampus, there was a strong upregulation of Quin-IR in all splenic compartments (**Figure 5B**). In the PALS, the number of strongly stained cells increased substantially, and staining also increased throughout all B cell follicles. Further, the number of strongly stained macrophages in the red pulp increased as well. On day 2 after LPS administration to the brain, Quin-IR was reduced as compared with day 1, but remained elevated in all three compartments (follicles, PALS, and red pulp; **Figure 5C**). Strong staining was observed in the central region of some follicles in probable dendritic cells. On day 3 after LPS, Quin-IR remained elevated in all compartments, but was somewhat attenuated as compared with day 2 (**Figure 5D**). Some follicles continued to harbor strongly stained dendritic cells. B cell follicles remained more immunoreactive than controls. On day 5 after LPS administration, Quin expression in all

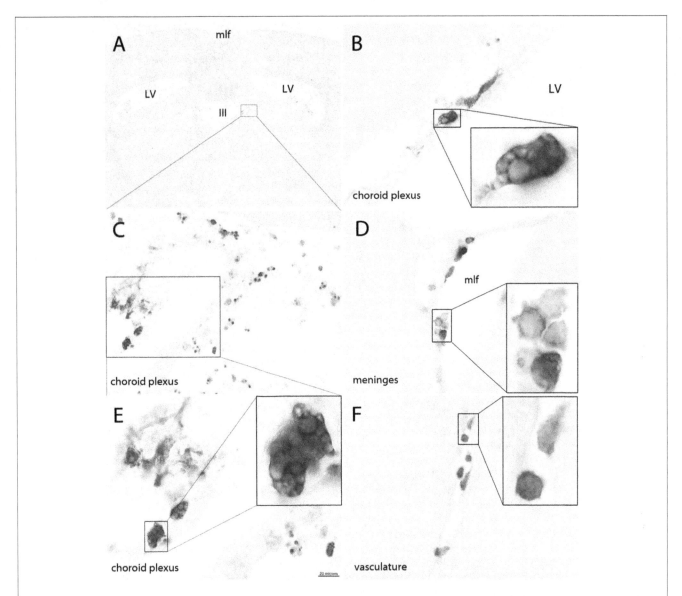

FIGURE 2 | The gerbil brain is shown stained for Quin 24 h after IP injection of PWM (500 μg). No Quin-IR cells were observed within the brain parenchyma **(A)**. The majority of Quin-IR cells were found in the choroid plexus **(B,C,E)**. Additional Quin-IR cells were observed in the meninges, for example, at the apex of the medial longitudinal fissure **(D)**. Quin-IR cells were also observed adherent to the interior surfaces of the brain vasculature **(F)**. Quin-IR cells ranged widely in morphology, and some appeared relatively unstained but contained Quin-IR phagosomes, which may have been phagocytized debris from apoptotic cells. Others appeared similar to so-called "foam cells," which are activated macrophages filled with lipid-containing vesicles (insets in **B,E**). Bar in **(E)**, 320 μm in **(A)**, 40 μm in **(C)**, 20 μm in **(B,D,E,F)**, and 6 μm in the insets. III, third ventricle; LV, lateral ventricles; mlf, medial longitudinal fissure.

compartments was again greater than in controls (**Figure 5E**). Diffuse staining in follicles was elevated and more strongly stained cells were present in the PALS and red pulp, as compared with controls. However, the concentration of strongly stained dendritic cells in the follicles was not as apparent by day 5. By day 7, Quin-IR was beginning to return to pre-LPS levels (**Figure 5F**). However, the number of stained cells scattered throughout the red pulp and PALS remained elevated relative to controls.

In general, the Quin-IR reaction at the center of follicles, where expression increased in apparent dendritic cells, persisted for at least 3 days. The increase in diffuse staining throughout

the B cell-containing follicles lasted for at least 5 days. Elevated numbers of strongly stained cells in the T cell containing PALS, as well as in the red pulp, continued for at least 7 days. These findings indicate a prolonged upregulation of the kynurenine pathway in specific cells of the rat spleen in response to LPS injection into the brain. The major cell types that responded with increased intracellular Quin levels included macrophages, dendritic cells, and B cells. Small, round cells of the T cell-rich PALS were the least immunoreactive for Quin at all-time points. These findings are consistent with macrophages and dendritic cells as major sources of kynurenines and Quin, and that T

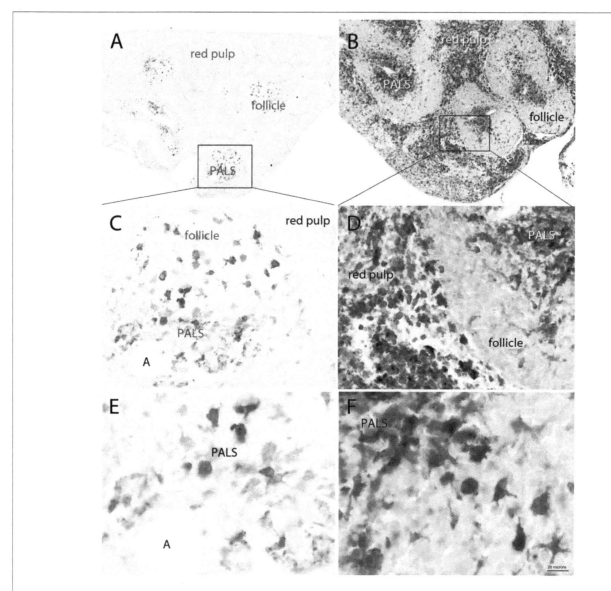

FIGURE 3 | Quin-IR in the gerbil spleen 24 h after IP injection of saline **(A,C,E)** or PWM **(B,D,F)**. Quin-IR was low in the saline group, with most stained cells being present in the periarteriolar lymphoid sheaths (PALS) where antigen presentation occurs between dendritic cells and T cells. Cells in the red pulp were unstained or very lightly stained. In contrast, after PWM administration, Quin-IR was dramatically increased in both the red pulp and PALS. The core of the PALS was strongly stained, suggesting that the Quin-IR cells were dendritic cells. Intense Quin-IR was observed in the red pulp of PWM stimulated gerbils. A in panels **(C,E)**—arteriole. Bar in **(F)**, 200 μm in **(A,B)**, 40 μm in **(C,D)**, and 20 μm in **(E,F)**.

cells are signaling targets of active tryptophan metabolites, rather than producers.

Quin-IR in Rat Brain

A 4-μg dose of LPS was injected into the hippocampus of rats and the brains were fixed with carbodiimide and prepared for immunohistochemistry at various time points. LPS is known to disrupt the blood–brain barrier (41) and injections into the hippocampus elicit strong immune cell infiltration and microglial activation over the course of 7 or more days (42). As expected, high-dose LPS injection into the hippocampus of rats elicited a dramatic, fulminant immune response that resulted in significant local tissue

destruction over the course of several days. LPS induced leukocyte recruitment, microglial activation, and astrogliosis. However, a minimal increase of Quin-IR was observed in the brain under these conditions. Twenty-four hours after LPS injection, scattered Quin-IR cells were observed in the meninges, choroid plexus, hippocampal fissure, and in the brain parenchyma in cortex and hippocampus (**Figures 6**, **7**). In the cortex, in the vicinity of the injection track, only scattered Quin-IR cells were present at 24 h (**Figure 6A**). Three days after LPS administration, the number of Quin-IR cells in the cortex peaked (**Figure 6C**). Quin-IR cells were observed in the ipsilateral and contralateral hemispheres and extended laterally into temporal cortex on the ipsilateral side. Even so, during

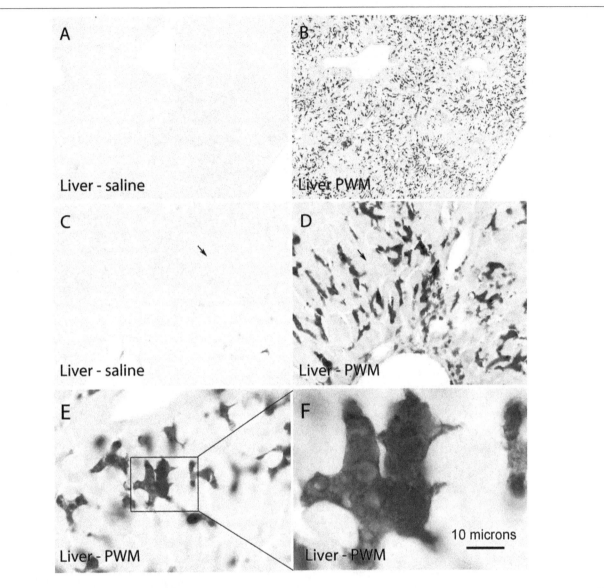

FIGURE 4 | Quin-IR in the gerbil liver 24 h after IP PWM injection (500 μg). Quin-IR was very low in the liver of saline-injected gerbils **(A,C)**. However, 24 h after PWM injection, very strong Quin-IR was observed in cells throughout the liver **(B)**. Morphologically, the cells were identified as resident hepatic macrophages known as Kupffer cells **(D,E,F)**. Quin-IR increased slightly in hepatocytes in the PWM-stimulated liver (arrows in **C,D**), but staining was substantially lower than in the presumptive Kupffer cells. Bar in **(F)**, 370 μm in **(A,B)**, 74 μm in **(C,D)**, 37 μm in **(E)**, and 10 μm in **(F)**.

this time period, the number of Quin-IR cells in the brain was dramatically exceeded by the number of lectin-stained macrophages and activated microglia (**Figures 6B, 7**). We also examined animals that had saline injected into the hippocampus as controls. In these animals, a very small number of Quin-IR cells were seen around the injection site on day 3 after the injection (**Figure 6D**), and astrocytes were reactive as shown by GFAP staining (**Figure 6F**). By 5 days after LPS injection, the number of Quin-IR in the brain had declined, and scar tissue started to form in the necrotic region around the injection site (**Figure 6E**).

In the hippocampus, the Quin-IR response was similar to that in cortex (**Figure 7**). Scattered Quin-IR cells were observed throughout the hippocampus 24 h after LPS (**Figure 7A**). The maximal Quin-IR response was observed by the third day after LPS injection (**Figure 7C**). In contrast to Quin expression, the increase in GSL-IB$_4$ staining was dramatic in the hippocampus by day 3 (**Figure 7E**). Lectin-stained cells were adherent to the luminal face of the vasculature (**Figure 7B**), indicating recruitment of leukocytes from the general circulation. Lectin-stained microglia throughout the hippocampus displayed an activated morphology (**Figure 7D**). In the necrotic zone around the injection site on day 3, many active phagocytes were strongly stained by GSL-IB$_4$ (**Figure 7F**). The vast majority of these lectin-stained cells were not immunoreactive for Quin (also see **Figure 9**, discussed below).

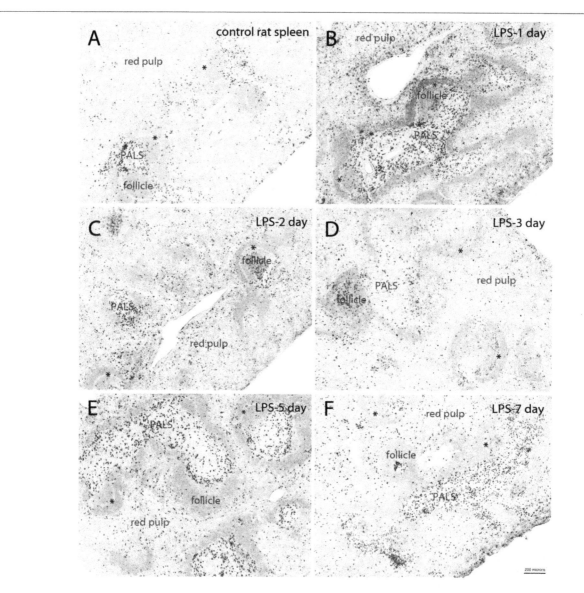

FIGURE 5 | Time course of Quin-IR in the rat spleen after intracerebral injection of LPS into the hippocampus **(A–F)**. Quin-IR was modest in the control rat spleen, but was substantially increased 1 day after injection of 4 μg of LPS into the hippocampus. Strong increases in Quin-IR occurred in all compartments of the spleen (red pulp, PALS, and follicles). Quin-IR remained elevated, but slowly diminished, over the next several days. By day 7, the Quin-IR was returning to near-control levels, but remained elevated. *, marginal sinus. Bar in **(F)**, 200 μm for all images.

The morphology of Quin-IR cells was highly variable. Many of the immunoreactive cells in the brain had membrane elaborations including lamellipodia and filopodia (**Figure 8**). These membrane extensions included knob-like structures (**Figure 8B**), short, spike-like protrusions (**Figure 8C**), broad, ruffled extensions (**Figure 8D**) and various combinations of these (**Figures 8E,F**). Based on our observations we conclude that most or all Quin-IR cells in the brain after LPS injection are highly motile macrophages. They were generally smaller in diameter than the lectin-stained phagocytic macrophages that occupied the necrotic area (see **Figure 9C**). Based on their clustering in and around blood vessels in the vicinity of the LPS injection (**Figures 8B,D**), their apparently motile morphology, as well

as their relatively small size, it is very likely that most or all Quin-IR cells observed in the brain were recruited from the peripheral circulation.

Double staining with Quin antibodies and GSL-IB$_4$ lectin in the brain after intracerebral LPS injection clearly showed that the strong immune response involving macrophages and reactive microglia was accompanied by relatively restricted Quin accumulation in motile macrophages (**Figure 9**). GSL-IB$_4$ binds to α-galactose residues and is a selective marker for rodent macrophages (43) and microglia (44), and also stained some endothelia. Lectin staining was observed throughout the hippocampus on day 3 after LPS injection (**Figure 9A**), with many strongly stained cells clustering around the vasculature

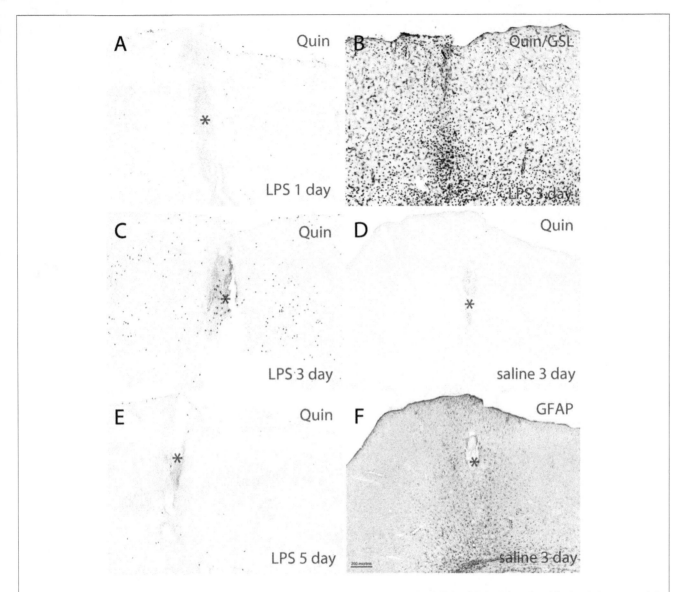

FIGURE 6 | Short-term time course of reactions in rat brain cortex after intracerebral injection of LPS. **(A,C,E)** Show Quin-IR around the injection site in cortex at 1, 3, and 5 days after LPS administration. **(B)** Shows staining for the lectin GSL-IB$_4$ (purple chromogen) and Quin (orange chromogen) 3 days after LPS injection, demonstrating the dramatic microglial and macrophage response at 3 days post-injection. **(D)** Shows Quin-IR at the injection site 3 days after saline injection into the hippocampus. **(F)** Shows a moderate astrocyte response (glial acidic fibrillary protein: GFAP) around the injection site 3 days after saline administration, given as control. In the LPS-injected rats, GFAP staining in the damaged area near the injection site was reduced due to astrocyte death. *Injection tract in cortex. Bar in **(F)**, 200 μm in all panels. The orange color in the injection tract is due to hemoglobin in red blood cells.

(**Figures 9B,D**). Lectin staining was extremely light in control rats, and was mainly seen in some blood vessels (data not shown). Ramified, resting microglia did not stain with the lectin. However, phagocytes (**Figure 9C**) and reactive microglia stained very strongly with GSL-IB$_4$ (**Figures 9D–F**). After LPS injection, Quin-IR cells were much less frequent than lectin-stained cells, but some Quin-IR cells were also stained at their periphery by GSL-IB$_4$ (**Figures 9E,F**).

Remarkably, some Quin-IR cells were observed within the corpus callosum as late as 30 days after LPS administration (**Figure 10**). The number of Quin-IR cells was very low

(**Figure 10A**), and GFAP staining remained elevated even at this late time point (**Figure 10B**). The Quin-IR cells appeared to be infiltrating from the peripheral circulation into the scar area around the injection site (**Figures 10C,D**). The stained cells again had the morphology of motile macrophages and displayed an array of membrane protrusions and extensions.

We expected to find Quin-IR microglia after direct LPS injection into the brain. This was not apparent, but we did observe some very faintly stained cells that had the morphology of reactive microglia. However, these cells were at the detection limit for immunohistochemistry. Based on the available evidence,

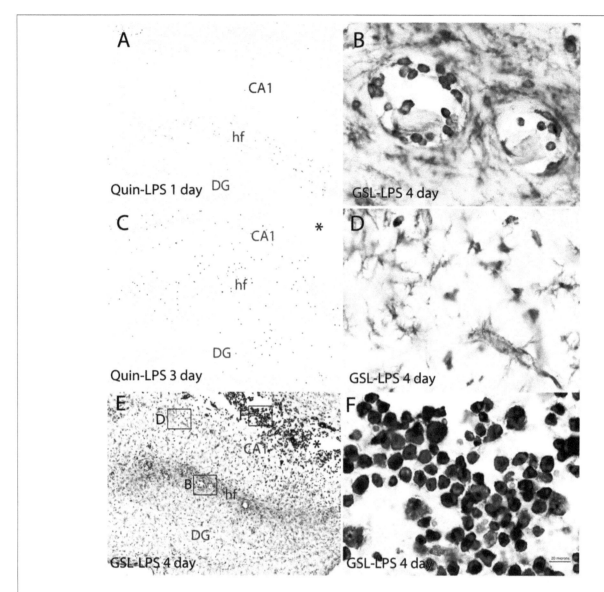

FIGURE 7 | Comparison of the Quin-IR and lectin (GSL) reactions in the hippocampus at several time points after LPS injection. Quin-IR at 1 and 3 days after LPS is shown in **(A,C)**. **(E)** Shows lectin staining for macrophages and activated microglia 4 days after LPS injection. **(B,D,F)** Show enlargements of the lectin staining in areas designated by the boxes in **(E)**. **(B)** Shows monocytes/macrophages adherent to the blood vessels in the hippocampal fissure. **(D)** Shows the strong activation of microglia in the CA1 region of hippocampus. **(F)** Shows the strong infiltration of phagocytes into the necrotic region (*) around the injection site. Bar in **(F)**, 200 μm in **(A,C,E)**; 20 μm in **(B,D,F)**. CA1, CA1 region of hippocampus; DG, dentate gyrus; hf, hippocampal fissure.

microglia do synthesize Quin under these conditions, but they clearly do not accumulate it in their cytoplasm to the same extent as some macrophages.

Based on these findings, we propose that Quin-IR is a useful biomarker for kynurenine pathway activation and metabolite formation up to the level of QPRT and ACMSD (see **Figure 1**), especially in the periphery. In the brain, the utility of Quin immunohistochemistry as a marker of kynurenine pathway flux is more limited. While it is likely that Quin-IR cells express active kynurenine pathway enzymes from IDO to QPRT, it is possible that not all cells require IDO expression. Our experiments involving tryptophan and kynurenine loading in rats indicate that many cells of the immune system avidly take up kynurenine and

convert it to Quin in <3 h (29). This suggests that cells such as fibroblasts that release kynurenine (45) may feed Quin synthesis and NAD$^+$ production in other cell types.

Effect of Kynurenine Administration on Protein Expression in the Mouse Spleen

We investigated the effects of high-dose acute and low-dose prolonged kynurenine loading using two administration methods in mice: IP injection (high-dose acute) and addition to drinking water (low-dose prolonged). For the acute group ($N = 3$ experimental and 3 control), we administered 300 mg/kg of L-kynurenine dissolved in sterile saline, or sterile saline alone, by IP injection 8 h before sacrifice. For the prolonged low-dose

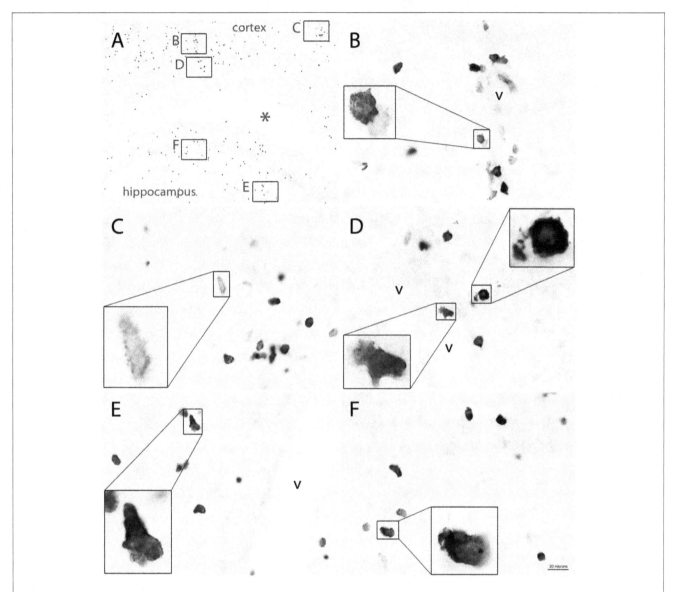

FIGURE 8 | Quin-IR in the vicinity of the injection site 3 days after intracerebral injection of LPS. Quin expression was maximal on day 3 after LPS injection. Immunoreactive cells exhibited highly variable morphology, including lamellipodia and filopodia. Membrane protrusions in the stained cells were very common, indicative of highly mobile cells. Quin-IR cells were scattered around the LPS-affected region **(A)**. Inset areas in **(A)** show magnified regions in **(B–F)**. Concentrated Quin-IR cells were observed around the vasculature (v) **(B,D,E,F)**. Some Quin-IR cells were stained at their periphery and had many membrane extensions **(C)**. *Necrotic region around injection site. Bar in **(F)**, 200 μm in **(A)**, 20 μm in **(C–F)**, and 5.5 μm in insets.

administration group, we included 5 mM kynurenine in the drinking water ($N = 3$) as compared with mice given plain water ($N = 3$) for 48 h.

We employed super-physiological doses of kynurenine to study the effects of maximal pathway throughput in the absence of increased TDO or IDO activity. The 300 mg/kg dose is equivalent to 40 mg for a 25-g mouse, which translates to 1.44 mM if distributed completely and uniformly, meaning that the levels in blood and some tissues may have been substantially higher for a short time. The 5 mM dose in drinking water would translate to a dose of approximately 5.2 mg/day/mouse assuming water consumption of 5 ml/day. The use of super-physiological

kynurenine doses was done for several reasons. First, we wanted to maximize kynurenine pathway throughput in the absence of immune stimulation or IDO activation. Second, we did not know what concentrations the downstream metabolites would reach in the spleen, especially under conditions where the downstream enzymes had not been activated. Finally, drug dosages for smaller animals often need to be increased relative to larger animals to achieve the same effects, depending on the pharmacodynamics. Nonetheless, we delivered a single IP dose, which would have been mostly cleared from the system during the 8-h post-injection period, and we monitored the proteins that remained altered in expression at 8 h. For the 5 mM dose in drinking water,

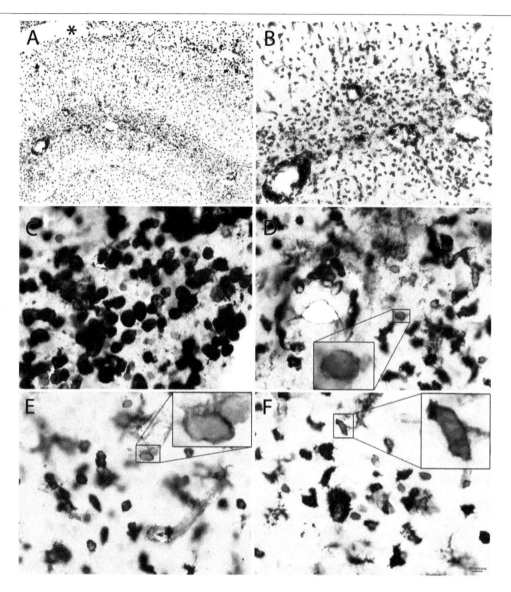

FIGURE 9 | Double staining for Quin-IR (orange chromogen) and GSL-IB$_4$ lectin staining (purple chromogen) in the hippocampus 3 days after LPS injection into the hippocampus. Lectin staining showed a massive reaction from phagocytes and microglia surrounding a necrotic region (*) between hippocampus and the overlying corpus callosum **(A)**. Many lectin-stained cells accumulated in and around the vasculature of the hippocampus **(B)**. In contrast to widespread lectin staining of activated microglia and phagocytes throughout the cortex and hippocampus, only a small number of Quin-IR cells was observed **(C–F)**. Some of the Quin-IR cells were stained lightly at their perimeter with the lectin (insets in **D–F**) but many did not have observable lectin staining. Bar in **(F)**, 100 µm in **(A)**, 40 µm in **(B)**, 10 µm in **(C–F)**, and 3 µm in insets.

the administration was intermittent during waking hours, and therefore would have remained elevated throughout that period.

One noteworthy feature of kynurenine loading is production of kynurenic acid, as the relevant kynurenine aminotransferase reaction (see **Figure 1**) is dependent on the high substrate concentrations due to the high Km of the enzyme for kynurenine (46). For example, intraperitoneal administration of kynurenine induces dose-dependent increases in rat brain cortical and striatal kynurenic acid concentrations and a dramatic elevation of its extracellular striatal levels (47, 48). As such, kynurenine loading with high doses would lead to saturation of pathway enzymes and increase kynurenic acid formation by kynurenine

aminotransferase. Kynurenic acid may be one of the more important ligands for activating the aryl hydrocarbon receptor (AHR; discussed below).

2D Gel Analysis

The quantitative fluorescent 2D-DIGE proteomic methods have been described previously (33) and involve labeling protein samples from control and experimental groups with distinct fluorescent dyes prior to 2D gel analysis (49). The experimental and control samples are mixed and run together on 2D gels along with an internal standard. Only protein spots that were altered in ratio in the same direction between all three

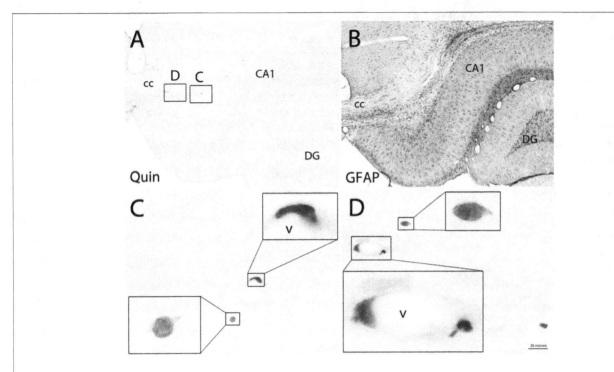

FIGURE 10 | Quin-IR cells in the brain 30 days after LPS injection into the hippocampus. Quin-IR cells were rare near the injection site 30 days after LPS injection **(A)** and were mostly associated with the vasculature (v). GFAP staining in a tissue section adjacent to that in **(A)** is shown in **(B)**. GFAP remained elevated around the injection site at 30 days. The Quin-IR cells exhibited many forms of membrane extension suggestive of diapedesis or migration through tissue **(C,D)**. CA1, area CA1 of hippocampus, cc = corpus callosum, DG = dentate gyrus of hippocampus. Bar in **(D)**, 200 μm in **(A,B)**, 20 μm in **(C,D)**, and 6 μm in panel insets.

experimental and control animals were considered. This system has been found to provide sensitive and reproducible results with low protein samples (50). In the current study, over 1,000 protein spots were resolved on the 2D gels at both time points (**Supplementary Figure 2**). In all, 115 protein spots were altered at the two time points that had significantly changed ratios ($p < 0.05$) between control and experimental groups, and among these, 92 proteins were identified by mass spectroscopy.

Mass Spectroscopy; Acute (8 h) Group

In mice given a single 300 mg/kg injection of L-kynurenine 8 h before sacrifice, a total of 69 protein spots were found to change in abundance relative to controls. Among these, 55 changes were statistically significant ($p < 0.05$), and 41 of the proteins were identified by mass spectroscopy (**Table 1**). Fourteen of the protein spots that had statistically significant variable ratios between experimental and control groups were not identified by mass spectroscopy.

Ten cytoskeletal protein spots were changed in abundance, six were expressed at higher levels, and four were reduced. Beta-actin was identified in six distinct spots on the gels, and the expression of this isoform of actin was increased in all six spots, with the experimental to control ratios ranging between +1.23 and +1.92. The mass fingerprint for gelsolin was found in three distinct spots on 2D gels, and all were increased relative to controls (average ratios of +1.23, +1.27 and +1.35). Two distinct protein spots representing radixin and moesin were both increased in the spleens of animals 8 h after kynurenine administration (ratios

of +1.18 and +1.24, respectively). Actin interacting protein 1 (also called WD repeat protein 1) was increased in abundance, with a ratio of +1.3, and coronin 1a was also increased, with a ratio of +1.37. In contrast, coronin 1b was decreased in abundance at 8 h, with a ratio of −1.26. Three isoforms of tubulin had decreased ratios, including tubulin beta-5 (−1.11), tubulin alpha3/alpha7 (−1.16), and tubulin alpha1 (−1.18). VCAM-1, a cell adhesion molecule that is involved in leukocyte adhesion and diapedesis, was increased 8 h after kynurenine administration (ratio of +1.42).

At the 8-h time point, several protein expression changes were notable. These included eukaryotic translation elongation factor 2 (EF-2, also EEF-2) (ratio +1.27), which positively regulates translation of certain proteins including heat shock protein 90 (HSP90) (51) and TNF-α (52). Also, valosin-containing protein (VCP, also known as transitional endoplasmic reticulum ATPase or p97) had an increased ratio of +1.30. VCP is involved in several processes including protein quality control (ERAD), autophagy, and autophagosome–lysosome fusion, among others (53). Interestingly, heat shock protein 90B1 (HSP90B1; also known as endoplasmin), which is associated with the HSP90 chaperone complex, was expressed at an increased ratio +1.43. Sorting nexin 5 (SNX5), which is involved in macropinocytosis and antigen processing, had a reduced ratio of −1.10 in the 8-h acute kynurenine group as compared with controls.

Two immune cell-specific proteins were upregulated at 8 h, including endoplasmic reticulum aminopeptidase 1 (ERAP1; increased average ratio of +1.40) and SAM domain- and HD

TABLE 1 | Identified protein spots from spleen that were significantly increased or decreased 8 h after IP kynurenine administration (300 mg/kg).

Protein name	Protein ID	Av. ratio	T-test
Actin, cytoplasmic 1 (Beta-actin)	ACTB_HUMAN	1.92	0.037
Actin, cytoplasmic 1 (Beta-actin)	P02570	1.62	0.025
Endoplasmin precursor	ENPL_MOUSE	1.43	0.003
Vascular cell adhesion protein 1 precursor (V-CAM1)	VCA1_MOUSE	1.42	0.00084
Adipocyte-derived leucine aminopeptidase precursor (ERAP1)	ART1_MOUSE	1.4	0.013
Coronin-like protein p57 (Coronin 1A)	CO1A_MOUSE	1.37	0.0072
Alpha-actinin 4 (Non-muscle alpha-actin 4)	P57780	1.35	0.019
Gelsolin precursor, plasma (Actin-depolymerizing factor)	GELS_MOUSE	1.35	0.048
Actin, cytoplasmic 1 (Beta-actin)	ACTB_HUMAN	1.33	0.018
Actin, cytoplasmic 1 (Beta-actin)	ACTB_HUMAN	1.33	0.017
Calreticulin precursor (CRP55) (Calregulin) (HACBP) (ERp60)	P14211	1.37	0.0033
SAM domain and HD domain-containing protein 1	SAD1_MOUSE	1.33	0.02
Actin, cytoplasmic 1 (Beta-actin)	ACTB_CRIGR	1.31	0.0027
Calreticulin precursor (CRP55) (Calregulin) (HACBP) (ERp60)	P14211	1.31	0.0027
WD-repeat protein 1 (Actin interacting protein 1)	WDR1_MOUSE	1.3	0.0041
Transitional endoplasmic reticulum ATPase (TER ATPase)	P46462	1.3	0.019
Gelsolin precursor, plasma (Actin-depolymerizing factor)	P13020	1.27	0.028
Elongation factor 2 (EF-2)	EF2_MOUSE	1.27	0.025
Actin, cytoplasmic 1 (Beta-actin)	P02570	1.24	0.00076
Moesin (Membrane-organizing extension spike protein)	P26041	1.24	0.0089
Heat shock protein HSP 90-alpha (HSP 86)	HS9A_MOUSE	1.24	0.024
Heat shock protein HSP 90-alpha (HSP 86)	P07901	1.24	0.018
Gelsolin precursor, plasma (Actin-depolymerizing factor)	GELS_MOUSE	1.23	0.0031
Peroxiredoxin 2 (EC 1.11.1.-) (Thioredoxin peroxidase 1)	Q61171	1.23	0.019
Pyruvate dehydrogenase E1 component beta subunit	ODPB_RAT	1.2	0.0032
Radixin	RADI_MOUSE	1.18	0.0031
Sorting nexin 5	Q9D8U8	−1.1	0.017
Tubulin beta-5 chain	P05218	−1.11	0.014
Glyceraldehyde 3-phosphate dehydrogenase (EC 1.2.1.12)	P16858	−1.14	0.0037
L-lactate dehydrogenase A chain (EC 1.1.1.27) (LDH-A)	P06151	−1.14	0.0043
Heterogeneous nuclear ribonucleoproteins A2/B1	O88569	−1.15	0.0066
Alpha enolase (EC 4.2.1.11)	ENOA_MOUSE	−1.15	0.015
Tubulin alpha-3/alpha-7 chain (Alpha-tubulin 3/7)	TBA3_MOUSE	−1.16	0.0071
Heterogeneous nuclear ribonucleoproteins A2/B1	O88569	−1.17	0.013
Tubulin alpha-1 chain	TBA1_MOUSE	−1.18	0.011
Hsp90 co-chaperone Cdc37 (Hsp90 chaperone protein)	CC37_MOUSE	−1.21	0.024
Adenylyl cyclase-associated protein 1 (CAP 1)	P40124	−1.23	0.02
Coronin 1B (Coronin 2)	CO1B_MOUSE	−1.26	0.035
Serum albumin precursor	P07724	−1.34	0.043
Heterogeneous nuclear ribonucleoprotein K	ROK_HUMAN	−1.36	0.044

All identified spots that were changed significantly are shown, including multiple spots with the same protein.

domain-containing protein 1 (ratio of +1.33). Mice lacking ERAP1 had reduced numbers of both Tr1-like regulatory T cells and tolerogenic dendritic cells (54), suggesting that increased ERAD1 expression could be associated with increased numbers of these tolerogenic cell types in the spleen in response to kynurenine administration. SAM and HD domain-containing protein 1 (SAMHD1) is involved in anti-viral responses (55).

Two ribonucleoproteins that have been associated with apoptosis were downregulated at 8 h, including heterogeneous nuclear ribonucleoproteins A2/B1 (reduced ratios of −1.17 and −1.15 in two spots) and heterogeneous nuclear ribonucleoprotein K (hnRNPK: reduced ratio of −1.36). hnRNPK is a DNA-binding protein that can act as a transcription enhancer or repressor (56).

One antioxidant enzyme, peroxyredoxin 2, was changed in abundance 8 h after kynurenine administration (ratio of +1.23). Additionally, three chaperone proteins were differentially expressed in experimental animals relative to controls, including

TABLE 2 | Protein expression changes in mouse spleen after mice were exposed to 5 mM kynurenine in drinking water for 48 h.

Protein name	Protein ID	Av. ratio	*T*-test
Moesin	MOES_MOUSE	1.88	0.00099
Gelsolin precursor, plasma	GELS_MOUSE	1.77	0.0067
Elongation factor 2 (EF-2)	EF2_RAT	1.69	0.00034
Gelsolin precursor, plasma	GELS_MOUSE	1.68	0.026
SAM domain and HD domain-containing protein	SAD1_MOUSE	1.62	0.0067
C-1-tetrahydrofolate synthase, cytoplasmic	C1TC_RAT	1.62	0.015
DNA replication licensing factor MCM7	MCM7_MOUSE	1.5	0.0095
Gelsolin precursor, plasma	GELS_MOUSE	1.5	0.013
Gelsolin precursor, plasma	GELS_MOUSE	1.49	0.029
Non-muscle caldesmon (CDM) (L-caldesmon)	CALD_RAT	1.48	0.015
Moesin	MOES_MOUSE	1.47	0.036
Ezrin (p81) (Cytovillin) (Villin 2)	EZRI_MOUSE	1.43	0.0064
Radixin (ESP10)	RADI_MOUSE	1.43	0.039
Radixin (ESP10)	RADI_MOUSE	1.4	0.024
Phosphatidylinositol 3-kinase regulator	P85A_MOUSE	1.38	0.00013
Endoplasmin precursor	ENPL_MOUSE	1.35	0.0077
Transketolase (EC 2.2.1.1) (TK) (P68)	TKT_MOUSE	1.33	0.012
Transketolase (EC 2.2.1.1) (TK) (P68)	TKT_RAT	1.33	0.031
Elongation factor 2 (EF-2)	EF2_MOUSE	1.33	0.017
Vacuolar protein sorting 35	VP35_MOUSE	1.32	0.019
Gelsolin precursor, plasma	GELS_MOUSE	1.31	0.027
Transketolase (EC 2.2.1.1) (TK) (P68)	TKT_MOUSE	1.31	0.0042
Osmotic stress protein 94	OS94_MOUSE	1.31	0.028
Keratin, type I cytoskeletal 10	K1CJ_MOUSE	1.29	0.017
Elongation factor 2 (EF-2)	EF2_MOUSE	1.29	0.015
Endoplasmin precursor	ENPL_MOUSE	1.28	0.0057
Heat shock 70-related protein APG-2	HS74_MOUSE	1.28	0.00048
Heat shock protein HSP 90-beta (HSP 84)	HS9B_RAT	1.26	0.0061
Alpha-actinin 4	AAC4_MOUSE	1.24	0.034
Elongation factor 2 (EF-2)	EF2_MOUSE	1.23	0.014
Structure-specific recognition protein 1	SSRP_MOUSE	1.22	0.044
Hematopoietic lineage cell specific protein	HS1_MOUSE	1.22	0.0075
Serum albumin	ALBU_RAT	1.22	0.033
Endoplasmin precursor	ENPL_MOUSE	1.21	0.035
14-3-3 protein epsilon	143E_HUMAN	1.06	0.02
Swiprosin 1	SWS1_MOUSE	−1.14	0.04
26S proteasome non-ATPase reg. subunit	PSDD_MOUSE	−1.14	0.0084
Keratin, type I cytoskeletal 10	K1CJ_MOUSE	−1.16	0.018
T-complex protein 1, theta subunit	TCPQ_MOUSE	−1.19	0.0098
Tubulin alpha-1 chain	TBA1_MOUSE	−1.19	0.016
Activator of 90 kDa heat shock protein	AHA1_MOUSE	−1.21	0.037
Actin, cytoplasmic 1 (Beta-actin)	ACTB_CRIGR	−1.21	0.014
Actin, cytoplasmic 1 (Beta-actin)	ACTB_CRIGR	−1.21	0.003
Thioredoxin domain containing protein 4	TXN4_MOUSE	−1.22	0.0051
Thioredoxin domain containing protein 4	TXN4_MOUSE	−1.25	0.011
Hsc70-interacting protein (Hip)	ST13_MOUSE	−1.27	0.023
60 kDa heat shock protein	CH60_MOUSE	−1.36	0.015
Heterogeneous nuclear ribonucleoprotein	ROK_HUMAN	−1.38	0.027
Actin, cytoplasmic 1 (Beta-actin)	ACTB_CRIGR	−1.97	0.0037
Ubiquitous tropomodulin (U-Tmod)	TMO3_MOUSE	−1.99	0.0095
14-3-3 protein zeta/delta (YWHAZ)	143Z_MOUSE	−2.31	0.0035

All identified proteins that were changed significantly are included, showing identification of multiple spots representing the same protein.

heat shock protein 90-alpha (HSP90-alpha; ratios of +1.24 in two distinct spots), calreticulin (calregulin; increased ratios of +1.37 and +1.31 in two spots), and HSP90 co-chaperone (CDC37, reduced ratio of −1.21).

Mass Spectroscopy; Prolonged (48 h) Group

In mice administered 5 mM kynurenine in their drinking water for 48 h, 60 protein spots were differentially expressed at significant levels ($p < 0.05$) of which 51 were identified by mass spectroscopy (**Table 2**). Nine additional spots that were significantly altered in expression could not be identified.

The suite of cytoskeletal protein changes at 48 h was somewhat different from that observed at 8 h. Ten cytoskeletal proteins were changed in abundance in the kynurenine group, with seven showing increased expression, and three having decreased expression. Gelsolin was upregulated in five distinct protein spots, with increased ratios ranging from +1.31 to +1.77. The important cytoskeletal regulatory proteins ezrin, radixin, and moesin were all upregulated in experimental animals, and both radixin and moesin were present in two distinct spots on gels. Alpha-actinin-4 showed an increased ratio of +1.24, and non-muscle caldesmon had an increased ratio of +1.48. There were four cytoskeletal proteins that were reduced in abundance 48 h after kynurenine administration, including tubulin alpha-1 chain (ratio reduced by −1.19), keratin type 1 (1 spot with a positive ratio of +1.29, and 1 spot with a negative ratio of −1.16), ubiquitous tropomodulin (negative ratio of −1.99), and beta-actin (3 spots with negative ratios of −1.97, −1.21, and −1.21).

Several proteins associated with apoptosis showed differential expression at 48 h, including 14-3-3 zeta/delta, which had a ratio of −2.31 (a >50% drop). This was the largest single change observed in the study. Also, 26S proteasome non-ATPase regulatory subunit 13 was slightly decreased in abundance (ratio −1.14). A number of other proteins that were altered 8 h after kynurenine administration have connections to the regulation of apoptosis. For example, ezrin is involved in apoptotic regulation by linking the actin cytoskeleton to CD95. Heterogeneous nuclear ribonuclear protein K has also been associated with apoptosis (57). Elongation factor 2 inhibition has been associated with apoptosis, but in the present study, we see increases in abundance of this protein (58).

Three immune system associated proteins were increased in the spleens of experimental animals at 48 h. SAM domain- and HD domain-containing protein, which was also elevated at 8 h, was further increased in abundance at 48 h (ratio +1.62). Hematopoietic lineage cell specific protein 1 (HS1) was increased (ratio +1.22), as was structure-specific recognition protein 1 (SSRP-1; ratio +1.22). HS1 induces actin polymerization and branching in hematopoietic cells by interacting with the ARP2/3 complex (59). HS1 is also a caspase target during apoptosis (60). SSRP-1 can act as either a transcriptional activator, or co-activator, and plays multiple roles in the regulation of transcription. However, it has been shown that overexpression

of SSRP1 with p63-gamma caused a ∼43% increase of apoptotic cells (61).

Several growth or protein translation/translocation associated proteins were increased in expression after 48 h of kynurenine administration. Elongation factor 2 (EF-2, also EEF-2), which is associated with protein chain elongation on ribosomes, was found at four spots on gels, and these had increased ratios of +1.23, +1.29, +1.33, and +1.69. Transketolase was present in three distinct spots on the gels, all of which showed increased ratios at 48 h (ratios of +1.33, +1.33, and +1.31). DNA replication licensing factor MCM7, which is associated with controlling cell cycle check points, was increased in abundance (ratio +1.5). Vacuolar protein sorting 35 was upregulated at 48 h (ratio +1.32).

Seven chaperone or heat shock-related proteins were differentially expressed after 48 h of kynurenine administration (3 increased, 4 decreased). Heat shock protein 90-beta (HSP90-beta) was increased (ratio +1.26), as were osmotic stress protein 94 (ratio +1.31) and heat shock 70-related protein APG-2 (ratio +1.28). The four proteins in this category that were decreased in abundance included T-complex protein 1-theta (ratio −1.19), heat shock protein 60 (HSP60, ratio −1.36), activator of 90 kDa heat shock protein (AHSA1, also AHA1; ratio −1.21), thioredoxin domain-containing protein 4 (two spots: ratios −1.22 and −1.25), and HSC70-interacting protein (ST13, also HIP; ratio −1.27). High expression levels of ST13 are associated with reduced cell migration and proliferation of colorectal cancer cells (62). Swiprosin 1, which is involved in cortical cytoskeleton dynamics among other functions (63, 64), was also decreased in the spleen after 48 h of kynurenine administration (ratio −1.14).

Only nine of the identified proteins that had altered ratios at 8 h were also changed at 48 h (**Figure 11**). Among these,

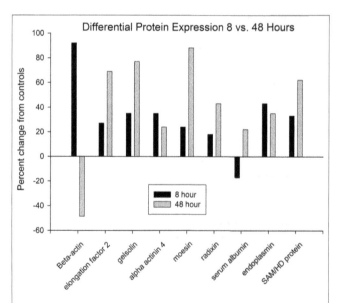

FIGURE 11 | Only nine proteins were identified that were differentially expressed at both time points. Seven of these increased at both time points, whereas two proteins displayed reversed expression patterns at the two time points. Beta-actin was increased at 8 h, but decreased at 48 h, whereas serum albumin was decreased at 8 h, but increased at 48 h.

seven of the protein expression changes at 8 and 48 h were in the same direction (upregulated). In contrast, two proteins, beta-actin and serum albumin, reversed expression levels between the two time points. Because both serum tryptophan and kynurenine are substantially albumin-bound (65), the observed changes in serum albumin levels would be expected to alter the free/bound tryptophan and kynurenine ratios, and downstream flux through the kynurenine pathway. At both time points, several proteins were observed in multiple positions on the gels. This was particularly true of the 48-h group, in which 16 identified proteins were present at two or more spots. This could have been due to increased apoptosis and caspase-mediated proteolysis, and/or due to post-translational modifications. Many of the protein expression changes observed after kynurenine administration were associated with the dynamic actin cytoskeleton, or with cell migration, proliferation or apoptosis.

DISCUSSION

The brain is an immune-privileged organ, with heightened barriers to peripheral immune cell trafficking, and therefore, it does not respond to immune challenges to the same degree as many peripheral organ systems [reviewed in (66)]. This was clearly observed with Quin immunohistochemistry in our models involving peripheral and central immune stimulation. Because the brain is less responsive to certain types of immune stimulation as compared with peripheral organ systems, there may be less need for the immunosuppressive kynurenine metabolites in the brain. Even though kynurenine pathway activity in the brain is lower than in the periphery, the kynurenine pathway has been shown to be critical for immune privilege in the brain (67). Limited Quin production in the brain remains a poorly understood aspect of the immune-privileged status. Microglia are fully capable of generating Quin if provided super-physiological levels of the immediate precursor (31), but we observed little or no Quin-IR in microglia after direct injection of LPS into the hippocampus. The LPS injection needles breached the meningeal and blood–brain barriers, resulting in a strong immune response that activated microglia and recruited peripheral immune cells. Most of the scattered Quin-IR cells in the brain after LPS injection appeared to be infiltrating monocytes/macrophages. The immunosuppressive effects of kynurenine pathway metabolites are important mechanisms employed by the immune system to prevent excess responses that harm the host, at least outside of the brain. But due to its immune privileged status, and the neurotoxic nature of Quin, the brain does not appear to task the kynurenine pathway with preventing excess activation of immune responses to the same extent as in the periphery. Instead, we propose that the brain channels kynurenine pathway metabolism to the synthesis of metabolites other than Quin, and the Quin that is generated is rapidly converted to NAD^+, rather than accumulated in the cytoplasm of cells.

In contrast to Quin immunohistochemistry, lectin staining showed a dramatic immune response in the brain after LPS injection involving microglia and infiltrating macrophages. The immune reaction to LPS was accompanied by extensive tissue damage to the hippocampus, corpus callosum, and cortex that was maximal at 3 days after LPS injection. The number of Quin-IR cells in the brain represented a very small fraction of the observed macrophages and activated microglia as shown by lectin histochemistry (see **Figures 6, 7, 9**). This clearly indicates that the vast majority of the macrophages, microglia, and other cells that responded to the LPS challenge were not immunoreactive for Quin. These results do not support a major role for excessive Quin formation as causative in the tissue damage that occurred in response to LPS injection into the hippocampus.

The Quin-IR response in the liver and spleen of gerbils after systemic PWM administration was dramatic (**Figures 3, 4**). Gerbils lack the apoenzyme form of tryptophan dioxygenase and therefore cortisol does not regulate tryptophan catabolism in the liver as it does in certain other species, including rats and humans (68). Thus, tryptophan catabolism in the gerbil liver is constitutive and systemic tryptophan levels are generally lower than in many other species. In the gerbil spleen, the red pulp transitioned from virtually no Quin-IR in the saline-treated animals to a strong and nearly ubiquitous distribution 24 h after PWM administration. In the white pulp, the PALS dramatically increased Quin expression, whereas staining in the B cell-containing follicles increased modestly. Based on morphology and location within the compartments of the spleen, the majority of Quin-IR cells were macrophages and dendritic cells. Much lower immunoreactivity was observed in areas rich in T and B cells.

In the brain of gerbils after peripheral PWM stimulation, Quin-IR cells were only observed in the choroid plexus, vasculature, and meninges. Some Quin-IR cells in the choroid plexus had the appearance of foam cells, and were filled with large intracellular inclusions (**Figures 2B,E**). Foam cells are lipid-laden macrophages that have taken up oxidized lipids, and this form of macrophage has been associated with disorders including atherosclerosis (69, 70). Similarly, in the liver of gerbils after PWM administration, some Kupffer cells were filled with many large intracellular inclusions that could represent phagolysosomes (**Figure 4F**). The kynurenine metabolite 3-hydroxyanthranilate has been found to affect foam cell formation by reducing uptake of oxidized low-density lipoprotein by macrophages (71, 72). These findings suggest that kynurenine pathway metabolites may be linked to phagocytosis.

The morphology of Quin-IR cells was varied in different tissues. Some cells in the follicles and PALS of the gerbil spleen after PWM administration had the appearance of dendritic cells (**Figure 3F**). In the rat spleen after LPS injection into the hippocampus, many Quin-IR cells could be identified as macrophages and dendritic cells based on location and morphology. In the rat brain after LPS injections, the cells tended to be relatively small, and often had membrane elaborations including lamellipodia and filopodia (**Figures 8, 9**). Overall, Quin-IR cells in the brain after LPS injection resembled motile macrophages [see (73)]. Many Quin-IR cells had multiple knob-like membrane protrusions that have been referred to as "blebs." We also observed Quin-IR cells with filopodia and lamellipodia.

Motile macrophages employ the cortical cytoskeleton to generate membrane protrusions that facilitate cell migration through tissues [reviewed in (74)]. We observed a wide array of membrane extensions in Quin-IR cells after LPS injection into the brain.

In our 2D-DIGE proteomics investigation, kynurenine pathway flux was engaged in the absence of immune stimulation, IDO induction, tryptophan depletion, or interferon-gamma administration. The significant spleen protein changes observed resulted from exposure to kynurenine pathway metabolites alone, further confirming that these molecules have modulatory and regulatory roles in leukocyte protein expression and function.

Selective induction of apoptosis is a frequently cited action of some kynurenine metabolites (75). In the current proteomic study, six protein spots that were significantly increased at 8 h and seven spots increased at 48 h were found to have the sequence of beta actin. These distinct spots containing related amino acid sequences might suggest that several post-translationally modified forms of actin were formed in response to kynurenine administration. However, cytoskeletal proteins are also important targets for caspase-mediated proteolysis during apoptosis, and the presence of beta-actin in multiple locations on gels could be due to proteolytic breakdown. A notable finding of the current study was that numerous protein targets of kynurenine catabolite action in the spleen were cytoskeletal including ERM proteins (ezrin, radixin, and moesin), gelsolin, WD repeat protein-1, and coronin-like protein p57, as well as actin and tubulin isoforms. A plausible explanation of these protein changes could be that kynurenine catabolites induce selective leukocyte apoptosis, because many of these cytoskeletal proteins are primary targets for caspase-3-mediated proteolysis (60, 76). However, these findings could also suggest that kynurenines may play a role in regulating the dynamics of the actin cytoskeleton in leukocytes based on the levels of kynurenine metabolites.

In leukocytes, ERM proteins are involved in cell polarization, extension of lamellipodia and filopodia, chemotaxis, formation of the immunological synapse, intracellular granule movement, and phagocytosis. ERM protein action is regulated by a system of kinases and phosphatases that control the level of phosphorylation in response to various signals. Phosphorylation is associated with ERM activation, association of ERM with the cortical actin cytoskeleton, and the formation of cellular microvilli. Proteomic data in the present study showed that ERM proteins were significantly increased at 48 h, and both moesin and radixin were present in two distinct protein spots with increased ratios. ERM proteins are critically involved in the formation of the immunological synapse between T cells and antigen-presenting cells (77), and their phosphorylation is associated with the exclusion of certain surface proteins from the contact zone between the two cell types. The finding that endoplasmic reticulum aminopeptidase I (gene ERAP1) was increased in abundance after kynurenine administration may relate to antigen presentation by APCs during the formation of the immunological synapse. Interestingly, the NAD^+-dependent deacetylase enzyme SIRT1 is required for lamellipodia extension and migration of melanoma cells (78). Sirtuins including SIRT1 consume NAD^+

and therefore it is possible that migrating cells benefit from an increased supply. This raises the possibility that local supply of NAD^+ at the leading edge of migrating cells could be generated from stored intracellular Quin if QPRT, NMNAT, and NADSYN1 are also expressed locally (see **Figure 1**).

Links between the kynurenines and cell motility come from research into the AHR and cancer. The AHR is a transcription factor that responds to a number of different signaling agents including several of the kynurenine pathway metabolites. In particular, kynurenine, kynurenic acid, and xanthurenic acid have been shown to activate the AHR (79–82). The AHR is the primary receptor system that kynurenine metabolites act through. Inactive AHR is retained in the cytoplasm bound to HSP90, and ligand binding dissociates AHR from HSP90 and exposes a nuclear localization signal. AHR is then transported to the nucleus where it forms a transcription factor complex and binds to specific DNA response elements [reviewed in (83)]. In the current study, we found a number of changes in HSP90-related protein levels [HSP90 reviewed in (84)]. HSP90-beta (HSP90AA1; HSP86) had an increased ratio of 1.24-fold 8 h after kynurenine administration, whereas HSP90 co-chaperone (CDC37) was decreased by −1.21-fold at this time point. HSP90-alpha (HSP90AB1; also known as HSP84) had an increased ratio of +1.26 after 48 h of kynurenine administration in drinking water. Also at 48 h, activator of 90 kDa heat shock protein (AHSA1, also AHA1) was decreased −1.21-fold. AHSA1 has been reported to regulate proliferation, apoptosis, migration, and invasion of osteosarcoma (85). Silencing of AHSA1 via siRNA significantly reduced migration of osteosarcoma cells in culture. Finally, at both time points, endoplasmin precursor (HSP90B1) was upregulated (see **Figure 11**). HSP90B1 overexpression has been associated with metastasis of breast cancer (86). Our results on the upregulation of HSP90 protein expression after kynurenine administration are consistent with the conclusion that the AHR/HSP90 system acts to regulate responses to kynurenine metabolites.

There are a number of published reports that indicate the AHR is somehow linked to cell motility and migration. For example, in human breast cancer cell lines, Novikov et al. found that a combination of 50 μM kynurenine and 10 μM xanthurenic acid exerted a maximal effect on promoting cell migration (80). This effect was mediated by the AHR system, but in the case of breast cancer cells, AHR activation was linked to increased TDO activity, rather than IDO. Activation of the AHR in epithelial cells led to morphological changes associated with cytoskeletal remodeling, increased interaction with the extracellular matrix, and reduced cell–cell contacts (87). AHR activation in lung fibroblasts significantly enhanced migration via generation of arachidonic acid metabolites (88). AHR agonists also significantly increased migration of squamous cell carcinoma cells in culture (89). Our data are consistent with these findings and suggest that kynurenine metabolites lead to changes in the expression levels of HSP90-related proteins that impact on cell motility and other cellular behaviors. We propose that kynurenine and its derivatives facilitate cell motility and cancer metastasis via activation of the AHR/HSP90 system, resulting in dissociation of the cytoplasmic complex and nuclear translocation of AHR, which activates genes that are involved in enhanced cytoskeletal dynamics and increased cell motility.

Hepatic vs. Immune Kynurenine Pathways and the Kynurenine Switch

Not all enzymes of the kynurenine pathway are present in all cells, so the complement of expressed enzymes is key to how tryptophan is catabolized in a particular cell type (see **Figure 1**). Hepatocytes express the full repertoire of kynurenine pathway enzymes including the NAD$^+$ synthetic and oxidation pathways. As such, the liver is the primary site of tryptophan metabolism under normal physiological conditions. The regulation of hepatic TDO and non-hepatic IDO kynurenine pathway activation is distinct. An important activator of TDO is cortisol, whereas interferon-γ is one of the more potent inducers of IDO activity (90, 91).

In hepatocytes, any tryptophan that is not required for protein synthesis can be converted to NAD$^+$ or oxidized internally to CO_2. As such, most systemic tryptophan that is in excess of current requirements will be fully metabolized in the liver. If there is ever a need to divert tryptophan metabolism from the liver to the periphery, especially to the immune system, then IDO would provide the necessary switch. We propose that strong IDO activation initiates a "kynurenine switch" that diverts a substantial proportion of downstream kynurenine pathway metabolism and NAD$^+$ synthesis from the liver to the immune system (**Figure 12**). Quoting from our Quin-IR studies on tryptophan and kynurenine loading: *"During immune system activation, the metabolite in the kynurenine pathway that reaches the highest concentration appears to be kynurenine itself, and tissues such as lung are significant producers of kynurenine* (92). *If kynurenine is taken up poorly by hepatocytes and avidly by leukocytes, as our results suggest, then one function of the extensive activation of IDO in tissues such as lung may be to shift tryptophan utilization from the liver to the immune system"* (29). The strong induction of IDO in many tissues during an immune response has not been satisfactorily explained. We propose that a primary function is to shift NAD$^+$ metabolism from centralized hepatic production to distributed immune system production. This local, on-demand substrate diversion for NAD$^+$ production would clearly be more efficient than relying on hepatic supplies of nicotinamide. This view ties together many themes on tryptophan metabolism and has greater explanatory power than the tryptophan depletion hypothesis. We suggest that the tryptophan utilization model provides a unifying conceptual framework for understanding the multiple roles played by IDO, kynurenines, and Quin in regulating immune system responsiveness, tolerance, and metabolism in cells of the immune system.

Quin release and uptake for use in NAD$^+$ synthesis is evolutionarily conserved in eukaryotes as it has been shown to occur in yeast. Quin is released by yeast cells and taken up by other yeast cells where it is converted to NAD$^+$ (93). It is not known to what extent this occurs in mammals. In mammalian systems, it is more likely that, upon immune stimulation, various cell types release excess kynurenine, which is then taken up and

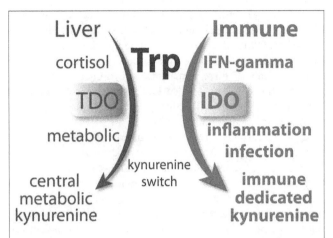

FIGURE 12 | Many researchers have hypothesized that the strong induction of IDO during infection was directed at reducing tryptophan levels in order to control pathogen replication or induce tolerance. We hypothesize that IDO, which is upregulated in many tissues by immune-activating agents such as INF-γ, initiates a system-wide diversion of tryptophan metabolism from the liver to the immune system. During normal metabolism, cortisol activates TDO in hepatocytes to metabolize tryptophan. During an immune response, INF-γ activates IDO in many cell types, converting tryptophan to kynurenine, which is then released to the circulation where it can be preferentially taken up by cells of the immune system. This enzyme-mediated kynurenine switch diverts tryptophan metabolism and NAD$^+$ synthesis from the liver to the immune system during an immune response.

converted to NAD$^+$ by cells of the immune system. As such, IDO activation in cells such as lung cells does not "deplete tryptophan," it initiates a biosynthetic pathway that generates excess systemic kynurenine, which can then be taken up and utilized preferentially by cells of the immune system.

In macrophages and other cells that utilize tryptophan or kynurenine to generate high internal concentrations of Quin, it is apparent that they slow or block further Quin utilization for at least two primary purposes, to stockpile an NAD$^+$ precursor for later use, and to increase the concentration and release of upstream kynurenine metabolites to regulate other immune cell's responses. Interestingly, extracellular tryptophan can be exchanged with intracellular kynurenine across the plasma membrane in cells in culture via the large neutral amino acid transporter SLC7A5, also called LAT1 (94). SLC7A5 is also involved in kynurenine uptake and is expressed in T cells (95), B cells (96), and monocytes/macrophages (97), indicating that all of these cell types are able to take up extracellular kynurenine.

Quin-IR in the Brain vs. Periphery

In humans, Quin is excreted in the urine and the level in urine increases with increasing oral doses of tryptophan (98). This suggests that when tryptophan availability is in excess of current needs, the kynurenine pathway provides an efficient means for metabolism and subsequent excretion via the kidneys (46). Quin levels rise in the bloodstream and in many tissues during infections and after stimulation with agents such as PWM (92), indicating that some cell types release Quin in response to pathogens or inflammatory signals. Both before and after PWM treatment, Quin levels are lowest in the brain and highest in the spleen (92), which is consistent with our current findings. Quin levels in normal mouse brain tissue are at detection limits by LC/MS-MS (99). In a comprehensive evaluation of the mechanisms controlling Quin levels in the brain, Morrison et al. showed that three primary factors maintained low brain concentrations. These included local synthesis, entry into the brain from the blood, and active Quin extrusion from brain by a probenecid-sensitive pump (100).

Quin is excluded from the brain to the extent possible, including during an immune response (28, 101). Quin levels in the brain are maintained below blood levels by barriers and transporters (100). During strong immune stimulation with LPS infusion into the brain, the extracellular Quin level, as measured by microdialysis, increased 66-fold (102). This was reportedly due to a combination of increased local synthesis and a decrease in the efflux/influx ratio. Normally, Quin synthesis in the brain is very low, but when super-physiological concentrations of 3-hydroxyanthranilate are provided, microglia produce significant quantities of Quin as shown by immunohistochemistry (31). During potent immune stimulation, Quin levels rise in many tissues, but brain levels remain low (92, 103). Further, in the current study, we induced a powerful and sustained immune response in the brain via LPS injection, and this only resulted in a minimal infiltration of Quin-positive cells (**Figures 6– 9**). Peripheral PWM administration resulted in splenomegaly and a dramatic increase in Quin-IR in the spleen and liver (**Figures 3, 4**), but no immunoreactive cells were observed in brain parenchyma (**Figure 2**).

The low number of Quin-IR cells in the brain after direct LPS administration and subsequent local tissue necrosis is noteworthy. Lectin-stained macrophages and activated microglia outnumbered Quin-IR macrophages by many fold. Kynurenine metabolism in the brain is reported to be complete and robust under various conditions of immune stimulation, and in the case of LPS infusion into the brain, 98% of kynurenine and Quin in the brain was derived from local synthesis rather than from the blood supply (104). But as we have shown here, unlike peripheral tissues, Quin accumulation does not occur in the vast majority of cells even after direct LPS injection into the brain. In fact, the lack of Quin production within the area of damage may have contributed to the uncontrolled immune response and tissue necrosis noted by day 3 after LPS injection. If the kynurenine pathway response to immune stimulation in the brain is diminished, as our results suggest, then its immunosuppressive effects may be attenuated and less effective, resulting in more extensive tissue damage.

Quin Accumulation in Cells of the Immune System

Because Quin is a neurotoxin, and has pro-apoptotic effects on some cell types, the accumulation of high intracellular levels in specific cells of the immune system is of significant interest. Numerous studies have shown that Quin accumulates in tissues and blood during infections or immune challenge, but very few methods allow researchers to look at Quin accumulation in various cell types throughout different tissues and organ systems. Quin immunohistochemistry provides a means to examine this question in detail. Immunohistochemistry is more useful at locating cells with high concentrations of the target molecule than it is at localizing trace amounts. Quin immunohistochemistry clearly shows that most cell types do not generate high intracellular levels. It is now clear that several immune system cell types are the most likely to accumulate substantial levels of cytosolic Quin including monocytes/macrophages, dendritic cells, microglia, Langerhans cells, and Kupffer cells, suggesting that phagocytes and antigen-presenting cells are major producers (26, 27, 31).

We have shown that Quin-IR is increased in a number of different conditions where the immune system is stimulated, in addition to those detailed here, including SIV in monkeys (105), human T-cell lymphotropic virus type 1 infection of human peripheral blood monocytes/macrophages (106), and in a murine AIDS model (107). Also, tryptophan and kynurenine loading in rats increased Quin-IR differentially in distinct cell types demonstrating selective uptake and utilization systems for these closely related metabolites (29). The plasma kynurenine to tryptophan ratio (Kyn/Trp) is often used as an indicator of IDO action and kynurenine pathway flux, despite its complications and limitations (65). Quin-IR provides a unique method for looking at kynurenine pathway throughput up to the point of Quin synthesis. Most of the active signaling metabolites are in the early segments of the kynurenine pathway initiated by IDO (see **Figure 1**). The metabolites in the remaining segments of the kynurenine pathway are destined for other metabolic fates, including NAD^+ synthesis or oxidation for energy derivation.

There could be many explanations for the observation that Quin is generated at high intracellular levels in certain immune cells. Foremost, halting the kynurenine pathway at QPRT and ACMSD in macrophages would result in stockpiling of Quin after strong IDO induction and allow for controlled release of upstream metabolites to modulate immune responses. It could also allow for sustained conversion to NAD^+. Other potential reasons for Quin stockpiling include the fact that many bacteria secrete NAD^+ glycohydrolases [e.g., tuberculosis necrotizing toxin or TNT, streptococcus pyogenes beta-NAD^+(+) glycohydrolase, known as SPN, etc.] that deplete intracellular NAD^+ levels in macrophages, leading to cell death (108–110). It is possible that some phagocytes accumulate Quin from tryptophan catabolism to replenish depleted NAD^+ resulting from pathogens that secrete NAD^+ hydrolase enzymes. In addition, endogenous NAD^+ degrading enzymes such as CD38 (111) may also favor increased NAD^+ synthesis from tryptophan. CD38 and CD157 are ectonucleotidase enzymes involved in immune tolerance that convert NAD^+ into ADP-ribose and cyclic-ADP-ribose (112). Overall, the increased requirements for NAD^+ synthesis during inflammation and infection include the PARP reaction, cell surface ADP ribosyltransferases, the respiratory burst, sirtuins, NAD^+ hydrolase activity, ectonucleotidase activity, and maintaining redox homeostasis and energy derivation (**Figure 13**). All of these actions are enhanced during an immune response.

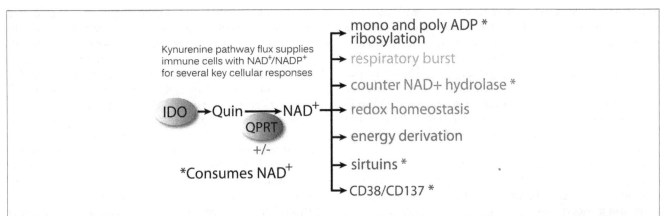

FIGURE 13 | The kynurenine pathway generates immune modulatory agents, but it also supplies Quin to be directed to NAD$^+$ synthesis in cells of the immune system. Regulation of the enzyme QPRT controls the flow of kynurenine pathway metabolism to NAD$^+$. Increased NAD$^+$ demand during inflammation and infection is driven by a number of cellular actions including energy derivation, the respiratory burst, and cellular redox homeostasis. In addition, there are a number of enzymatic reactions that use NAD$^+$ as cosubstrate, and these reactions consume NAD$^+$. These include the PARP reaction for DNA repair (poly-ADP ribosylation) and mono-ADP ribosylases, such as tankerases TNKS1 and 2. Increased NAD$^+$ demand may also come from infections by bacteria that employ NAD$^+$ hydrolases to deprive phagocytes of intracellular NAD$^+$. NAD$^+$ is also consumed by the NAD$^+$-dependent deacetylases known as sirtuins, which regulate metabolism. Certain host enzymes/receptors also have NAD$^+$ hydrolase activity including CD38 and CD157, which are ADP-ribosyl cyclases and hydrolases.

Most kynurenine pathway metabolites increase in blood plasma during infection or after administration of immune stimulants such as LPS, PWM, or INF-γ. Cells that have high levels of Quin are those that contain the enzymes of the kynurenine pathway up to QPRT and ACMSD (see **Figure 1**). It is likely that restriction at the level of QPRT is one reason why certain cells of the immune system show up strongly in Quin immunohistochemistry. QPRT activity is low in unstimulated monocytes, but is increased significantly after IFN-γ treatment (113). The Km of QPRT is 100 times greater than the normal levels of Quin in the liver, but the Vmax of the enzyme is low, meaning that during times of high tryptophan throughput, some degree of Quin accumulation would be expected (114). Therefore, when cells of the immune system are activated by cytokines such as INF-γ and IDO activity is greatly increased, the rapid tryptophan catabolism would be expected to cause some degree of Quin accumulation. High-dose administration of tryptophan in rats leads to more than a doubling of the Quin levels in the liver (114). We observed a modest increase in Quin-IR in the liver after high-dose tryptophan (29). The increase in Quin staining in liver after tryptophan or kynurenine administration indicates that Quin IHC can detect transiently increased levels in cells that express QPRT such as hepatocytes. Therefore, similar effects should be seen in leukocytes that further process Quin to NAD$^+$, such as macrophages. Using Quin immunohistochemistry, several cell types showed mild to moderate levels of Quin staining, including B cells in splenic follicles after LPS injection into the hippocampus, and in gerbil hepatocytes after IP PWM injection.

How Much NAD$^+$ Is Synthesized From Quin Outside the Liver?

Adequate diets supply substantial amounts of NAD$^+$ precursors including nicotinic acid and nicotinamide (collectively known as niacin). However, the tryptophan-to-NAD$^+$ pathway operates independently of niacin supply (115). When tryptophan is required for NAD$^+$ synthesis due to a poor diet or prolonged fasting, the liver activates TDO and tryptophan is catabolized through the kynurenine pathway to NAD$^+$ (116). NAD$^+$ is then broken down to nicotinamide and ADP ribose, and the nicotinamide is released to the circulation to be used by other cells throughout the body. However, less information is available on how much NAD$^+$ is synthesized from Quin in cells of the immune system, especially during various immune responses and during the types of oxidative and metabolic stress that would be encountered during an injury or infection. Based on work with TDO-deficient mice and niacin-controlled diets, Terakata et al. proposed that the TDO-deficient mice could develop normally on a niacin-deficient diet because extra hepatic cells released kynurenine, which the liver took up and converted to Quin and then NAD$^+$ (117). These findings highlight the fact that kynurenine synthesis via IDO and release from various cell types provides sufficient substrate for NAD$^+$ synthesis to meet both developmental and nutritive needs. Kynurenine released to the bloodstream effectively bypasses the rate-limiting enzymes TDO and IDO in any cell type that is capable of kynurenine uptake (23, 29).

IDO, KMO and QPRT (see **Figure 1**) are all upregulated in human peripheral blood monocytes by IFN-γ (113), and this is consistent with the potential for extra hepatic NAD$^+$ synthesis in macrophages. It was reported by Grant that INF-γ increases IDO and in turn increases NAD$^+$ synthesis from tryptophan in RAW264.7 macrophages (13). In these studies, it was also shown that inhibition of the PARP reaction increased intracellular NAD$^+$ levels by 35% over controls, whereas PARP inhibition along with INF-γ treatment resulted in an 84% increase in NAD$^+$ content. Tryptophan was required for the effect and IDO inhibition reduced NAD$^+$ levels. These findings indicate that the PARP reaction is a major utilizer of intracellular NAD$^+$, and that IDO catabolism of tryptophan does replenish NAD$^+$ supplies.

NAD^+ utilized for redox reactions is not consumed, but many enzyme systems such as the PARP reaction utilize NAD^+ as cosubstrate and convert it to nicotinamide and ADP-ribose, thus depleting intracellular supplies (118). Recently, studies on NAD^+ synthesis from tryptophan were repeated in primary human monocytes where it was found that induction of kynurenine metabolism by INF-γ was more robust in macrophages than in undifferentiated monocytes (14). INF-γ increased IDO activity as well as kynurenine and Quin levels in the culture media. Quin levels in the culture media after INF-γ treatment were an order of magnitude lower than the kynurenine levels, indicating that kynurenine is greatly favored over Quin for export from activated macrophages. Interestingly, the effect of INF-γ alone on human monocytes and macrophages was to cause a decrease in NAD^+ levels because INF-γ also strongly activated PARP. However, a PARP inhibitor resulted in an increase in NAD^+ levels in macrophages and INF-γ plus the PARP inhibitor further increased NAD^+ levels (14).

In one of the first comprehensive studies of the contribution of the kynurenine pathway to *de novo* NAD^+ synthesis, Minhas et al. investigated the importance of the IDO-mediated pathway in macrophages. They confirmed *de novo* NAD^+ synthesis using mass labeled kynurenine, and showed that human monocyte-derived macrophages generated 40% of their NAD^+ from kynurenine, rather than from the salvage pathway (15). Blockade of the salvage pathway resulted in over 90% of NAD^+ synthesis coming from the kynurenine pathway. $QPRT^{-/-}$ mice did not incorporate mass labeled tryptophan or kynurenine into NAD^+. Loss of QPRT activity also affected mitochondrial oxidative phosphorylation in macrophages and reduced phagocytosis. A major finding by Minhas and coworkers was that LPS resulted in strong activation of the kynurenine pathway in macrophages, but that it also decreased QPRT expression, resulting in a bottleneck in NAD^+ synthetic capacity. This maintained the macrophages in an inflammatory state with reduced phagocytosis. Overexpression of QPRT overcame the bottleneck and restored homeostasis. The authors suggested that QPRT represents a functional switch between pro-inflammatory and anti-inflammatory macrophage phenotypes.

Clearly, regulation of the expression and activity QPRT is the primary control point in the switch from Quin accumulation and release of kynurenines to NAD^+ synthesis. As such, Quin immunohistochemistry provides a useful tool for determining which particular cell types are accumulating Quin during various immune challenges. It can be assumed that the Quin-IR cells have high IDO and relatively low QPRT activity. This may also explain the lack of Quin-IR in the vast majority of phagocytes in the brain after intracerebral LPS injection. During the transition from an active, inflammatory state to an anti-inflammatory, phagocytic state, macrophages upregulate QPRT activity and consume their intracellular Quin to restore their NAD^+ supplies.

CONCLUSIONS

Something interesting is going on with tryptophan during inflammatory and immune responses. It is now well-established that various kynurenine pathway metabolites are involved in regulating immune responses to various pathogens and pathologies, as well as acting to limit responses to self-antigens. The fact that the kynurenine pathway is evolutionarily conserved clearly indicates that it serves important biological functions. When this system works as intended, it confers survival advantages, but when it goes awry, there are substantial deleterious consequences. Maintaining this balance appears to involve a number of signaling systems, and the expression and regulation of various enzymes in the kynurenine pathway in different cell types. Further, diet may turn out to have an influence on the pro-survival benefits conferred by kynurenine pathway metabolism in the hepatic and immune systems, wherein excess protein in a calorie dense diet may exaggerate deleterious effects of strong kynurenine pathway activation and alter the course of inflammatory disorders or cancer. Humans require ~250 mg of tryptophan per day to maintain nitrogen balance, but modern diets rich in dairy products and meat contain 3–4 times as much or more (119). Interestingly, studies indicate that high protein diets have a negative impact on plasma NAD^+ levels (120). It is possible that prolonged dietary tryptophan excess during a strong immune response may turn out to be an exacerbating factor in certain inflammatory conditions, shifting kynurenine pathway flux from a net positive to an overall negative effect. The effects of excessive kynurenine flux on cancer cell evasion may be another pathology associated with excess tryptophan in the diet (121).

Quin immunohistochemistry provides a unique window on kynurenine pathway throughput by highlighting cells that accumulate high intracellular levels of Quin. This intracellular stockpiling effect would not be apparent by most other analytical methods, but becomes obvious using Quin immunohistochemistry. Cells that are constitutively capable of synthesizing NAD^+ from Quin such as hepatocytes do not demonstrate strong Quin stockpiling, but they do show a moderate, transient increase in Quin-IR after tryptophan loading or immune stimulation. In contrast, cells of the immune system including macrophages, dendritic cells, Langerhans cells, Kupffer cells, and others generate high, sustained levels of intracellular Quin in response to various immune stimulants. Because Quin is present at very high concentrations in the cytoplasm of these cells, they did not release all of their kynurenine metabolites, nor did they fully metabolize Quin to NAD^+ or CO_2. The most obvious conclusion is that intensely stained Quin-IR cells catabolized tryptophan through the pathway up to the point of QPRT and ACMSD. There is a bottleneck at these enzymatic steps, either via regulatory mechanisms that temporarily limit further metabolism of Quin, or enzyme saturation. Our initial impression on viewing this Quin stockpiling effect in 1994 was that it was associated with at least two functions: the production of immune signaling agents and increased NAD^+ synthesis in the immune system (26). Further research will be required to fully answer the question of whether kynurenine pathway metabolism from kynurenine to NAD^+ has a net positive or negative effect on outcomes in various pathological conditions. We expect that under many circumstances, the kynurenine-to-NAD^+ pathway will turn out to be essential for host cell protection while also regulating the response to and resolution of various infectious or inflammatory conditions.

We hypothesize that kynurenine metabolites will also turn out to facilitate or regulate the motility of certain immune cell types, including lamellipodia formation and movement through tissues, which could be important for connections between IDO, kynurenines, and cancer metastasis. Kynurenines may also be involved in regulating or facilitating phagocytosis. Overall, we predict that kynurenine pathway activation during immune responses to various pathogens and stimuli will turn out to be protective of cells in the immune system and facilitate pathogen clearance and resolution of the immune response. The balance between killing pathogens or cancer cells and sparing host cells is delicate, and the chances for dysregulation under physiological stress are significant. Most research is currently focused on the negative effects of activation of the kynurenine pathway via IDO, especially in the nervous system and in cancer. However, it is likely that research focused on the protective functions of this pathway, including the release of metabolites that modulate the interplay between immunogenic and tolerogenic responses, as well as the diversion of NAD^+ metabolism from the liver to the immune cells and concomitant extra-hepatic production of NAD^+, will provide further insights into the evolutionary conservation of this metabolic signaling pathway in the immune system.

AUTHOR CONTRIBUTIONS

JM, AN, and PA conceived the study and conducted the studies. JM, AN, PA, JI, NP, AB, and RV analyzed the data and wrote the paper.

FUNDING

This work was supported by NIH grant NS084206, CHIRP grant APG-70-3917, and grant EY09085 from the National Eye Institute.

ACKNOWLEDGMENTS

We would like to thank Dr. Kuniaki Saito for expert assistance in the gerbil PWM model.

REFERENCES

1. Henderson LM. Quinolinic acid metabolism; replacement of nicotinic acid for the growth of the rat and Neurospora. *J Biol Chem.* (1949) 181:677–85.

2. Mehler AH, Yano K, MAY EL. Nicotinic acid biosynthesis: control by an enzyme that competes with a spontaneous reaction. *Science.* (1964) 145:817–9. doi: 10.1126/science.145.3634.817

3. Campbell BM, Charych E, Lee AW, Moller T. Kynurenines in CNS disease: regulation by inflammatory cytokines. *Front Neurosci.* (2014) 8:12. doi: 10.3389/fnins.2014.00012

4. Lovelace MD, Varney B, Sundaram G, Lennon MJ, Lim CK, Jacobs K, et al. Recent evidence for an expanded role of the kynurenine pathway of tryptophan metabolism in neurological diseases. *Neuropharmacology.* (2017) 112:373–88. doi: 10.1016/j.neuropharm.2016.03.024

5. Savitz J. The kynurenine pathway: a finger in every pie. *Mol Psychiatry.* (2019) 25:131–47. doi: 10.1038/s41380-019-0414-4

6. Schwarcz R, Foster AC, French ED, Whetsell WO Jr, Köhler C. Excitotoxic models for neurodegenerative disorders. *Life Sci.* (1984) 35:19–32. doi: 10.1016/0024-3205(84)90148-6

7. Schwarcz R, Bruno JP, Muchowski PJ, Wu HQ. Kynurenines in the mammalian brain: when physiology meets pathology. *Nat Rev Neurosci.* (2012) 13:465–77. doi: 10.1038/nrn3257

8. Stone TW, Mackay GM, Forrest CM, Clark CJ, Darlington LG. Tryptophan metabolites and brain disorders. *Clin Chem Lab Med.* (2003) 41:852–9. doi: 10.1515/CCLM.2003.129

9. Stone TW, Forrest CM, Mackay GM, Stoy N, Darlington LG. Tryptophan, adenosine, neurodegeneration and neuroprotection. *Metab Brain Dis.* (2007) 22:337–52. doi: 10.1007/s11011-007-9064-3

10. Fallarino F, Grohmann U, Puccetti P. Indoleamine 2,3-dioxygenase: from catalyst to signaling function. *Eur J Immunol.* (2012) 42:1932–7. doi: 10.1002/eji.201242572

11. Munn DH, Mellor AL. IDO in the tumor microenvironment: inflammation, counter-regulation, and tolerance, trends. *Immunology.* (2016) 37:193–207. doi: 10.1016/j.it.2016.01.002

12. Massudi H, Grant R, Guillemin GJ, Braidy N. NAD^+ metabolism and oxidative stress: the golden nucleotide on a crown of thorns. *Redox Rep.* (2012) 17:28–46. doi: 10.1179/1351000212Y.0000000001

13. Grant RS, Passey R, Matanovic G, Smythe G, Kapoor V. Evidence for increased *de novo* synthesis of NAD in immune-activated RAW264.7 macrophages: a self-protective mechanism? *Arch Biochem Biophys.* (1999) 372:1–7. doi: 10.1006/abbi.1999.1381

14. Grant RS. Indoleamine 2,3-dioxygenase activity increases NAD^+ production in IFN-gamma-stimulated human primary mononuclear cells. *Int J Tryptophan Res.* (2018) 11:1178646917751636. doi: 10.1177/1178646917751636

15. Minhas PS, Liu L, Moon PK, Joshi AU, Dove C, Mhatre S, et al. Macrophage *de novo* NAD(+) synthesis specifies immune function in aging and inflammation. *Nat Immunol.* (2019) 20:50–63. doi: 10.1038/s41590-018-0255-3

16. Rodriguez Cetina BH, Vasudevan A, Elkhal A. Aspects of tryptophan and nicotinamide adenine dinucleotide in immunity: a new twist in an old tale. *Int J Tryptophan Res.* (2017) 10:1178646917713491. doi: 10.1177/1178646917713491

17. Badawy AA. Tryptophan metabolism: a versatile area providing multiple targets for pharmacological intervention, Egypt. *J Basic Clin Pharmacol.* (2019) 9:1–30. doi: 10.32527/2019/101415

18. Ball HJ, Jusof FF, Bakmiwewa SM, Hunt NH, Yuasa HJ. Tryptophan-catabolizing enzymes - party of three. *Front Immunol.* (2014) 5:485. doi: 10.3389/fimmu.2014.00485

19. Hayaishi O. My life with tryptophan–never a dull moment. *Protein Sci.* (1993) 2:472–5. doi: 10.1002/pro.5560020320

20. Yuasa HJ, Takubo M, Takahashi A, Hasegawa T, Noma H, Suzuki T. Evolution of vertebrate indoleamine 2,3-dioxygenases. *J Mol Evol.* (2007) 65:705–14. doi: 10.1007/s00239-007-9049-1

21. Yuasa HJ, Ball HJ, Ho YF, Austin CJ, Whittington CM, Belov K, et al. Characterization and evolution of vertebrate indoleamine 2, 3-dioxygenases IDOs from monotremes and marsupials. *Comp Biochem Physiol B Biochem Mol Biol.* (2009) 153:137–44. doi: 10.1016/j.cbpb.2009.02.002

22. Badawy AA, Namboodiri AM, Moffett JR. The end of the road for the tryptophan depletion concept in pregnancy and infection. *Clin Sci.* (2016) 130:1327–33. doi: 10.1042/CS20160153

23. Moffett JR, Namboodiri MA. Tryptophan and the immune response. *Immunol Cell Biol.* (2003) 81:247–65. doi: 10.1046/j.1440-1711.2003.t01-1-01177.x

24. Espey MG, Moffett JR, Namboodiri MA. Temporal and spatial changes of quinolinic acid immunoreactivity in the immune system of lipopolysaccharide-stimulated mice. *J Leukoc Biol.* (1995) 57:199–206. doi: 10.1002/jlb.57.2.199

25. Moffett JR, Espey MG, Gaudet SJ, Namboodiri MA. Antibodies to quinolinic acid reveal localization in select immune cells rather than neurons or astroglia. *Brain Res.* (1993) 623:337–40. doi: 10.1016/0006-8993(93)91450-7

26. Moffett JR, Espey MG, Namboodiri MA. Antibodies to quinolinic acid and the determination of its cellular distribution within the rat immune system. *Cell Tissue Res.* (1994) 278:461–9. doi: 10.1007/BF00331364

27. Moffett JR, Els T, Espey MG, Walter SA, Streit WJ, Namboodiri MA. Quinolinate immunoreactivity in experimental rat brain tumors is present in macrophages but not in astrocytes. *Exp Neurol.* (1997) 144:287–301. doi: 10.1006/exnr.1996.6365

28. Moffett JR, Espey MG, Saito K, Namboodiri MA. Quinolinic acid immunoreactivity in cells within the choroid plexus, leptomeninges and brain vasculature of the immune stimulated gerbil. *J Neuroimmunol.* (1994) 54:69–73. doi: 10.1016/0165-5728(94)90232-1

29. Moffett JR, Blinder KL, Venkateshan CN, Namboodiri MA. Differential effects of kynurenine and tryptophan treatment on quinolinate immunoreactivity in rat lymphoid and non-lymphoid organs. *Cell Tissue Res.* (1998) 293:525–34. doi: 10.1007/s004410051145

30. Moffett JR, Namboodiri MA, Neale JH. Enhanced carbodiimide fixation for immunohistochemistry: application to the comparative distributions of N-acetylaspartylglutamate and N-acetylaspartate immunoreactivities in rat brain. *J Histochem Cytochem.* (1993) 41:559–70. doi: 10.1177/41.4.8450195

31. Lehrmann E, Molinari A, Speciale C, Schwarcz R. Immunohistochemical visualization of newly formed quinolinate in the normal and excitotoxically lesioned rat striatum. *Exp Brain Res.* (2001) 141:389–97. doi: 10.1007/s002210100887

32. Dixon LJ, Barnes M, Tang H, Pritchard MT, Nagy LE. Kupffer cells in the liver. *Compr Physiol.* (2013) 3:785–97. doi: 10.1002/cphy.c120026

33. Somiari RI, Sullivan A, Russell S, Somiari S, Hu H, Jordan R, et al. High-throughput proteomic analysis of human infiltrating ductal carcinoma of the breast. *Proteomics.* (2003) 3:1863–73. doi: 10.1002/pmic.200300560

34. Marouga R, David S, Hawkins E. The development of the DIGE system: 2D fluorescence difference gel analysis technology. *Anal. Bioanal Chem.* (2005) 382:669–78. doi: 10.1007/s00216-005-3126-3

35. Fodor IK, Nelson DO, Alegria-Hartman M, Robbins K, Langlois RG, Turteltaub KW, et al. Statistical challenges in the analysis of two-dimensional difference gel electrophoresis experiments using DeCyder. *Bioinformatics.* (2005) 21:3733–40. doi: 10.1093/bioinformatics/bti612

36. Chiarugi A, Moroni F. Quinolinic acid formation in immune-activated mice: studies with (m-nitrobenzoyl)-alanine (mNBA) and 3,4-dimethoxy-[-N-4-(-3-nitrophenyl)thiazol-2yl]-benzenesul fonamide (Ro 61-8048), two potent and selective inhibitors of kynurenine hydroxylase. *Neuropharmacology.* (1999) 38:1225–33. doi: 10.1016/S0028-3908(99)00048-9

37. Nam JH, Choi H, Cha B, Kim HD, Park JY, Abekura F, et al. Mitogen-induced interferon gamma production in human whole blood: the effect of heat and cations. *Curr Pharm Biotechnol.* (2019). doi: 10.2174/1389201020666190528093432

38. McLaren JE, Michael DR, Ashlin TG, Ramji DP. Cytokines, macrophage lipid metabolism and foam cells: implications for cardiovascular disease therapy. *Prog Lipid Res.* (2011) 50:331–47. doi: 10.1016/j.plipres.2011.04.002

39. Guillot A, Tacke F. Liver Macrophages: old dogmas and new insights. *Hepatol Commun.* (2019) 3:730–43. doi: 10.1002/hep4.1356

40. Yan ML, Wang YD, Tian YF, Lai ZD, Yan LN. Inhibition of allogeneic T-cell response by Kupffer cells expressing indoleamine 2,3-dioxygenase. *World J Gastroenterol.* (2010) 16:636–40. doi: 10.3748/wjg.v16.i5.636

41. Johanson CE, Johanson NL. Choroid plexus blood-CSF barrier: major player in brain disease modeling and neuromedicine. *J Neurol Neuromedicine.* (2018) 3:39–58. doi: 10.29245/2572.942X/2018/4.1194

42. Andersson PB, Perry VH, Gordon S. (1992). The acute inflammatory response to lipopolysaccharide in CNS parenchyma differs from that in other body tissues. *Neuroscience.* (2018) 48:169–86. doi: 10.1016/0306-4522(92)90347-5

43. Honda T, Schulte BA, Spicer SS. Glycoconjugate with terminal galactose. A selective property of macrophages in developing rat lung, *Histochemistry.* (1989) 91:61–7. doi: 10.1007/BF00501913

44. Pinteaux E, Inoue W, Schmidt L, Molina-Holgado F, Rothwell NJ, Luheshi GN. Leptin induces interleukin-1beta release from rat microglial cells through a caspas(2007). e 1 independent mechanism. *J Neurochem.* (2007) 102:826–33. doi: 10.1111/j.1471-4159.2007.04559.x

45. Chen JY, Li CF, Kuo CC, Tsai KK, Hou MF, Hung WC. Cancer/stroma interplay via cyclooxygenase-2 and indoleamine 2,3-dioxygenase promotes breast cancer progression. *Breast Cancer Res.* (2014) 16:410. doi: 10.1186/s13058-014-0410-1

46. Badawy AA. Kynurenine pathway of tryptophan metabolism: regulatory and functional aspects. *Int J Tryptophan Res.* (2017) 10:1178646917691938. doi: 10.1177/1178646917691938.

47. Miller JM, MacGarvey U, Beal MF. The effect of peripheral loading with kynurenine and probenecid on extracellular striatal kynurenic acid concentrations. *Neurosci Lett.* (1992) 146:115–8. doi: 10.1016/0304-3940(92)90186-B

48. Vecsei L, Miller J, MacGarvey U, Beal MF. Kynurenine and probenecid inhibit pentylenetetrazol- and NMDLA-induced seizures and increase kynurenic acid concentrations in the brain. *Brain Res Bull.* (1992) 28:233–8. doi: 10.1016/0361-9230(92)90184-Y

49. Alban A, David SO, Bjorkesten L, Andersson C, Sloge E, Lewis S, et al. A novel experimental design for comparative two-dimensional gel analysis: two-dimensional difference gel electrophoresis incorporating a pooled internal standard. *Proteomics.* (2003) 3:36–44. doi: 10.1002/pmic.200390006

50. Gharbi S, Gaffney P, Yang A, Zvelebil MJ, Cramer R, Waterfield MD, et al. Evaluation of two-dimensional differential gel electrophoresis for proteomic expression analysis of a model breast cancer cell system. *Mol Cell Proteomics.* (2002) 1:91–8. doi: 10.1074/mcp.T100007-MCP200

51. Xie J, Van DP, Fang D, Proud CG. Ablation of elongation factor 2 kinase enhances heat-shock protein 90 chaperone expression and protects cells under proteotoxic stress. *J Biol Chem.* (2019) 294:7169–76. doi: 10.1074/jbc.AC119.008036

52. Gonzalez-Teran B, Cortes JR, Manieri E, Matesanz N, Verdugo A, Rodriguez ME, et al. Eukaryotic elongation factor 2 controls TNF-alpha translation in LPS-induced hepatitis. *J Clin Invest.* (2013) 123:164–78. doi: 10.1172/JCI65124

53. Yamanaka K, Sasagawa Y, Ogura T. Recent advances in p97/VCP/Cdc48 cellular functions. *Biochim Biophys Acta.* (2012) 1823:130–7. doi: 10.1016/j.bbamcr.2011.07.001

54. Pepelyayeva Y, Rastall DPW, Aldhamen YA, O'Connell P, Raehtz S, Alyaqoub FS, et al. ERAP1 deficient mice have reduced Type 1 regulatory T cells and develop skeletal and intestinal features of ankylosing spondylitis. *Sci Rep.* (2018) 8:12464. doi: 10.1038/s41598-018-30159-5

55. Li M, Zhang D, Zhu M, Shen Y, Wei W, Ying S, et al. Roles of SAMHD1 in antiviral defense, autoimmunity and cancer. *Rev Med Virol.* (2017) 27:e1931. doi: 10.1002/rmv.1931

56. Wang Z, Qiu H, He J, Liu L, Xue W, Fox A, et al. The emerging roles of hnRNPK. *J Cell Physiol.* (2020) 235:1995–2008. doi: 10.1002/jcp.29186

57. Verrills NM, Walsh BJ, Cobon GS, Hains PG, Kavallaris M. Proteome analysis of vinca alkaloid response and resistance in acute lymphoblastic leukemia reveals novel cytoskeletal alterations. *J Biol Chem.* (2003) 278:45082–93. doi: 10.1074/jbc.M303378200

58. Keppler-Hafkemeyer A, Brinkmann U, Pastan I. Role of caspases in immunotoxin-induced apoptosis of cancer cells. *Biochemistry*. (1998) 37:16934–42. doi: 10.1021/bi980995m

59. Uruno T, Zhang P, Liu J Hao JJ, Zhan X. Haematopoietic lineage cell-specific protein 1 (HS1) promotes actin-related protein (Arp) 2/3 complex-mediated actin polymerization. *Biochem J*. (2003) 371:485–93. doi: 10.1042/bj20021791

60. Chen YR, Kori R, John B, Tan TH. Caspase-mediated cleavage of actin-binding and SH3-domain-containing proteins cortactin, HS1, and HIP-55 during apoptosis. *Biochem Biophys Res Commun*. (2001) 288:981–9. doi: 10.1006/bbrc.2001.5862

61. Zeng SX, Dai MS, Keller DM, Lu H. SSRP1 functions as a co-activator of the transcriptional activator p63. *EMBO J*. (2002) 21:5487–97. doi: 10.1093/emboj/cdf540

62. Bai R, Shi Z, Zhang JW, Li D, Zhu YL, Zheng S. ST13, a proliferation regulator, inhibits growth and migration of colorectal cancer cell lines. *J Zhejiang. Univ Sci B*. (2012) 13:884–93. doi: 10.1631/jzus.B1200037

63. Kwon MS, Park KR, Kim YD, Na BR, Kim HR, Choi HJ, et al. Swiprosin-1 is a novel actin bundling protein that regulates cell spreading and migration. *PLoS ONE*. (2013) 8:e71626. doi: 10.1371/journal.pone.0071626

64. Thylur RP, Gowda R, Mishra S, Jun CD. Swiprosin-1: its expression and diverse biological functions. *J Cell Biochem*. (2018) 119:150–6. doi: 10.1002/jcb.26199

65. Badawy AA, Guillemin G. The Plasma [Kynurenine]/[Tryptophan] ratio and indoleamine 2,3-dioxygenase: time for appraisal. *Int J Tryptophan Res*. (2019) 12:1–10. doi: 10.1177/1178646919868978

66. Engelhardt B, Vajkoczy P, Weller RO. The movers and shapers in immune privilege of the CNS. *Nat Immunol*. (2017) 18:123–31. doi: 10.1038/ni.3666

67. Routy JP, Routy B, Graziani GM, Mehraj V. The kynurenine pathway is a double-edged sword in immune-privileged sites and in cancer: implications for immunotherapy. *Int J Tryptophan Res*. (2016) 9:67–77. doi: 10.4137/IJTR.S38355

68. Badawy AA, Evans M. Animal liver tryptophan pyrrolases: absence of apoenzyme and of hormonal induction mechanism from species sensitive to tryptophan toxicity. *Biochem J*. (1976) 158:79–88. doi: 10.1042/bj1580079

69. He J, Zhang G, Pang Q, Yu C, Xiong J, Zhu J, et al. SIRT6 reduces macrophage foam cell formation by inducing autophagy and cholesterol efflux under ox-LDL condition. *FEBS J*. (2017) 284:1324–37. doi: 10.1111/febs.14055

70. Kunjathoor VV, Febbraio M, Podrez EA, Moore KJ, Andersson L, Koehn S, et al. Scavenger receptors class A-I/II and CD36 are the principal receptors responsible for the uptake of modified low density lipoprotein leading to lipid loading in macrophages. *J Biol Chem*. (2002) 277:49982–8. doi: 10.1074/jbc.M209649200

71. Polyzos KA, Ketelhuth DF. The role of the kynurenine pathway of tryptophan metabolism in cardiovascular disease. An emerging field. *Hamostaseologie*. (2015) 35:128–36. doi: 10.5482/HAMO-14-10-0052

72. Zhang L, Ovchinnikova O, Jonsson A, Lundberg AM, Berg M, Hansson GK, et al. The tryptophan metabolite 3-hydroxyanthranilic acid lowers plasma lipids and decreases atherosclerosis in hypercholesterolaemic mice. *Eur Heart J*. (2012) 33:2025–34. doi: 10.1093/eurheartj/ehs175

73. Ma M, Baumgartner M. Filopodia and membrane blebs drive efficient matrix invasion of macrophages transformed by the intracellular parasite *Theileria annulata*. *PLoS ONE*. (2013) 8:e75577. doi: 10.1371/journal.pone.0075577

74. Blanchoin L, Boujemaa-Paterski R, Sykes C, Plastino J. Actin dynamics, architecture, and mechanics in cell motility. *Physiol Rev*. (2014) 94:235–63. doi: 10.1152/physrev.00018.2013

75. Fallarino F, Grohmann U, Vacca C, Bianchi R, Orabona C, Spreca A, et al. T cell apoptosis by tryptophan catabolism. *Cell Death. Differ*. (2002) 9:1069–77. doi: 10.1038/sj.cdd.4401073

76. Geng YJ, Azuma T, Tang JX, Hartwig JH, Muszynski M, Wu Q, et al. Caspase-3-induced gelsolin fragmentation contributes to actin cytoskeletal collapse, nucleolysis, and apoptosis of vascular smooth muscle cells exposed to proinflammatory cytokines. *Eur J Cell Biol*. (1998) 77:294–302. doi: 10.1016/S0171-9335(98)80088-5

77. Faure S, Salazar-Fontana LI, Semichon M, Tybulewicz VL, Bismuth G, Trautmann A, et al. ERM proteins regulate cytoskeleton relaxation promoting T cell-APC conjugation. *Nat Immunol*. (2004) 5:272–9. doi: 10.1038/ni1039

78. Kunimoto R, Jimbow K, Tanimura A, Sato M, Horimoto K, Hayashi T, et al. SIRT1 regulates lamellipodium extension and migration of melanoma cells. *J Invest Dermatol*. (2014) 134:1693–700. doi: 10.1038/jid.2014.50

79. DiNatale BC, Murray IA, Schroeder JC, Flaveny CA, Lahoti TS, Laurenzana EM, et al. Kynurenic acid is a potent endogenous aryl hydrocarbon receptor ligand that synergistically induces interleukin-6 in the presence of inflammatory signaling. *Toxicol Sci*. (2010) 115:89–97. doi: 10.1093/toxsci/kfq024

80. Novikov O, Wang Z, Stanford EA, Parks AJ, Ramirez-Cardenas A, Landesman E, et al. An aryl hydrocarbon receptor-mediated amplification loop that enforces cell migration in ER-/PR-/Her2- human breast cancer cells. *Mol Pharmacol*. (2016) 90:674–88. doi: 10.1124/mol.116.105361

81. Opitz CA, Litzenburger UM, Sahm F, Ott M, Tritschler I, Trump S, et al. An endogenous tumour-promoting ligand of the human aryl hydrocarbon receptor. *Nature*. (2011) 478:197–203. doi: 10.1038/nature10491

82. Seok SH, Ma ZX, Feltenberger JB, Chen H, Chen H, Scarlett C, et al. Trace derivatives of kynurenine potently activate the aryl hydrocarbon receptor (AHR). *J Biol Chem*. (2018) 293:1994–2005. doi: 10.1074/jbc.RA117.000631

83. Shinde R, McGaha TL. The aryl hydrocarbon receptor: connecting immunity to the microenvironment. *Trends Immunol*. (2018) 39:1005–20. doi: 10.1016/j.it.2018.10.010

84. Schopf FH, Biebl MM, Buchner J. The HSP90 chaperone machinery. *Nat Rev Mol Cell Biol*. (2017) 18:345–60. doi: 10.1038/nrm.2017.20

85. Shao J, Wang L, Zhong C, Qi R, Li Y. AHSA1 regulates proliferation, apoptosis, migration, and invasion of osteosarcoma. *Biomed Pharmacother*. (2016) 77:45–51. doi: 10.1016/j.biopha.2015.11.008

86. Cawthorn TR, Moreno JC, Dharsee M, Tran-Thanh D, Ackloo S, Zhu PH, et al. Proteomic analyses reveal high expression of decorin and endoplasmin (HSP90B1) are associated with breast cancer metastasis and decreased survival. *PLoS ONE*. (2012) 7:e30992. doi: 10.1371/journal.pone.0030992

87. Diry M, Tomkiewicz C, Koehle C, Coumoul X, Bock KW, Barouki R, et al. Activation of the dioxin/aryl hydrocarbon receptor (AhR) modulates cell plasticity through a JNK-dependent mechanism. *Oncogenet*. (2006) 25:5570–4. doi: 10.1038/sj.onc.1209553

88. Su HH, Lin HT, Suen JL, Sheu CC, Yokoyama KK, Huang SK, et al. Aryl hydrocarbon receptor-ligand axis mediates pulmonary fibroblast migration and differentiation through increased arachidonic acid metabolism. *Toxicology*. (2016) 370:116–26. doi: 10.1016/j.tox.2016.09.019

89. Stanford EA, Ramirez-Cardenas A, Wang Z, Novikov O, Alamoud K, Koutrakis P, et al. Role for the aryl hydrocarbon receptor and diverse ligands in oral squamous cell carcinoma migration and tumorigenesis. *Mol Cancer Res*. (2016) 14:696–706. doi: 10.1158/1541-7786.MCR-16-0069

90. Yoshida R, Imanishi J, Oku T, Kishida T, Hayaishi O. Induction of pulmonary indoleamine 2,3-dioxygenase by interferon. *Proc Natl Acad Sci USA*. (1981) 78:129–32. doi: 10.1073/pnas.78.1.129

91. Yoshida R, Oku T, Imanishi J, Kishida T, Hayaishi O. Interferon: a mediator of indoleamine 2,3-dioxygenase induction by lipopolysaccharide, poly(I) X poly(C), and pokeweed mitogen in mouse lung. *Arch Biochem Biophys*. (1986) 249:596–604. doi: 10.1016/0003-9861(86)90038-X

92. Saito K, Crowley JS, Markey SP, Heyes MP. A mechanism for increased quinolinic acid formation following acute systemic immune stimulation. *J Biol Chem*. (1993) 268:15496–503.

93. Ohashi K, Kawai S, Murata K. Secretion of quinolinic acid, an intermediate in the kynurenine pathway, for utilization in NAD$^+$ biosynthesis in the yeast *Saccharomyces cerevisiae*. *Eukaryot Cell*. (2013) 12:648–53. doi: 10.1128/EC.00339-12

94. Kaper T, Looger LL, Takanaga H, Platten M, Steinman L, Frommer WB. Nanosensor detection of an immunoregulatory tryptophan Influx/Kynurenine Efflux cycle. *PLoS. Biol*. (2007) 5:e257. doi: 10.1371/journal.pbio.0050257

95. Sinclair LV, Neyens D, Ramsay G, Taylor PM, Cantrell DA. Single cell analysis of kynurenine and system L amino acid transport in T cells. *Nat Commun*. (2018) 9:1981. doi: 10.1038/s41467-018-04366-7

96. Torigoe M, Maeshima K, Ozaki T, Omura Y, Gotoh K, Tanaka Y, et al. l-Leucine influx through Slc7a5 regulates inflammatory responses of human B cells via mammalian target of rapamycin complex 1 signaling. *Mod Rheumatol*. (2019) 29:885–91. doi: 10.1080/14397595.2018.1510822

97. Yoon BR, Oh YJ, Kang SW, Lee EB, Lee WW. Role of SLC7A5 in metabolic reprogramming of human monocyte/macrophage immune responses. *Front Immunol.* (2018) 9:53. doi: 10.3389/fimmu.2018.00053

98. Sarett HP. Quinolinic acid excretion and metabolism in man. *J Biol Chem.* (1951) 193:627–34.

99. Fuertig R, Ceci A, Camus SM, Bezard E, Luippold AH, Hengerer B. LC-MS/MS-based quantification of kynurenine metabolites, tryptophan, monoamines and neopterin in plasma, cerebrospinal fluid and brain. *Bioanalysis.* (2016) 8:1903–17. doi: 10.4155/bio-2016-0111

100. Morrison PF, Morishige GM, Beagles KE, Heyes MP. Quinolinic acid is extruded from the brain by a probenecid-sensitive carrier system: a quantitative analysis. *J Neurochem.* (1999) 72:2135–44. doi: 10.1046/j.1471-4159.1999.0722135.x

101. Foster AC, Miller LP, Oldendorf WH, Schwarcz R. Studies on the disposition of quinolinic acid after intracerebral or systemic administration in the rat. *Exp Neurol.* (1984) 84:428–40. doi: 10.1016/0014-4886(84)90239-5

102. Beagles KE, Morrison PF, Heyes MP. Quinolinic acid *in vivo* synthesis rates, extracellular concentrations, and intercompartmental distributions in normal and immune-activated brain as determined by multiple-isotope microdialysis. *J Neurochem.* (1998) 70:281–91. doi: 10.1046/j.1471-4159.1998.70010281.x

103. Saito K, Markey SP, Heyes MP. Effects of immune activation on quinolinic acid and neuroactive kynurenines in the mouse. *Neuroscience.* (1992) 51:25–39. doi: 10.1016/0306-4522(92)90467-G

104. Kita T, Morrison PF, Heyes MP, Markey SP. Effects of systemic and central nervous system localized inflammation on the contributions of metabolic precursors to the L-kynurenine and quinolinic acid pools in brain. *J Neurochem.* (2002) 82:258–68. doi: 10.1046/j.1471-4159.2002.00955.x

105. Namboodiri MA, Venkateshan CN, Narayanan R, Blinder K, Moffett JR, Gajdusek DC, et al. Increased quinolinate immunoreactivity in the peripheral blood monocytes/macrophages from SIV-infected monkeys. *J Neurovirol.* (1996) 2:433–8. doi: 10.3109/13550289609146910

106. Venkateshan CN, Narayanan R, Espey MG, Moffett JR, Gajdusek DC, Gibbs CJ, et al. Immunocytochemical localization of the endogenous neuroexcitotoxin quinolinate in human peripheral blood monocytes/macrophages and the effect of human T-cell lymphotropic virus type I infection. *Proc Natl Acad Sci USA.* (1996) 93:1636–41. doi: 10.1073/pnas.93.4.1636

107. Espey MG, Tang Y, Morse HC, Moffett JR, Namboodiri MA. Localization of quinolinic acid in the murine AIDS model of retrovirus-induced immunodeficiency: implications for neurotoxicity and dendritic cell immunopathogenesis. *AIDS.* (1996) 10:151–8. doi: 10.1097/00002030-199602000-00004

108. Hsieh CL, Huang HM, Hsieh SY, Zheng PX, Lin YS, Chiang-Ni C, et al. NAD-glycohydrolase depletes intracellular NAD(+) and inhibits acidification of autophagosomes to enhance multiplication of group A streptococcus in endothelial cells. *Front Microbiol.* (2018) 9:1733. doi: 10.3389/fmicb.2018.01733

109. Pajuelo D, Gonzalez-Juarbe N, Tak U, Sun J, Orihuela CJ, Niederweis M. NAD(+) depletion triggers macrophage necroptosis, a cell death pathway exploited by *Mycobacterium tuberculosis. Cell Rep.* (2018) 24:429–40. doi: 10.1016/j.celrep.2018.06.042

110. Smith CL, Ghosh J, Elam JS, Pinkner JS, Hultgren SJ, Caparon MG, et al. Structural basis of Streptococcus pyogenes immunity to its NAD$^+$ glycohydrolase toxin. *Structure.* (2011) 19:192–202. doi: 10.1016/j.str.2010.12.013

111. Camacho-Pereira J, Tarrago MG, Chini CCS, Nin V, Escande C, Warner GM, et al. CD38 dictates age-related NAD decline and mitochondrial dysfunction through an SIRT3-dependent mechanism. *Cell Metab.* (2016) 23:1127–39. doi: 10.1016/j.cmet.2016.05.006

112. Bahri R, Bollinger A, Bollinger T, Orinska Z, Bulfone-Paus S. Ectonucleotidase CD38 demarcates regulatory, memory-like CD8+ T cells with IFN-gamma-mediated suppressor activities. *PLoS ONE.* (2012) 7:e45234. doi: 10.1371/journal.pone.0045234

113. Jones SP, Franco NF, Varney B, Sundaram G, Brown DA, de Bie J, et al. Expression of the kynurenine pathway in human peripheral blood mononuclear cells: implications for inflammatory and neurodegenerative disease. *PLoS ONE.* (2015) 10:e0131389. doi: 10.1371/journal.pone.0131389

114. Bender DA, Magboul BI, Wynick D. Probable mechanisms of regulation of the utilization of dietary tryptophan, nicotinamide and nicotinic acid as precursors of nicotinamide nucleotides in the rat. *Br J Nutr.* (1982) 48:119–27. doi: 10.1079/BJN19820094

115. Fukuwatari T, Shibata K. Effect of nicotinamide administration on the tryptophan-nicotinamide pathway in humans. *Int J Vitam Nutr Res.* (2007) 77:255–62. doi: 10.1024/0300-9831.77.4.255

116. Shibata K, Kondo T, Miki A. Increased conversion ratio of tryptophan to niacin in severe food restriction. *Biosci Biotechnol Biochem.* (1998) 62:580–3. doi: 10.1271/bbb.62.580

117. Terakata M, Fukuwatari T, Kadota E, Sano M, Kanai M, Nakamura T, et al. The niacin required for optimum growth can be synthesized from L-tryptophan in growing mice lacking tryptophan-2,3-dioxygenase. *J Nutr* (2013) 143:1046–51. doi: 10.3945/jn.113.176875

118. Opitz CA, Heiland I. Dynamics of NAD-metabolism: everything but constant. *Biochem Soc Trans.* (2015) 43:1127–32. doi: 10.1042/BST20150133

119. Sainio EL, Pulkki K, Young SN. L-tryptophan: biochemical, nutritional and pharmacological aspects. *Amino Acids.* (1996) 10:21–47. doi: 10.1007/BF00806091

120. Seyedsadjadi N, Berg J, Bilgin AA, Braidy N, Salonikas C, Grant R. High protein intake is associated with low plasma NAD$^+$ levels in a healthy human cohort. *PLoS ONE.* (2018) 13:e0201968. doi: 10.1371/journal.pone.0201968

121. Audrito V, Manago A, Gaudino F, Sorci L, Messana VG, Raffaelli N, et al. NAD-biosynthetic and consuming enzymes as central players of metabolic regulation of innate and adaptive immune responses in cancer. *Front Immunol.* (2019) 10:1720. doi: 10.3389/fimmu.2019.01720

6

Pharmacologic Induction of Endotoxin Tolerance in Dendritic Cells by L-Kynurenine

Giorgia Manni[†], Giada Mondanelli[†], Giulia Scalisi, Maria Teresa Pallotta, Dario Nardi,
Eleonora Padiglioni, Rita Romani, Vincenzo Nicola Talesa, Paolo Puccetti,
Francesca Fallarino*[‡] and Marco Gargaro*[‡]

Department of Experimental Medicine, University of Perugia, Perugia, Italy

*Correspondence:
Francesca Fallarino
Francesca.fallrino@unipg.it
Marco Gargaro
marco.gargaro@unipg.it

*[†] These authors have contributed
equally to this work*

*[‡] These authors share senior
authorship*

Endotoxin tolerance aims at opposing hyperinflammatory responses to lipopolysaccharide (LPS) exposure. The aryl hydrocarbon receptor (AhR) participates in protection against LPS-mediated tissue damage, as it plays a necessary role in restraining the proinflammatory action of IL-1β and TNF-α while fostering the expression of protective TGF-β. TGF-β, in turn, promotes durable expression of the immune regulatory enzyme indoleamine 2,3-dioxygenase 1 (IDO1). IDO1 degrades L-tryptophan to L-kynurenine—an activating ligand for AhR—thus establishing a feed-forward loop. In this study, we further demonstrate that L-kynurenine also promotes the dissociation of the Src kinase–AhR cytosolic complex, leading to the activation of both genomic and non-genomic events in conventional dendritic cells (cDCs) primed with LPS. Specifically, the Src kinase, by phosphorylating the downstream target IDO1, triggers IDO1's signaling ability, which results in enhanced production of TGF-β, an event key to establishing full endotoxin tolerance. We demonstrated that exogenous L-kynurenine can substitute for the effects of continued or repeated LPS exposure and that the AhR–Src–IDO1 axis represents a critical step for the transition from endotoxin susceptibility to tolerance. Moreover, much like fully endotoxin-tolerant dendritic cells (DCs) (i.e., treated twice with LPS *in vitro*), DCs—treated once with LPS *in vitro* and then with kynurenine—confer resistance on naïve recipients to an otherwise lethal LPS challenge. This may have clinical implications under conditions in which pharmacologically induced onset of endotoxin tolerance is a therapeutically desirable event.

Keywords: L-kynurenine, dendritic cells, endotoxin tolerance, aryl hydrocarbon receptor, indoleamine (2,3)-dioxygenase

INTRODUCTION

A first exposure to lipopolysaccharide (LPS) makes mice resistant to shock caused by a subsequent LPS injection, an occurrence known as LPS or endotoxin tolerance. In particular, a low amount of LPS causes a long-lived state of cell refractoriness to a second LPS challenge that prevents excessive inflammatory responses. Appropriate modulation of LPS-responsive genes to foster the onset of endotoxin tolerance would be beneficial in clinical settings dominated by acute hyperinflammatory responses to infection (1, 2).

In infection resistance and disease tolerance to microbial insult, the ligand-activated transcription factor aryl hydrocarbon receptor (AhR) adaptively balances aggressive immune responses ("resistance") with the host's ability to withstand the negative effects of infection, namely, immunopathology or damage due to pathogen metabolism and virulence factors ("tolerance") (3, 4).

AhR is a heterodimeric transcriptional regulator. Broadly present in a variety of animal species as well as in humans, AhR has constitutive functions that are only now being appreciated in their intricacies. The main interest is now shifting from the role of AhR in the hepatic metabolism—and thus inactivation—of potentially toxic xenobiotics toward the nature of its physiological ligands as well as its mode of action in response to functionally distinct molecules, which are remarkably different in nature as to their endogenous source and chemical structure. Among physiologically relevant ligands, tryptophan metabolites, including L-kynurenine, act as activating molecules for the receptor (3, 5).

Animal and human data indicate that AhR is key to multiple signaling pathways critical to cellular and tissue homeostasis, which relates apparently disparate aspects of physiology, including cell proliferation and differentiation, gene regulation, cell motility and migration, inflammation, and neoplasia (6–9).

In its inactive state, AhR is complexed with two heat-shock proteins 90 (Hsp90), p23, the AhR-interacting protein (AIP), and the non-receptor tyrosine kinase c-Src (10). Upon ligand binding, the chaperones are released, and AhR shuttles to the nucleus, where it heterodimerizes with the AhR nuclear translocator (ARNT) at promoter recognition sequences of target genes.

Beside these genomic events, AhR mediates non-canonical signaling pathways. AhR can indeed participate in the phosphorylation of multiple target proteins through the release of c-Src from the cytoplasmic complex (11), and it can also regulate protein turnover thanks to its E3 ubiquitin ligase activity (12). The immunoregulatory enzyme indoleamine 2,3-dioxygenase (IDO1) has been identified as one of the c-Src targets (13). In particular, double exposure of splenic dendritic cells (DCs) to LPS triggers AhR–Src kinase-dependent IDO1 phosphorylation and TGF-β production, and IDO1 expression by DCs further increases L-kynurenine production, the main tryptophan byproduct (3). Based on these data, we investigated whether exogenous L-kynurenine might be able to replace the second LPS exposure for the transition from endotoxin susceptibility to tolerance. Here we found that L-kynurenine can replace a second exposure to LPS in triggering genomic and non-genomic, AhR-dependent effects capable of rendering conventional DCs (cDCs) suitable for transferring endotoxin tolerance onto naïve recipients. In clinical settings where onset of endotoxin tolerance is therapeutically desirable, replacing the LPS stimulus by a pharmacological means such as L-kynurenine would represent an undoubtful advantage in terms of patients' safety and possible side effects.

MATERIALS AND METHODS

Mice

Eight- to 10-week-old male C57BL/6 mice were obtained from Charles River Breeding Laboratories. IDO1-deficient mice ($Ido1^{-/-}$) were purchased from The Jackson Laboratory. B6.129-Ahrtm1Bra/J Ahr-deficient ($Ahr^{-/-}$) mice were kindly supplied

by B. Stockinger (MRC National Institute for Medical Research, London, United Kingdom). All *in vivo* studies were in compliance with national (Italian Parliament DL 116/92) and Perugia University Animal Care and Use Committee guidelines, and the overall study was approved by the Bioethics Committee of the University of Perugia.

Cell Lines and Cell Culture

The mouse fibroblast line, SYF, was obtained from ATCC, and cells were cultured in DMEM (Gibco) supplemented with 10% FBS at 37°C. This cell line was transfected to over-express c-Src and AhR and used for immunoprecipitation assays and as a source of nuclear extracts, as described below. Mouse embryonic fibroblasts (MEFs) were obtained according to the guidelines of the University of Perugia Ethical Committee and the European Communities Council Directive 2010/63/EU. MEFs and $Ahr^{-/-}$ MEFs were prepared as described (14). Briefly, pregnant mice were sacrificed at 13.5 days post-coitum (dpc) by cervical dislocation. The embryos were separated from placenta and membranes and were placed in 10 cm culture dishes in sterile phosphate-buffered saline. Then, the liver, heart, and brain were removed and discarded. The remaining part of each embryo was washed and minced with cool razor blades and incubated 20 min at 37°C with trypsin-EDTA (500 mg L^{-1}). The minced tissues were chopped by repeated pipetting, and then the cell suspension was plated on 10 cm tissue culture dishes, and DMEM medium (10 ml) containing 10% FBS (Euroclone) was added. Electroporation was used to transfect MEFs.

DC Preparation

Dendritic cells were isolated from bone marrows of C57BL/6 mice by crushing tibias, femurs, and hips in MACS buffer as previously described (15). Extracted cells were filtered through a 40 μm cell strainer and centrifuged at $300 \times g$ for 5 min. Cells were re-suspended in red blood cell lysis buffer to remove erythrocytes. For DC differentiation, BM cells were cultured at a density of 2×10^6/ml in culture media (IMDM from Gibco) conditioned with 5% Flt-3l for 9 days at 37°C with 7% CO$_2$. At the end of the culture, 25–30 million/mouse total DCs were obtained. Purification of cDCs was performed by MACS column (Miltenyi) and biotin antibodies (Biolegend). Total DCs were incubated with biotin mouse monoclonal antibodies against B220 (a marker of pDCs and B cells). After this, cells were incubated with MagniSort Streptavidin Negative Selection Beads (Thermo Fisher) followed by depletion of B220$^+$ cells. We collected the B220$^-$ cell fraction and used this to verify cell purity. cDCs were stained with fluorescent antibodies, identified as B220$^-$ CD3$^-$ and MHC-II$^+$ CD11c$^+$ CD24$^+$ CD172$^+$ by cytofluorimetric analysis by LSRFortessa (BD BioSciences), and analyzed by flowJo data analysis software. Cell purity was more than 90%. Cells (1×10^6/ml) were primed with 250 ng/ml LPS (055:B5 Sigma-Aldrich) overnight before treating with II° LPS (1 μg/ml) or 50 μM L-kynurenine (Sigma-Aldrich) for 24 h.

Cytokine Production

Purified DCs were re-suspended at 1×10^6/ml in fresh media in the presence or absence of LPS and L-kynurenine for a total of 36 h; supernatants were collected and analyzed for TGF-β by ELISA according to the manufacturer's instructions (R&D system). DCs treated with LPS with either LPS or L-kynurenine were analyzed by ELISA for IL-10 and TGF-β contents according to the manufacturer's instructions (R&D system) (16).

Real-Time PCR

Real-time PCR (for mouse *Ido1*, *Ido2*, and *Tdo2* expressions) analyses were carried out as described (17) using the specific primers listed in **Supplementary Table S1**. In all figures depicting RT-PCR data, bars represent the ratio of the relevant gene to β-actin-encoding gene expression, as determined by the relative quantification method ($\Delta\Delta$CT; means ± SD of triplicate determinations).

Co-immunoprecipitation

SYF cells expressing c-Src kinase and LPS-primed cDCs were stimulated with L-kynurenine at 50 μM for different lengths of time (0.5, 1, and 2 h). Nuclear and cytoplasmic fractions were prepared from cells lysed on ice with Buffer N (15 mM Tris–HCl, pH 7.5, 15 mM NaCl, 60 mM KCl, 5 mM MgCl$_2$, 25 mM sucrose, 0.6% Non-idet P-40, 1 mM DTT, 2 mM Na$_3$VO$_4$). Lysates were then immunoprecipitated by means of sheep polyclonal antibody recognizing AhR, previously complexed with G Dynabeads (Invitrogen). Alternatively, cytosolic and nuclear lysates were run directly on SDS/PAGE.

Western Blotting

IDO1 and pIDO1 expressions were investigated in cDCs by immunoblot with a rabbit monoclonal anti-mouse IDO1 antibody (cv152) or a rabbit polyclonal antibody to the phosphorylated immunoreceptor tyrosine-based inhibitory motifs (ITIM) motif of IDO1, respectively, both raised in our laboratory (18). c-Src and its phosphorylated form were revealed by specific anti-Src and -pSrc antibodies (Tyr416; Cell Signaling Technology). Anti-AhR antibody was from R&D system. Anti-β-actin and β-tubulin antibodies (Sigma-Aldrich) were used as a normalizer. Anti-lamininB antibody (Thermo Fisher) was used as a nuclear extract control. Whole-cell extracts, immunoprecipitates, and nuclear and cytosolic extracts were denatured in Laemmli sample buffer at 95°C for 5 min. Samples were run on a gel and transferred onto a nitrocellulose membrane (Bio-Rad). Immunoblots were blocked in TBS containing 3% BSA or 5% non-fat milk and 0.1% Tween 20 at room temperature for 1 h and then incubated with primary antibody overnight at 4°C. After washing, membranes were incubated with goat anti-rabbit, goat anti-mouse IgG or anti-sheep IgG conjugated to horseradish peroxidase (Jackson ImmunoResearch Laboratories, Inc) for 1 h at room temperature in 5% non-fat milk and 0.1% Tween 20 TBS. Then, membranes were washed and developed with ECL BioRad.

cDC–T-Cell Co-culture

LPS-unprimed and LPS-primed cDCs treated or not with L-kynurenine, as described above, were cultured with CD4$^+$ T cells isolated from the spleens of Foxp3^{YFP} mice. Briefly, CD4$^+$ T cells were isolated via cell separation by two steps. A first step was meant to enrich the CD3$^+$ cell fraction, using biotin mouse monoclonal antibodies against B220 (a marker of pDCs and B cells) and CD11c (a marker of DCs). After this step, cells were incubated with MagniSort Streptavidin Negative Selection Beads (Thermo Fisher) followed by depletion of B220$^+$CD11c$^+$. B220$^-$ CD11c$^-$ collected cell fractions were incubated with magnetic anti-mouse CD4 beads (Miltenyi Biotec) to select CD4$^+$ T cells. The purity of CD4$^+$ T cells was verified by FACS analysis by cell staining with anti-B220, anti-CD3, anti-CD11c, anti-CD4, and anti-CD8 specific antibodies. CD4$^+$ T cells (2 × 10^5) were activated with 5 μg/ml anti-CD3 mAb (clone OKT3) and co-cultured for 4 days with unprimed and primed cDCs (5 × 10^4) treated or not with L-kynurenine for 36 h (19). Treg cells were evaluated by FACS, analyzing the induction of Foxp3 expressing YFP.

Endotoxin Tolerance Mouse Model and Histology

In the induction of primary endotoxemia, mice of the different genotypes (WT, *Ahr*$^{-/-}$, and *Ido1*$^{-/-}$) were randomly grouped (10 per group) and injected intravenously with 1 × 10^6 cDCs, primed or not with LPS and treated or not with L-kynurenine, as described above. After 48 h, mice were injected intraperitoneally with a lethal dose of LPS (40 mg/kg). Vehicle-treated groups (no cDCs) were used as controls. Animals were monitored daily for 1 week for mortality or the presence of signs of moribundity, including lack of responsiveness to manual stimulation, immobility, and inability to eat or drink.

For histology, morphological analysis of paraffin-embedded lung sections (4 μm) from mice treated as above included stained with H&E at 48 h after challenge and examination by light microscopy, using representative specimens from one of three experiments.

Statistical Analysis

For animal studies, randomization consisted of generating a random permutation of a sequence and selecting random numbers. On assessing outcomes involving scores, the investigator was totally blinded to group allocation. The log-rank test was used for paired data analyses of Kaplan–Meier survival curves. All *in vitro* determinations are means ± SD from three independent experiments and were evaluated by two-way and one-way ANOVA. GraphPad Prism version 6.0 (San Diego, CA, United States) was used for all analyses and graph preparation.

RESULTS

L-Kynurenine Potentiates IDO1 Induction and TGF-β Production in LPS-Primed cDCs via AhR

Unlike a single LPS stimulation, repeated exposure *in vitro* of splenic cDCs to endotoxin significantly induces IDO1 protein expression and L-kynurenine production, the main

IDO1 enzymatic product. Such conditioned cDCs protect mice from lethal endotoxemia, and this effect requires that the cDCs be competent for IDO1 and TGF-β production (17). We here examined whether L-kynurenine could substitute for the second LPS challenge in mimicking an endotoxin-tolerant state in cDCs. We preliminarily set up cultures of bone marrow-derived cDCs (**Supplementary Figure S1A**). Then, IDO1 induction was assessed in these cells after priming with LPS overnight, followed by treatment with LPS or L-kynurenine for an additional 24 h, and unprimed cDCs were used as control. Priming with LPS alone modestly induced IDO1 at both transcript and protein levels; however, sequential treatment with LPS and L-kynurenine significantly enhanced this effect. In LPS-primed cDCs derived from AhR-deficient mice, IDO1 induction by L-kynurenine as a second stimulus was instead lost (**Figures 1A,B**). Under the same conditions, the expressions of the IDO1 paralog, *Ido2*, and of *Tdo2* were not significantly affected by the treatment with LPS and L-kynurenine. Of note, *Ido2* expression was induced by LPS alone on first exposure but not by a subsequent exposure to L-kynurenine or LPS as a repeated stimulus (**Supplementary Figure S1B**). Treatment of cDCs with L-kynurenine in the absence of prior LPS did not affect *Ido1* expression (**Figure 1A**), implying that early TLR4-dependent events are necessary for initiating the loop whereby L-kynurenine will later reinforce AhR-dependent *Ido1* transcription. The transition from endotoxin susceptibility to tolerance in cDCs is marked by an increased TGF-b secretion (3). We found that in unprimed cDCs, L-kynurenine alone treatment would increase TGF-β production according to a slower kinetic pattern than when used after LPS pre-conditioning. The ideal conditions for TGF-β production for the former involved removing L-kynurenine by extensive washing, followed by additional culturing for 48 h in medium alone (**Figure 1C**). Yet, production of the cytokine was strongly enhanced by previous LPS conditioning (**Figure 1C**). As expected, TGF-β production was unaffected by LPS + L-kynurenine treatment in cDCs derived from $Ahr^{-/-}$ and $Ido1^{-/-}$ mice.

Based on the finding that L-kynurenine binds AhR on the Gln377 residue, and in order to validate the ability of L-kynurenine to induce IDO1 *via* AhR in cDCs, we reconstituted AhR-deficient cDCs with a vector encoding the mutated form of AhR where Gln at position 377 is replaced by an Ala residue (Q377A) as described (3). The engineered cDCs were primed with LPS and then treated with L-kynurenine. Cells, either reconstituted with empty vector or the Q377A mutant, failed to express IDO1 (**Figures 1D,E**) and to produce TGF-β (**Figure 1F**). While confirming the binding mode of L-kynurenine to the Gln377 domain of the PAS-B domain of AhR, these results showed a crucial requirement for the Gln377 residue of AhR in L-kynurenine-mediated induction of IDO1 in LPS-primed cDCs, and for reprogramming those cells toward a tolerogenic phenotype. Overall, these data suggest that, *in vitro*, externally added L-kynurenine contributes to reprogramming gene expression—including *Ido1*'s—in endotoxin tolerance via effects involving AhR.

L-Kynurenine Induces AhR/Src-Dependent Phosphorylation of IDO1

Phosphorylation of a specific domain in IDO1 is involved in its non-enzymatic function leading to reprogramming gene expression and the induction of a stable regulatory phenotype in splenic plasmacytoid DCs that will produce less IL-6 and more TGF-β in response to TLR signaling (20). We investigated whether IDO1 phosphorylation occurs in LPS-primed, IDO1-competent cDCs upon L-kynurenine exposure. We found that phosphorylation of IDO1 occurs after 30 min of L-kynurenine treatment in wild type cDCs but not in AhR-deficient cells (**Figure 2A**). The inhibition of c-Src—the most widely represented kinase in mouse cDCs (13)—with PP2 (but not its inactive analog PP3) negated IDO1 phosphorylation in LPS-primed cDCs exposed to L-kynurenine (**Figure 2A**).

It has been previously demonstrated that several AhR ligands can promote the activation of c-Src (21). We thus assessed c-Src activity by measuring the phosphorylation status of the kinase in LPS-primed cDCs upon challenge with L-kynurenine. Western blot analysis showed that c-Src activity increased at 5 and 15 min of L-kynurenine exposure (**Figure 2B**), an effect that was contingent on AhR activation in that it was lost in AhR-deficient cDCs. Moreover, we found that induction of c-Src activity by L-kynurenine is necessary for TGF-β production (**Figure 2C**). Overall, these data indicated that L-kynurenine can mimic the effects of a second LPS challenge in inducing an endotoxin-tolerant state. In particular, L-kynurenine promotes the activation of c-Src and the subsequent phosphorylation of IDO1 in AhR-competent cDCs.

L-Kynurenine Favors the Dissociation of c-Src From the AhR Complex in cDCs

The c-Src protein may exist in at least two different conformations (namely, inactive and active), whose relative stability determines the overall activity of the enzyme (22). Post-translational modifications, as well as binding of regulatory substrates and ligands, may alter this equilibrium by favoring one conformational population over the other and thus change the overall kinase activity. Several lines of evidence have shown that, upon tetrachlorodibenzo-*p*-dioxin (TCDD) binding, the kinase is released from the AhR complex and becomes activated (21). We thus investigated whether c-Src kinase activation mediated by L-kynurenine would require the dissociation from the AhR complex. SYF cells (i.e., a fibroblast cell line that does not express the ubiquitous c-Src, c-Fyn, and c-Yes kinases) were reconstituted with a vector coding for c-Src and exposed to L-kynurenine for different lengths of time. By co-immunoprecipitation assays, we found that AhR interacts with c-Src kinase and that L-kynurenine significantly reduces this association (**Figure 3A**). Moreover, by analyzing the cellular fractions of cells exposed to L-kynurenine, we observed that AhR localizes to the nucleus, while Src is mostly present in the cytosol in its active state (**Figure 3B**).

Co-immunoprecipitation and cellular fractionation studies confirmed that these molecular events (i.e., Src disjunction from

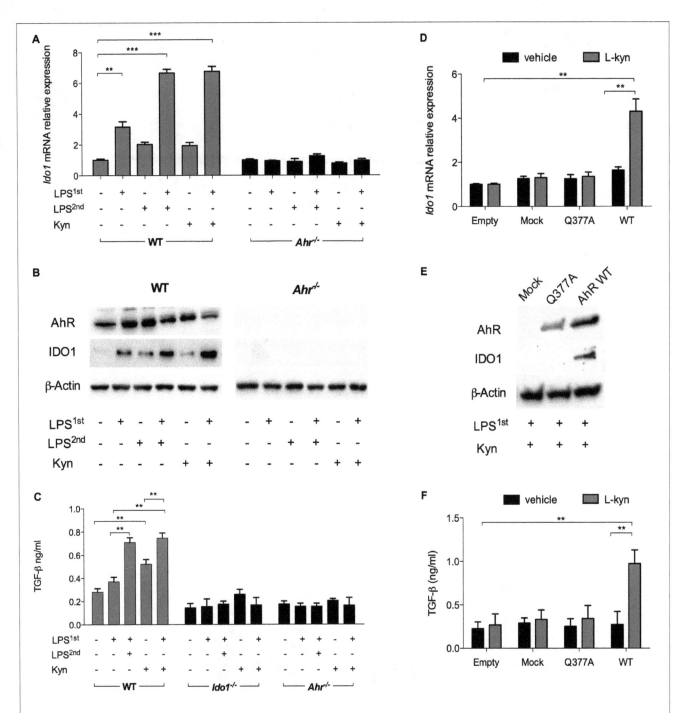

FIGURE 1 | L-Kynurenine induces indoleamine 2,3-dioxygenase 1 (IDO1) and TGF-β in lipopolysaccharide (LPS)-primed conventional dendritic cells (cDCs) *via* aryl hydrocarbon receptor (AhR). **(A)** Real-time PCR analysis of *Ido1* mRNA expression in WT and *Ahr*$^{-/-}$ BMDCs, either unprimed or primed with LPS (250 ng/ml) overnight (LPS1st) and then treated with a second dose of LPS (1 μg/ml) (LPS2nd) or L-kynurenine (50 mM) for an additional 24 h. Data (mean ± SD of three experiments) are represented as normalized transcript expression in the samples relative to normalized transcript expression in control cultures. **(B)** Western blotting analysis of IDO1 and AhR protein expression in cells treated as in A. β-Actin was used as a loading control. **(C)** TGF-β content was measured in 48 h culture supernatants from either WT, *Ido1*$^{-/-}$, or *Ahr*$^{-/-}$ cDCs stimulated as in A, after removing the stimuli by extensive washing, followed by additional culturing for 48 h in medium alone. **(D)** Real-time PCR analysis of *Ido1* mRNA expression in AhR-deficient cDCs reconstituted with mutated AhR (bearing the Q377A mutation) or the empty vector (mock). Cells were primed with LPS, followed by L-kynurenine treatment or vehicle alone. Data (mean ± SD of three experiments) are represented as normalized transcript expression in the samples relative to normalized transcript expression in control cultures. **(E)** Western blotting analysis of IDO1 and AhR protein expression in cells treated as in **(D)**. β-Actin was used as a loading control. **(F)** TGF-β production was measured in cells treated as in **(D)**. **P < 0.01, ***P < 0.001 (two-way ANOVA).

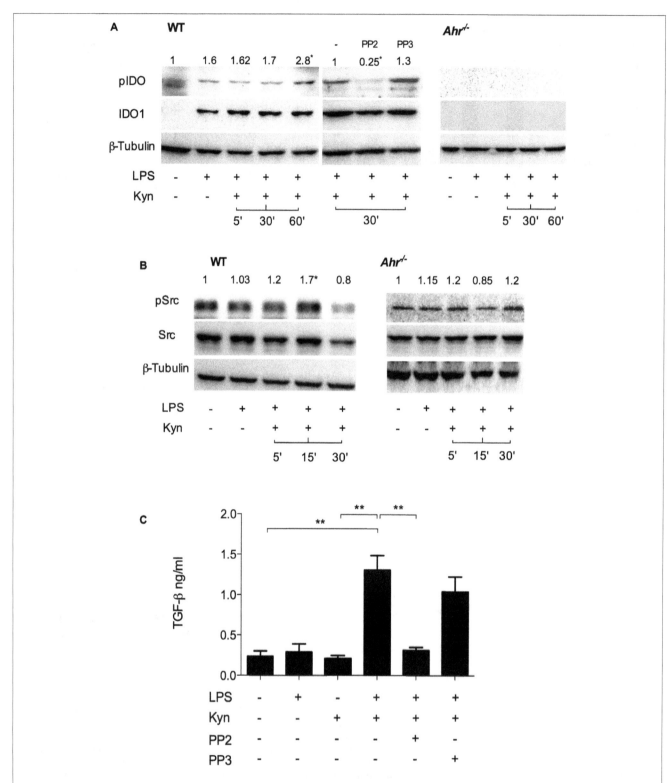

FIGURE 2 | L-Kynurenine induces IDO1 phosphorylation in AhR- and Src-dependent manner. **(A)** Western blotting analysis of IDO1 phosphorylation in WT and AhR-deficient cDCs, either unprimed or primed with LPS and then treated with L-kynurenine alone or with L-kynurenine plus PP2 or PP3 (i.e., a c-Src kinase inhibitor and its inactive analog, respectively). One experiment of three is shown. pIDO/tubulin ratios were obtained by densitometric quantification of the relevant bands and are expressed relative to untreated cells **(B)**. Immunoblot analysis of Src and phosphorylated Src-Y416 (pSrc) in WT and AhR-deficient cDCs treated as in **(A)**. One experiment of three is shown. pSrc/tubulin ratios were obtained by densitometric quantification of the relevant bands and are expressed relative to untreated cells **(C)**. Production of TGF-β by cDCs treated as in **(A)**. Means ± SD from three experiments. **P < 0.01 (two-way ANOVA).

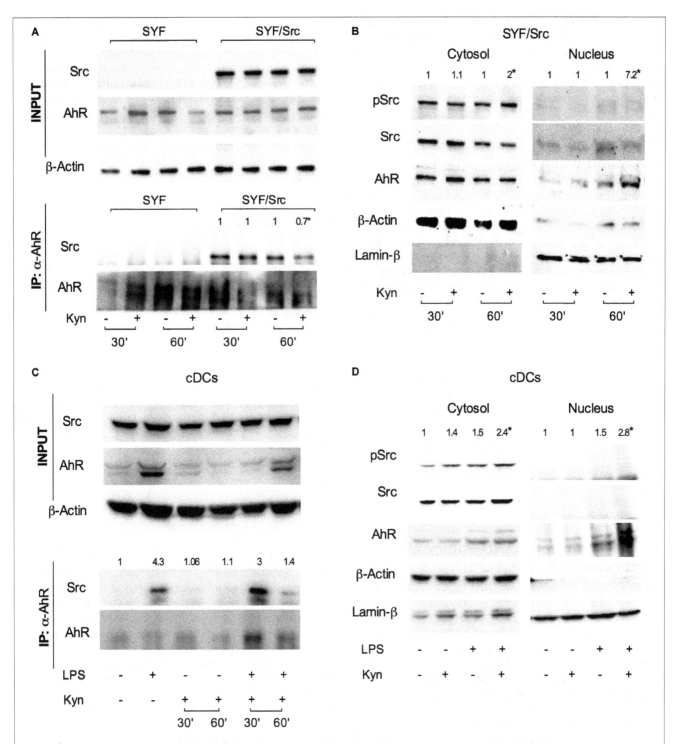

FIGURE 3 | L-kynurenine promotes the activation of c-Src via AhR. **(A)** Immunoprecipitation of AhR from SYF cells, either reconstituted with c-Src or empty vector, and detection of Src and AhR by sequential immunoblotting with specific antibodies. Cells were treated with L-kynurenine for 30 and 60 min before lysis. Input refers to whole-cell lysates used as control of protein expression. One representative immunoblot of three is shown. **(B)** Expression of pSrc, Src, and AhR in nuclear and cytoplasmatic extracts from SYF cells expressing Src and treated as in **(A)**. Lamin-β and β-actin were used as loading control of nuclear and cytoplasmic extracts, respectively. One representative experiment of three is shown. **(C)** Immunoprecipitation of AhR from cDCs either unprimed or primed with LPS and then exposed to L-kynurenine for 30 and 60 min. Src and AhR protein expression were analyzed by sequential immunoblotting with specific antibodies. Input refers to whole-cell lysates used as control of protein expression. One representative experiment of three is shown. **(D)** Expression of pSrc, Src, and AhR in nuclear and cytoplasmatic extracts from cDCs treated as in **(C)** for 60 min. Lamin-β and β-actin were used as loading control of nuclear and cytoplasmic extracts, respectively. One representative experiment of three is shown. Src/AhR ratio **(A,C)** is calculated by densitometric quantification of the specific bands and is reported as fold change against untreated cells. pSrc/Src ratio [**(B,D)**; left panel, cytosol] and Ahr/Lamin-β ratio [**(B,D)**; right panel, nucleus] are measured by densitometric quantification of the specific bands and are expressed relative to untreated cells. Ratios are means from the three experiments. *$P < 0.05$ (one-way ANOVA).

the complex and AhR shuttling to the nucleus) occur in LPS-primed cDCs exposed to L-kynurenine as well (**Figures 3C,D**). Overall, these data demonstrated that L-kynurenine can indirectly regulate c-Src kinase activity. By binding AhR, L-kynurenine promotes the receptor's conformational changes required for the release of c-Src, which then becomes activated and capable of phosphorylating downstream target proteins.

L-Kynurenine-Primed cDCs Promote *in vitro* Induction of LAP⁺ T Cells

IDO1⁺ cDCs are known to be involved in the regulation of hyperinflammatory conditions *via* the generation of regulatory T cells (23). In particular, cDC co-treatment with LPS and L-kynurenine promotes TGF-β release in an AhR- and IDO1-dependent manner (**Figure 2C**) that is essential for Treg cell differentiation *in vitro* and *in vivo*.

To evaluate if the combined effects of L-kynurenine and LPS promoted functional regulatory cDCs, those cells—either unprimed or primed with LP—were incubated with L-kynurenine and cultured with naïve CD4⁺CD25⁻ T cells, after removing the stimuli by extensive washing. L-Kynurenine, either alone or in combination with LPS, significantly increased LAP expression on the T-cell surface relative to control samples (**Figures 4A,B**). By contrast, when the cDCs had been derived from AhR- and IDO1-deficient mice, this effect was abolished (**Figures 4A,B**). Foxp3 expression was evaluated in the same co-cultures. We failed to observe any differences between samples (data not shown). Moreover, the primed cDCs further treated with L-kynurenine decreased TNFα production as well as increased IL-10 secretion by the T cells in AhR- and IDO1-dependent fashion (**Figure 4C**). Overall, these findings validate the hypothesis that L-kynurenine progressively suppresses T CD4⁺ cell effector function, favoring instead the emergence of a regulatory T-cell phenotype.

Adoptive Transfer of LPS-Primed cDCs Conditioned With L-Kynurenine *in vitro* Protects Mice From Lethal Endotoxemia

Because cDCs stimulated twice *in vitro* with LPS protect mice from a primary, otherwise lethal LPS challenge (3), we investigated whether the combined effects of LPS and L-kynurenine treatment *in vitro* would confer a protective potential on those cells *in vivo*. We established an adoptive transfer model using Flt-3L-induced, BM-derived cDCs (**Supplementary Figure S1A**). LPS-primed or unprimed cDCs, treated or not with L-kynurenine, were transferred i.v., into naïve mice to be challenged at 48 h with a lethal i.p., dose of LPS (**Figure 5A**). We found that all vehicle-treated control animals died within 48–72 h after LPS challenge. Among mice treated with differentially treated DCs, we found that as many as 80% mice receiving LPS + L-kynurenine-treated DCs survived challenge over 200 h (**Figure 5B**). To further assess the effects of cDCs *in vivo*, groups of mice were sacrificed at 48 h of LPS challenge, and lung injury—a typical feature of septic shock and endotoxemia—was sought for on gross pathology. Interestingly, lungs of mice receiving primed cDCs further conditioned by L-kynurenine were characterized by reduced inflammatory cell infiltration and vascular congestion

relative to control or to the other DC treated groups (**Figure 5C**). Based on *in vitro* evidence of AhR and IDO1 dependence for pharmacologic induction of endotoxin tolerance by LPS and L-kynurenine in cDCs, the same experiment was performed using LPS-primed or unprimed cDCs, treated or not with L-kynurenine from AhR- and IDO1-deficient mice. The protective effect of the double (LPS + L-kynurenine) pulsed cDCs on recipient mice was lost when the transferred cells were not competent for AhR and IDO1 (**Figure 5D**). Thus, successful transfer of endotoxin tolerance by fully tolerogenic DCs requires that AhR and IDO1 be fully functional.

DISCUSSION

In the present studies, we expand upon our previous observations that endotoxin tolerance *in vivo*—a condition clinically desirable to prevent the detrimental effect endotoxemia—may be transferred to naïve hosts by adoptive transfer of cDCs repeatedly exposed to LPS *in vitro* (3, 17). In particular, our previous studies had shown markedly differential (and even dichotomic) effects of single vs. repeated exposure of cDCs to LPS *in vitro*. Namely, a single exposure to LPS failed to upregulate IDO1—one of the mediators of anti-inflammatory functions of DCs—and it was instead associated with high IL-6, which promotes inflammation and IDO1 ubiquitin degradation. In contrast, cDCs stimulated twice with LPS expressed high levels of IDO1 and of TGF-β. Adoptive transfer of double LPS-treated cDCs greatly improved the outcome of an otherwise lethal LPS challenge *in vivo*, Such protective effect required that the *in vivo* transferred cDCs be fully competent for IDO1 and the host for TGF-β production.

Here we found that L-kynurenine can replace a second exposure to LPS in triggering genomic and non-genomic, AhR-dependent effects, making cDCs suitable for transferring endotoxin tolerance onto naïve recipients. The effect of externally added L-kynurenine to LPS-conditioned cDCs resulted in the promotion *Ido1* transcriptional expression and in IDO1 phosphorylation and TGF-β production. One major finding in this study was that L-kynurenine, by binding AhR, will promote the release/activation of c-Src kinase, thus triggering IDO1 signaling ability in cDCs.

Our initial experiments along this direction provided evidence that L-kynurenine potentiates IDO1 induction and TGF-β production in LPS-primed cDCs *via* AhR. AhR-deficient cDCs transfected with a vector encoding a mutated form of AhR incapable of binding L-kynurenine (3) failed to express IDO1 and to produce TGF-β when sequentially treated with LPS and L-kynurenine *in vitro*. Next, we demonstrated that one major effect of the latter was to induce AhR/Src-dependent phosphorylation of IDO1. IDO1, indeed, exerts both short-term and long-term effects in the regulation of immune homeostasis and in preventing both (hyper)acute and chronic inflammatory responses (4, 24). IDO1 contains ITIMs that, once phosphorylated, bind protein tyrosine phosphatases (SHP-1 and SHP-2) and thus activate an immunoregulatory signaling in DCs. This mechanism promotes sustained IDO1 expression, which

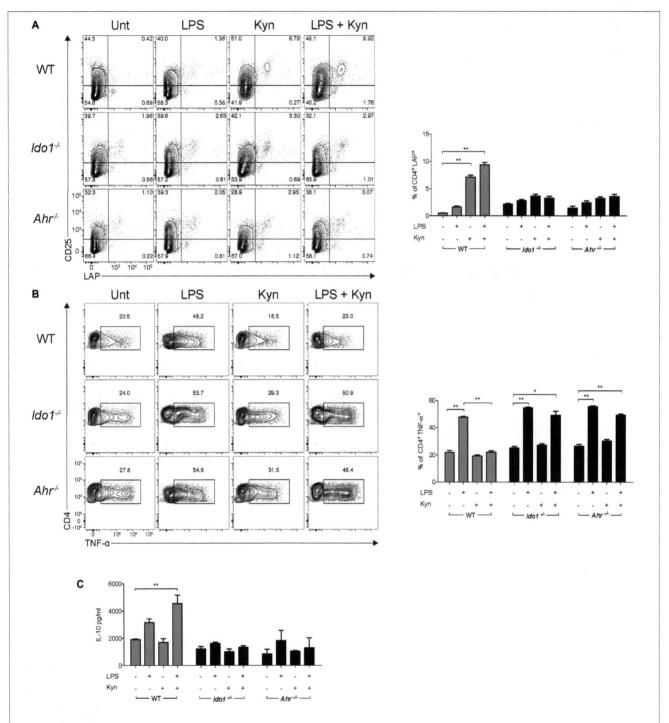

FIGURE 4 | L-Kynurenine-primed cDCs promote *in vitro* induction of LAP⁺ T cells. Representative cytofluorimetric dot plots and relative analysis of percent expression of LAP **(A)** and TNF-α **(B)** coexpression in CD4⁺ cells co-cultured for 96 h with cDCs either unprimed or LPS-primed and then incubated for 24 h with Kyn at 50 μM. A mouse IgG2a antibody was used as isotype control. Shown in upper right quadrants are percentages of double-positive cells. **(C)** IL-10 production was measured in cells treated as in **(A)**. Data are means ± SD of three independent experiments. *P < 0.05, **P < 0.01 (two-way ANOVA).

is particularly important in restraining chronic inflammation and autoimmunity. This dual—shorter term and longer term—IDO1 ability to restrain inflammation is thus to be traced to two distinct functions of the IDO1 protein, one enzymatic in nature (i.e., tryptophan degradation to kynurenine) and the other

independent of its enzymic function. As mentioned above, once phosphorylated in a specific ITIM (namely, ITIM1) domain, IDO1 becomes capable of signaling ability and long-term genomic effects restraining the production of proinflammatory mediators and the emergence of regulatory T cells (25, 26).

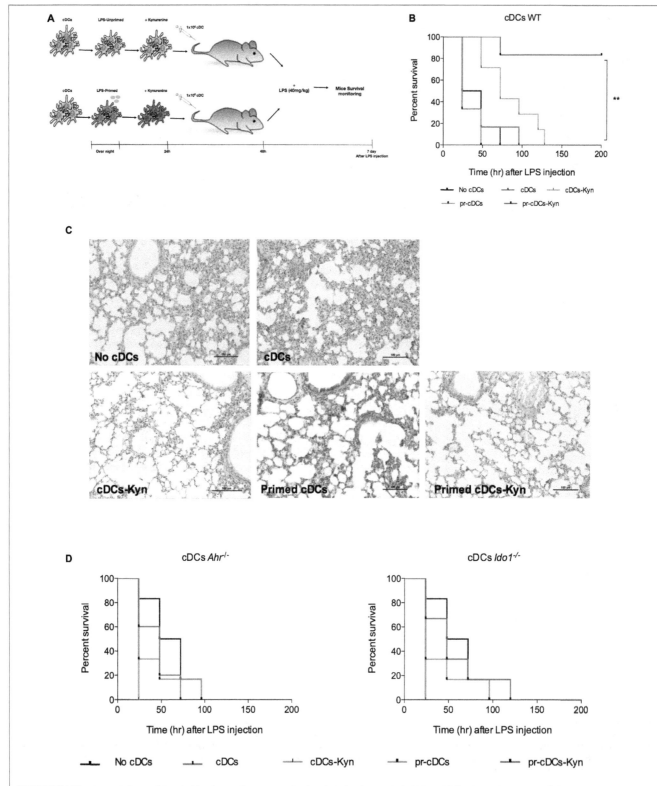

FIGURE 5 | LPS-primed cDCs conditioned with L-kynurenine protect mice from lethal endotoxemia in AhR and IDO1-dependent manner. **(A)** Representative scheme of adoptive transfer mouse model. **(B)** Survival curves of WT mice receiving an otherwise lethal 40 mg/kg LPS challenge after transfer of cDCs. Mice were transferred with AhR-competent cDCs (1.5×10^6/mouse), either unprimed (cDCs) or primed *in vitro* with LPS (1 μg/ml) and then stimulated with 50 μM kyn (pr-cDC–kyn) or medium (pr-cDCs) for an additional 24 h. Survival was monitored every 12 h through day 8 of LPS challenge. **(C)** Histopathology of lung obtained from mice treated as in **(B)**. Scale bar, 100 μm. **(D)** Survival curves of $Ahr^{-/-}$ and $Ido1^{-/-}$ mice receiving an otherwise lethal 40 mg/kg LPS challenge after transfer of cDCs *in vitro* treated as in **(A)**. n = 8–10 per group per experiment. One experiment representative of three. **P < 0.01 (log-rank test).

Of particular interest in this study was the finding that L-kynurenine favors the dissociation of c-Src from the AhR complex in cDCs, allowing the former to phosphorylate the IDO1's ITIM2 domain and promoting the generation of T cells with a regulatory phenotype. Finally, we found that—much like double LPS-pulsed DCs—adoptive transfer of LPS-primed cDCs conditioned with L-kynurenine *in vitro* protected mice from lethal endotoxemia.

Overall, the combined effects of LPS and L-kynurenine on cDCs initiates a feed-forward loop—triggered by L-kynurenine and sustained by the combined actions of IDO1, AhR, and TGF-β—which represents a key event in preventing mortality in endotoxin tolerance *in vivo*. Pharmacologically induced endotoxin tolerance, i.e., by means of kynurenine-based immunotherapy, may thus be considered a clinical option in the control of hyperinflammatory responses.

AUTHOR CONTRIBUTIONS

GMa and FF designed and supervised the study as a whole. MG and GMo performed the majority of experiments. MP, RR, and EP helped with some experiments. GS and DN helped with the generation of gene constructs and with the *in vivo* experiments. VT provided some tools. MG, FF, and PP wrote the manuscript.

FUNDING

This work was supported by the Italian Association for Cancer Research (AIRC 19903 to FF and AIRC 16851 to PP), Telethon (GGP17094 to FF), and the research projects of National Interest (Prin 2017BZEREZ to FF).

REFERENCES

1. Quintana FJ, Bohannon JK, Hernandez A, Enkhbaatar P, Adams WL, Sherwood ER. The immunobiology of toll-like receptor 4 agonists: from endotoxin tolerance to immunoadjuvants. *Shock.* (2013) 40:451–62. doi: 10.1097/SHK.0000000000000042
2. O'Carroll C, Fagan A, Shanahan F, Carmody RJ. Identification of a unique hybrid macrophage-polarization state following recovery from lipopolysaccharide tolerance. *J Immunol.* (2014) 192:427–36. doi: 10.4049/jimmunol.1301722
3. Bessede A, Gargaro M, Pallotta MT, Matino D, Servillo G, Brunacci C, et al. Aryl hydrocarbon receptor control of a disease tolerance defence pathway. *Nature.* (2014) 511:184–90. doi: 10.1038/nature13323
4. Gargaro M, Pirro M, Romani R, Zelante T, Fallarino F. Aryl hydrocarbon receptor-dependent pathways in immune regulation. *Am J Transplant.* (2016) 16:2270–6. doi: 10.1111/ajt.13716
5. Zelante T, Iannitti RG, Cunha C, De Luca A, Giovannini G, Pieraccini G, et al. Tryptophan catabolites from microbiota engage aryl hydrocarbon receptor and balance mucosal reactivity via interleukin-22. *Immunity.* (2013) 39:372–85. doi: 10.1016/j.immuni.2013.08.003
6. Quintana FJ, Sherr DH. Aryl hydrocarbon receptor control of adaptive immunity. *Pharmacol Rev.* (2013) 65:1148–61. doi: 10.1124/pr.113.007823
7. Stockinger B, Di Meglio P, Gialitakis M, Duarte JH. The aryl hydrocarbon receptor: multitasking in the immune system. *Annu Rev Immunol.* (2014) 32:403–32. doi: 10.1146/annurev-immunol-032713-120245
8. Wu PY, Yu IS, Lin YC, Chang YT, Chen CC, Lin KH, et al. Activation of aryl hydrocarbon receptor by kynurenine impairs progression and metastasis of neuroblastoma. *Cancer Res.* (2019) 79:5550–62. doi: 10.1158/0008-5472.CAN-18-3272
9. Gargaro M, Pirro M, Manni G, De Luca A, Zelante T, Fallarino F. Aryl hydrocarbon receptor: an environmental sensor in control of allergy outcomes. In: Schmidt-Weber C editor. *Allergy Prevention and Exacerbation. Birkhäuser Advances in Infectious Diseases.* Cham: Springer (2017). p. 167–89.
10. Gutiérrez-Vázquez C, Quintana FJ. Regulation of the immune response by the aryl hydrocarbon receptor. *Immunity.* (2018) 48:19–33. doi: 10.1016/j.immuni.2017.12.012
11. Ghotbaddini M, Cisse K, Carey A, Powell JB. Simultaneous inhibition of aryl hydrocarbon receptor (AhR) and Src abolishes androgen receptor signaling. *PLoS One.* (2017) 12:e0179844. doi: 10.1371/journal.pone.0179844
12. Ohtake F, Baba A, Takada I, Okada M, Iwasaki K, Miki H, et al. Dioxin receptor is a ligand dependent E3 ubiquitin ligase. *Nature.* (2007) 446:562–6. doi: 10.1038/nature05683
13. Mondanelli G, Bianchi R, Pallotta MT, Orabona C, Albini E, Iacono A, et al. A relay pathway between arginine and tryptophan metabolism confers immunosuppressive properties on dendritic cells. *Immunity.* (2017) 46:233–44. doi: 10.1016/j.immuni
14. Dolciami D, Gargaro M, Cerra B, Scalisi G, Bagnoli L, Servillo G, et al. Binding mode and structure-activity relationships of ITE as an aryl hydrocarbon receptor (AhR) agonist. *ChemMedChem.* (2018) 13:270–9. doi: 10.1002/cmdc.201700669
15. Durai V, Bagadia P, Briseño CG, Theisen DJ, Iwata A, Davidson JT IV, et al. Altered compensatory cytokine signaling underlies the discrepancy between Flt3$^{-/-}$ and Flt3l$^{-/-}$ mice. *J Exp Med.* (2018) 215:1417–35. doi: 10.1084/jem.20171784
16. Romani R, Manni G, Donati C, Pirisinu I, Bernacchioni C, Gargaro M, et al. S1P promotes migration, differentiation and immune regulatory activity in amniotic-fluid-derived stem cells. *Eur J Pharmacol.* (2018) 833:173–82. doi: 10.1016/j.ejphar.2018.06.005
17. Fallarino F, Pallotta MT, Matino D, Gargaro M, Orabona C, Vacca C, et al. LPS-conditioned dendritic cells confer endotoxin tolerance contingent on tryptophan catabolism. *Immunobiology.* (2015) 220:315–21. doi: 10.1016/j.imbio.2014.09.017
18. Volpi C, Mondanelli G, Pallotta MT, Vacca C, Iacono A, Gargaro M, et al. Allosteric modulation of metabotropic glutamate receptor 4 activates IDO1-dependent, immunoregulatory signaling in dendritic cells. *Neuropharmacology.* (2016) 102:59–71. doi: 10.1016/j.neuropharm
19. Gargaro M, Vacca C, Massari S, Scalisi G, Manni G, Mondanelli G, et al. Engagement of nuclear coactivator 7 by 3-hydroxyanthranilic acid enhances activation of aryl hydrocarbon receptor in immunoregulatory dendritic cells. *Front Immunol.* (2019) 10:1973. doi: 10.3389/fimmu.2019.01973
20. Volpi C, Fallarino F, Bianchi R, Orabona C, De Luca A, Vacca C, et al. A GpC-rich oligonucleotide acts on plasmacytoid dendritic cells to promote immune suppression. *J Immunol.* (2012) 189:2283–9. doi: 10.4049/jimmunol.1200497
21. Dong B, Cheng W, Li W, Zheng J, Wu D, Matsumura F, et al. FRET analysis of protein tyrosine kinase c-Src activation mediated via aryl hydrocarbon receptor. *Biochim Biophys Acta.* (2011) 1810:427–31. doi: 10.1016/j.bbagen.2010.11.007
22. Roskoski R Jr. Src protein-tyrosine kinase structure, mechanism, and small molecule inhibitors. *Pharmacol Res.* (2015) 94:9–25. doi: 10.1016/j.phrs.2015.01.003
23. Grohmann U, Puccetti P. The coevolution of IDO1 and AhR in the emergence of regulatory T-cells in mammals. *Front Immunol.* (2015) 6:58. doi: 10.3389/fimmu.2015.00058

24. Mondanelli G, Iacono A, Allegrucci M, Puccetti P, Grohmann U. Immunoregulatory interplay between arginine and tryptophan metabolism in health and disease. *Front Immunol.* (2019) 10:1565. doi: 10.3389/fimmu.2019. 01565

25. Pallotta MT, Orabona C, Volpi C, Vacca C, Belladonna ML, Bianchi R, et al. Indoleamine 2,3-dioxygenase is a signaling protein in long-term tolerance by dendritic cells. *Nat Immunol.* (2011) 12:870–8. doi: 10.1038/ni.2077

26. Orabona C, Pallotta MT, Volpi C, Fallarino F, Vacca C, Bianchi R, et al. SOCS3 drives proteasomal degradation of indoleamine 2,3-dioxygenase (IDO) and antagonizes IDO-dependent tolerogenesis. *Proc Natl Acad Sci USA.* (2008) 105:20828–33. doi: 10.1073/pnas.0810278105

Immune and Neuroendocrine Trait and State Markers in Psychotic Illness: Decreased Kynurenines Marking Psychotic Exacerbations

Livia De Picker [1,2]*, Erik Fransen [3], Violette Coppens [1,2], Maarten Timmers [4,5], Peter de Boer [4], Herbert Oberacher [6], Dietmar Fuchs [7], Robert Verkerk [8], Bernard Sabbe [1,2] and Manuel Morrens [1,2]

[1] Faculty of Medicine and Health Sciences, Collaborative Antwerp Psychiatric Research Institute, University of Antwerp, Antwerp, Belgium, [2] University Department of Psychiatry, Campus Duffel, Antwerp, Belgium, [3] StatUa Center for Statistics, University of Antwerp, Antwerp, Belgium, [4] Janssen Research and Development, Janssen Pharmaceutica N.V., Beerse, Belgium, [5] Reference Center for Biological Markers of Dementia (BIODEM), Institute Born-Bunge, University of Antwerp, Antwerp, Belgium, [6] Core Facility Metabolomics, Institute of Legal Medicine, Medical University of Innsbruck, Innsbruck, Austria, [7] Biocenter, Division of Biological Chemistry, Medical University of Innsbruck, Innsbruck, Austria, [8] Department of Pharmaceutical Sciences, University of Antwerp, Antwerp, Belgium

*Correspondence:
Livia De Picker
livia.depicker@uantwerp.be

Objective: Different patterns of immune system upregulation are present in the acute vs. post-treatment states of psychotic illness. We explored the existence of state and trait markers in the peripheral immune system and two immune-associated neuroendocrine pathways (IDO and GTP-CH1 pathway) in a longitudinal sample of psychosis patients. We also evaluated the association of these markers with neuropsychiatric symptomatology.

Method: Plasma concentrations of peripheral blood markers were measured in a transdiagnostic group of 49 inpatients with acute psychosis and 52 matched healthy control subjects. Samples were obtained in patients within 48 h after hospital admission for an acute psychotic episode (before initiation of antipsychotics), after 1–2 weeks and again after 8 weeks of treatment. Kynurenine, kynurenic acid (KA), 3-hydroxykynurenine (3-HK), quinolinic acid (QA), phenylalanine, tyrosine, nitrite, and neopterin were measured using HPLC and LC-MS/MS analysis. Concentrations of CRP, CCL2 (MCP1) and cytokines were determined with multiplex immunoassay. PANSS interviews and cognitive tests were performed at baseline and follow-up. Mixed model analyses were used to identify trait and state markers.

Results: Patients had significantly higher plasma concentrations of CRP, CCL2, IL1RA, and lower concentrations of KA and KA/Kyn at all time points (F7.5–17.5, all $p < 0.001$). Increased concentrations of IL6, IL8, IL1RA, TNFα, and CCL2 and decreased QA and 3-HK (F8.7–21.0, all $p < 0.005$) were found in the acute psychotic state and normalized after treatment. Low nitrite concentrations at admission rose sharply after initiation of antipsychotic medication (F42.4, $p < 0.001$). PANSS positive scale scores during the acute episode correlated with pro-inflammatory immune markers ($r \geq |0.5|$), while negative scale scores correlated inversely with IDO pathway markers ($r \geq |0.4|$). Normalization of KA and 3-HK levels between admission and follow-up corresponded to a larger improvement of negative symptoms ($r = 0.5$, $p < 0.030$) A reverse association was found between relative improvement of SDST scores and decreasing KA levels ($r = 0.5$, $p < 0.010$).

Conclusion: The acute psychotic state is marked by state-specific increases of immune markers and decreases in peripheral IDO pathway markers. Increased CRP, CCL2, and IL1RA, and decreased KA and KA/Kyn are trait markers of psychotic illness.

Keywords: psychosis, schizophrenia, cytokines, kynurenines, kynurenic acid, inflammation, immune, biomarkers

INTRODUCTION

Premorbid dysregulation of the immune system has been identified as an important factor of vulnerability for schizophrenia (1–3). Immune system activation could also be involved in schizophrenia symptom development by upregulating two neuroendocrine pathways which affect the biological availability of the two main monoamine neurotransmitter precursors: tryptophan (Trp) and tyrosine (Tyr) (cfr. **Figure 1**).

Stimulation by inflammatory molecules, particularly IFNγ, strongly activates indoleamine-2,3-dioxygenase (IDO) and the closely related tryptophan 2,3-dioxygenase 2 (TDO2), the first and rate-limiting enzymes of tryptophan breakdown into kynurenine (Kyn). In particular IDO has been linked to immune functioning: the enzyme is found in a variety of immune cells, including microglia in the central nervous system (CNS), and is often upregulated when the immune response is activated (4). Kynurenine is further degraded into downstream metabolites such as 3-hydroxykynurenine (3-HK), quinolinic acid (QA), and kynurenic acid (KA), which directly affect neuronal functioning. KA is an endogenous antagonist of all ionotropic excitatory amino acid receptor activities and therefore considered a protective metabolite against neurotoxic NMDA receptor agonist QA (5). However, abnormal accumulation of KA could lead to glutamatergic hypofunctioning and induce psychotomimetic effects (6, 7). In animal models, elevated KA levels are associated with sensory gating deficits and schizophrenia-like cognitive dysfunctions (e.g., deficits in set-shifting tasks, spatial working memory, hippocampal long-term potentiation, and attentional processing of environmental stimuli) (8–12).

A second neuroendocrine pathway which is upregulated by proinflammatory cytokines runs through GTP cyclohydrolase 1 (GTP-CH1), producing neopterin and tetrahydrobiopterin (BH4). BH4 is an essential cofactor of phenylalanine-hydroxylase (PHA), tyrosine-hydroxylase, tryptophan-hydroxylase, and nitric oxide synthases (NOS) and plays a fundamental role in the synthesis of monoamine neurotransmitters (13). Neopterin is released by activated human monocytic cells at the expense of BH4 activity. BH4 is particularly sensitive to oxidative stress and BH4 deficiencies have been reported in patients afflicted with various chronic inflammatory conditions as well as schizophrenia (14–16). In summary, the IDO and GTP-CH1 pathways may represent a neuroendocrine link between the immune system abnormalities and neuropsychiatric symptoms of psychosis patients.

Meta-analyses have confirmed peripheral changes in the levels of cytokines, chemokines, lymphocytes, and oxidative stress markers of patients with schizophrenia during acute exacerbations (acute psychotic relapse or first psychotic episode), which normalize with antipsychotic treatment (summarized in De Picker et al.) (17). These "state" markers are differentiated from other "trait" markers that remain significantly altered throughout the disorder (18, 19). Thus, different patterns of immune system upregulation are present in the acute vs. post-treatment states of psychotic illness. We hypothesized similar state-dependent changes to exist in the immune-associated neuroendocrine pathways.

The aim of this study was to identify *state* and *trait* IDO and GTP-CH1 pathway markers together with immune system markers in a longitudinal sample of patients during acute psychotic exacerbation, and to evaluate the association of these markers with neuropsychiatric symptomatology.

MATERIALS AND METHODS
Participants

We recruited a transdiagnostic group of 49 inpatients fulfilling the Diagnostic and Statistical Manual of Mental Disorders (DSM−5) criteria for a diagnosis within the spectrum of primary psychotic illnesses (DSM-5 #295.1–295.6, 295.9, 298.9). Patients were newly admitted to one of three major psychiatric hospitals in the Antwerp region of Belgium (University Psychiatric Hospital Antwerp Campus Duffel, Multiversum Campus Alexianen, and Campus Amedeus) for first-episode psychosis or for acute relapse of psychosis, as defined by Positive and Negative Syndrome Scale (PANSS) interview scores (20), and were antipsychotics-naïve or–free for at least 4 weeks prior to hospital admission. Additionally, 52 healthy age-, gender-, and BMI-matched controls from the same area were enrolled. All controls were considered healthy based on clinical evaluation with vital signs and laboratory tests (including liver enzymes, hematology, HBV, HCV, and HIV serology, and urinalysis). Individuals with a personal medical history of (1) auto-immune disorders or any chronic or recent acute physical illnesses associated with abnormal immune changes or who used anti-inflammatory or immunomodulating drugs or systemic corticosteroids within the last 3 weeks; or (2) substance use disorders according to DSM-5 criteria (except nicotine or caffeine) within the last 3 months were excluded. Control subjects with a personal history of any psychiatric disorders or family

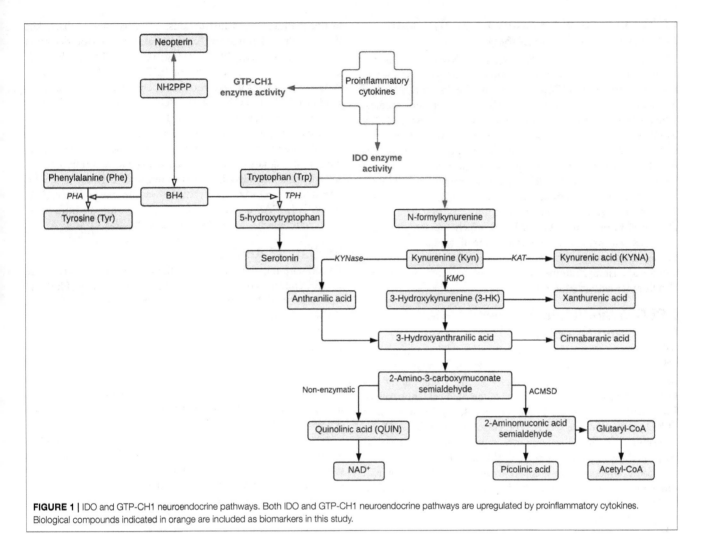

FIGURE 1 | IDO and GTP-CH1 neuroendocrine pathways. Both IDO and GTP-CH1 neuroendocrine pathways are upregulated by proinflammatory cytokines. Biological compounds indicated in orange are included as biomarkers in this study.

history (first degree relatives) of psychotic or bipolar disorders were also excluded.

Patients' symptom severity was measured using the Positive and Negative Syndrome Scale (PANSS). Psychotic exacerbations were defined by a total score of ≥14 on the positive scale of the PANSS and at least a score of 5 on one item or a score of 4 on two "psychotic" PANSS items P1, P3, P5, or G9 at Screening (20, 21). PANSS interviews were conducted with patients during the acute psychotic state and at follow-up (within 1 week of each blood sampling) by a trained interviewer. Together with the interviews, cognitive measures (Symbol-Digit Substitution Task Test and WAIS IV Letter-Number Sequencing Task) were obtained.

The study procedures were described in detail to all participants, who gave written informed consent. The local ethics committees of University Hospital Antwerp, Emmaüs, Brothers of Charity, and Spes et Fides approved the study.

Blood Sampling
Non-fasting blood samples were obtained from all participants in a standardized manner at three different occasions in

patients and two occasions in controls. Whenever possible, a first (*Unmedicated Psychosis; UMP*) sample was obtained from patients within 48 h of hospital admission (available for 37 of 49 patients), after which antipsychotic medication was initiated as determined by clinical needs. Subsequently, a sample was obtained during the first 2 weeks of hospitalization (*Psychosis*, in some patients this represented the first study sample; mean 10.2 ± 5.6 days after *UMP* sample) together with the first PANSS interview and cognitive tests. Finally, the last (*Follow-up*) sample was obtained after at least 8 weeks of treatment (mean 81.2 ± 25.9 days after *Psychosis* sample) together with the second PANSS interview and cognitive tests. In controls, two samples were drawn at the same time of day at least 6 weeks apart (mean 77.1 ± 43.2 days). Blood samples were collected from January 2014 to May 2016 without any dietary or fasting protocols and drawn via a forearm vein in EDTA and citrate containing tubes. See **Supplementary Figure 1** for timing of blood draws. Blood samples were transferred to the laboratory (<30 min) on cold packs and centrifuged for 10 min at 4°C immediately after arrival. The resulting plasma was aliquoted into Eppendorf tubes which were frozen immediately at −80°C and kept frozen until analysis.

LCMS Quantitative Analysis of Trp, Kyn, QA, and KA by LC-MS/MS

IDO pathway analytes Trp, Kyn, QA, and KA were measured in citrate plasma samples using liquid chromatography–tandem mass spectrometry (LCMS) analysis at the Institute of Legal Medicine and Core Facility Metabolomics of the Medical University of Innsbruck, Austria as described elsewhere (22). Samples were shipped frozen to Innsbruck where they were stored at $-20°C$ until analysis. Samples were processed in batches of 20–30 samples. Additionally, two quality control samples were analyzed with each batch of patient samples added to each batch. These plasma samples were kindly donated by the blood bank of the Medical University of Innsbruck. They were stored at $-20°C$ prior to use. The order in which the samples were processed was pre-specified to make sure all samples belonging to the same participant were in the same batch, and each batch contained a similar number of patient and control samples (see also **Supplementary Material**).

HPLC Quantitative Analysis of Phe, Tyr, Nitrite, and Neopterin

Free concentrations of phenylalanine (Phe), Tyr, nitrite, and neopterin were measured in EDTA plasma samples by high performance liquid chromatography (HPLC) analysis at the Center of Chemistry & Biomedicine of the Medical University of Innsbruck, Austria as described elsewhere (4, 13). For an estimate of NO production, the stable NO metabolite nitrite ($NO2^-$) was determined in the cell-free culture supernatants by the Griess reaction assay (Promega, Madison, Wisconsin).

Plasma aliquots were shipped frozen to Innsbruck at two different timepoints (6 months interval) and were stored at $-20°C$ until analysis. They were processed in batches of 20–30 samples with a pre-specified order, as above.

HPLC Quantitative Analysis of 3-HK

3-hydroxykynurenine (3-HK) was measured at the University of Antwerp Department of Pharmaceutical Sciences by HPLC with electrochemical detection as described elsewhere (23). Two hundred milliliters of citrate plasma sample was deproteinized with 40 ml of 0.23 M perchloric acid. To 120 ml of deproteinized sample was added a solution of 20 g/l sodium decane sulphonate and 1 g/l EDTA in acetonitrile:water (40:60) and injected into a HPLC system equipped with a Chromolith Performance 3.0 × 100 mm column with a Chromolith guard cartridge. Elution solvent was 2.0 g/l decane sulphonic acid, 100 mg EDTA, and 5.9 ml phosphoric acid in 1,250 ml of water and 130 ml ACN. pH is brought to 3.5 with trimethylamine. Flow was 1.7 ml/min. Detection was coulometrically using an ESA electrochemical detector at 350 mV. Recovery of 3-HK was more than 95%. Within-assay CV was 4.7%, between-assay CV was 14.7%. Specificity was checked by observing retention by changing solvent composition.

Quantitative Immunoassays

Immune markers of interest were measured in duplicate in EDTA plasma by an electrochemiluminescence immunoassay technique developed by Mesoscale Discovery (Rockville, USA), according to the manufacturer's instructions. We used standardized kits V-PLEX Proinflammatory Panel 1 Human Kit (for detection of IFNγ, IL10, IL12p70, IL1B, IL6, IL8, and TNFα), V-PLEX Cytokine Panel 1 Human Kit (for IL17A), V-PLEX Chemokine Panel 1 Human Kit (for monocyte chemoattractant protein-1, MCP1/CCL2) and V-PLEX Vascular Injury Panel 2 Human Kit (for C-reactive protein, CRP). Additionally, IL-1RA was detected using a custom 4-Spot Prototype Human IL-1RA kit. Concentrations for each cytokine were calculated by fitting the sample signals on a 4-parametric logistic calibration curve. Assays were excluded if concentrations were below detection threshold in >50% of participants (as was the case for IFNγ, IL10, IL12p70, IL17A), as well as all data points with an intra-assay coefficient of variation >15% (cfr. **Table 2**).

Statistical Analysis

To estimate the activity of PHA, the ratio of the substrate Phe vs. the concentrations of the enzyme product Tyr (Phe/Tyr) was calculated. A similar ratio was calculated for Kyn/Trp and KA/Kyn as indices of IDO and KAT, respectively.

All statistical analyses were performed in JMP version 13 and Review Manager 5.3. Non-normally distributed markers were log normalized prior to the use of parametric statistics (IL1RA, IL6, IL8, CCL2, TNFα, CRP, QA, QA/KA). We applied a reflected transformation to the distribution of neopterin because of negative skew. Outlier plasma concentrations of markers (>3 × z-score) were excluded from analysis.

Baseline differences in clinical and demographic parameters between cohorts were examined by two-tailed independent t-tests for continuous variables and Pearson chi-square test for categorical variables. Pearson correlation analyses tested the association between different markers and symptom severity. All medium-to-high strength correlations ($r > |0.3|$) are reported. All data are presented as mean ± SD unless otherwise indicated.

A series of linear mixed model restricted maximum likelihood (REML) analyses were performed with the different immune and neuroendocrine markers as the dependent variables. To model trait differences in peripheral immune and neuroendocrine markers between the cohorts as well as differences related to the acute psychotic state vs. post-treatment state in patients, Subject was included as random effect and Cohort, State (i.e., the psychotic state, including both UMP, and Psychosis timepoints) nested in Cohort and Batch as fixed effects (marker = [SubjID] + Cohort + State[Cohort] + Batch). Because the graphical presentation of the identified markers (demonstrated in **Figure 2**) indicated distinct results for the samples taken at admission (during Unmedicated Psychosis; UMP), the above linear mixed model for each marker was repeated using UMP as State. Dependent variables which demonstrated significant effects for State [Cohort] in either of two mixed models were considered *state* markers, whereas variables for which Cohort was significant in both mixed model analyses were considered *trait* markers. Subsequently, the models were adjusted for sex, age, BMI, and smoking.

All significance levels are reported as two-sided P-values, corrected for multiple testing using the Benjamini-Hochberg implementation (24) of the False Discovery Rate

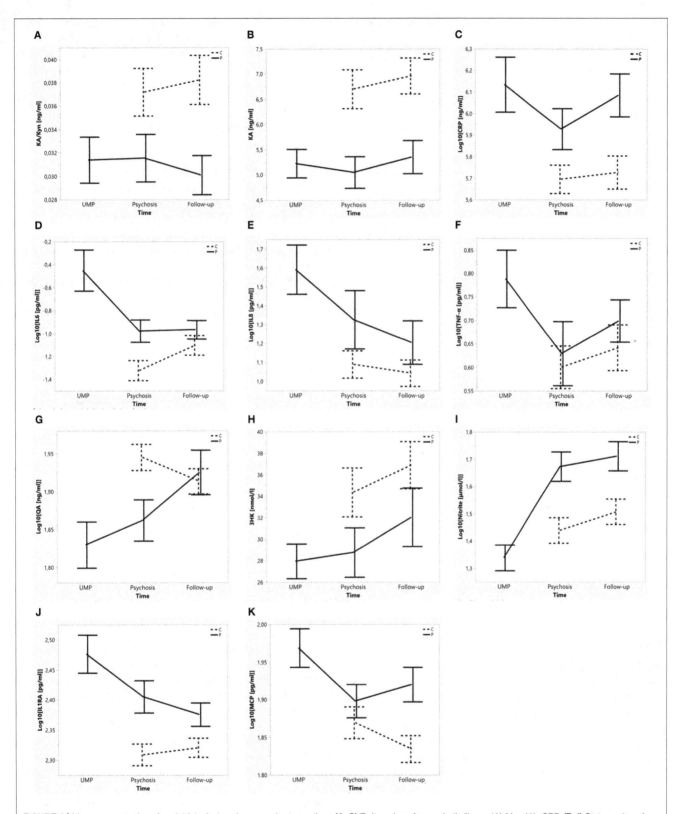

FIGURE 2 | Mean concentration of each biological marker per cohort over time. **(A–C)** Trait markers for psychotic illness: KA/Kyn, KA, CRP. **(D–I)** State markers for the acute psychotic state: IL6, IL8, TNFα, QA, 3HK, Nitrite. **(J,K)** Trait ánd state markers for psychotic illness and the acute psychotic state: IL1RA, CCL2/MCP1. Error bars represent mean ± SE. Dotted lines indicate control subjects, full lines patients. "UMP" (unmedicated psychosis) represents the first blood sampling in patients; "Psychosis" represents the second blood sampling in patients and the first blood sampling in controls; "Follow-up" represents the last timepoint in patients and controls.

TABLE 1 | Demographics, PANSS interview, and cognitive test results at baseline and follow-up.

	Patients	Controls	Test statistic
N	49	52	
Age range	19–49 years	18–47 years	
Age mean + SD	32.4 ± 7.5 years	28.5 ± 7.0 years	t2.66, df99, $p = 0.010$
M:F (absolute)	42:7	39:13	
M:F (pct)	86:14	75:25	χ1.82, $p = 0.177$
BMI mean + SD	24.9 ± 4.0	23.9 ± 3.7	t1.29, $p = 0.201$
Smoking	63.8%	5.9%	χ36.77, $p < 0.001$
THC use prior to study (heavy use defined as more than three times per week)	18.8% light 20.8% heavy	3.9% light	χ19.5, $p < 0.001$
Duration of illness	6.1 ± 5.9 years		
1st episode	26.1%		

	Acute psychosis (n = 46)	At follow-up (n = 39)	
PANSS total score	83.4 ± 14.6	59.1 ± 12.1	t10.9, df37, $p < 0.001$
PANSS positive scale score	24.8 ± 5.0	10.8 ± 2.9	t17.9, df37, $p < 0.001$
PANSS negative scale score	18.4 ± 7.4	17.2 ± 7.0	t1.3, df37, $p = 0.197$
PANSS general psychopathology scale score	40.6 ± 7.9	30.9 ± 7.1	t6.9, df37, $p < 0.001$
SDST score (numbers correct)	44.0 ± 12.0	48.0 ± 11.7	t2.84, df37, $p = 0.008$
LNS adjusted score	5.0 ± 2.2	5.2 ± 2.4	t0.77, df37, $p = 0.446$

Data are expressed as mean values ± SD.

(FDR) correction. An FDR adjusted p-value of 0.05 was used as cutoff for significance (significant p-values are indicated by *).

RESULTS

Demographics

We enrolled 52 controls and 49 patients, of whom seven dropped out of the study prior to the last timepoint. The first unmedicated UMP blood sample was available for 37 out of 49 patients. Demographic information and patients' PANSS scores are presented in **Table 1**. PANSS scores were not available for analysis in three patients. Patients' baseline PANSS total scores, positive subscale and general psychopathology subscale scores were significantly higher than at follow-up.

Trait and State Markers of Psychosis

Increased concentrations of IL6, IL8, TNFα, CCL2, and decreased Nitrite were identified as markers of the unmedicated acute psychotic state [State(Cohort) for UMP: all $F = 8.68$–42.36; $p = \leq 0.001$–0.004], whereas increased IL1RA ($F =$

8.33; $p = 0.005$) and decreased 3-HK ($F = 12.81$; $p = 0.001$) and QA ($F = 16.07$; $p < 0.001$) were state markers of the whole acute psychotic episode, both before and after initiation of antipsychotic medication. We identified increased IL1RA, CRP, and CCL2 and decreased KA and KA/Kyn as trait markers (Cohort: all $F = 5.96$–17.39; $p = \leq 0.001$–0.017) (see **Figure 2**). No significant differences were identified for Trp, Phe, Tyr, Phe/Tyr, and Neopterin. Results of the analyses are summarized in **Table 2** and **Supplementary Table 1**.

Adjustment for Confounders

The above analyses were adjusted for the effects of sex, BMI, smoking, and age: (1) A significant interaction between cohort and sex existed in KA ($F = 17.39$; $p < 0.001$) and KA/Kyn ($F = 13.64$; $p < 0.001$), with male controls demonstrating higher KA and male patients demonstrating lower KA; (2) Nitrite levels were lower in men compared to women in both cohorts ($F = 12.0$, $p < 0.001$); (3) Higher BMI significantly increased concentrations of CRP, IL1RA, and QA in both cohorts; (4) The effect of smoking was not significant; (5) A significant interaction between cohort and age was found for IL1B ($F = 7.96$; $p = 0.006$) and Kyn/Trp ($F = 8.94$; $p = 0.004$) and a significant main effect of age for IL6 ($F = 7.45$; $p = 0.008$). Results are summarized in **Supplementary Table 1**.

Relationship Between Immune and Neuroendocrine Markers

TNFα concentrations in patients but not controls correlated with Kyn ($r = 0.310$–0.509), Kyn/Trp ($r = 0.361$–0.451), QA ($r = 0.432$–0.481), and QA/KA ($r = 0.349$–0.518), but not with KA at each of the three timepoints. In contrast, in controls CRP and IL1RA concentrations correlated with IDO pathway metabolites. Results are summarized in **Supplementary Table 2**.

Relationship With Clinical Symptoms and Patient Characteristics

PANSS positive scale scores during the acute psychotic state correlated with concentrations of IL1B ($r = 0.463$, $p = 0.026$), IL6 ($r = 0.541$, $p = 0.008$), and CRP ($r = 0.507$, $p = 0.014$) and correlated inversely with Neopterin ($r = -0.427$, $p = 0.021$), whereas PANSS negative scale scores correlated with Kyn ($r = 0.458$, $p = 0.013$), QA/KA ($r = 0.379$, $p = 0.040$) and inversely with KA/Kyn ($r = -0.400$, $p = 0.032$). Furthermore, the relative change in PANSS negative scale scores between the acute and post-treatment states [(acute–post-treatment)/acute] correlated inversely with the relative change in KA ($r = -0.470$, $p = 0.024$) as well as 3-HK ($r = -0.465$, $p = 0.026$).

Both groups improved between the first and second rounds of cognitive testing but patients performed significantly poorer compared to controls (SDST controls 70.0 ± 12.1, vs. patients 45.6 ± 12.1, within-pairs $F = 0.76$, $p = 0.386$, among-pairs $F = 85.0$, $p < 0.001$; LNS controls 9.96 ± 2.9 vs. patients 5.10 ± 2.3, within-pairs $F = 5.6$, $p = 0.020$, among-pairs $F = 85.4$, $p < 0.001$). The relative change in SDST performance over time in patients [(acute–post-treatment)/acute] correlated inversely with the relative change in KA ($r = -0.489$, $p = 0.010$) and KA/Kyn ($r = -0.358$, $p = 0.067$).

DISCUSSION

Trait and State Markers of Psychotic Illness

In the present study, we tested the hypothesis that state or trait increases in levels of pro-inflammatory cytokines may be accompanied by state-specific IDO and GTP-CH1 pathway abnormalities in schizophrenia spectrum disorders. We defined five immune (IL1RA, IL6, IL8, TNF, CCL2) and three neuroendocrine (QA, 3-HK, Nitrite) *state* markers of acute exacerbations which normalized after treatment with antipsychotics. Five *trait* markers (IL1RA, CRP, CCL2, KA, KA/Kyn) differentiated between patients and controls at any of the timepoints. IL1RA and CCL2 were both state and trait markers, distinguishing patients from controls as well as patients during a psychotic episode from those at post-treatment follow-up. Kyn/Trp was a trait marker only in participants older than 30 years of age.

Our findings confirm the association of schizophrenia and the acute psychotic state with increased peripheral (pro-inflammatory) immune markers, as described earlier by Miller et al. in two meta-analyses of blood cytokine and CRP levels. Miller et al. identified IL1B, IL6, and TGFβ as state markers for acute exacerbations, while IL12, IFNγ, TNFα, sIL2R, and CRP were trait markers. IFNγ and IL12p70 were measured in our study but did not meet quality control criteria required for further analysis. CCL2 was also identified as a trait marker (defined here as elevated in both first- and multiple-episode schizophrenia patients irrespective of treatment) in another recent meta-analysis (25).

However, although our patients exhibited state and trait immune activation, the GTP-CH1 pathway did not differentiate patients from controls (except for nitrite) and the IDO pathway appeared overall downregulated in patients vs. controls. Although this finding contradicts our original hypothesis of immune-activated IDO upregulation, it is in line with results from two recent amino-acid profiling studies (one cross-sectional study in 208 first episode psychosis patients and one 7-month follow-up study in 38 schizophrenia patients) in which tryptophan and kynurenine were decreased in participants with schizophrenia vs. controls (26, 27).

Furthermore, subgroup analyses of a recent meta-analysis by Plitman et al. of 13 studies in schizophrenia demonstrated that KA levels were increased centrally (cerebrospinal fluid and brain tissue, $n = 7$ studies) but not peripherally ($n = 5$ studies) (28). However, two studies of peripheral IDO pathway metabolites which have emerged since then suggest a relative decrease in KA even in the presence of a pro-inflammatory state (29, 30). We therefore repeated this meta-analysis using the same methods, while adding the data of the two newer studies plus our own findings. Significant study heterogeneity existed in the main analysis ($I^2 = 90\%$), with the funnel plot indicating the smallest and oldest study (31) acted as an outlier, influencing the overall result. When this study was excluded, the meta-analysis of the remaining seven studies indicated KA levels were mildly but significantly decreased in the blood of patients with schizophrenia compared to controls (standardized mean difference -0.35, $p = 0.020$) (cfr. **Figure 3**).

Our study has specifically looked at state-specific changes of neuroendocrine markers. Only a few other studies have longitudinally investigated IDO pathway metabolite concentrations in both arms downstream from kynurenine in psychosis patients. Myint et al. (32) studied 53 medication-free patients with schizophrenia admitted to hospital with psychotic symptoms and treated with antipsychotic medication over 6 weeks. They also identified decreased KA and KA/Kyn as trait markers, but found increased 3-HK at admission, which normalized after 6 weeks of treatment (32). Fazio et al. (33) found decreased QA and 3-HK in first- and multiple-episode schizophrenia patients, the latter of which increased significantly in first-episode patients after 1 year of treatment. KA levels were found to be increased in their study, however this result may have been confounded by a gender imbalance in this study (69% male in patients vs. 44% in controls), considering KA levels are lower in females than males (33, 34). Szymona et al. (30) analyzed blood levels of KA and 3-HK in 51 chronic schizophrenia patients during acute relapse, after 4 weeks of therapy and at remission. KA levels were significantly lower in comparison with controls throughout the study, whereas 3-HK did not differ from controls at admission and during therapy but increased at remission and correlated negatively with the improvement of negative symptoms (SANS scores) at discharge–matching our findings for PANSS negative scale scores. Finally, Wurfel et al. demonstrated reductions in serum KA and KA/QA in acutely ill inpatients with affective psychosis.

Age and Sex Effects

The term "inflammaging" (35) has been coined to indicate significant relationships between aging and circulating concentrations of immune markers such as IL-6 and neopterin, as well as increased tryptophan breakdown in the presence of immune activation in the elderly (36). Moreover, we have recently demonstrated important age effects on microglial activity during psychosis in a subpopulation of our current sample, in whom TSPO radioligand uptake was measured using Positron Emission Tomography (37, 38).

In the current study, we observed that state and trait increases in IL1RA and IL6 became more pronounced in older patients, while state-dependent changes of QA and 3-HK were more pronounced in younger patients. Not unimportantly given the sexual dimorphism in age of onset and progression of schizophrenia, a significant interaction between cohort and sex existed in KA.

Limitations

There are some noteworthy limitations to the present study. Firstly, the number of samples obtained was not the same in all patients. Our aim was to obtain blood samples at the earliest possible time during the acute psychotic episode. Therefore, some patients were enrolled in the study within 48 h of being admitted to hospital and before the initiation of antipsychotic medication (UMP timepoint), whereas others only entered the study at a later timepoint (Psychosis, timepoint) within the first 2 weeks of hospitalization. We therefore preferred methods of analyses which are less affected by missing or unbalanced data, such as

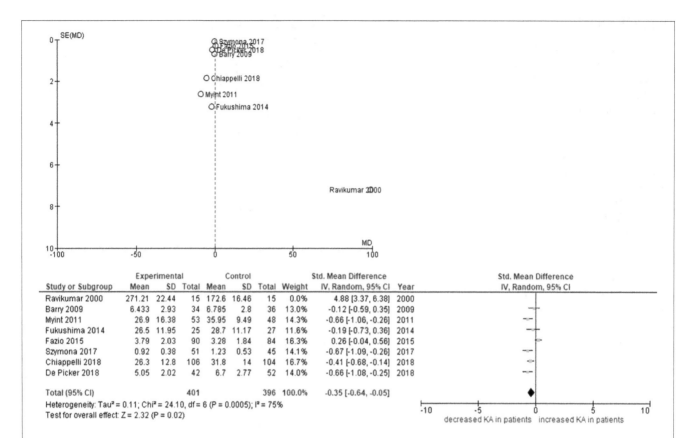

FIGURE 3 | Funnel and forest plots of studies on peripheral KA levels. Funnel plot depicts standardized mean differences (SMDs) of studies on peripheral KA levels. Forest plot excludes Ravikumar et al. from analysis.

TABLE 2 | Concentrations of different immune markers at the different timepoints.

Compound	UMP (at admission)	Psychosis (<2 weeks in hospital)	Follow-up (>8 weeks treatment)	Control	Datapoints excluded or missing
IL6 (pg/ml)	3.09 ± 6.83	0.38 ± 1.12	0.20 ± 0.21	0.16 ± 0.26	N = 11
IL8 (ng/ml)	0.98 ± 4.17	1.30 ± 4.61	0.20 ± 0.77	0.03 ± 0.08	N = 4
IL1RA (ng/ml)	0.33 ± 0.16	0.28 ± 0.15	0.25 ± 0.07	0.22 ± 0.07	N = 16
IL1B (pg/ml)	0.07 ± 0.29	0.03 ± 0.08	0.02 ± 0.08	0.27 ± 1.86	N = 25
TNFα (pg/ml)	8.01 ± 5.55	6.23 ± 5.51	6.35 ± 6.41	5.44 ± 4.02	N = 41
CRP (µg/ml)	4.03 ± 6.22	2.18 ± 3.10	2.20 ± 1.99	1.00 ± 1.22	N = 4
CCL2 (pg/ml)	99.12 ± 36.96	82.99 ± 24.80	88.85 ± 36.06	75.17 ± 27.46	N = 3
Trp (µg/ml)	10.68 ± 2.66	10.57 ± 2.19	10.21 ± 1.93	10.88 ± 1.76	N = 0
Kyn (ng/ml)	172.30 ± 36.58	165.64 ± 40.45	179.38 ± 43.41	185.16 ± 47.09	N = 0
KA (ng/ml)	5.22 ± 1.62	5.05 ± 2.03	5.35 ± 1.99	6.83 ± 2.66	N = 0
QA (ng/ml)	72.39 ± 24.79	78.55 ± 30.59	91.43 ± 38.88	88.39 ± 25.17	N = 0
3-HK (nmol/l)	27.95 ± 8.98	28.77 ± 14.55	32.04 ± 16.09	35.69 ± 15.53	N = 16
Nitrite	26.16 ± 15.86	59.86 ± 34.151	63.64 ± 34.25	39.47 ± 30.16	N = 6
Neopterin	5.80 ± 2.07	5.44 ± 2.31	6.50 ± 5.15	5.56 ± 2.74	N = 6

Data are expressed as mean values ± SD. Phe and Tyr are not represented due to significant batch effects.

linear mixed models. Secondly, our naturalistic study design does not allow us to differentiate to which extent changes between the different illness states can be accounted for by effects of treatment with antipsychotic medication, non-specific aspects

of being hospitalized or natural illness course. Furthermore, although there is a significant reduction between baseline and follow-up PANSS total and positive subscale scores, our follow-up period of 8 weeks may still have been too short for the immune markers to normalize. A longitudinal study with longer follow-up period would be needed to monitor the evolution of state makers and to verify if the trait markers indeed remain altered in patients irrespective of their clinical course (39).

All patients in our study were started on a regimen of antipsychotic treatment during the follow-up period. Unfortunately, our data did not allow us to compare neuroimmune markers against the type and dose of antipsychotic treatment. Antipsychotics in general have been suggested to increase nitric oxide plasma levels, which would explain the sharp increase in nitrite levels in patients after antipsychotics were initiated (40). Thirdly, our findings concern peripheral measures which cannot be generalized to the central nervous system and are susceptible to confounding by factors which affect peripheral bioavailability. We repeated our analysis controlled for albumin concentration which did not alter our findings. All samples were taken in non-fasting conditions, except UMP which were usually drawn together with routine clinical sampling in early morning fasting conditions—as plasma kynurenine is typically lower in non-fasting conditions, it is unlikely this would explain our findings (41). Our IDO pathway results were very consistent despite having been generated in two different labs (University of Antwerp and University of Innsbruck) and with two different methods (LC-MS/MS vs. HPLC). In contrast, the GTP-CH1 pathway results were subject to considerable batch effects which could have nullified any biological differences in Phe, Tyr, and Neopterin.

The importance of IDO pathway metabolites is usually linked to their actions in the central nervous system. TRP, KYN, and 3-HK readily cross the blood-brain barrier while KA and QA cannot (42). Human brain kynurenines are not autonomous but are linked to, and influenced by, the peripheral IDO pathway (5). Sixty to eighty percentage of cerebral KYN—the predominant source of downstream cerebral IDO pathway metabolites—is contributed from the periphery, where the highly regulated IDO pathway accounts for $\sim$80% of non-protein-bound Trp metabolism (43, 44). During inflammation and enhanced tryptophan breakdown, increased amounts of peripheral KYN are transported across the blood-brain barrier and become available for further downstream metabolization in astrocytes and microglia of the central nervous system. Finally, while our work has focused on IDO-initiated kynurenine metabolism, it is worth pointing out the existence of an alternative—albeit less well-studied—route catalyzed by TDO2. While TDO2 expression in mammals is mostly restricted to the liver, one study has demonstrated a 1.6-fold increase in TDO2 mRNA as well as increased density of TDO2-immunopositive astrocytes in postmortem tissue of patients with schizophrenia (45). Clearly further work is needed to elucidate the differential pathophysiological roles of IDO- vs. TDO2-mediated kynurenine metabolism in pro-inflammatory states.

Clinical Relevance and Recommendations for Future Research

After adjustment for potential confounders and multiple testing we find that immune and neuroendocrine profiles of patients differ throughout the course of a psychotic episode. Future studies evaluating these compounds in both exploratory or interventional designs should therefore carefully select or differentiate between patients in different illness stages.

While positive symptom scores during the acute episode correlated mostly with markers of the pro-inflammatory state, IDO pathway markers were associated with negative symptom scores. Normalization of KA and 3-HK levels between admission and follow-up corresponded to a larger improvement of negative symptoms. A reverse association was found between relative improvement of SDST scores and decreased KA levels, which could represent the first evidence in humans of the preclinical findings that sudden increases in brain kynurenic acid impair cognitive flexibility (8). More comprehensive research in larger samples would be needed to further explore this relationship.

Clearly, the most unexpected finding of this study is the global downregulation of both arms of the IDO pathway in psychosis. The IDO or kynurenine pathway has been of interest to schizophrenia research because of its strong relation to the immune system as well as the fact that KA tightly controls glutamatergic and dopaminergic neurotransmission and influences behavior in animals (46). In humans, exogenous glutamate receptor antagonists induce schizophrenia-like phenomena in healthy controls.

Based on our findings, which are echoed by recently published evidence on decreased peripheral KA concentrations, a critical re-evaluation of the kynurenic acid hypothesis is needed. Alternative hypotheses to identify the origins of the IDO pathway abnormalities in schizophrenia, their relation to treatment responses and in particular the striking discrepancies between central and peripheral findings should be considered (29). Similar to a mechanism proposed in glioblastoma patients, in whom plasma concentrations of Trp, Kyn, KA, and QA were found to be decreased compared with healthy controls in the context of CNS IDO1 upregulation (47), decreased peripheral KA could be indicative of an increased demand for and transfer of Trp or Kyn through the blood–brain barrier to serve as substrate for local synthesis of KA in brain tissue. This corresponds to increased KA concentrations in the CSF of patients with schizophrenia (48). This hypothesis however does not explain why KA remains decreased throughout the illness course as trait marker while, especially in younger patients, 3-HK and QA concentrations increase post-treatment. Nor does it clarify why we found Kyn, 3-HK, and QA concentrations to correlate with TNFα concentrations in patients while KA levels did not.

Despite several decades of increased attention for kynurenines in the field of mental health research, many basic issues about their pathophysiology remain unsettled as recently extensively reviewed by Schwarcz and Stone (42). The effect of persistent up- or downregulation of kynurenine pathway metabolism in the periphery on the dynamics of blood-brain barrier transport have not yet been studied. Future work is needed to clarify the functional dynamics of IDO pathway metabolism in the CNS as well as the implications of peripheral kynurenine changes. Ideally future studies in psychosis patients should look at both kynurenine pathway arms, comparing both CSF and plasma and longitudinally following patients throughout the course of their illness.

CONCLUSION

To our knowledge, this is the first study to comprehensively and longitudinally evaluate state and trait changes of IDO and GTP-CH1 pathway metabolites in parallel to immune markers in psychosis patients. Our study confirmed that the acutely psychotic (and unmedicated) state is marked by specific state increases of immune markers (IL6, IL8, TNFα, CCL2, IL1RA) and decreased Nitrite. We also demonstrated these increases in peripheral pro-inflammatory immune markers are accompanied by state-specific decreases in peripheral 3-HK and QA. Trait markers which differentiate psychosis patients from healthy controls throughout the illness course were increased CRP, CCL2, and IL1RA, and decreased KA and KA/Kyn. While PANSS positive scale scores during the acute episode correlated with pro-inflammatory immune markers, IDO pathway markers were associated with negative scale scores and normalization of KA and 3-HK levels between admission and follow-up corresponded to a larger improvement of negative symptoms. A reverse association was found between relative improvement of SDST scores and decreasing KA levels.

AUTHOR CONTRIBUTIONS

LDP, PB, MT, BS, and MM devised the project, the main conceptual ideas, and proof outline. LDP, RV, VC, DF, and HO carried out the experiments. EF verified the statistical analysis methods. LDP wrote the manuscript with support from MM, VC, and BS. All authors discussed the results and contributed to the final manuscript.

FUNDING

This study was in part funded by research grants from the Flanders' Agency for Innovation by Science and Technology (IWT-SB 121373) and Janssen Research and Development, a division of Janssen Pharmaceutica N.V. Neither funding body was responsible for the design, collection and analysis of data or the decision to publish.

ACKNOWLEDGMENTS

The authors are thankful to J. Schuermans, D. Ooms, and G. Koppen for support with the MSD multiplex procedures. The authors are equally thankful to I. Vanderplas, S. Apers, L. Claes, and S. Debruyne for their support with all patient-related procedures. Finally, we would like to express our gratitude to all the participants of this study.

REFERENCES

1. Borglum AD, Demontis D, Grove J, Pallesen J, Hollegaard MV, Pedersen CB, et al. Genome-wide study of association and interaction with maternal cytomegalovirus infection suggests new schizophrenia loci. *Mol Psychiatry*. (2014) 19:325–33. doi: 10.1038/mp. 2013.2

2. Demontis D, Nyegaard M, Buttenschon HN, Hedemand A, Pedersen CB, Grove J, et al. Association of GRIN1 and GRIN2A-D with schizophrenia and genetic interaction with maternal herpes simplex virus-2 infection affecting disease risk. *Am J Med Genet Part B, Neuropsychiatr Genet*. (2011) 156B:913–22. doi: 10.1002/ajmg.b. 31234

3. Clarke MC, Tanskanen A, Huttunen M, Whittaker JC, Cannon M. Evidence for an interaction between familial liability and prenatal exposure to infection in the causation of schizophrenia. *Am J Psychiatry*. (2009) 166:1025–30. doi: 10.1176/appi.ajp.2009.080 10031

4. Widner B, Werner ER, Schennach H, Wachter H, Fuchs D. Simultaneous measurement of serum tryptophan and kynurenine by HPLC. *Clin Chem*. (1997) 43:2424–6.

5. Schwarcz R, Bruno JP, Muchowski PJ, Wu HQ. Kynurenines in the mammalian brain: when physiology meets pathology. *Nat Rev Neurosci*. (2012) 13:465–77. doi: 10.1038/nrn3257

6. Javitt DC, Zukin SR. Recent advances in the phencyclidine model of schizophrenia. *Am J Psychiatry*. (1991) 148:1301–8. doi: 10.1176/ajp.148. 10.1301

7. Moghaddam B, Krystal JH. Capturing the angel in "angel dust": twenty years of translational neuroscience studies of NMDA receptor antagonists in animals and humans. *Schizophr Bull*. (2012) 38:942–9. doi: 10.1093/schbul/sbs075

8. Alexander KS, Wu HQ, Schwarcz R, Bruno JP. Acute elevations of brain kynurenic acid impair cognitive flexibility: normalization by the alpha7 positive modulator galantamine. *Psychopharmacology*. (2012) 220:627–37. doi: 10.1007/s00213-011-2539-2

9. Erhardt S, Schwieler L, Emanuelsson C, Geyer M. Endogenous kynurenic acid disrupts prepulse inhibition. *Biol Psychiatry*. (2004) 56:255–60. doi: 10.1016/j.biopsych.2004. 06.006

10. DeAngeli NE, Todd TP, Chang SE, Yeh HH, Yeh PW, Bucci DJ. Exposure to kynurenic acid during adolescence increases sign-tracking and impairs long-term potentiation in adulthood. *Front Behav Neurosci*. (2014) 8:451. doi: 10.3389/fnbeh.2014.00451

11. Chess AC, Bucci DJ. Increased concentration of cerebral kynurenic acid alters stimulus processing and conditioned responding. *Behav Brain Res*. (2006) 170:326–32. doi: 10.1016/j.bbr.2006. 03.006

12. Chess AC, Simoni MK, Alling TE, Bucci DJ. Elevations of endogenous kynurenic acid produce spatial working memory deficits. *Schizophr Bull*. (2007) 33:797–804. doi: 10.1093/schbul/sbl033

13. Neurauter G, Scholl-Burgi S, Haara A, Geisler S, Mayersbach P, Schennach H, et al. Simultaneous measurement of phenylalanine and tyrosine by high performance liquid chromatography (HPLC) with fluorescence detection. *Clin Biochem*. (2013) 46:1848–51. doi: 10.1016/j.clinbiochem.2013.10.015

14. Neurauter G, Schrocksnadel K, Scholl-Burgi S, Sperner-Unterweger B, Schubert C, Ledochowski M, et al. Chronic immune stimulation correlates with reduced phenylalanine turnover. *Curr Drug Metabol*. (2008) 9:622–7. doi: 10.2174/1389200087858 21738

15. Zangerle R, Kurz K, Neurauter G, Kitchen M, Sarcletti M, Fuchs D. Increased blood phenylalanine to tyrosine ratio in HIV-1 infection and correction following effective antiretroviral therapy. *Brain Behav Immun.* (2010) 24:403–8. doi: 10.1016/j.bbi.2009.11.004

16. Richardson MA, Read LL, Reilly MA, Clelland JD, Clelland CL. Analysis of plasma biopterin levels in psychiatric disorders suggests a common BH4 deficit in schizophrenia and schizoaffective disorder. *Neurochem Res.* (2007) 32:107–13. doi: 10.1007/s11064-006-9233-5

17. De Picker LJ, Morrens M, Chance SA, Boche D. Microglia and brain plasticity in acute psychosis and schizophrenia illness course: a meta-review. *Front Psychiatry.* (2017) 8:238. doi: 10.3389/fpsyt.2017.00238

18. Miller BJ, Buckley P, Seabolt W, Mellor A, Kirkpatrick B. Meta-analysis of cytokine alterations in schizophrenia: clinical status and antipsychotic effects. *Biol Psychiatry.* (2011) 70:663–71. doi: 10.1016/j.biopsych.2011.04.013

19. Flatow J, Buckley P, Miller BJ. Meta-analysis of oxidative stress in schizophrenia. *Biol Psychiatry.* (2013) 74:400–9. doi: 10.1016/j.biopsych.2013.03.018

20. Kay SR, Fiszbein A, Opler LA. The positive and negative syndrome scale (PANSS) for schizophrenia. *Schizophr Bull.* (1987) 13:261–76. doi: 10.1093/schbul/13.2.261

21. Wallwork RS, Fortgang R, Hashimoto R, Weinberger DR, Dickinson D. Searching for a consensus five-factor model of the Positive and Negative Syndrome Scale for schizophrenia. *Schizophr Res.* (2012) 137:246–50. doi: 10.1016/j.schres.2012.01.031

22. Arnhard K, Pitterl F, Sperner-Unterweger B, Fuchs D, Koal T, Oberacher H. A validated liquid chromatography-high resolution-tandem mass spectrometry method for the simultaneous quantitation of tryptophan, kynurenine, kynurenic acid, and quinolinic acid in human plasma. *Electrophoresis.* (2018) 39:1171–80. doi: 10.1002/elps.201700400

23. Heyes MP, Quearry BJ. Quantification of 3-hydroxykynurenine in brain by high-performance liquid chromatography and electrochemical detection. *J Chromatogr.* (1988) 428:340–4. doi: 10.1016/S0378-4347(00)83925-0

24. Benjamini Y, Hochberg Y. Controlling the false discovery rate: a practical and powerful approach to multiple testing. *J R Stat Soc Ser B.* (1995) 57:289–300. doi: 10.1111/j.2517-6161.1995.tb02031.x

25. Frydecka D, Krzystek-Korpacka M, Lubeiro A, Stramecki F, Stanczykiewicz B, Beszlej JA, et al. Profiling inflammatory signatures of schizophrenia: a cross-sectional and meta-analysis study. *Brain Behav Immun.* (2018) 71:28–36. doi: 10.1016/j.bbi.2018.05.002

26. Cao B, Wang D, Brietzke E, McIntyre RS, Pan Z, Cha D, et al. Characterizing amino-acid biosignatures amongst individuals with schizophrenia: a case-control study. *Amino Acids.* (2018) 50:1013–23. doi: 10.1007/s00726-018-2579-6

27. Leppik L, Kriisa K, Koido K, Koch K, Kajalaid K, Haring L, et al. Profiling of amino acids and their derivatives biogenic amines before and after antipsychotic treatment in first-episode psychosis. *Front Psychiatry.* (2018) 9:155. doi: 10.3389/fpsyt.2018.00155

28. Plitman E, Iwata Y, Caravaggio F, Nakajima S, Chung JK, Gerretsen P, et al. Kynurenic acid in schizophrenia: a systematic review and meta-analysis. *Schizophr Bull.* (2017) 43:764–77. doi: 10.1093/schbul/sbw221

29. Chiappelli J, Notarangelo FM, Pocivavsek A, Thomas MAR, Rowland LM, Schwarcz R, et al. Influence of plasma cytokines on kynurenine and kynurenic acid in schizophrenia. *Neuropsychopharmacology.* (2018) 43:1675–80. doi: 10.1038/s41386-018-0038-4

30. Szymona K, Zdzisinska B, Karakula-Juchnowicz H, Kocki T, Kandefer-Szerszen M, Flis M, et al. Correlations of kynurenic acid, 3-hydroxykynurenine, sIL-2R, IFN-alpha, and IL-4 with clinical symptoms during acute relapse of schizophrenia. *Neurotox Res.* (2017) 32:17–26. doi: 10.1007/s12640-017-9714-0

31. Ravikumar A, Deepadevi KV, Arun P, Manojkumar V, Kurup PA. Tryptophan and tyrosine catabolic pattern in neuropsychiatric disorders. *Neurol India.* (2000) 48:231–8.

32. Myint AM, Schwarz MJ, Verkerk R, Mueller HH, Zach J, Scharpe S, et al. Reversal of imbalance between kynurenic acid and 3-hydroxykynurenine by antipsychotics in medication-naive and medication-free schizophrenic patients. *Brain Behav Immun.* (2011) 25:1576–81. doi: 10.1016/j.bbi.2011.05.005

33. Fazio F, Lionetto L, Curto M, Iacovelli L, Cavallari M, Zappulla C, et al. Xanthurenic acid activates mGlu2/3 metabotropic glutamate receptors and is a potential trait marker for schizophrenia. *Sci Rep.* (2015) 5:17799. doi: 10.1038/srep17799

34. Meier TB, Drevets WC, Teague TK, Wurfel BE, Mueller SC, Bodurka J, et al. Kynurenic acid is reduced in females and oral contraceptive users: Implications for depression. *Brain Behav Immun.* (2018) 67:59–64. doi: 10.1016/j.bbi.2017.08.024

35. Franceschi C, Capri M, Monti D, Giunta S, Olivieri F, Sevini F, et al. Inflammaging and anti-inflammaging: a systemic perspective on aging and longevity emerged from studies in humans. *Mech Ageing Dev.* (2007) 128:92–105. doi: 10.1016/j.mad.2006.11.016

36. Capuron L, Schroecksnadel S, Feart C, Aubert A, Higueret D, Barberger-Gateau P, et al. Chronic low-grade inflammation in elderly persons is associated with altered tryptophan and tyrosine metabolism: role in neuropsychiatric symptoms. *Biol Psychiatry.* (2011) 70:175–82. doi: 10.1016/j.biopsych.2010.12.006

37. De Picker L, Ottoy J, Verhaeghe J, Deleye S, Wyffels L, Fransen E, et al. State-associated changes in longitudinal [18F]-PBR111 TSPO PET Imaging of psychosis patients: evidence for the accelerated ageing hypothesis? *Brain Behav Immun.* (2018) 77:46–54. doi: 10.1016/j.bbi.2018.11.318

38. Ottoy J, De Picker L, Verhaeghe J, Deleye S, Wyffels L, Kosten L, et al. [(18)F]PBR111 PET imaging in healthy controls and schizophrenia: test - retest reproducibility and quantification of neuroinflammation. *J Nucl Med.* 59:1267–74. doi: 10.2967/jnumed.117.203315

39. Savitz J, Drevets WC, Wurfel BE, Ford BN, Bellgowan PS, Victor TA, et al. Reduction of kynurenic acid to quinolinic acid ratio in both the depressed and remitted phases of major depressive disorder. *Brain Behav Immun.* (2015) 46:55–9. doi: 10.1016/j.bbi.2015.02.007

40. Maia-de-Oliveira JP, Trzesniak C, Oliveira IR, Kempton MJ, Rezende TM, Iego S, et al. Nitric oxide plasma/serum levels in patients with schizophrenia: a systematic review and meta-analysis. *Rev Bras Psiquiatr.* (2012) 34(Suppl 2):S149–55. doi: 10.1016/j.rbp.2012.07.001

41. Badawy AA, Doughrty DM, Marsh-Richard DM, Steptoe A. Activation of liver tryptophan pyrrolase mediates the decrease in tryptophan availability to the brain after acute alcohol consumption by normal subjects. *Alcohol Alcohol.* (2009) 44:267–71. doi: 10.1093/alcalc/agp005

42. Schwarcz R, Stone TW. The kynurenine pathway and the brain: challenges, controversies and promises. *Neuropharmacology.* (2017) 112(Pt B):237–47. doi: 10.1016/j.neuropharm.2016.08.003

43. Allegri G, Bertazzo A, Biasiolo M, Costa CV, Ragazzi E. Kynurenine pathway enzymes in different species of animals. *Adv Exp Med Biol.* (2003) 527:455–63. doi: 10.1007/978-1-4615-0135-0_53

44. Gal EM, Sherman AD. L-kynurenine: its synthesis and possible regulatory function in brain. *Neurochem Res.* (1980) 5:223–39. doi: 10.1007/BF00964611

45. Miller CL, Llenos IC, Dulay JR, Barillo MM, Yolken RH, Weis S. Expression of the kynurenine pathway enzyme tryptophan 2,3-dioxygenase is increased

in the frontal cortex of individuals with schizophrenia. *Neurobiol Dis.* (2004) 15:618–29. doi: 10.1016/j.nbd.2003.12.015

46. Erhardt S, Schwieler L, Imbeault S, Engberg G. The kynurenine pathway in schizophrenia and bipolar disorder. *Neuropharmacology.* (2017) 112(Pt B):297–306. doi: 10.1016/j.neuropharm.2016.05.020

47. Adams S, Teo C, McDonald KL, Zinger A, Bustamante S, Lim CK, et al. Involvement of the kynurenine pathway in human glioma pathophysiology. *PLoS ONE.* (2014) 9:e112945. doi: 10.1371/journal.pone.0112945

48. Wirthgen E, Hoeflich A, Rebl A, Gunther J. Kynurenic acid: the janus-faced role of an immunomodulatory tryptophan metabolite and its link to pathological conditions. *Front Immunol.* (2017) 8:1957. doi: 10.3389/fimmu.2017.01957

8

Activation of the Kynurenine Pathway in Human Malignancies can be Suppressed by the Cyclin-Dependent Kinase Inhibitor Dinaciclib

Christin Riess [1,2,3], Björn Schneider [4], Hanna Kehnscherper [3], Julia Gesche [3], Nina Irmscher [3], Fatemeh Shokraie [1], Carl Friedrich Classen [1], Elisa Wirthgen [1], Grazyna Domanska [5], Annette Zimpfer [4], Daniel Strüder [6], Christian Junghanss [3] and Claudia Maletzki [3]*

[1] University Children's Hospital, Rostock University Medical Centre, Rostock, Germany, [2] Institute for Medical Microbiology, Virology, and Hygiene, Rostock University Medical Centre, Rostock, Germany, [3] Medical Clinic III - Hematology, Oncology, Palliative Care, Department of Internal Medicine, Rostock University Medical Center, Rostock, Germany, [4] Institute of Pathology, Rostock University Medical Center, University of Rostock, Rostock, Germany, [5] Institute of Immunology and Transfusion Medicine, University of Greifswald, Greifswald, Germany, [6] Department of Otorhinolaryngology, Head and Neck Surgery "Otto Koerner", Rostock University Medical Center, Rostock, Germany

*Correspondence:
Claudia Maletzki
claudia.maletzki@med.uni-rostock.de

Indoleamine 2,3-dioxygenase (IDO) and tryptophan 2,3-dioxygenase (TDO2) are the key enzymes of tryptophan (TRP) metabolism in the kynurenine pathway (KP). Both enzymes function as indicators of immunosuppression and poor survival in cancer patients. Direct or indirect targeting of either of these substances seems thus reasonable to improve therapy options for patients. In this study, glioblastoma multiforme (GBM) as well as head and neck squamous cell carcinomas (HNSCC) were examined because of their different mechanisms of spontaneous and treatment-induced immune escape. Effects on gene expression and protein levels were examined. Accompanying assessment of TRP metabolites from treated GBM cell culture supernatants was conducted. Our results show a heterogeneous and inversely correlated expression profile of TRP-metabolizing genes among GBM and HNSCC cells, with low, but inducible *IDO1* expression upon IFNγ treatment. *TDO2* expression was higher in GBM cells, while genes encoding kynurenine aminotransferases were mainly confined to HNSCC cells. These data indicate that the KP is active in both entities, with however different enzymes involved in TRP catabolism. Upon treatment with Temozolomide, the standard of care for GBM patients, *IDO1* was upregulated. Comparable, although less pronounced effects were seen in HNSCC upon Cetuximab and conventional drugs (i.e., 5-fluorouracil, Gemcitabine). Here, *IDO1* and additional genes of the KP (*KYAT1*, *KYAT2*, and *KMO*) were induced. Vice versa, the novel yet experimental cyclin-dependent kinase inhibitor Dinaciclib suppressed KP in both entities. Our comprehensive data imply inhibition of the TRP catabolism by Dinaciclib, while conventional chemotherapeutics tend to activate this pathway. These data point to limitations of conventional therapy and highlight the potential of targeted therapies to interfere with the cells' metabolism more than anticipated.

Keywords: targeted therapy, solid tumor models, tryptophan metabolites, IDO1, chemotherapy

INTRODUCTION

Tumor cells release immunosuppressive factors that shape a tolerogenic environment and enable progression and invasion. Indoleamine 2,3-dioxygenase (IDO1) is an intracellular monomeric, immune-checkpoint molecule that degrades the essential amino acid l-tryptophan along the kynurenine pathway (KP) (1, 2). Like other immune checkpoints, including programmed cell death protein 1 and cytotoxic T-lymphocyte-associated protein 4, IDO suppresses the hosts' antitumor immunity by inducing apoptosis in T- and natural killer cells (3). As a direct consequence of this, many cancer and cancer-associated cells express IDO1 (mesenchymal stromal cells, myeloid-derived suppressor cells, dendritic cells, endothelial cells, tumor-associated macrophages, and fibroblasts) (3–6). IDO1 is influenced by interferon-γ (IFNγ) (7–9), nitric oxide (10), pro- [interleukin (IL)-1β, tumor necrosis factor α] and anti-inflammatory (IL4, IL10, transforming growth factor β) cytokines. IDO1 activity inhibits T-cell activation and proliferation and even mediates regulatory T-cell recruitment to the tumor microenvironment, provoking local immune tolerance. In head and neck squamous cell carcinomas (HNSCCs), IDO1 inversely correlates with programmed cell death protein ligand 1, which constitutes an important prognostic biomarker for immune-checkpoint inhibition (11). The increased IDO1 activation decreases intratumoral TRP levels, resulting in tumor starvation and increase in kynurenine (KYN) metabolites (which are toxic to lymphocytes) (12). This immune exhaustion may be further boosted by conventional chemotherapeutics, leading to decreased efficacy. Therefore, IDO1 overexpression in the tumor microenvironment intimately impairs patients' outcome and may serve as a future prognostic predictor and drug target (13–18).

In the KP, most studies focused on IDO1 because this molecule is amenable to pharmacological intervention (19–22), and a couple of specific and global IDO inhibitors [including natural compounds (17, 23, 24)] already entered clinical trials, mostly reporting safe application and efficacy (stable disease at best outcome) (25). Current trials are evaluating the efficacy of IDO1 inhibitors in combination with chemotherapy, radiotherapy, and other immunotherapies including cytotoxic T-lymphocyte-associated protein 4 blockade (11, 22). The latter is based on the observation of an enhanced lytic ability of tumor-antigen-specific T cells upon IDO1 inhibition and decreased numbers of local immunosuppressive cells such as regulatory T cells and myeloid-derived suppressor cells (20, 26). The efficacy and toxicity data from recent clinical trials with IDO1 inhibitors is reviewed in Yentz and Smith (27). In most cases, however, overall survival was not significantly improved, leaving the future role for this combination therapy in question (28). More key enzymes are involved in TRP metabolism: tryptophan 2.3-dioxygenase (TDO2), a member of the oxidoreductases family, catalyzes the same initial step of the KP as IDO1 (2). Thus, TDO2 has been shown to be constitutively and highly expressed in various cancer cells such as malignant glioma and HNSCC (29, 30). More importantly, TDO2 also has immunomodulatory functions by promoting immune tolerance. This, in turn, promotes survival, growth, invasion, and metastasis and decreases patients' survival (just like IDO1) (13, 22, 31, 32).

In this study, we performed a comprehensive analysis on the expression status of genes belonging to the KP. HNSCC and glioblastoma multiforme (GBM) were picked as prime examples for different spontaneous and treatment-induced immune escape mechanisms. Therefore, expression changes were determined under standard and targeted therapy, and results were compared among each other.

MATERIALS AND METHODS

Tumor Cell Lines and Culture Conditions

Patient-derived GBM cell lines (N = 13; HROG02, HROG04, HROG05, HROG06, HROG10, HROG15, HROG24, HROG36, HROG38, HROG52, HROG63, HROG73, HROG75) and HNSCC cell lines (N = 6; FADU, Detroit-562, Cal-33, PE/CA/PJ-15, UT-SCC-14, UT-SCC-15) were either established and basically characterized in our lab or originally obtained from the German collection of cell cultures (DSMZ; Braunschweig, Germany). UT-SCC14 and UT-SCC15 cells were kindly provided by Prof. R. Grenman [University of Turku, Finland (33)]. All cells were routinely cultured in our lab and maintained in full medium: Dulbecco's modified Eagle Medium/HamsF12 supplemented with 10% fetal calf serum, glutamine (2 mmol/L), and antibiotics (medium and supplements were purchased from PAA, Cölbe, Germany). For functional analysis, cell lines from each tumor entity were chosen, and all subsequent experiments were performed with these lines only.

IFNγ Stimulation

Cells were cultured in six-well plates or ibidi chamber slides, incubated overnight and treated with IFNγ (50 ng/ml, Immunotools, Friesoythe, Germany) for 24 and 72 h, respectively. Thereafter, cells were harvested and further processed.

Cytostatic Drugs and Targeted Substance

Cytostatics used in this study included 5-fluorouracil (5-FU) (2.5 μM), Cisplatin (0.2 μM), Gemcitabine (0.0002 μM), and Cetuximab (0.34 μM) for HNSCC, as well as Temozolomide (10 μM, TMZ) for GBM (pharmacy of the University Hospital Rostock). CDKi Dinaciclib (10 or 100 nM) was used as experimental targeted drug. All substances were used in doses below the IC_{50} as determined before.

Apoptosis/Necrosis Assay

A Yo-Pro-1/PI-based assay for discriminating early apoptotic, late apoptotic, and necrotic cells was applied as described before (34).

Hemolysis Assay

Hemolytic activity of Dinaciclib was determined by hemoglobin release from whole blood cells after 2 h of incubation. Briefly,

---

Abbreviations: CDKi, cyclin-dependent kinase inhibitor; GBM, glioblastoma multiforme; HNSCC, head and neck squamous cell carcinoma; IDO1, indoleamine 2,3-dioxygenase; IFN, interferon; KYAT, kynurenine aminotransferase; KP, kynurenine pathway; PBMC, peripheral blood mononuclear cells; SCC, squamous cell carcinoma; TDO2, tryptophan 2,3-dioxygenase.

whole blood of healthy donors ($N = 5$) was seeded in 96-well plates and treated with increasing Dinaciclib doses (ranging from 1, 5, and $10 \mu M$). Negative controls were left untreated, and positive controls (=maximum lysis) were treated with 1% sodium dodecyl sulfate. Following the incubation period, cell-free supernatants were transferred into a new 96-well plate, and absorption was measured on a plate reader at 560 nm (reference wave length, 750 nm). Hemolytic activity was quantified according to the following formula and corrected for spontaneous hemolysis (=untreated controls):

$$\%\text{Hemolysis} = ((OD_{560nm}\text{sample}$$
$$-OD_{560nm}\text{buffer})/OD_{560nm}\text{max} - OD_{560nm}\text{buffer}) \times 100$$

In addition, peripheral blood mononuclear cells' (PBMC) viability ($N = 5$) were determined by Calcein AM staining. This was done upon 24 h incubation at the above-mentioned doses. Fluorescence measurement and quantification were done as described (34).

IDO1 Immunofluorescence

Tumor cells were treated with 50 ng/ml of IFNγ (Immunotools), TMZ, Cetuximab, or Dinaciclib for 24 h in chamber slides, respectively. Cells were washed with phosphate-buffered saline, fixed in 4% paraformaldehyde w/o methanol (Thermo Scientific, Darmstadt, Germany) for 20 min, washed again, followed by cell permeabilization in 0.3% Triton X−100/5% normal bovine serum in phosphate-buffered saline for 60 min. Cells were then incubated overnight at 4°C in monoclonal rabbit IDO1 primary antibody (1:100; Cell Signaling Technology, Frankfurt/Main, Germany). Cells were washed, labeled with fluorochrome-conjugated secondary antibody using goat antirabbit secondary antibody (1:250, Boster Biological Technology, Pleasanton CA, USA), and incubated in the dark for 2 h. Cell nuclei were stained with 4′,6-diamidino-2-phenylindole (DAPI), and cells were analyzed with a Zeiss LSM-780 Confocal Laser Microscope (Zeiss, Jena, Germany). Quantification of staining intensity was done using the ImageJ software. Therefore, channels were split into red, green, and blue. Subsequently, integrated density profiles of the same size were measured in the green channel.

IDO1 Immunohistochemistry on Patients' Tumor Samples

Primary antibody against IDO1 (rabbit IgG, clone D5J4E, Cell Signaling Technology, dilution 1:200) was used. All samples were pretreated for 20 min at 97°C and pH 6.9. Standard immunoperoxidase technique was applied using an automated immunostainer (DAKO link) with diaminobenzidine as chromogen. IDO1 expression was defined as cytoplasmatic and membranous staining in >1% inflammatory cells.

Quantification of Tryptophan, Kynurenine, and Kynurenic Acid in Cell Culture Supernatant by Liquid Chromatography Tandem Mass Spectrometry System

The basis for the measurement was the method of Fuertig et al. which was adapted to the system used here (35).

Sample Preparation

Cell culture supernatant was mixed 1:1 with internal standards [$10 \mu M$ D5-kynurenic acid (Buchem BV, Apeldoorn, Netherlands), $10 \mu M$ D5-phenylalanine (Cambridge Isotope Laboratories, Inc. Andover, MA, United States), $5 \mu M$ D4-kynurenine (Cambridge Isotope Laboratories), $10 \mu M$ D5-tryptophan (Sigma Aldrich, Hamburg, Germany), $10 \mu M$ D3-quinolinic acid (Buchem BV), 5.5 nM 15N5-8-hydroxy-2-deoxyguanosine (Cambridge Isotope Laboratories)], and with 10 μl of mobile phase (0.4% formic acid, 1% acetonitrile in water). Reagents were gently shaken on a mixer, and 150 μl of ice-cold methanol was added. Samples were incubated overnight at −20°C to allow protein precipitation. On the following day, samples were centrifugated at 0°C and $18,000 \times g$ for 15 min. Supernatants were transferred to a new tube, and the liquid phase was removed by evaporation at 30°C among vacuum. Solid samples were stored until measurement at −20°C. Afterwards, dried extracts were reconstituted in 100 μl of acidified mobile phase. Samples were incubated at 40°C (1 h), centrifuged (4°C, $18,000 \times g$, 5 min), and clear supernatant (100 μl) was transferred onto a 96-well plate.

Liquid Chromatography Tandem Mass Spectrometry

Measurements were performed on an AB Sciex 5500 QTrap™ mass spectrometer (AB SCIEX, Darmstadt, Germany) with electrospray ionization in positive mode combined with a high-performance liquid chromatography system (Agilent 1260 Infinity Binary LC, Santa Clara, United States) including a degasser unit, column oven, autosampler, and a binary pump. Twenty microliters of the supernatant was injected and separated using a VisionHT C18 column (100 × 2.1 mm; particle size, 3 μm; Grace, MD, United States). To prevent contamination, a precolumn (VisionHT C18, Guard 5 × 2 mm) was used additionally. The temperature of the column oven was set at 15°C. The flowrate was set to 0.4 ml/min, and the sample was separated in a total run time of 11 min using solution A (water + 0.1% formic acid + 0.01% trifluoroacetic acid) and solution B (MeOH + 0.1% formic acid + 0.01% trifluoroacetic acid) with the following gradient: 0–2.8 min, 97% A, 3% B; 2.8–3.3 min, 70% A, 30% B; 3.3–4.4, 40% A, 60% B; 4.5–5.0 min, 40% A, 60% B; 5.0–5.5, 5% A, 95% B; 5.5–6.9 min, 5% A, 95% B; 6.9–7.0 min, 97% A, 3% B; 7.0–11.0 min, 97% A, 3% B.

The eluate between 0.5 and 9 min was introduced into the mass spectrometer and analyzed in MRM mode. The ion spray voltage (IS) was 4,000 V, the curtain gas flow was 40.0 psi, and the ion source temperature were set at 550°C.

Internal standards were used for metabolite quantification (**Table 1**). Data analysis, including peak integration and concentration determination, was performed with Analyst software (Version 1.5.1, AB Sciex, Darmstadt, Germany).

RNA Isolation, cDNA Synthesis, and Quantitative Real-Time PCR

Total RNA was isolated with RNeasy Mini Kit (Qiagen, Hilden, Germany) according to the manufacturers' instructions. RNA was reverse transcribed into complementary DNA (cDNA) from

1 µg RNA using 1 µl dNTP mix (10 mM), oligo (dT)15 primer (50 ng/µl), 1 µl reverse transcriptase (100 U), and 4 µl 5× reverse transcription buffer complete (all purchased from Bioron GmbH, Ludwigshafen, Germany). Final reaction volume was 20 µl (filled with RNAse free water). cDNA synthesis conditions were as follows: 70°C for 10 min, 45°C for 120 min, and 70°C for 10 min. Target cDNA levels of human cell lines were analyzed by quantitative real-time PCR using TaqMan Universal PCR Master Mix and self-designed TaqMan gene expression assays either labeled with 6-FAM-3′ BHQ-1 or 5′ HEX−3′ BHQ-1 to be used as duplex: *IDO1*, *TDO2*, *KMO*, *HAAO*, *KYAT1/2/3/4*, *KYNU*, *QPRT*, and *GAPDH*

or *β-actin* were used as housekeeping genes. Reaction was performed in the light cycler Viia7 (Applied Biosystems, Foster City, USA) with the following PCR conditions: 95°C for 10 min, 40 cycles of 15 s at 95°C, and 1 min at 60°C. All reactions were run in triplicates. The messenger RNA (mRNA) levels of target genes were normalized to *GAPDH/β-actin*. Reactions were performed in triplicate wells and repeated four times. The general expression level of each sample was considered by calculating $2^{-\Delta CT}$ ($\Delta Ct = Ct_{target} - Ct_{Housekeeping\ genes}$).

Statistical Analysis

All values are reported as mean ± SD. After proving the assumption of normality, differences between controls and treated cells were determined using the unpaired Student's *t*-test. If normality failed, the non-parametric Mann-Whitney *U*-test was applied. Statistical evaluation was performed using GraphPad PRISM software, version 5.02 (GraphPad Software, San Diego, CA, USA). In case of multiple comparisons, two- or one-way ANOVA on ranks (Bonferroni's multiple comparison test) was used. The criterion for significance was taken to be $p < 0.05$.

TABLE 1 | Internal standards.

Analyte	Q1 mass (m/z)	Q3 mass (m/z)	CE (V)	DP (V)
Tryptophan	205.1	118.0	28.0	39.0
d5-Tryptophan	210.1	122.1	37.0	31.0
Kynurenine	209.1	94.1	19.6	41.0
d4-Kynurenine	213.1	140.1	21.0	39.0
Kynurenic acid	190.1	162.0	24.0	65.0
d5-Kynurenic acid	195.1	167.1	24.0	65.0

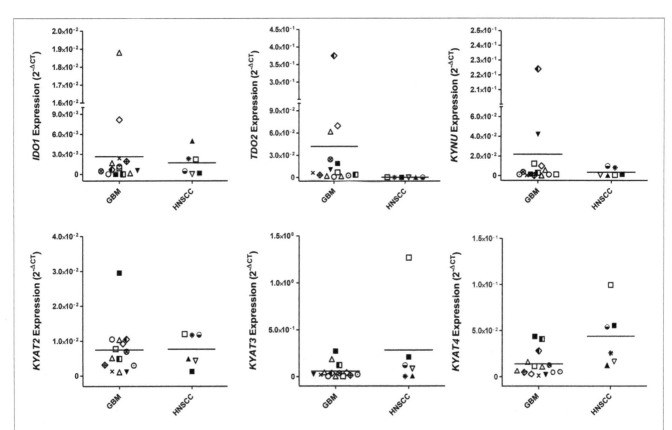

FIGURE 1 | Relative messenger RNA (mRNA) expression of IDO1, TDO2, KYNU, KYAT2, KYAT3, and KYAT4 in glioblastoma multiforme (GBM) and head and neck squamous cell carcinoma cells (HNSCC). The graphs indicate the mRNA expression normalized to the housekeeping genes ($2^{-\Delta CT}$). GBM (N = 13, HROG02, HROG04, HROG05, HROG06, HROG10, HROG15, HROG24, HROG36, HROG38, HROG52, HROG63, HROG73, HROG75) and HNSCC cell lines [N = 6; FADU, Detroit-562, Cal-33, PE/CA/PJ-15, UT-SCC14, UT-SCC-15 (33)].

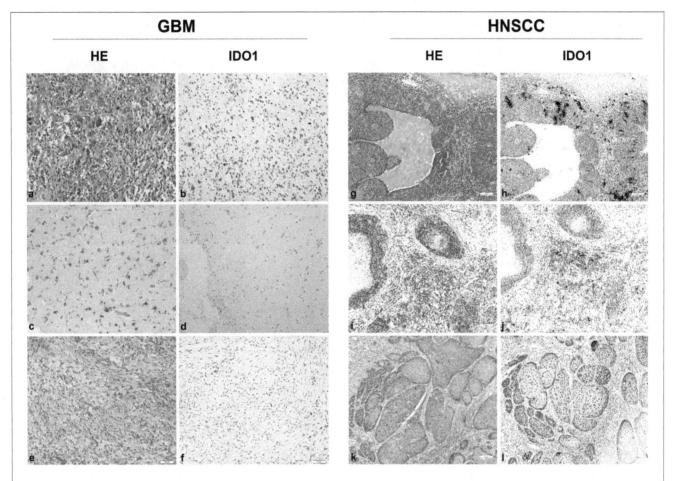

FIGURE 2 | IDO1 immunohistochemistry. Representative images of primary glioblastoma multiforme (GBM) [HROG36 **(a,b)**, HROG63 **(c,d)**, and HROG73 **(e,f)**] and head and neck squamous cell carcinoma (HNSCC) [HNSCC06 **(g,h)**, HNSCC02 **(i,j)**, HNSCC01 **(k,l)**] samples. Left panel: Routine HE staining. Right panel: Note the focal IDO1 expression on tumor-infiltrating lymphocytes exclusively in HNSCC cases. HNSCC case 1 **(g,h)**: tonsil (HPV[positive]); case 2 **(i,j)**: mouth base (HPV[negative], relapse); case 3 **(k,l)**: larynx (HPV[negative]). Pictures were taken at 20× and 10× magnification, respectively.

RESULTS

Basal IDO1 and Related Genes in GBM and HNSCC Cell Lines

While IDO1 itself is not the only mechanism by which tumors can resist immune-mediated killing, we studied the expression status of different KP-related genes on a panel of human GBM and HNSCC cell lines. These experiments revealed not only differences between both entities but also a heterogeneous profile of all tested genes among cell lines (**Figure 1**). *IDO1* was differently expressed by most glioma samples (11/13) analyzed. In general, *IDO1* was only detectable at very low levels (**Figure 1**). *TDO2*, the other rate-limiting enzyme of the KP (36), was constitutively expressed by all glioma samples, and expression was even higher in comparison to *IDO1*. Generally, expression status for *TDO2* and kynurenine hydrolase (*KYNU*) was higher in GBM, while HNSCC expressed more kynurenine aminotransferases (*KYAT*) (**Figure 1**). Hence, these data indicate that the KP is active in both entities, with however different enzymes being involved in TRP catabolism.

Still, tumor cell lines grown *in vitro* not necessarily represent the *in vivo* situation; we therefore analyzed the IDO1 abundance in clinical resection specimens (**Figure 2**). In GBM, IDO1 was detectable in one of three cases (representative images are shown in **Figure 2**). By contrast, HNSCC samples presented with IDO1 but only on a small fraction of tumor-infiltrating lymphocytes (**Figure 2**). Although not analyzed systematically, the only HPV[positive] case in this small cohort showed highest IDO1 abundance, nicely reflecting the tumors' immunogenicity (11, 37).

Gene Expression and Protein Changes Upon IFNγ Stimulation

IDO1 is an IFNγ-inducible enzyme. Upon stimulation, the KP is activated to induce immunosuppression. *In vitro* stimulation with IFNγ mimics the *in vivo* situation of an inflammatory microenvironment. Hence, upon immune-mediated inflammation, IDO1-negative tumor cells may upregulate *IDO1* as resistance mechanism.

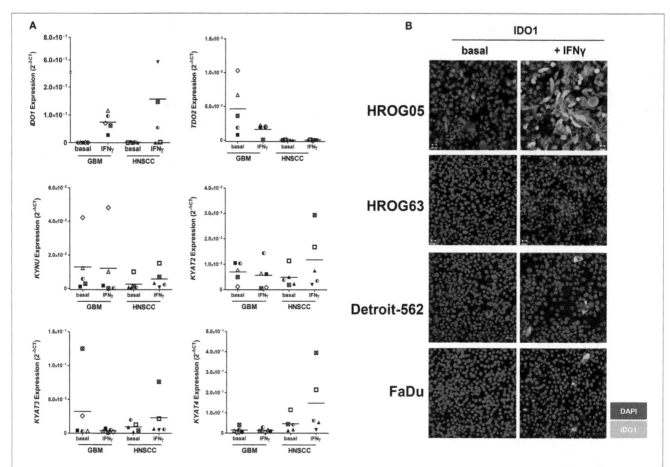

FIGURE 3 | Relative messenger RNA (mRNA) expression of *IDO1, TDO2, KYNU, KYAT2, KYAT3,* and *KYAT4* as well as IDO1 protein abundance following interferon-γ (IFNγ) stimulation in glioblastoma multiforme (GBM) and head and neck squamous cell carcinoma (HNSCC) cells. The cell cultures were either untreated or treated with IFNγ (50 ng/ml) for 24 h. **(A)** The graphs indicate the mRNA expression normalized to the housekeeping genes ($2^{-\Delta CT}$). GBM $N = 5$ cell lines (HROG02, HROG05, HROG52, HROG63, HROG75); HNSCC, $N = 4$ cell lines (FADU, Detroit-562, Cal-33, PE/CA/PJ-15). **(B)** IDO1 immunofluorescence in selected cell lines. Cell nuclei were stained with DAPI, and IDO1 was depicted by monoclonal rabbit IDO1 primary antibody (1:100; Cell Signaling Technology), followed by secondary antibody (1:250, Boster Biological Technology Pleasanton, CA, United States) labeling. Cells were analyzed with a Zeiss LSM-780 Confocal Laser Microscope. Original magnification 20×.

Using five individual GBM cell lines, *IDO1* expression was inducible in all cases (**Figure 3A**). Upregulation of *IDO1* was high on protein levels in HROG05 cells and marginal in HROG63 (**Figure 3B**). *TDO2* and *KYAT3* were suppressed upon IFNγ stimulation in three of five samples and hardly detectable in one cell line, supporting data from a recent publication (38). *KYNU* was not affected by IFNγ stimulation (**Figure 3A**).

Just as in GBM, *IDO1* was inducible in HNSCC cells (**Figure 3A**). Immunofluorescence revealed focal expression of singular cells with different intensity (**Figure 3B**). Of note, IFNγ stimulation even induced upregulation of *KYAT1, KYAT2, KYAT3,* and *KYAT4* (**Figure 3A** and data not shown), most likely constituting a compensatory mechanism as described before in experimental autochthonous tumor models (39).

Interference With the KP of Cytostatic and Targeted Therapies

Next, we examined whether cytostatic and targeted drugs have an influence on the KP. For GBM, TMZ was chosen, and for HNSCC, 5-FU, Cisplatin, Gemcitabine, as well as Cetuximab were used. As a targeted yet still experimental agent, the potent and specific CDKi Dinaciclib was applied to cells of both entities.

Before this experiment, drug doses were carefully tested in dose-response analyses (data not shown) along with discrimination of apoptosis and necrosis. Generally, drugs used in this study tended to induce necrosis, while apoptosis, if present, was only detectable at early time points. Exemplary results for the HNSCC cell line Detroit-562 are given in **Supplementary Figures 1A,B**. While cytostatics are well-known to affect normal cells' viability, the impact of the CDKi Dinaciclib on immune and red blood cells is less clear. We therefore performed a hemolysis and leukocyte viability assay. In this experiment, no toxicity was seen against normal cells (**Supplementary Figure 1C**). Even at high concentrations, Dinaciclib impaired cellular viability/integrity only marginally (**Supplementary Figure 1C**).

TMZ is an oral alkylating agent that methylates DNA at the O^6 position of guanine causing cell cycle arrest at G2/M. It is used as standard of care for GBM. However, acquired resistance, a process not fully understood, leads to

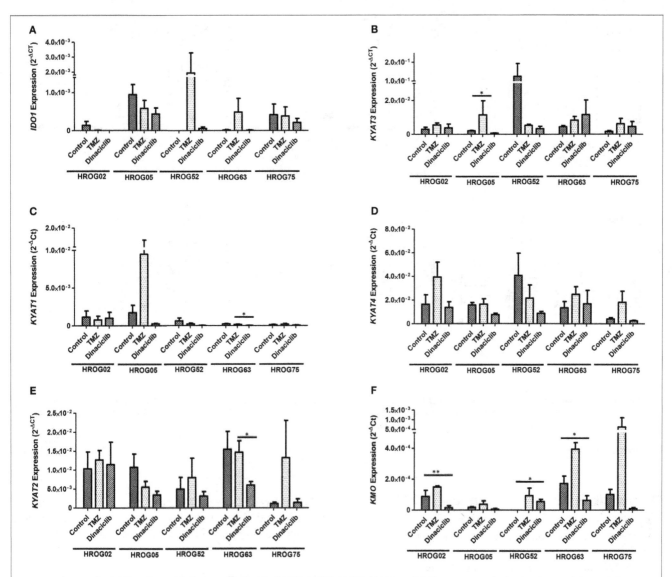

FIGURE 4 | Relative messenger RNA (mRNA) expression of *IDO1, KYAT1, KYAT2, KYAT3, KYAT4,* and KMO upon cytostatic drugs and targeted therapy in glioblastoma multiforme (GBM) cells. Graphs indicate the mRNA expression of selected kynurenine pathway (KP)-related genes normalized to the housekeeping genes ($2^{-\Delta CT}$). Results show data of three independent experiments. *$p < 0.05$; **$p < 0.01$ vs. control. Two-way ANOVA.

major limitations in treatment. Here, TMZ downregulated *IDO1* in three of five GBM cell lines but led to increased expression in HROG52 and HROG63—a paired GBM cell line established from the very same patient (primary lesion and upon relapse) (**Figure 4**). Gene expression of *KYAT2, KYAT4,* and *KMO* was heterogeneous. Generally, there was a trend toward higher expression of those genes but with cell-line-specific differences (e.g., *KYAT3*: $p < 0.05$ vs. control in HROG05 cells; **Figure 4**). *KYNU* expression was not affected by TMZ (data not shown). Interestingly, the combination of IFNγ and TMZ that mimics the *in vivo* situation led to similar or even stronger *IDO1* upregulation compared to IFNγ alone in two out of four glioma samples (**Figure 5**). Adding Dinaciclib to either IFNγ or TMZ lowered the mRNA expression of *IDO1* massively. Other KP-related genes like

TDO2 and *KYAT1-4* were similarly downregulated (**Figure 5**). **Supplementary Table for Figure 5** provides a detailed statistical analysis of each cell line in relation to the individual treatment regimens.

In HNSCC cells, Cetuximab was the only *IDO1*-inducing substance (exemplary results for Detroit-562 cells are given in **Figure 6**). Beyond that, the cytostatics as well as Cetuximab induced at least one of the KP-related genes ($p < 0.05$ vs. control), implicating activation of this pathway *via* different effectors. By adding Dinaciclib to cytostatic drugs, this effect was abrogated, even in the presence of IFNγ (**Figure 6** and data not shown). Of note, Dinaciclib alone as well as in combination with other substances effectively suppressed all KP-related genes, implying inhibition of the TRP catabolism by this CDKi.

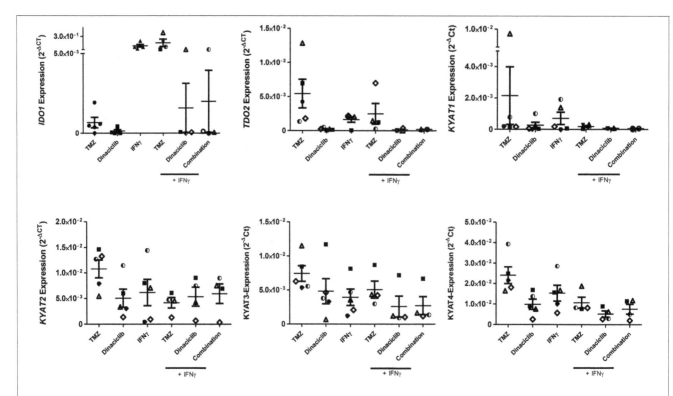

FIGURE 5 | Relative messenger RNA (mRNA) expression of *IDO1, TDO2, KYAT1, KYAT2, KYAT3,* and *KYAT4* upon concomitant treatment with interferon-γ (IFNγ) and cytostatic drugs in glioblastoma multiforme (GBM) cells. The cell cultures (*N* = 5, HROG02, HROG05, HROG52, HROG63, HROG75) were either left untreated or treated with IFNγ (50 ng/ml) for 24 h. Treatments were performed simultaneously, i.e., IFNγ ± TMZ, and/or Dinaciclib. Graphs indicate the mRNA expression of selected KP-related genes normalized to the housekeeping genes ($2^{-\Delta CT}$). Results show data of three independent experiments. A statistical report is given in **Supplementary Table for Figure 5**.

Dinaciclib Blocks IFNγ-Induced IDO1 Expression in GBM and HNSCC Cells

Considering the active downregulation of KP-related genes by Dinaciclib, we investigated whether this CDKi is able to inhibit or reverse IFNγ-induced IDO1 upregulation in GBM and HNSCC cells on a protein level. TMZ and Cetuximab were included as active inductors of *IDO1* and associated KP-related genes.

IFNγ and selected drugs were added simultaneously for 72 h. Dinaciclib effectively blocked IFNγ-induced IDO1 protein in both entities, while TMZ alone as well as the combination with IFNγ strongly enhanced IDO1 protein level (**Figure 7**). Hence, mRNA expression data were nicely confirmed.

When Dinaciclib was combined with IFNγ and TMZ, the IDO1-inducing stimulus of these latter substances was far too strong to be suppressed (**Figure 7**). However, the low number of residual cells in this combination hints toward additive or even synergistic effects independent from IDO1 (**Figures 7A,B**).

While IDO1 was highly inducible in GBM cells only, we then determined protein level upon IFNγ-prestimulation approaching the *in vivo* situation. The cytotoxic effect of Dinaciclib was preserved; however, levels of IDO1 enzyme were not significantly altered (**Supplementary Figures 2A,B**). Comparable results were obtained for TMZ. Virtually, all residual cells showed positive staining; still there was a trend toward lower intensity in monotherapy and in combination (**Supplementary Figure 2B**).

Taken together, the CDKi Dinaciclib is able to block IFNγ-mediated and thus most likely even chemotherapy-induced *IDO1* upregulation in GBM and HNSCC cells. However, blunt interference with this TRP-metabolizing enzyme is unlikely.

Treatment Induced Influence on KP-Related Metabolites

Our data revealed IDO1 induction by TMZ, which is reversible by Dinaciclib. Thus, we examined the influence on KP-related metabolites in GBM cell lines.

TRP, KYN, and the downstream metabolite kynurenic acid (KYNA) were quantified by MS using cell culture supernatants of GBM cell lines (**Figures 8A,B**). TRP was catabolized after 24 h from all cell lines among all treatment regimens. Adding TMZ or Dinaciclib in monotherapy marginally affected TRP consumption as well as KYN and KYNA production. Stimulation with either IFNγ or a combination of TMZ resulted in greatly enhanced TRP depletion and increased KYN levels, although to varying degrees in the different cell lines (**Figure 8A**). Small amounts of KYNA were produced constitutively and to a greater extent after IFNγ mono- and TMZ combination in all cell lines (**Figure 8A**). In contrast, KYNA level remained unchanged upon Dinaciclib in combination with IFNγ, confirming immunofluorescence results (please see **Figure 7** for details). The same was true for the KYN/TRP ratio, being only

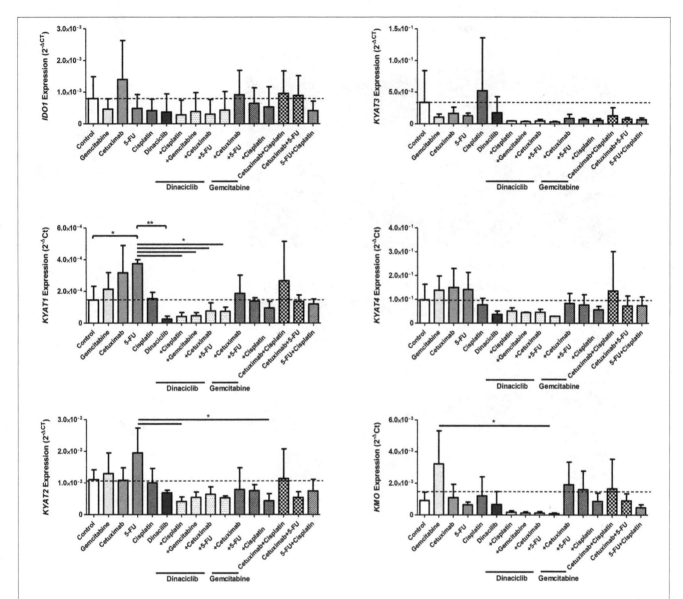

FIGURE 6 | Relative messenger RNA (mRNA) expression of *IDO1, KYAT1, KYAT2, KYAT3, KYAT4,* and KMO upon cytostatic drugs and targeted therapy in head and neck squamous cell carcinoma (HNSCC) cells. Graphs indicate the mRNA expression of selected KP-related genes normalized to the housekeeping genes ($2^{-\Delta CT}$). Results show data of three independent experiments using HNSCC cell line Detroit-562. *$p < 0.05$; **$p < 0.01$. One-way ANOVA (Bonferroni's multiple comparison test).

affected in samples treated with IFNγ as well as the combination of IFNγ and TMZ (**Figure 8B**).

These data underline our gene and protein expression data. The CDKi Dinaciclib is directly or indirectly capable of blocking the KP. TMZ particularly in combination with the proinflammatory cytokine IFNγ accelerates TRP consumption accompanied by KYN and KYNA production in GBM cells.

DISCUSSION

The finding that high *IDO1* expression is associated with shorter survival in cancer patients made IDO1 a promising target either by specific inhibitors or indirectly by immunomodulation.

A recent study described dramatically suppressed tumor growth upon *IDO1* knockdown by increasing the number of CD4+ and CD8+ T cells in murine GBM models (9). However, the exact mechanisms underlying IDO1 and thus TRP metabolism along the KP remain unclear. Therefore, we focused on the expression of *IDO1* and *IDO*-related KP genes and their potential involvement in immune evasion in experimental models of HNSCC and GBM.

We were able to show that the KP is active in both entities, with different enzymes involved in TRP catabolism. Of note, basal *IDO1* expression was low and inversely correlated with *TDO2*. In the only prior study on primary GBM cultures, similar results were described with constitutive *TDO2* expression in

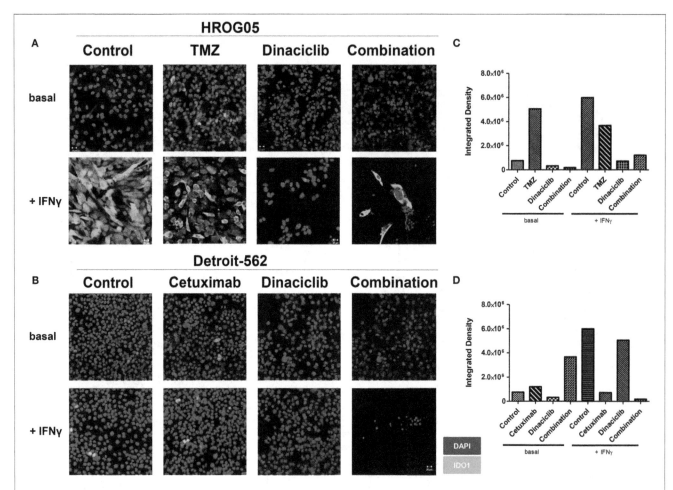

FIGURE 7 | Indoleamine 2,3-dioxygenase (IDO1) protein abundance in selected glioblastoma multiforme (GBM) and head and neck squamous cell carcinoma (HNSCC) cells upon cytostatic drugs and targeted therapy. The cell cultures [(A) GBM: HROG05; (B) HNSCC: Detroit-562] were either left untreated or treated with IFNγ (50 ng/ml) for 24 h. Treatments were performed simultaneously, i.e., IFNγ ± TMZ, Cetuximab, and/or Dinaciclib. Cell nuclei were stained with DAPI. Original magnification 20×. (C,D) Quantification was done to score staining intensity in untreated and treated HROG05 and Detroit-562 cells. This was carried out using ImageJ software as described in Material and Methods.

most GBM cell cultures (29). In here, TDO2 likely promotes tumor growth by suppressing antitumor immune responses (2, 31). KP products are considered as therapeutic targets because *IDO1* and other genes of the TRP metabolism are not expressed in healthy brain tissue, but gradually increase with GBM dedifferentiation (low vs. high grade GBM). In HNSCC, different results on *IDO1* are documented, and expression is heterogeneous among different HNSCC cell lines. Of note, IDO1 abundance of primary resection specimen and cultured cells seems to be independent from anatomical site and HPV status (40). Still, IDO1 is a useful marker for progression of in oral squamous cell carcinoma (41). In esophageal squamous cell carcinoma, progression and metastasis correlates with strong inflammation at the tumors' invasive front and disturbed TRP metabolism (42). These cumulative data highlight the biological relevance of the KP in malignancies and may explain why IDO1 is barely detectable upon long-term *in vitro* culture. By mimicking the inflamed microenvironment and thus taking a step closer to the *in vivo* situation, IFNγ was added as strong IDO1 inductor

(43). While GBM cells responded with the expected *IDO1* upregulation on mRNA expression and protein level as well as accelerated TRP consumption, this molecule was barely inducible in HNSCC cells. It is conceivable that this is due to the duration of *in vitro* culture. GBM cells were established recently and thus used in defined low passages (<P40), whereas half of the HNSCC cell lines were long-term cultures with more or less unknown passage [Detroit-562 as well as UT-SCC14 and UT-SCC15 (44) are the only exceptions; <P40]. Cell lines may acquire additional mutations overtime changing their protein expression. Another *in vitro* limitation is that experiments were conducted without immunological pressure. *In vivo* studies are desirable to verify the results.

Indirect effects of TRP metabolism include interference with other biological functions like migration, angiogenesis, and cell growth regulation (18, 40). To investigate the influence of anticancer drugs on TRP catabolism, we performed a comprehensive analysis using conventional chemotherapy (TMZ, 5-FU, Cisplatin, Gemcitabine) and targeted drugs

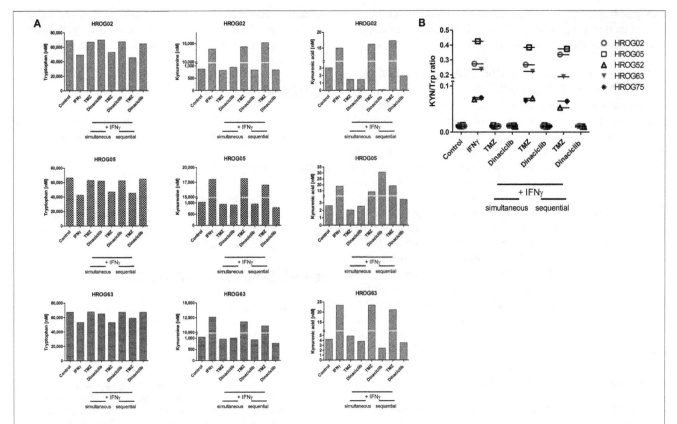

FIGURE 8 | Indoleamine 2,3-dioxygenase (IDO) protein abundance in glioblastoma multiforme (GBM) and head and neck squamous cell carcinoma (HNSCC) cells as well as kynurenine pathway (KP) metabolite levels in GBM cells upon cytostatic drugs and targeted therapy. Treatments were performed sequentially, i.e., interferon-γ (IFNγ) pretreatment for IDO1 induction, followed by Temozolomide (TMZ) and/or Dinaciclib. **(A)** KP metabolites changed upon TMZ but not Dinaciclib treatment. The combination of TMZ and IFNγ accelerates tryptophan (TRP) consumption accompanied by kynurenine (KYN) and kynurenic acid (KYNA) production **(B)**. KYN/TRP ratios in GBM cells were determined dividing KYN values by TRP values. Results show data of a single measurement.

(Cetuximab, Dinaciclib). The KP-related gene expression and metabolites were determined in residual cells. In GBM, the standard of care drug TMZ was applied either with or without IFNγ stimulation. While this substance affected *IDO1* on the expression level, the amount of the resulting protein increased. This may be explained by either increased protein's half-life due to a reduced rate of degradation or the preferential translation during cellular stress. In previous studies, exposure of several cultured human malignant glioma cell lines, primary neurons, and a neuroblastoma cell line to IFNγ reduced TRP levels in culture medium accompanied by increased *IDO1* expression and KYN production (29, 45). Our results confirm these data, and in addition, we were able to demonstrate that IFNγ stimulation in combination with TMZ stimulated KYN and KYNA production and TRP catabolism in GBM cell cultures. The increase in TRP catabolism and KYN production (KYN/TRP ratio) is widely used as indirect indicator of the cumulative activities of TDO2, IDO1, and IDO-2 (38, 46). The KP in brain tumors is likely triggered by IFNγ from immediate surrounding tissue (29, 47, 48). Thus, *IDO1* expression in brain tumor cells is likely to be triggered when IFNγ is produced from activated T cells and/or microglia and neurons. Furthermore, gliomas and glioneuronal tumors have an elevated tryptophan uptake and catabolism *in vivo* (49).

Given our observation on a further enhanced KP activity upon TMZ treatment, this might provide an explanation of (acquired) drug resistance and final relapse. Hence, IDO1 blocking agents should be investigated in TMZ-tailored therapeutic approaches.

In HNSCC cells, KP activation was different. KP-related genes were exclusively induced by standard drugs, and only Cetuximab induced *IDO1*. Additional upregulated genes involved kynurenine aminotransferases, responsible for synthesizing a neuroprotectant, and KMO. While the specific biochemical activity of these molecules and biological relevance in cancer is barely examined, we interpret this result as one possible mechanism of resistance upon therapy—a finding quite common after conventional chemotherapy and usually also being associated with poor response toward neoadjuvant therapy in other entities (50).

Mechanistically, this can be attributed to the secretion of proinflammatory substances, such as prostaglandin E2 or high-mobility group protein B1 by dying tumor cells, secondary contributing to KP activation. By accumulating TRP, toxic metabolites of tumor cells actively shape an immunosuppressive microenvironment. Breaking down this shield is one of the main objectives in pharmacological inhibition of KP. Questions remain why most inhibitors failed in clinical trials, and mechanisms are only just beginning to become clear. A fact worth mentioning is the functional redundancy of IDO1, IDO-2, and TDO2 (51), augmenting the risk of mechanistic bypass.

Dinaciclib is a potent and specific CDK inhibitor of CDK1, CDK2, CDK5, and CDK9. Preclinical studies showed that this inhibitor is capable of decelerating tumor growth in numerous cancer entities via cell cycle arrest and apoptosis induction (52, 53). In our study, Dinaciclib was the only KP-inhibiting substance tested here. Of note, impairment of the KP was independent from the combination partner, and this CDKi effectively suppressed IFNγ-induced *IDO1* upregulation after simultaneous treatment. While this result was completely unexpected and has—to the best of our knowledge—not been described previously, our data do not support the idea of blunt interference with the KP. GBM cells with strong *IDO1* expression showed only marginally reduced IDO1 protein level after Dinaciclib treatment. This effect might be boosted after long or repeated treatment cycles. In line with these findings, several preclinical studies already proposed synergistic effects of selective and unselective IDO1 inhibitors when administered in conjunction with chemo- and/or radiotherapy (4). This may finally have impact for second- or third-line immunotherapeutic approaches. Therefore, the late KYN/TRP index is indeed a relevant clinical benchmark providing prognostic value for GBM patients (54).

Summarizing our findings, we provide evidence for the relevance of TRP catabolism in malignancies especially in the context of standard therapy. The CDKi Dinaciclib was identified as indirect KP inhibitor. Lastly, specific KP inhibition may increase the efficacy of standard drugs by restoring immune function and thus improve patients' outcome.

AUTHOR CONTRIBUTIONS

CR performed experiments, analyzed data, and participated in manuscript writing. BS and AZ performed immunohistochemistry and analysis, and provided images. HK, JG, NI, and FS performed experiments and analyzed data. GD performed LC-MS analyses. CC and CJ participated in paper finalization and critically revised the manuscript. DS and EW critically revised the manuscript. CM designed study, the outline of the manuscript, performed data interpretation, and wrote the manuscript.

FUNDING

CM was supported by grants from the Deutsche Forschungsgemeinschaft (MA5799/2-1 and MA5799/2-2).

ACKNOWLEDGMENTS

The authors are also grateful to Susanne Neumeister and Dr. Ann-Kristin Henning from the Institute of Clinical Chemistry and Laboratory Medicine, University of Greifswald, for assisting with the quantification of TRP metabolites.

SUPPLEMENTARY MATERIAL

Supplementary Figure 1 | Quantitative analysis of cell death in Detroit-562 HNSCC cells upon cytostatic drugs and targeted therapy. The cells were treated with the given substances for 24 and 72 h. Thereafter, cells were harvested and stained with Yo-Pro-1 to detect early and late apoptotic cells, as well as propidium iodide for necrosis determination. Apoptosis/necrosis discrimination was done on a flow cytometer (BD FACSVerse™) as described in material and methods. **(A)** Quantitative analysis of cell death after 24 and 72 h, respectively. *$p < 0.05$ vs. control; **$p < 0.01$ vs. control. t-test. **(B)** Representative dot plots showing elevated numbers of necrotic cells upon treatment. **(C)** Hemolysis and viability of PBMC upon treatment with Dinaciclib. Therefore, whole blood and PBMC were cultured in the presence of increasing Dinaciclib concentrations (1, 5, and 10 μM) for 2 and 24 h, respectively. Hemolytic activity was determined from cell-free supernatants (red blood cell lysis), Calcein AM was used for quantifying viability of PBMC. Mean + SD, $N = 5$ individual donors.

Supplementary Figure 2 | IDO1 protein abundance in HROG05 GBM cells upon cytostatic drugs and targeted therapy. The cells were pretreated with IFNγ (50 ng/ml) for 24 h. Thereafter TMZ, Dinaciclib and the combination of both substances was added to see whether IFNγ-induced upregulation of IDO1 is reversible. **(A)** None of these substances downregulated IDO1 in the sequential setting. Cell nuclei were stained with DAPI. Original magnification 20x. **(B)** Quantification was done to score staining intensity in untreated and treated HROG05 cells. This was carried out by using ImageJ software as described in material and methods.

Supplementary Table for Figure 5 | Statistical analysis of individual treatment regimens, depicted for each cell line, and genes analyzed.

REFERENCES

1. Liu M, Wang X, Wang L, Ma X, Gong Z, Zhang S, et al. Targeting the IDO1 pathway in cancer: from bench to bedside. *J Hematol Oncol.* (2018) 11:100. doi: 10.1186/s13045-018-0644-y
2. Platten M, Wick W, Van den Eynde BJ. Tryptophan catabolism in cancer: beyond IDO and tryptophan depletion. *Cancer Res.* (2012) 72:5435–40. doi: 10.1158/0008-5472.CAN-12-0569
3. Gajewski TF, Schreiber H, Fu Y-X. Innate and adaptive immune cells in the tumor microenvironment. *Nat Immunol.* (2013) 14:1014–22. doi: 10.1038/ni.2703

4. Muller AJ, DuHadaway JB, Donover PS, Sutanto-Ward E, Prendergast GC. Inhibition of indoleamine 2,3-dioxygenase, an immunoregulatory target of the cancer suppression gene Bin1, potentiates cancer chemotherapy. *Nat Med.* (2005) 11:312–9. doi: 10.1038/nm1196
5. Moon YW, Hajjar J, Hwu P, Naing A. Targeting the indoleamine 2,3-dioxygenase pathway in cancer. *J Immunother Cancer.* (2015) 3:51. doi: 10.1186/s40425-015-0094-9
6. Munn DH, Mellor AL. IDO in the tumor microenvironment: inflammation, counter-regulation, and tolerance. *Trends Immunol.* (2016) 37:193–207. doi: 10.1016/j.it.2016.01.002

7. Avril T, Saikali S, Vauleon E, Jary A, Hamlat A, De Tayrac M, et al. Distinct effects of human glioblastoma immunoregulatory molecules programmed cell death ligand-1 (PDL-1) and indoleamine 2,3-dioxygenase (IDO) on tumour-specific T cell functions. *J Neuroimmunol.* (2010) 225:22–33. doi: 10.1016/j.jneuroim.2010.04.003

8. Wainwright DA, Chang AL, Dey M, Balyasnikova IV, Kim CK, Tobias A, et al. Durable therapeutic efficacy utilizing combinatorial blockade against IDO, CTLA-4, and PD-L1 in mice with brain tumors. *Clin Cancer Res.* (2014) 20:5290–301. doi: 10.1158/1078-0432.CCR-14-0514

9. Hanihara M, Kawataki T, Oh-Oka K, Mitsuka K, Nakao A, Kinouchi H. Synergistic antitumor effect with indoleamine 2,3-dioxygenase inhibition and temozolomide in a murine glioma model. *J Neurosurg.* (2016) 124:1594–601. doi: 10.3171/2015.5.JNS141901

10. Badawy AAB. Kynurenine pathway of tryptophan metabolism: regulatory and functional aspects. *Int J Tryptophan Res.* (2017) 10:1178646917691938. doi: 10.1177/1178646917691938

11. Solomon B, Young RJ, Rischin D. Head and neck squamous cell carcinoma: genomics and emerging biomarkers for immunomodulatory cancer treatments. *Semin Cancer Biol.* (2018) 52:228–40. doi: 10.1016/j.semcancer.2018.01.008

12. Acovic A, Gazdic M, Jovicic N, Harrell CR, Fellabaum C, Arsenijevic N, et al. Role of indoleamine 2,3-dioxygenase in pathology of the gastrointestinal tract. *Therap Adv Gastroenterol.* (2018) 11:1756284818815334. doi: 10.1177/1756284818815334

13. Sordillo PP, Sordillo LA, Helson L. The kynurenine pathway: a primary resistance mechanism in patients with glioblastoma. *Anticancer Res.* (2017) 37:2159–71. doi: 10.21873/anticanres.11551

14. Zamanakou M, Germenis AE, Karanikas V. Tumor immune escape mediated by indoleamine 2,3-dioxygenase. *Immunol Lett.* (2007) 111:69–75. doi: 10.1016/j.imlet.2007.06.001

15. Ma W-J, Wang X, Yan W-T, Zhou Z-G, Pan Z-Z, Chen G, et al. Indoleamine-2,3-dioxygenase 1/cyclooxygenase 2 expression prediction for adverse prognosis in colorectal cancer. *World J Gastroenterol.* (2018) 24:2181–90. doi: 10.3748/wjg.v24.i20.2181

16. Brandacher G, Perathoner A, Ladurner R, Schneeberger S, Obrist P, Winkler C, et al. Prognostic value of indoleamine 2,3-dioxygenase expression in colorectal cancer: effect on tumor-infiltrating T cells. *Clin Cancer Res.* (2006) 12:1144–51. doi: 10.1158/1078-0432.CCR-05-1966

17. Jeong Y-I, Kim SW, Jung ID, Lee JS, Chang JH, Lee C-M, et al. Curcumin suppresses the induction of indoleamine 2,3-dioxygenase by blocking the Janus-activated kinase-protein kinase Cdelta-STAT1 signaling pathway in interferon-gamma-stimulated murine dendritic cells. *J Biol Chem.* (2009) 284:3700–8. doi: 10.1074/jbc.M807328200

18. Platten M, von Knebel Doeberitz N, Oezen I, Wick W, Ochs K. Cancer immunotherapy by targeting IDO1/TDO and their downstream effectors. *Front Immunol.* (2014) 5:673. doi: 10.3389/fimmu.2014.00673

19. Uyttenhove C, Pilotte L, Theate I, Stroobant V, Colau D, Parmentier N, et al. Evidence for a tumoral immune resistance mechanism based on tryptophan degradation by indoleamine 2,3-dioxygenase. *Nat Med.* (2003) 9:1269–74. doi: 10.1038/nm934

20. Fox E, Oliver T, Rowe M, Thomas S, Zakharia Y, Gilman PB, et al. Indoximod: an immunometabolic adjuvant that empowers T cell activity in cancer. *Front Oncol.* (2018) 8:370. doi: 10.3389/fonc.2018.00370

21. Beatty GL, O'Dwyer PJ, Clark J, Shi JG, Bowman KJ, Scherle PA, et al. First-in-human phase I study of the oral inhibitor of indoleamine 2,3-dioxygenase-1 epacadostat (INCB024360) in patients with advanced solid malignancies. *Clin Cancer Res.* (2017) 23:3269–76. doi: 10.1158/1078-0432.CCR-16-2272

22. Platten M, Nollen EAA, Röhrig UF, Fallarino F, Opitz CA. Tryptophan metabolism as a common therapeutic target in cancer, neurodegeneration and beyond. *Nat Rev Drug Discov.* (2019) 18:379–401. doi: 10.1038/s41573-019-0016-5

23. Kanai M, Yoshimura K, Asada M, Imaizumi A, Suzuki C, Matsumoto S, et al. A phase I/II study of gemcitabine-based chemotherapy plus curcumin for patients with gemcitabine-resistant pancreatic cancer. *Cancer Chemother Pharmacol.* (2011) 68:157–64. doi: 10.1007/s00280-010-1470-2

24. Maletzki C, Scheinpflug P, Witt A, Klar E, Linnebacher M. Targeting immune-related molecules in cancer therapy: a comprehensive *in vitro* analysis on patient-derived tumor models. *Biomed Res Int.* (2019) 2019:4938285. doi: 10.1155/2019/4938285

25. Vacchelli E, Aranda F, Eggermont A, Sautes-Fridman C, Tartour E, Kennedy EP, et al. Trial watch: IDO inhibitors in cancer therapy. *Oncoimmunology.* (2014) 3:e957994. doi: 10.4161/21624011.2014.957994

26. Schafer CC, Wang Y, Hough KP, Sawant A, Grant SC, Thannickal VJ, et al. Indoleamine 2,3-dioxygenase regulates anti-tumor immunity in lung cancer by metabolic reprogramming of immune cells in the tumor microenvironment. *Oncotarget.* (2016) 7:75407–24. doi: 10.18632/oncotarget.12249

27. Yentz S, Smith D. Indoleamine 2,3-dioxygenase (IDO) inhibition as a strategy to augment cancer immunotherapy. *BioDrugs.* (2018) 32:311–7. doi: 10.1007/s40259-018-0291-4

28. Long GV, Dummer R, Hamid O, Gajewski TF, Caglevic C, Dalle S, et al. Epacadostat plus pembrolizumab versus placebo plus pembrolizumab in patients with unresectable or metastatic melanoma (ECHO-301/KEYNOTE-252): a phase 3, randomised, double-blind study. *Lancet Oncol.* (2019) 20:1083–97. doi: 10.1016/S1470-2045(19)30274-8

29. Adams S, Teo C, McDonald KL, Zinger A, Bustamante S, Lim CK, et al. Involvement of the kynurenine pathway in human glioma pathophysiology. *PLoS ONE.* (2014) 9:e112945. doi: 10.1371/journal.pone.0112945

30. Ball HJ, Jusof FF, Bakmiwewa SM, Hunt NH, Yuasa HJ. Tryptophan-catabolizing enzymes—party of three. *Front Immunol.* (2014) 5:485. doi: 10.3389/fimmu.2014.00485

31. Pilotte L, Larrieu P, Stroobant V, Colau D, Dolusic E, Frederick R, et al. Reversal of tumoral immune resistance by inhibition of tryptophan 2,3-dioxygenase. *Proc Natl Acad Sci USA.* (2012) 109:2497–502. doi: 10.1073/pnas.1113873109

32. Abdel-Magid AF. Targeting the inhibition of tryptophan 2,3-dioxygenase (TDO-2) for cancer treatment. *ACS Med Chem Lett.* (2017) 8:11–3. doi: 10.1021/acsmedchemlett.6b00458

33. Jamieson SM, Tsai P, Kondratyev MK, Budhani P, Liu A, Senzer NN, et al. Evofosfamide for the treatment of human papillomavirus-negative head and neck squamous cell carcinoma. *JCI Insight.* (2018) 3:122204. doi: 10.1172/jci.insight.122204

34. Maletzki C, Klier U, Marinkovic S, Klar E, Andrä J, Linnebacher M. Host defense peptides for treatment of colorectal carcinoma-a comparative *in vitro* and *in vivo* analysis. *Oncotarget.* (2014) 5:4467–79. doi: 10.18632/oncotarget.2039

35. Fuertig R, Ceci A, Camus SM, Bezard E, Luippold AH, Hengerer B. LC-MS/MS-based quantification of kynurenine metabolites, tryptophan, monoamines and neopterin in plasma, cerebrospinal fluid, and brain. *Bioanalysis.* (2016) 8:1903–17. doi: 10.4155/bio-2016-0111

36. Opitz CA, Litzenburger UM, Sahm F, Ott M, Tritschler I, Trump S, et al. An endogenous tumour-promoting ligand of the human aryl hydrocarbon receptor. *Nature.* (2011) 478:197–203. doi: 10.1038/nature10491

37. Guo T, Califano JA. Molecular biology and immunology of head & neck cancer. *Surg Oncol Clin N Am.* (2015) 24:397–407. doi: 10.1016/j.soc.2015.03.002

38. Adam I, Dewi DL, Mooiweer J, Sadik A, Mohapatra SR, Berdel B, et al. Upregulation of tryptophanyl-tRNA synthetase adapts human cancer cells to nutritional stress caused by tryptophan degradation. *Oncoimmunology.* (2018) 7:e1486353. doi: 10.1080/2162402X.2018.1486353

39. Smith C, Chang MY, Parker KH, Beury DW, DuHadaway JB, Flick HE, et al. IDO is a nodal pathogenic driver of lung cancer and metastasis development. *Cancer Discov.* (2012) 2:722–35. doi: 10.1158/2159-8290.CD-12-0014

40. Bates AM, Gomez Hernandez MP, Lanzel EA, Qian F, Brogden KA. Matrix metalloproteinase (MMP) and immunosuppressive biomarker profiles of seven head and neck squamous cell carcinoma (HNSCC) cell lines. *Transl Cancer Res.* (2018) 7:533–42. doi: 10.21037/tcr.2018.05.09

41. Seppala M, Halme E, Tiilikainen L, Luukkainen A, Laranne J, Rautiainen M, et al. The expression and prognostic relevance of indoleamine 2,3-dioxygenase in tongue squamous cell carcinoma. *Acta Otolaryngol.* (2016) 136:729–35. doi: 10.3109/00016489.2016.1152631

42. Cheng J, Jin H, Hou X, Lv J, Gao X, Zheng G. Disturbed tryptophan metabolism correlating to progression and metastasis of esophageal squamous cell carcinoma. *Biochem Biophys Res Commun.* (2017) 486:781–7. doi: 10.1016/j.bbrc.2017.03.120

43. Grant RS, Naif H, Espinosa M, Kapoor V. IDO induction in IFN-gamma activated astroglia: a role in improving cell viability during oxidative stress. *Redox Rep.* (2000) 5:101–4. doi: 10.1179/135100000101535357

44. Tonlaar N, Galoforo S, Thibodeau BJ, Ahmed S, Wilson TG, Yumpo Cardenas P, et al. Antitumor activity of the dual PI3K/MTOR inhibitor, PF-04691502, in combination with radiation in head and neck cancer. *Radiother Oncol.* (2017) 124:504–12. doi: 10.1016/j.radonc.2017.08.001

45. Miyazaki T, Moritake K, Yamada K, Hara N, Osago H, Shibata T, et al. Indoleamine 2,3-dioxygenase as a new target for malignant glioma therapy. Laboratory investigation. *J Neurosurg.* (2009) 111:230–7. doi: 10.3171/2008.10.JNS081141

46. Suzuki Y, Suda T, Asada K, Miwa S, Suzuki M, Fujie M, et al. Serum indoleamine 2,3-dioxygenase activity predicts prognosis of pulmonary tuberculosis. *Clin Vaccine Immunol.* (2012) 19:436–42. doi: 10.1128/CVI.05402-11

47. Guillemin GJ, Smythe G, Takikawa O, Brew BJ. Expression of indoleamine 2,3-dioxygenase and production of quinolinic acid by human microglia, astrocytes, and neurons. *Glia.* (2005) 49:15–23. doi: 10.1002/glia.20090

48. Adams S, Braidy N, Bessede A, Brew BJ, Grant R, Teo C, et al. The kynurenine pathway in brain tumor pathogenesis. *Cancer Res.* (2012) 72:5649–57. doi: 10.1158/0008-5472.CAN-12-0549

49. Juhasz C, Chugani DC, Muzik O, Wu D, Sloan AE, Barger G, et al. *In vivo* uptake and metabolism of alpha-[11C]methyl-L-tryptophan in human brain tumors. *J Cereb Blood Flow Metab.* (2006) 26:345–57. doi: 10.1038/sj.jcbfm.9600199

50. Li F, Wei L, Li S, Liu J. Indoleamine-2,3-dioxygenase and Interleukin-6 associated with tumor response to neoadjuvant chemotherapy in breast cancer. *Oncotarget.* (2017) 8:107844–58. doi: 10.18632/oncotarget.22253

51. Muller AJ, Manfredi MG, Zakharia Y, Prendergast GC. Inhibiting IDO pathways to treat cancer: lessons from the ECHO-301 trial and beyond. *Semin Immunopathol.* (2019) 41:41–8. doi: 10.1007/s00281-018-0702-0

52. Parry D, Guzi T, Shanahan F, Davis N, Prabhavalkar D, Wiswell D, et al. Dinaciclib (SCH 727965), a novel and potent cyclin-dependent kinase inhibitor. *Mol Cancer Ther.* (2010) 9:2344–53. doi: 10.1158/1535-7163.MCT-10-0324

53. Lin SF, Lin JD, Hsueh C, Chou TC, Wong RJ. A cyclin-dependent kinase inhibitor, dinaciclib in preclinical treatment models of thyroid cancer. *PLoS ONE.* (2017) 12:e172315. doi: 10.1371/journal.pone.0172315

54. Zhai L, Dey M, Lauing KL, Gritsina G, Kaur R, Lukas RV, et al. The kynurenine to tryptophan ratio as a prognostic tool for glioblastoma patients enrolling in immunotherapy. *J Clin Neurosci.* (2015) 22:1964–8. doi: 10.1016/j.jocn.2015.06.018

9

Constitutive Expression of the Immunosuppressive Tryptophan Dioxygenase TDO2 in Glioblastoma is Driven by the Transcription Factor C/EBPβ

Takumi Kudo[1,2,3], Mirja T. Prentzell[4], Soumya R. Mohapatra[4], Felix Sahm[1,5], Zhongliang Zhao[6], Ingrid Grummt[6], Wolfgang Wick[7,8], Christiane A. Opitz[4,8], Michael Platten[1,2]* and Edward W. Green[1,2]*

[1] DKTK CCU Neuroimmunology and Brain Tumor Immunology, German Cancer Research Center (DKFZ), Heidelberg, Germany, [2] Department of Neurology, Medical Faculty Mannheim, Heidelberg University, Mannheim, Germany, [3] Department of Neurosurgery, Tokyo Medical and Dental University, Tokyo, Japan, [4] DKTK Brain Cancer Metabolism Group, German Cancer Research Center (DKFZ), Heidelberg, Germany, [5] Department of Neuropathology, Institute of Pathology, University Hospital Heidelberg, Heidelberg, Germany, [6] DKTK Division Molecular Biology of the Cell, German Cancer Research Center (DKFZ), Heidelberg, Germany, [7] DKTK CCU Neurooncology, German Cancer Research Center (DKFZ), Heidelberg, Germany, [8] Neurology Clinic and National Center for Tumor Diseases, University Hospital of Heidelberg, Heidelberg, Germany

Correspondence:
Michael Platten
m.platten@dkfz.de
Edward W. Green
e.green@dkfz.de

Catabolism of the essential amino acid tryptophan is a key metabolic pathway contributing to the immunosuppressive tumor microenvironment and therefore a viable drug target for cancer immunotherapy. In addition to the rate-limiting enzyme indoleamine-2,3-dioxygenase-1 (IDO1), tryptophan catabolism via tryptophan-2,3-dioxygenase (TDO2) is a feature of many tumors, particularly malignant gliomas. The pathways regulating TDO2 in tumors are poorly understood; using unbiased promoter and gene expression analyses, we identify a distinct CCAAT/enhancer-binding protein β (C/EBPβ) binding site in the promoter of TDO2 essential for driving constitutive TDO2 expression in glioblastoma cells. Using The Cancer Genome Atlas (TCGA) data, we find that C/EBPβ expression is correlated with TDO2, and both are enriched in malignant glioma of the mesenchymal subtype and associated with poor patient outcome. We determine that TDO2 expression is sustained mainly by the LAP isoform of CEBPB and interleukin-1β, which activates TDO2 via C/EBPβ in a mitogen-activated protein kinase (MAPK) kinase-dependent fashion. In summary, we provide evidence for a novel regulatory and therapeutically targetable pathway of immunosuppressive tryptophan degradation in a subtype of glioblastoma with a particularly poor prognosis.

Keywords: TDO2, glioblastoma, regulation, CEBPB, tryptophan, IL1B

INTRODUCTION

Malignant gliomas are characterized by profound local and systemic immunosuppression (1), which blunts the efficacy of the novel immunotherapeutic treatments for malignant gliomas (2). Overcoming the immunosuppressive glioma microenvironment is therefore an important challenge (3). The enzymatic degradation of tryptophan (Trp) to kynurenine (Kyn), mediated by indoleamine-2,3-dioxygenase-1 (IDO1) or tryptophan-2,3-dioxygenase (TDO2), is a key immunosuppressive pathway operative in gliomas and other types of tumors (4–8), and an emerging drug target in cancer immunotherapy (9–11). Trp metabolism promotes local immune tolerance by both inducing anergy and apoptosis of CD8-positive T cells, and activating regulatory T (Treg) cells, mainly through accumulation of immunosuppressive Kyn (12, 13). IDO1 is known to be overexpressed in many tumors – including gliomas – with both tumor and stromal cells contributing to IDO1 activity (5, 14–16). More recently, TDO2 has been shown to be expressed in many tumors and to promote tumor growth by suppressing antitumor immune responses in a similar fashion (17–20) (**Supplementary Figure S1**). In contrast to IDO1, whose regulation has been thoroughly characterized and involves tumor suppressor genes (21), oncogenes (22), growth factor/cytokine signaling pathways (23), and epigenetic mechanisms (24), the regulation of TDO2 in gliomas is not well understood. Here, we employed an unbiased approach to identify transcriptional regulators of TDO2.

MATERIALS AND METHODS

Cell Culture
The human malignant glioma cell line T98G was obtained from the American Type Culture Collection (ATCC), and cultured in Dulbecco's modified Eagle's medium (DMEM) containing 10% fetal bovine serum (Gibco), penicillin (100 U/mL), and streptomycin (100 µg/mL) (Gibco). Interleukin-1β (IL-1β) was purchased from R&D Systems (201-LB-005); SB203580 was purchased from AdipoGen (AG-CR1-0030-M001).

TDO2 Expression, Reporter Cloning and Luciferase Experiments
Fragments of the human TDO2 enhancer were amplified from T98G cells using the primers listed in **Supplementary Table S1** and ligated into the minimal promoter vector pGL4.26[luc2/minP/Hygro] (Promega E8441) using BglII–XhoI restriction sites. Reporter constructs were transfected into T98G cells using FuGene HD (Promega E2311), and cells were simultaneously co-transfected with a constitutively active renilla luciferase-expressing plasmid (pRL-TK, Promega E2231) as a transfection control. Forty-eight hours after transfection, reporter assays were performed according to the manufacturers' protocol using the Promega Dual-Luciferase Reporter Assay System (Promega E1910) and a PHERAstar FS instrument (BMG Labtech). Firefly luciferase was normalized to renilla luciferase expression. The CEBPB consensus sequence deletion construct was made using the Q5® Site-Directed Mutagenesis Kit (New England Biolabs E0554S) using primers listed in **Supplementary Table S1**.

Enhancer Binding Site Analysis
The enhancer region of TDO2 (−130 to −92 bp) was screened for putative transcription factor binding sites using an online implementation of TFBIND[1]. TFBIND identifies putative transcription factor binding sites by identifying regions similar to those of transcription factor consensus binding motifs, using transcription factor-specific similarity cutoffs derived from the TRANSFAC database (R3.4). The TRANSFAC consensus motif identified for CEBPB in the TDO2 promoter was V$CEBPB_01, consensus motif "RNRTKNNGMAAKNN" with a score of 0.84 (exceeding the cutoff score of 0.81).

Chromatin Immunoprecipitation
Cells were fixed by adding formaldehyde directly to culture medium for 10 min (final concentration 1.0%). The reaction was quenched using glycine (final concentration 125 mM). Cells were washed twice with phosphate-buffered saline (PBS) before being resuspended in buffer A [100 mM of Tris-HCl at pH 8.0, and 10 mM of dithiothreitol (DTT)] on ice for 15 min, followed by vortexing and incubation at 30°C for 15 min. Cells were then spun down and resuspended iteratively in buffer B [10 mM of HEPES at pH 7.5, 10 mM of EDTA, 0.5 mM of EGTA, and 0.25% (w/v) Triton X-100], buffer C (10 mM of HEPES at pH 7.5, 10 mM of EDTA, 0.5 mM of EGTA, and 200 mM of NaCl), and finally buffer D [50 mM of Tris-HCl at pH 8.0, 10 mM of EDTA, 1% sodium dodecyl sulfate (SDS), and 0.5% proteinase inhibitor cocktail]. Samples were sonicated for 10 min, spun down, and sonicated for a further 10 min to generate fragments of 300–500 bp of length. DNA fragments were spun down and resuspended 1:5 with immunoprecipitation (IP) buffer [15 mM of Tris-HCl at pH 8.0, 1.2 mM of EDTA, 180 mM of NaCl, and 1.2% (w/v) Triton X-100]. Ten µL of blocked Protein A/G sepharose beads were added per mL of IP buffer, and the samples were incubated at 4°C for 1 h to pre-clear chromatin. One mL of supernatant was then incubated overnight at 4°C with 1–3 µg of antibody. A further 10 µL of blocked Protein A/G sepharose beads was added to each sample and incubated at 4°C for 1 h. Beads were then washed twice with 1 mL of each of the following buffers: low salt wash buffer [20 mM of Tris-HCl at pH 8.0, 2 mM of EDTA, 150 mM of NaCl, 0.1% (w/v) SDS, 1% (w/v) Triton X-100], High salt wash buffer (20 mM of Tris-HCl at pH 8.0, 2 mM of EDTA, 500 mM of NaCl, 0.1% (w/v) SDS, and 1% (w/v) Triton X-100), LiCl wash buffer [10 mM of Tris-HCl at pH 8.0, 1 mM of EDTA, 250 mM of LiCl, 1% (w/v) NP40, and 1% (w/v) deoxycholate], and Tris-EDTA (TE) buffer (pH 8.0). One hundred µL of 10% slurry was added to the beads. Samples were then boiled for 10 min, followed by 30 min incubation at 52°C with 40 µg of Protein K, and a further 10 min boiling. Beads were spun down, and the supernatant containing the precipitated DNA was analyzed by PCR using the primers in **Supplementary Table S1**.

CEBPB Overexpression
A custom codon-optimized cDNA of CEBPB in pDONR221 was purchased from Thermo Fisher Scientific (full sequence listed in **Supplementary Table S1**). LAP and LIP isoforms of CEBPB were generated by site-directed mutagenesis (New England Biolabs E0554S) using primers listed in **Supplementary Table S1**.

---

[1] http://tfbind.hgc.jp

Isoforms were cloned into the pMXs-GW-IRES-puro destination vector using Gateway™ cloning technology (Invitrogen). Cells were transfected using FuGene HD following the manufacturer's protocols (Promega). Expression values were compared using two-way ANOVA with Tukey's correction for multiple comparisons testing.

Bioinformatic Analysis of the Cancer Genome Atlas (TCGA) data, Survival Curves, and Gene Association

Expression data, overall survival data, and Spearman's correlation coefficients for glioblastoma (GBM) patients in The Cancer Genome Atlas (TCGA) study was downloaded from cBioportal[2] and Firebrowse[3]. Rank product was calculated as geometric mean of each rank. Subtype-specific analyses were performed on TCGA data downloaded using Firebrowse[3] followed by statistical analysis in R. For overall survival analysis, 525 GBM patients were divided into two groups according to CEBPB mRNA expression. p-value was calculated using the log-rank test in R.

Immunohistochemistry

Formalin-fixed paraffin-embedded GBM tissue was obtained from the archives of the Department of Neuropathology, Institute of Pathology, Heidelberg. For immunohistochemistry, sections cut into 3 μm were incubated and processed with rabbit anti-human TDO antibody (25) and rabbit anti-human C/EBPβ antibody (C-19, Santa Cruz Biotechnology) on a Ventana BenchMark XT immunostainer (Ventana Medical Systems, Tucson, AZ, United States). The Ventana staining procedure included pre-treatment with cell conditioner 1 (pH 6.0) for 60 min and followed by antibody incubation at 37°C for 32 min. Incubation was followed by Ventana standard signal amplification, UltraWash, counter−staining with one drop of hematoxylin for 4 min and one drop of bluing reagent for 4 min. For visualization, ultraViewUniversal DAB Detection Kit (Ventana Medical Systems) was used. For quantification of C/EBPβ and TDO protein levels, histo-scores with relative expression levels were calculated, and correlation was assessed using Spearman's rank correlation coefficient.

Quantitative Reverse Transcription PCR

Total RNA was extracted with RNeasy mini kit (Qiagen) followed by cDNA synthesis using the Applied Biosystems reverse transcription kit (Thermo Fisher). mRNA from biological triplicate experiments was measured by quantitative reverse transcription (qRT) PCR using primaQUANT SYBR Green reagents (Steinbrenner Laborsysteme GmbH) on a LightCycler 480 instrument (Roche). The primers for qRT-PCR were CAAATCCTCTGGGAGTTGGA (human TDO2 Fw), GTCCAAGGCTGTCATCGTCT (human TDO2 Rv), AAGCACAGCGACGAGTACAA (human CEBPB Fw), GTGAGCTCCAGGACCTTGTG (human CEBPB Rv),

CCCCGGTTTCTATAAATTGAGC (human GAPDH Fw), and CACCTTCCCCATGGTGTCT (human GAPDH Rv). Levels of TDO2 and CEBPB were calculated relative to GAPDH, with each reaction performed as a technical triplicate, and the results were normalized to TDO2 or CEBPB levels in respective control samples. Two-way ANOVA statistical analysis was performed using Prism 8.0, followed by Tukey's multiple comparisons tests, where appropriate.

Small Interfering RNA Experiments

Small interfering RNAs (siRNA) targeting CEBPB were ordered from Dharmacon (SMART-pool L-006423-00-0005), together with the ON-TARGET plus non-targeting pool control siRNAs (D-001810-10-05). siRNA target sequences were CCUCGCAGGUCAAGAGCAA, CUGCUU GGCUGCUGCGUAC, GCGCUUACCUCGGCUACCA, GCAC CCUGCGGAACUUGUU (human CEBPB) and UGGUUUAC AUGUCGACUAA, UGGUUUACAUGUUGUGUGA, UGGUU UACAUGUUUUCUGA, UGGUUUACAUGUUUUCCUA (non-targeting pool). Transfection of T98G cells was performed with Lipofectamine RNAiMAX (Invitrogen) according to the manufacturer's protocol, and knockdown efficiency was verified by either qRT-PCR or Western blot.

Western Blotting

Whole cell lysates were lysed with radioimmunoprecipitation assay (RIPA) buffer [50 mM/l of Tris-HCl (pH 8.0), 150 mM/l of sodium chloride, 0.5% (w/v) sodium deoxycholate, 0.1% (w/v) SDS, and 1.0% (w/v) NP-40 substitute] with complete protease inhibitor (Roche) for 20 min on ice and then centrifuged for 10 min (4°C, 13,000 rpm). Protein concentrations were measured by the Bio-Rad protein assay (Bio-Rad). Twenty μg of each samples was loaded on SDS–polyacrylamide gel electrophoresis (PAGE) and transferred to nitrocellulose membrane following immunoblotting using anti-C/EBPβ rabbit monoclonal (clone C-19, Santa Cruz) or anti-GAPDH goat polygclonal (LINARIS Biologische Produkte GmbH #LAH1064) antibodies. Pierce enhanced chemiluminescence (ECL) western blotting substrate was used to detect chemiluminescence using a ChemiDoc XRS + camera. Raw images taken were processed with Image Lab (version 5.2.1) and exported for publication as TIFF files with 600 dpi resolution. Quantification was performed using Image Lab; pixel values of each lane were normalized to the average value of all lanes and then normalized to the loading control GAPDH.

Kynurenine High-Performance Liquid Chromatography

High-performance liquid chromatography (HPLC) measurement of Kyn was performed in cell culture supernatants collected from each treatment type. One mL of supernatant sample was first treated with 168.6 μL of 72% trichloroacetic acid to precipitate out dissolved proteins; subsequently, samples were centrifuged at maximum speed for 10 min, and the resulting protein-free supernatants were transferred into glass HPLC vials for further HPLC analysis. Chromatographic

[2]http://www.cbioportal.org/
[3]http://firebrowse.org/

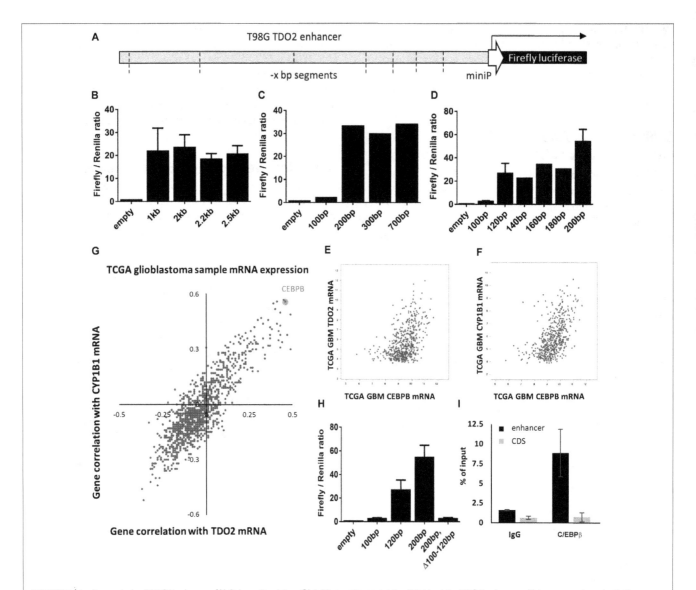

FIGURE 1 | *In vitro* analysis of TDO2 enhancer. **(A)** Schematic of the pGL4.26 reporter containing 2.5 kb of the TDO2 enhancer driving expression of a firefly luciferase gene. **(B–D)** Iterative deletion of the TDO2 enhancer defines a region between −100 and −120 bp as essential for TDO2 expression. Values are the mean of technical triplicates; standard error bars represent repeat experiments [n = 2 for B, n = 3 for selected constructs in panel **(D)**]. **(E)** Spearman's correlation coefficient was calculated between each gene expressed in The Cancer Genome Atlas (TCGA) glioblastoma (GBM) patients and both TDO2 and TDO2-induced aryl hydrocarbon receptor (AHR) target gene CYP1B1. **(F)** Correlation between CEBPB and TDO2 expression in TCGA GBM patients (Spearman: 0.47). **(G)** Correlation between CEBPB and CYP1B1 expression in TCGA GBM patients (Spearman: 0.56). **(H)** Deletion of the C/EBPβ binding site in the −100 to −120 bp enhancer region abrogates TDO2 expression. **(I)** Chromatin precipitation assay confirms an interaction between the TDO2 enhancer and C/EBPβ protein. Data are expressed ± standard deviation.

separation of Kyn was achieved on a Dionex Ultimate® 3000 UHPLC (Thermo Scientific) on a reversed-phase Accucore™ aQ column (Thermo Scientific™) with 2.6-μm particle size. The mobile phase gradient consisted of 0.1% trifluoroacetic acid (TFA) in water (A) and 0.1% TFA in acetonitrile (B). Standards for all analytes were utilized to determine the retention time and UV emission spectrum at 365 nm for Kyn. Analyte concentration in samples was analyzed by comparison with the respective standards using the Chromeleon™ 7.2 Chromatography Data System (Thermo Scientific™ Dionex™).

RESULTS

Identification of the Enhancer Motif Essential for Constitutive TDO2 Expression in T98G Glioma Cells

To identify the enhancer elements essential for the transcription of TDO2, 2.5 kb of enhancer sequence 5' of the TDO2 transcriptional start site was cloned from the constitutively TDO2-expressing T98G glioma cell line (18, 26). Insertion of this sequence into the pGL4.26 firefly luciferase reporter vector

TABLE 1 | TFBIND analysis of TDO2 enhancer.

Transcription factor	Number of sites	Mean site similarity score
AP1	6	0.805
AP2	1	0.796
AP4	2	0.797
CAAT	1	0.983
CAP	3	0.894
CEBPB	1	0.823
COMP1	1	0.809
CREB	3	0.808
CREBP1	1	0.789
GATA1	3	0.882
GATA2	3	0.845
GATA3	1	0.853
MYOD	1	0.813
NFY	2	0.950
OCT1	1	0.829
P53	4	0.856
S8	1	0.829
SP1	1	0.831
STAF	1	0.762
TAXCREB	1	0.751
VMAF	2	0.808

Transcription factors with binding sites overlapping the −100 to −120 bp human TDO2 enhancer region are essential for constitutive TDO2 expression in T98G cells.

TABLE 2 | TDO2-targeting transcription factors with correlations to both TDO2 and CYP1B1, ordered by rank product.

No.	TF	Correlation with		Rank
		TDO2	CYP1B1	Product
1	VDR	0.45	0.57	2.2
2	CEBPB	0.46	0.56	3.2
3	MAFB	0.49	0.49	3.2
4	FBN1	0.41	0.56	5.8
5	ELF4	0.43	0.50	7.1
6	STAT6	0.39	0.55	8.0
7	PLEK	0.47	0.38	8.1
8	BNC2	0.40	0.52	8.7
9	PLEK2	0.49	0.30	9.6
10	BATF	0.43	0.43	10.5

abolished TDO2 reporter activity in T98G cells, indicating that C/EBPβ is responsible for the constitutive TDO2 expression in this cell line. We then experimentally confirmed that C/EBPβ bound the TDO2 enhancer in T98G cells using a chromatin immunoprecipitation (ChIP) assay, showing that C/EBPβ precipitated significantly more TDO2 enhancer than did TDO2 gene body (**Figure 1I**).

C/EBPβ and TDO2 Protein Levels Are Correlated in Glioblastoma Samples and Are Associated With Poor Prognosis

C/EBPβ is a member of the *CCAAT/enhancer-binding proteins* (C/EBPs) family of leucine-zipper transcription factors that regulate gene expression controlling inflammation, differentiation, proliferation, and metabolism. In the context of glioma, C/EBPβ was reported as an initiator and master regulator of the GBM mesenchymal transition (28). To confirm that C/EBPβ-mediated expression of TDO2 was not a unique feature of T98G cells, we further examined the TCGA GBM gene expression database, finding both CEBPB and TDO2 to be enriched in the mesenchymal subtype of GBM (**Figure 2A**). We obtained slides of mesenchymal GBM tumors and confirmed that the correlation between CEBPB/TDO2 held true at the protein level using immunohistochemistry ($R^2 = 0.26$, **Figure 2B**). Finally, we examined the effect on patient survival using Cox regression modeling and log-rank testing, finding that GBM expressing high CEBPB showed modestly, but significantly, shorter overall survival in the TCGA dataset (log-rank $p = 0.0497$, **Figure 2C**).

CEBPB Expression Is Driven by IL-1β in Glioblastoma

As CEBPB is constitutively expressed, with higher levels in mesenchymal GBMs, we next aimed to delineate the signaling events responsible for constitutive CEBPB expression. IL-1β is a key cytokine produced by GBMs that stimulates C/EBPβ transcriptional activity (29, 30). Similar to TDO2 and CEBPB, IL1B was enriched in the mesenchymal subtype of GBM patients in the TCGA dataset (**Figure 3A**), and as expected, the expression

and transfection of this vector into T98G cells was confirmed to result in luciferase expression (**Figure 1A**). Iterative deletion of regions of the TDO2 enhancer (**Figures 1B–D**) revealed that motifs located between −100 and −120 bp from the transcriptional start site were essential for complete activation of the reporter construct, while the region between −180 and −200 bp contributed to high levels of TDO2 expression.

We used the TFBIND database (27) to identify 21 transcription factors with putative binding sites that would be disrupted by a deletion in the essential −100 and −120 bp region (**Table 1**). To narrow down this list to transcription factors driving TDO2 expression in gliomas, we interrogated TCGA dataset to find transcription factors showing strong transcriptional correlations with TDO2 (**Table 2**). TDO2 protein catalyzes the conversion of Trp to Kyn, activating the aryl hydrocarbon receptor (AHR) and leading to the upregulation of AHR target genes such as *cytochrome P450 oxygenase 1B1* (CYP1B1); therefore, we also determined correlations with CYP1B1 expression (**Table 2**) (18).

These analyses suggested that only *CCAAT/enhancer-binding protein β* (C/EBPβ) was predicted both to bind within the −92 to −130 bp of TDO2 enhancer essential region and to display a strong positive correlation with the expression of TDO2 (**Figure 1E**, Spearman: 0.47) and CYP1B1 (**Figure 1F**, Spearman: 0.56, **Figure 1G**) in TCGA GBM microarray data. We therefore deleted the putative binding motif of C/EBPβ in the TDO2 enhancer (ACCCTGCATCAGCC, −116 to −103 bp) and repeated the measurements of reporter activity (**Figure 1H**). We found that deletion of the C/EBPβ binding sequence

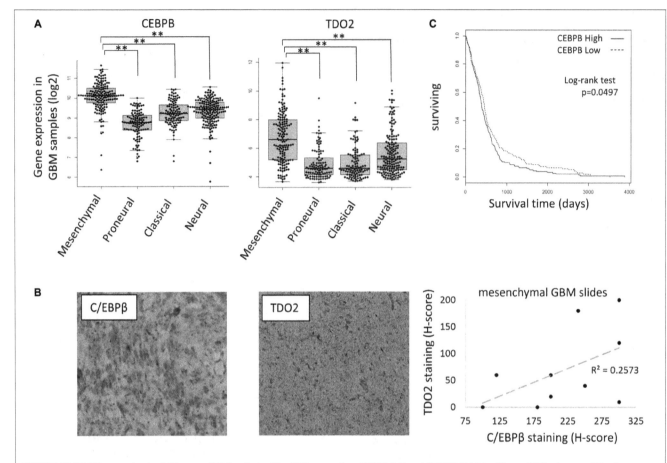

FIGURE 2 | CEBPB expression in glioblastoma (GBM) patients. **(A)** mRNA expression of TDO2 (left) and CEBPB (right) in different GBM subtypes of The Cancer Genome Atlas (TCGA) dataset. **(B)** Immunohistochemical staining confirms a correlation between C/EBPβ and TDO2 protein levels in pathologist-determined mesenchymal subtype GBM tumor sections. **(C)** Kaplan–Meier analysis of overall survival in GBM patients (all subtypes) according to CEBPB mRNA expression (log-rank $p = 0.0497$, high $n = 263$, low $n = 262$). *$p < 0.05$, **$p < 0.01$, ***$p < 0.001$, and ****$p < 0.0001$.

of IL1B positively correlated with TDO2 as well as CYP1B1 in GBM (**Figure 3B**). Log-rank testing showed that GBM patients with high IL1B expression showed significantly shorter overall survival (**Figure 3C**, $p = 0.034$), similar to patients expressing high CEBPB (**Figure 2C**, $p = 0.0497$).

Using T98G cells, we were able to show that TDO2 expression as well as Kyn production was increased by IL-1β treatment and that this effect was completely abolished by C/EBPβ knockdown (**Figure 3D**). Phosphorylation of C/EBPβ is important for its transcriptional activity, and p38 MAPK is reported to phosphorylate C/EBPβ (31). We confirmed that the IL-1β-induced, C/EBPβ-mediated increase in TDO2 expression and concomitant Kyn production were inhibited by the p38 MAPK inhibitor SB203580 (**Figure 3E**).

CEBPB mRNA can produce at least three protein isoforms – 38 (LAP*), 35 (LAP), and 20 kDa (LIP) – with the LAP and the LIP forms being the major polypeptides produced in cells (32). Because the LIP protein isoform lacks activation domains, LIP has been thought to repress transcription by competing for C/EBPβ consensus binding sites (33); however, emerging evidence suggests that LIP can also function as a transcriptional activator (34). In T98G cells, only

overexpression of the LAP isoform resulted in statistically significant increases in TDO2 mRNA ($p < 0.0001$) and Kyn ($p < 0.0001$), whereas LIP overexpression increased Kyn levels ($p = 0.0009$) and resulted in a non-significant increase in TDO2 mRNA ($p = 0.0846$) (**Figures 3F,G**). Treatment of CEBPB-transduced T98G cells with IL-1β increased TDO2 expression and Kyn production in LIP overexpressing T98G cells, but not LAP overexpressing cells, suggesting that IL-1β typically induces the LAP isoform and that this had already reached saturating levels in LAP overexpressing T98G cells (**Figure 3G**).

DISCUSSION

Solid tumors such as melanoma, breast, lung, and colon cancers constitutively express the Trp degrading enzyme IDO1. TDO2, which is constitutively present in the liver and responsible for regulating systemic Trp levels, has only recently been found to be expressed in cancers and capable of producing Kyn (18–20, 35). In contrast to IDO1, little is known about the regulation of TDO2 in cancer. Previous studies

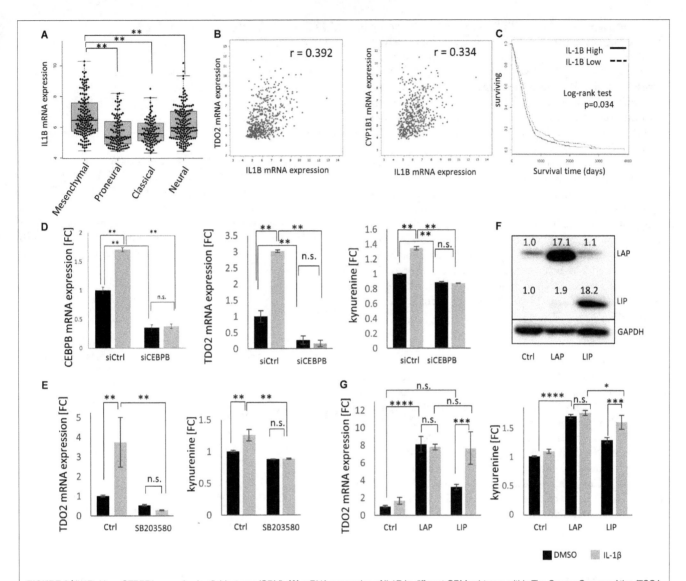

FIGURE 3 | IL1B drives CEBPB expression in glioblastoma (GBM). **(A)** mRNA expression of IL1B in different GBM subtypes within The Cancer Genome Atlas (TCGA dataset. **(B)** mRNA expression of IL1B correlated with TDO2 (left) and CYP1B1 (right) in GBM samples. **(C)** Kaplan–Meier analysis of overall survival of GBM patients according to the expression of IL1B (log-rank $p = 0.034$, high $n = 263$, low $n = 262$). **(D)** siRNA-mediated knockdown of CEBPB in T98G cells results in a decrease of CEBPB mRNA levels, as well as a decrease in TDO2 mRNA expression and concomitant kynurenine (Kyn) levels. **(E)** The CEBPB-driven increase in TDO2 expression (left) and Kyn levels (right) mediated by IL-1β treatment is blocked by the MAPK inhibitor SB203580. **(F)** Stably transfected T98G cells overexpressing CEBPB LIP or LAP isoforms show higher levels of the respective CEBPβ protein isoform. **(G)** TDO2 mRNA expression (left) and Kyn production (right) in T98G cells overexpressing CEBPB LAP or LIP in response to IL-1β treatment. *$p < 0.05$, **$p < 0.01$, ***$p < 0.001$, and ****$p < 0.0001$.

have shown that whereas in hepatocytes TDO2 expression and protein stability is induced by glucocorticoids (36), in GBM cell glucocorticoid signaling suppresses TDO2 expression (37). We have recently demonstrated that prostaglandins, chiefly prostaglandin E2 (PGE2), enhance TDO2 expression and enzymatic activity in malignant gliomas via activation of the prostaglandin E receptor-4 (EP4) (38).

In contrast to previous approaches, here, we used an unbiased search for regulators of constitutive TDO2 expression in a GBM cell line using iteratively deleted TDO2 reporter constructs to show that C/EBPβ plays an important role

in driving TDO2 expression in glioma cells. We confirmed our results by using the TCGA database to show strong transcriptional correlations between CEBPB and TDO2 itself, as well as between CEBPB and genes upregulated by TDO2 protein activity such as the AHR target gene CYP1B1 (18). We confirmed that this association holds true at the protein level using immunohistochemistry staining of mesenchymal GBM samples, a GBM subtype in which TDO2 expression is particularly elevated, although in the absence of a tumor cell stain in **Figure 2B**, we cannot exclude that the CEBP/β staining arises from infiltrating CEBPB-expressing macrophages.

We further showed that CEBPB expression is driven by IL-1β, and we confirmed that CEBPB-mediated upregulation of TDO2 requires the phosphorylation of C/EBPβ, which can be antagonized by the p38 MAPK inhibitor SB203580. Our data suggest that the IL-1β-driven increase in TDO2 expression acts predominantly through the LAP isoform of CEBPB, as previously reported in studies of IL-1β-mediated induction of CEBPB in SW1353 cells (39) and in accordance with the classical view of LAP as a transcriptional activator (32). One caveat to our data was that in some cases we observed a reduced sensitivity to IL-1β in cells held a long time in culture (see low induction of TDO2 mRNA in controls in **Figure 3G**), although whether this is due to genetic drift at high passage number or other factors is unclear. In line with our interpretation of these data, while preparing this manuscript, Yang and colleagues showed that the livers of mice kept under hypoxic conditions had more of the LAP isoform of CEBPB mRNA as well as more TDO2 protein and that knockdown of CEBPB precluded this increase in TDO2 protein (40).

Our approach demonstrates the value of combining experimental data with database-driven analyses, adding a molecular dimension to the work of Yang and colleagues and uncovering a novel role for this regulatory pathway driving the expression of the TDO2 enzyme in GBM. Given the key role that TDO2 plays in establishing the tryptophan-poor, immunosuppressive tumor microenvironment evident in the mesenchymal subtype of GBM – in which patient prognosis is particularly poor – our work uncovers a potential new target for therapeutic intervention.

AUTHOR CONTRIBUTIONS

TK, MTP, SM, FS, and ZZ generated the data. TK, MP, and EG conceived the experiments and wrote the manuscript. IG, WW, CO, MP, and EG supervised the work.

FUNDING

This work was supported by grants from the Chica and Heinz Schaller Foundation, the German Cancer Aid (110392), and the Helmholtz Association (VH−NG−306) to MP and the German Research Foundation (Deutsche Forschungsgemeinschaft SFB 938 TP K) to MP, CO, and WW. TK was supported by the Japan Society for the Promotion of Science (JSPS) KAKENHI Grant Number JP17K16630. EG was supported by a Marie Curie Intra-European Fellowship.

ACKNOWLEDGMENTS

The pMXs-GW-IRES-puro vector was a gift from Stefan Pusch. Thomas Hielscher provided assistance in performing statistical tests on TCGA data.

SUPPLEMENTARY MATERIAL

FIGURE S1 | IDO1 and TDO2 expression in TCGA GBM samples. Tryptophan degrading enzymes IDO1 and TDO2 are expressed in a subset of GBM tumors within the TCGA dataset.

TABLE S1 | Table of supplementary information regarding experimental materials used in this study, including DNA sequences of primers and transgenic contructs, and antibody clone numbers.

REFERENCES

1. Platten M, Ochs K, Lemke D, Opitz C, Wick W. Microenvironmental clues for glioma immunotherapy. *Curr Neurol Neurosci Rep.* (2014) 14:440. doi: 10.1007/s11910-014-0440-1
2. Platten M, Reardon DA. Concepts for Immunotherapies in Gliomas. *Semin Neurol.* (2018) 38:62–72. doi: 10.1055/s-0037-1620274
3. Mildenberger I, Bunse L, Ochs K, Platten M. The promises of immunotherapy in gliomas. *Curr Opin Neurol.* (2017) 30:650–8. doi: 10.1097/WCO.0000000000000491
4. Platten M, von Knebel Doeberitz N, Oezen I, Wick W, Ochs K. Cancer immunotherapy by targeting IDO1/TDO and their downstream effectors. *Front Immunol.* (2014) 5:673. doi: 10.3389/fimmu.2014.00673
5. Platten M, Wick W, Van den Eynde B. Tryptophan catabolism in Cancer: beyond IDO and tryptophan depletion. *Cancer Res.* (2012) 72:5435–40. doi: 10.1158/0008-5472.CAN-12-0569
6. Gabriely G, Wheeler MA, Takenaka MC, Quintana FJ. Role of AHR and HIF-1alpha in glioblastoma metabolism. *Trends Endocrinol Metab.* (2017) 28:428–36. doi: 10.1016/j.tem.2017.02.009

7. Zhai L, Ladomersky E, Lenzen A, Nguyen B, Patel R, Lauing KL, et al. IDO1 in cancer: a Gemini of immune checkpoints. *Cell Mol Immunol.* (2018) 15:447–57. doi: 10.1038/cmi.2017.143
8. Adams S, Teo C, McDonald KL, Zinger A, Bustamante S, Lim CK, et al. Involvement of the kynurenine pathway in human glioma pathophysiology. *PLoS One.* (2014) 9:e112945. doi: 10.1371/journal.pone.0112945
9. Lemos H, Huang L, Prendergast GC, Mellor AL. Immune control by amino acid catabolism during tumorigenesis and therapy. *Nat Rev Cancer.* (2019) 19:162–75. doi: 10.1038/s41568-019-0106-z
10. Labadie BW, Bao R, Luke JJ. Reimagining IDO pathway inhibition in cancer immunotherapy via downstream focus on the tryptophan-kynurenine-Aryl hydrocarbon axis. *Clin Cancer Res.* (2018) 25:1462–71. doi: 10.1158/1078-0432.CCR-18-2882
11. Prendergast GC, Mondal A, Dey S, Laury-Kleintop LD, Muller AJ. Inflammatory reprogramming with IDO1 inhibitors: turning immunologically unresponsive 'Cold' Tumors 'Hot'. *Trends Cancer.* (2018) 4:38–58. doi: 10.1016/j.trecan.2017.11.005
12. Cervenka I, Agudelo LZ, Ruas JL. Kynurenines: tryptophan's metabolites in exercise, inflammation, and mental health. *Science.* (2017) 357:eaaf9794. doi: 10.1126/science.aaf9794

13. Triplett TA, Garrison KC, Marshall N, Donkor M, Blazeck J, Lamb C, et al. Reversal of indoleamine 2,3-dioxygenase-mediated cancer immune suppression by systemic kynurenine depletion with a therapeutic enzyme. *Nat Biotechnol.* (2018) 36:758–64. doi: 10.1038/nbt.4180

14. Munn DH, Mellor AL. IDO in the Tumor microenvironment: inflammation, counter-regulation, and tolerance. *Trends Immunol.* (2016) 37:193–207. doi: 10.1016/j.it.2016.01.002

15. Prendergast GC, Smith C, Thomas S, Mandik-Nayak L, Laury-Kleintop L, Metz R, et al. Indoleamine 2,3-dioxygenase pathways of pathogenic inflammation and immune escape in cancer. *Cancer Immunol Immunother.* (2014) 63:721–35. doi: 10.1007/s00262-014-1549-4

16. Zhai L, Spranger S, Binder DC, Gritsina G, Lauing KL, Giles FJ, et al. Molecular pathways: targeting IDO1 and other tryptophan dioxygenases for cancer immunotherapy. *Clin Cancer Res.* (2015) 21:5427–33. doi: 10.1158/1078-0432.CCR-15-0420

17. Greene LI, Bruno TC, Christenson JL, D'Alessandro A, Culp-Hill R, Torkko K, et al. A role for tryptophan-2,3-dioxygenase in CD8 T-cell suppression and evidence of tryptophan catabolism in breast cancer patient plasma. *Mol Cancer Res.* (2019) 17:131–9. doi: 10.1158/1541-7786.MCR-18-0362

18. Opitz CA, Litzenburger UM, Sahm F, Ott M, Tritschler I, Trump S, et al. An endogenous tumour-promoting ligand of the human aryl hydrocarbon receptor. *Nature.* (2011) 478:197–203. doi: 10.1038/nature10491

19. Pilotte L, Larrieu P, Stroobant V, Colau D, Dolusic E, Frederick R, et al. Reversal of tumoral immune resistance by inhibition of tryptophan 2,3-dioxygenase. *Proc Natl Acad Sci USA.* (2012) 109:2497–502. doi: 10.1073/pnas.1113873109

20. D'Amato NC, Rogers TJ, Gordon MA, Greene LI, Cochrane DR, Spoelstra NS, et al. A TDO2-AhR signaling axis facilitates anoikis resistance and metastasis in triple-negative breast cancer. *Cancer Res.* (2015) 75:4651–64. doi: 10.1158/0008-5472.CAN-15-2011

21. Muller AJ, DuHadaway JB, Donover PS, Sutanto-Ward E, Prendergast GC. Inhibition of indoleamine 2,3-dioxygenase, an immunoregulatory target of the cancer suppression gene Bin1, potentiates cancer chemotherapy. *Nat Med.* (2005) 11:312–9.

22. Balachandran VP, Cavnar MJ, Zeng S, Bamboat ZM, Ocuin LM, Obaid H, et al. Imatinib potentiates antitumor T cell responses in gastrointestinal stromal tumor through the inhibition of Ido. *Nat Med.* (2011) 17:1094–100. doi: 10.1038/nm.2438

23. Litzenburger UM, Opitz CA, Sahm F, Rauschenbach KJ, Trump S, Winter M, et al. Constitutive IDO expression in human cancer is sustained by an autocrine signaling loop involving IL-6, STAT3 and the AHR. *Oncotarget.* (2014) 5:1038–51.

24. Dewi DL, Mohapatra SR, Blanco Cabanes S, Adam I, Somarribas Patterson LF, Berdel B, et al. Suppression of indoleamine-2,3-dioxygenase 1 expression by promoter hypermethylation in ER-positive breast cancer. *Oncoimmunology.* (2017) 6:e1274477. doi: 10.1080/2162402X.2016.1274477

25. Miller CL, Llenos IC, Dulay JR, Barillo MM, Yolken RH, Weis S. Expression of the kynurenine pathway enzyme tryptophan 2,3-dioxygenase is increased in the frontal cortex of individuals with schizophrenia. *Neurobiol Dis.* (2004) 15:618–29.

26. Schulte KW, Green E, Wilz A, Platten M, Daumke O. Structural basis for Aryl hydrocarbon receptor-mediated gene activation. *Structure.* (2017) 25:1025–33.e3. doi: 10.1016/j.str.2017.05.008

27. Tsunoda T, Takagi T. Estimating transcription factor bindability on DNA. *Bioinformatics.* (1999) 15:622–30.

28. Carro MS, Lim WK, Alvarez MJ, Bollo RJ, Zhao X, Snyder EY, et al. The transcriptional network for mesenchymal transformation of brain tumours. *Nature.* (2010) 463:318–25. doi: 10.1038/nature08712

29. Tarassishin L, Casper D, Lee SC. Aberrant expression of interleukin-1beta and inflammasome activation in human malignant gliomas. *PLoS One.* (2014) 9:e103432. doi: 10.1371/journal.pone.0103432

30. Gurgis FM, Yeung YT, Tang MX, Heng B, Buckland M, Ammit AJ, et al. The p38-MK2-HuR pathway potentiates EGFRvIII-IL1Beta-driven IL-6 secretion in glioblastoma cells. *Oncogene.* (2015) 34:2934–42. doi: 10.1038/onc.2014.225

31. Cesena TI, Cui TX, Piwien-Pilipuk G, Kaplani J, Calinescu AA, Huo JS, et al. Multiple mechanisms of growth hormone-regulated gene transcription. *Mol Genet Metab.* (2007) 90:126–33. doi: 10.1016/j.ymgme.2006.10.006

32. Zahnow CA, Younes P, Laucirica R, Rosen JM. Overexpression of C/EBPbeta-LIP, a naturally occurring, dominant-negative transcription factor, in human breast cancer. *J Natl Cancer Inst.* (1997) 89:1887–91. doi: 10.1093/jnci/89.24.1887

33. Descombes P, Schibler U. A liver-enriched transcriptional activator protein, LAP, and a transcriptional inhibitory protein, LIP, are translated from the same mRNA. *Cell.* (1991) 67:569–79.

34. Zahnow CA. CCAAT / enhancer-binding protein beta: its role in breast cancer and associations with receptor tyrosine kinases. *Expert Rev Mol Med.* (2009) 11:e12. doi: 10.1017/S1462399409001033

35. Sahm F, Oezen I, Opitz CA, Radlwimmer B, von Deimling A, Ahrendt T, et al. The endogenous tryptophan metabolite and NAD+ precursor quinolinic acid confers resistance of gliomas to oxidative stress. *Cancer Res.* (2013) 73:3225–34. doi: 10.1158/0008-5472.CAN-12-3831

36. Nakamura T, Niimi S, Nawa K, Noda C, Ichihara A, Takagi Y, et al. Multihormonal regulation of transcription of the tryptophan 2,3-dioxygenase gene in primary cultures of adult rat hepatocytes with special reference to the presence of a transcriptional protein mediating the action of glucocorticoids. *J Biol Chem.* (1987) 262:727–33.

37. Ott M, Litzenburger UM, Rauschenbach KJ, Bunse L, Ochs K, Sahm F, et al. Suppression of TDO-mediated tryptophan catabolism in glioblastoma cells by a steroid-responsive FKBP52-dependent pathway. *Glia.* (2015) 63:78–90. doi: 10.1002/glia.22734

38. Ochs K, Ott M, Rauschenbach KJ, Deumelandt K, Sahm F, Opitz CA, et al. Tryptophan-2,3-dioxygenase is regulated by prostaglandin E2 in malignant glioma via a positive signaling loop involving prostaglandin E receptor-4. *J Neurochem.* (2015) 136:1142–54. doi: 10.1111/jnc.13503

39. Petrella BL, Armstrong DA, Vincent MP. CCAAT-enhancer-binding protein beta activation of MMP-1 gene expression in SW1353 Cells: independent roles of extracellular signal-regulated and p90/ribosomal S6 kinases. *J Cell Physiol.* (2011) 226:3349–54. doi: 10.1002/jcp.22693

40. Yang F, Zhou L, Song J, WangJinMei A, Yang Y, Tang ZW, et al. Liver CEBPβ modulates the kynurenine metabolism and mediates the motility for hypoxia-induced central fatigue in mice. *Front Physiol.* (2019) 14:243. doi: 10.3389/fphys.2019.00243

10

Tryptophan Metabolic Pathways are Altered in Obesity and are Associated with Systemic Inflammation

Sofia Cussotto[1†], Inês Delgado[1†], Andrea Anesi[2], Sandra Dexpert[1], Agnès Aubert[1], Cédric Beau[3], Damien Forestier[3], Patrick Ledaguenel[3], Eric Magne[3], Fulvio Mattivi[2,4] and Lucile Capuron[1*]

[1] University of Bordeaux, INRAE, Bordeaux INP, NutriNeuro, UMR 1286, Bordeaux, France, [2] Department of Food Quality and Nutrition, Research and Innovation Centre, Fondazione Edmund Mach (FEM), San Michele all'Adige, Italy, [3] Service de Chirurgie Digestive et Parietale, Clinique Tivoli, Bordeaux, and Clinique Jean Villar, Bruges, France, [4] Department of Cellular, Computational and Integrative Biology (CIBIO), University of Trento, Trento, Italy

*Correspondence:
Lucile Capuron
lucile.capuron@inrae.fr

[†] These authors have contributed equally to this work

Background: Obesity is a condition with a complex pathophysiology characterized by both chronic low-grade inflammation and changes in the gut microbial ecosystem. These alterations can affect the metabolism of tryptophan (TRP), an essential amino acid and precursor of serotonin (5-HT), kynurenine (KYN), and indoles. This study aimed to investigate alterations in KYN and microbiota-mediated indole routes of TRP metabolism in obese subjects relatively to non-obese controls and to determine their relationship with systemic inflammation.

Methods: Eighty-five obese adults (avg. BMI = 40.48) and 42 non-obese control individuals (avg. BMI = 24.03) were recruited. Plasma levels of TRP catabolites were assessed using Ultra High Performance Liquid Chromatography-ElectroSpray-Ionization-Tandem Mass Spectrometry. High-sensitive C-reactive protein (hsCRP) and high-sensitive interleukin 6 (hsIL-6) were measured in the serum as markers of systemic inflammation using enzyme-linked immunosorbent assay.

Results: Both KYN and microbiota-mediated indole routes of TRP metabolism were altered in obese subjects, as reflected in higher KYN/TRP ratio and lower 5-HT and indoles levels, relatively to non-obese controls. HsIL-6 and hsCRP were increased in obesity and were overall associated with TRP metabolic pathways alterations.

Conclusion: These results indicate for the first time that KYN and indole TRP metabolic pathways are concomitantly altered in obese subjects and highlight their respective associations with obesity-related systemic inflammation.

Keywords: obesity, inflammation, tryptophan, kynurenine, indoles

INTRODUCTION

Obesity is a metabolic disorder characterized by a chronic low-grade inflammatory state, as reflected in increased levels of circulating inflammatory markers, including pro-inflammatory cytokines and the acute phase protein C-reactive protein (CRP) (1–4). Systemic inflammation in obesity originates primarily from the adipose tissue, in which adipocytes and infiltrated immune cells accumulate and secrete inflammatory factors (2–5). Additionally, changes in the gut microbiota composition and permeability that have been highly documented in obesity (6–9), were also found to play a role in obesity-related inflammation (10, 11).

A growing body of evidence indicates that inflammation is associated with alterations in the metabolism of tryptophan (TRP) (12, 13), an essential amino acid and biochemical precursor of serotonin (5-HT), kynurenine (KYN) and indoles (14). One mechanism likely to be involved in this effect relies on the induction of the enzyme indoleamine-2,3-dioxygenase (IDO) by pro-inflammatory cytokines (13, 15). IDO is responsible for the catabolism of TRP along the KYN pathway, likely resulting in reduced 5-HT synthesis. Consistent with this notion, activation of the KYN pathway has been documented in several studies conducted in obese subjects (16–19). Alterations in TRP metabolism in obese subjects may also arise from the gut microbiota, which has been shown to be disrupted both at compositional and functional levels in obesity (20–22). Accordingly, a greater ratio of Firmicutes/Bacteroidetes, along with disrupted intestinal permeability and increased endotoxemia have been repeatedly documented in obese subjects (6–9). Diet and nutritional habits represent the main contributors to obesity-related alterations in the gut microbiota given their major role in shaping intestinal bacteria environment. In the gut, TRP is metabolized by specific intestinal bacteria (23) into indole, indole-3-acetic acid (IAA), indole-3-acrylic acid (IA), indole-3-carboxalaldehyde (ICAld), indole-3-lactic acid (ILA), indole-3-propionic acid (IPA), indole-3-ethanol (IE), indole-3-acetonitrile (IACN), and indole-3-carboxylic acid (ICA) (24). In adults, the most abundant catabolite is indole, followed by IAA and IPA (25–27). Despite strong evidence of gut microbiota changes in obesity, little is known on the impact of these alterations on gut-derived TRP metabolism along the indole pathway.

Altogether, these data suggest that obesity may contribute to concomitant alterations in TRP metabolism, through parallel pathways, involving both inflammation and the microbiota. Moreover, the relationship between these two pathways remains to be determined, in particular the possibility that inflammatory processes relate to indoles production. Supporting this scenario, gut-derived inflammatory processes, including endotoxemia (9), in obesity could disrupt gut homeostasis and function leading thus to substantial alterations in the metabolism of indoles. In addition, indoles represent potent modulators of immune function. They can act as ligands of the aryl hydrocarbon receptor (AHR), a transcription factor widely expressed by cells in the immune system and whose activation can alter innate and adaptive immune responses (28, 29). For instance, ICAld produced by *Lactobacillus* spp. was found to attenuate intestinal inflammation by regulating IL-22 mucosal homeostasis via an AHR-dependant mechanism (30).

The aim of the present study was to investigate the KYN and indole pathways of TRP metabolism in obese subjects relatively to non-obese controls and to determine their relationship with systemic inflammation.

METHODS
Study Participants
Obese Subjects
Eighty-five adult obese subjects with severe or morbid obesity, awaiting a gastric surgery, were recruited from the services of digestive and parietal surgery of two private clinics (Tivoli and Jean-Villar) in Bordeaux, France. Participants met criteria for obesity surgery, i.e., BMI $\geq$ 40 kg/m^2 or $\geq$ 35 kg/m^2 with at least one comorbidity [e.g., hypertension [HT], type-2 diabetes [T2D], obstructive sleep apnea [OSA], dysthyroidism].

Non-obese Controls
Forty-two non-obese volunteers (BMI < 30 kg/m^2) with no acute or chronic immune/inflammatory condition were included as control participants. A level of high-sensitive (hs) CRP above 5 mg/L, indicative of low-grade inflammation (31), was considered as an exclusion criterion in this group of participants. Control subjects were recruited by phone interview conducted by the contract research organization CEN Nutriment (Dijon, France).

In both groups, exclusion criteria were: age > 65 years old; acute or chronic inflammatory conditions (other than obesity or obesity-related comorbidities); diagnosis of severe or uncontrolled medical illness; and current treatment with anti-inflammatory agents. All participants provided written informed consent after reading a complete description of the study. The study was approved by the Institutional Committee of Protection of Persons (CPP; registration numbers 2010/36 and 2016/40 for obese and non-obese subjects, respectively).

Measurements
Socio-Demographic and Clinical Characteristics
Socio-demographic and clinical characteristics, including anthropometric data, medical history and current treatment, were collected by trained professionals for all participants at inclusion. BMI was calculated as weight (kg)/height (m)^2.

Biological Measurements
The same day as clinical assessments, fasting blood samples were collected in plain or EDTA-containing tubes for serum and plasma, respectively. After 30–45 min at room temperature, samples were centrifuged (4,000 rpm, 20 min at 4°C for plasma and 3,200 rpm, 10 min at 4°C for serum) and stored at −80°C until further analysis.

Inflammatory Markers
Serum concentrations of hsCRP and high-sensitive interleukin 6 (hsIL-6) were determined by enzyme-linked immunosorbent assay (ELISA) according to the manufacturer's specifications (hsCRP: CYT298, Millipore, Billerica, Massachusetts; hsIL-6: R&D Systems, Minneapolis, Minnesota). Assays sensitivity and intra-/inter-assay variability were, respectively, 0.20 ng/mL, $\pm$ 4.6% and $\pm$ 6.0% for hsCRP and 0.031 pg/mL, $\pm$ 4.1% and $\pm$ 3.9% for hsIL-6.

Tryptophan Metabolites
Plasma concentrations of free TRP, 5-HT, 5-hydroxyindole-3-acetic acid (5-HIAA), KYN, IAA, ICAld, ILA, IPA, and

indoxyl sulfate (IS) were determined by Ultra High Performance Liquid Chromatography-ElectroSpay-Ionization-Tandem Mass Spectrometry (UHPLC-ESI-MS/MS), as described in detail elsewhere (32). This technique was developed and validated for the targeted quantification of TRP and tyrosine derived metabolites in human plasma and urine. The ratio KYN/TRP was calculated as an index of TRP breakdown along the KYN pathway indicative of IDO activation.

Data Analysis

Raw values for serum inflammatory markers as well as for plasma levels of TRP, 5-HT, 5-HIAA, IAA, ICAld, ILA, IPA, and IS were log-transformed due to non-normality, as assessed by the Shapiro-Wilk test. Extreme values (>3SD above the mean) were observed for IL-6 ($N = 1$ non-obese participant), 5-HIAA ($N = 1$ obese participant) and IAA ($N = 2$ obese participants). Accordingly, these values were considered outliers and were individually excluded from data analyses performed on biological markers. Of note, values for hsIL-6 were missing in two non-obese controls. Socio-demographic and clinical characteristics of the two experimental groups were compared using Student's t-tests for continuous variables or Chi-square tests for categorical variables. Levels of hsCRP, hsIL-6, TRP, and markers of its metabolic pathways were compared between the two groups using analyses of covariance (ANCOVAs) controlling for age, gender, and comorbidities. The relationship between inflammatory markers, BMI, and TRP metabolism (KYN/TRP and indoles) was estimated in the whole population under study and separately in the obese group using multiple regression analyses, adjusted for age, gender, and comorbidities. Statistical analyses were performed with SPSS Statistics version 25. All probabilities were two-sided with the degree of significance set at $p < 0.05$.

RESULTS

Socio-Demographic and Clinical Characteristics of Study Participants

Socio-demographic and clinical characteristics of study participants are presented in **Table 1**. There were no significant differences between obese subjects and non-obese controls in terms of age ($t = 0.410$, $p = 0.683$) and gender (Chi$^2 = 0.144$, $p = 0.705$). As expected, BMI and weight were significantly higher in the obese group compared to the non-obese one (BMI: $t = 22.48$, $p < 0.0001$; weight: $t = 16.62$, $p < 0.0001$). Similarly, the prevalence of HT was higher in obese subjects (Chi$^2 = 8.451$, $p =0.004$), as well as T2D and OSA that were only present in the obese population.

TRP Metabolic Pathways Are Altered in Obese Subjects Compared to Healthy Participants

Compared to non-obese controls, obese subjects exhibited decreased circulating levels of TRP [$F_{(1,122)} = 37.79$, $p < 0.0001$] together with increased KYN/TRP ratio [$F_{(1,122)} = 9.77$, $p < 0.01$], indicative of IDO activation and TRP breakdown along

TABLE 1 | Characteristics of study participants.

	Non-obese participants	Obese participants	p
Sample size, n	42	85	
Age, years (SD)	37.74 (7.48)	38.52 (111.14)	0.683
Women, n (%)	35 (83.33)	73 (85.88)	0.705
BMI, kg/m² (SD)	24.03 (3.52)	40.48 (4.05)	<0.0001
Weight, kg (SD)	68.18 (11.55)	111.20 (14.68)	<0.0001
Comorbidities			
HTA, n (%)	1 (2.38)	19 (22.35)	0.004
T2D, n (%)	0 (0)	10 (11.77)	0.021
Dyst, n (%)	1 (2.38)	9 (10.59)	0.106
OSA, n (%)	0 (0)	27 (45.0)	<0.001

Continuous variables are presented as mean and standard deviation and compared using Student's t-test, whereas categorical variables are presented as n (%) and compared by chi-square test. BMI, body mass index; HTA, hypertension; T2D, type 2 diabetes; Dyst, dysthyroidism; OSA, obstructive sleep apnea.

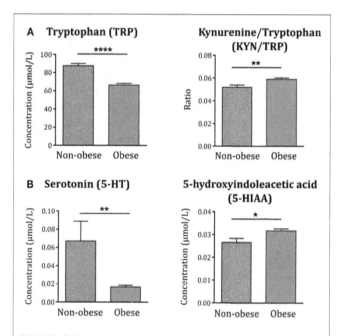

FIGURE 1 | TRP metabolism along the KYN and 5-HT pathways in obese subjects compared to non-obese controls. **(A)** Plasma levels of TRP were decreased whereas the KYN/TRP ratio was increased in obese subjects ($n = 85$) compared to non-obese controls ($n = 42$). **(B)** Similarly, plasma levels of 5-HT were decreased whereas 5-HIAA was increased in obese subjects ($n = 84–85$). Statistical analyses were performed on log-transformed data using ANCOVA controlling for age, gender and comorbidities. Data are expressed as mean + SEM. ****$p < 0.0001$, **$p < 0.01$, *$p < 0.05$.

the KYN pathway (**Figure 1A**). In line with the impact of this pathway on 5-HT synthesis, plasma levels of 5-HT were significantly decreased in obese subjects [$F_{(1,122)} = 10.83$, $p < 0.01$] whereas levels of 5-HIAA [$F_{(1,121)} = 5.57$, $p < 0.05$] were increased (**Figure 1B**).

Moreover, levels of IAA, ILA and IPA were all significantly decreased in obese subjects compared to non-obese controls [IAA: $F_{(1,120)} = 19.53$, $p < 0.0001$; ILA: $F_{(1,122)} = 64.34$, $p <$

0.0001; IPA: $F_{(1,122)} = 13.89$, $p < 0.001$] (**Figure 2**). In contrast, levels of ICAld were not altered [$F_{(1,122)} = 0.29$, $p = 0.59$]. IS, an indole-derived metabolite produced in the liver from free indole, was also significantly decreased in the obese group [($F_{(1,122)} = 21.83$, $p < 0.0001$].

Consistent with these results, BMI was positively associated with KYN/TRP ratio and 5-HIAA, but negatively correlated with levels of IAA, ILA, IPA, IS, TRP, and 5-HT in the whole population under study (data not shown).

Systemic Inflammation Correlates With Alterations in TRP Metabolic Pathways

As expected, serum levels of hsCRP [$F_{(1,122)} = 102.50$, $p < 0.0001$] and hsIL-6 [$F_{(1,119)} = 54.71$, $p < 0.0001$] were increased in obese subjects compared to non-obese controls (**Figure 3**). In line with this, hsCRP and hsIL-6 were positively associated with BMI in the whole population under study and were correlated to each other (data not shown). Increased levels of hsCRP and hsIL-6 were associated with reduced levels of TRP together with increased KYN/TRP ratios in the whole population, consistent with the inflammatory characteristic of this pathway. No significant correlations were found between inflammation and markers of 5-HT pathway (**Table 2**).

Interestingly, both hsCRP and hsIL-6 levels were negatively associated with plasma levels of IAA, ILA, IPA, and IS (**Table 2**). While no significant correlations were observed between inflammatory markers and ICAld levels in the whole population

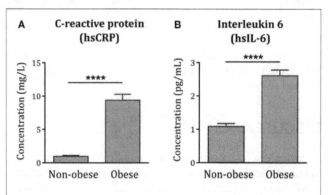

FIGURE 3 | Systemic inflammation in obese subjects compared to non-obese controls. Serum levels of hsCRP and hsIL-6 were significantly increased in the obese population ($n = 85$) compared to non-obese controls ($n = 39$–42). Statistical analyses were performed on log-transformed data using ANCOVA controlling for age, gender and comorbidities. Data are expressed as mean + SEM. ****$p < 0.0001$. *hsCRP*, high-sensitive C-reactive protein; *hsIL-6*, high-sensitive interleukin-6.

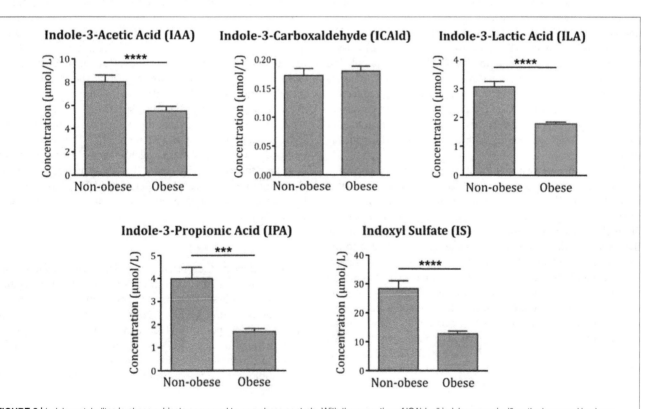

FIGURE 2 | Indole metabolites in obese subjects compared to non-obese controls. With the exception of ICAld, all indoles were significantly decreased in obese subjects ($n = 83$–85) compared to non-obese controls ($n = 42$). Statistical analyses were performed on log-transformed data using ANCOVA controlling for age, gender and comorbidities. Data are expressed as mean + SEM. ****$p < 0.0001$; ***$p < 0.001$.

TABLE 2 | Association between hsCRP, hsIL-6, and markers of tryptophan metabolism in the whole population.

	TRP	KYN/TRP	5-HT	5-HIAA	IAA	ICAld	ILA	IPA	IS
hsCRP	−0.397****	0.190*	−0.088	0.133	−0.332***	−0.078	−0.501****	−0.268**	−0.339***
hsIL-6	−0.380****	0.300**	−0.158	0.068	−0.290**	−0.108	−0.397****	−0.244**	−0.304***

Multiple regression analyses controlling for gender, age and comorbidities (β coefficient). IAA, indole-3-acetic acid; ICAld, indole-3-carboxaldehyde; ILA, indole-3-lactic acid; IPA, indole-3-propionic acid; IS, indoxyl sulfate; KYN/TRP, kynurenine/tryptophan; 5-HT, serotonin; 5-HIAA, 5-hydroxyindole-3-acetic acid. ****p < 0.0001, ***p < 0.001, **p < 0.01, *p < 0.05.

under study, this metabolite was significantly correlated with hsIL-6 levels in the group of obese subjects ($\beta = -0.261, p < 0.05$, data not shown).

DISCUSSION

There is an increasing emphasis on the interplay between obesity, inflammation, and TRP metabolism. While most of the research in inflammatory conditions has been focused on the KYN route of TRP metabolism, notably through activation of the enzyme IDO, here we assessed whether obesity-related inflammation may also impact the microbial route of TRP metabolism. To our knowledge, this is the first study showing concomitant alterations in the KYN and indole pathways of TRP metabolism in obesity.

In line with previous reports (17, 19), obese subjects exhibited higher serum levels of inflammatory markers together with reduced plasma levels of TRP and increased KYN/TRP ratio, indicative of inflammation-driven IDO activation. Interestingly, and consistent with the inflammatory component of the KYN pathway, the ratio of KYN/TRP was significantly associated with levels of systemic inflammation in the whole population under study. Alterations were also found in plasmatic markers of the 5-HT pathway, with obese subjects exhibiting reduced 5-HT and increased 5-HIAA levels. These findings are consistent with the hypothesis of an IDO-driven shift of TRP degradation toward the KYN pathway at the detriment of 5-HT pathway in obesity.

In addition, our results indicate that obesity is associated with significant reductions in microbial-derived indoles, notably IAA, ILA, and IPA. These alterations may rely on changes in microbiota composition and function, as described in obesity. Similarly, IS, an indole-derived metabolite produced in the liver, was also decreased in obese subjects, probably due to the low availability of its substrate, indole. Supporting this notion, reduced indole levels have been documented in children with class II-III obesity when compared to their healthy counterparts (33). Interestingly, findings from the present study reveal significant relationships between circulating levels of indoles and inflammatory markers. In particular, plasma levels of IPA, IAA, ILA, and IS were negatively correlated with serum levels of hsCRP and hsIL-6 in the whole population under study. Noteworthy, ICAld was the only indole metabolite that was

not affected by obesity *per se* but showed an association with inflammatory markers, especially hsIL-6, in the group of obese subjects. The nature of this association needs to be disentangled in future studies. To our knowledge, this report is the first to demonstrate a concomitant alteration of host (KYN) and microbial (indole) TRP metabolic pathways, both relating on systemic inflammation, in obesity. While inflammation is known to induce KYN pathway activation (13, 34), the direction of its relationship with the indole pathway is unclear and remains to be investigated in future studies. Data from the literature is heterogeneous and suggests that this relationship may be bidirectional. Not only indoles have been described as potent regulators of immune/inflammatory processes (30, 35, 36) but also gut inflammation, often described in obesity (6–9), is likely to modify microbiota-driven indoles production.

The present study bears some limitations. First, we did not assess fecal levels of indoles nor perform a microbiota characterization of study participants, which would add an important piece of data to this work. Second, only hsCRP and hsIL-6 were measured as markers of systemic inflammation. Although those markers are probably the most used in the literature to evaluate chronic low-grade inflammation 37), a more comprehensive spectrum of inflammatory factors is needed to assess the influence of obesity-related inflammation on microbial TRP metabolism. Finally, no record on food consumption was available in the study. Since diet is a key source of TRP (38), this information would help clarifying to what extent the differences in TRP levels observed between obese and non-obese subjects are linked to different dietary habits.

In conclusion, the present study demonstrates for the first time concomitant alterations in KYN and indole TRP metabolic pathways in obese subjects and highlights their respective associations with obesity-related systemic inflammation. These findings point to TRP metabolism as an important component of obesity. While the relevance of this mechanism to the pathophysiology and management of obesity and its comorbidities remains to be determined, this opens new avenues for future research.

AUTHOR CONTRIBUTIONS

SC, ID, and LC contributed to the conception and/or design of the study and were involved in writing the manuscript. CB, DF, PL, and EM enrolled obese participants in the study and performed the medical examinations. SD performed study inclusions and was involved in patients' follow up. ID and AAu conducted the biological experiments. SC and ID performed data analysis. AAn and FM assisted with the target metabolomics and interpretation of results. All authors critically revised the manuscript and approved the final version.

FUNDING

This work was supported by grants from the JPI HDHL Nutrition and Cognitive Function (AMBROSIAC, French National Research Agency, ANR-15-HDHL-0001-03, LC) and from the JPI HDHL Biomarkers for Nutrition and Health (HEALTHMARK, French National Research Agency, ANR-16-HDHL-0003-03, LC; and Italian Ministry of Education, University and Research, MIUR, CUP D43C17000100006, FM).

REFERENCES

1. Lasselin J, Capuron L. Chronic low-grade inflammation in metabolic disorders: relevance for behavioral symptoms. *Neuroimmunomodulation.* (2014) 21:95–101. doi: 10.1159/000356535
2. Lasselin J, Magne E, Beau C, Ledaguenel P, Dexpert S, Aubert A, et al. Adipose inflammation in obesity: relationship with circulating levels of inflammatory markers and association with surgery-induced weight loss. *J Clin Endocrinol Metab.* (2014) 99:E53–61. doi: 10.1210/jc.2013-2673
3. Ellulu MS, Patimah I, Khaza'ai H, Rahmat A, Abed Y. Obesity and inflammation: the linking mechanism and the complications. *Arch Med Sci.* (2017) 13:851–63. doi: 10.5114/aoms.2016.58928
4. Reilly SM, Saltiel AR. Adapting to obesity with adipose tissue inflammation. *Nat Rev Endocrinol.* (2017) 13:633–43. doi: 10.1038/nrendo.2017.90
5. Wellen KE, Hotamisligil GS. Obesity-induced inflammatory changes in adipose tissue. *J Clin Invest.* (2003) 112:1785–8. doi: 10.1172/JCI20514
6. Ley RE, Backhed F, Turnbaugh P, Lozupone CA, Knight RD, Gordon JI. Obesity alters gut microbial ecology. *Proc Natl Acad Sci USA.* (2005) 102:11070–5. doi: 10.1073/pnas.0504978102
7. Turnbaugh PJ, Hamady M, Yatsunenko T, Cantarel BL, Duncan A, Ley RE, et al. A core gut microbiome in obese and lean twins. *Nature.* (2009) 457:480–4. doi: 10.1038/nature07540
8. Patterson E, Ryan PM, Cryan JF, Dinan TG, Ross RP, Fitzgerald GF, et al. Gut microbiota, obesity and diabetes. *Postgrad Med J.* (2016) 92:286–300. doi: 10.1136/postgradmedj-2015-133285
9. Torres-Fuentes C, Schellekens H, Dinan TG, Cryan JF. The microbiota-gut-brain axis in obesity. *Lancet Gastroenterol Hepatol.* (2017) 2:747–56. doi: 10.1016/S2468-1253(17)30147-4
10. Cani PD, Osto M, Geurts L, Everard A. Involvement of gut microbiota in the development of low-grade inflammation and type 2 diabetes associated with obesity. *Gut Microbes.* (2012) 3:279–88. doi: 10.4161/gmic.19625
11. Mulders RJ, de Git KCG, Schele E, Dickson SL, Sanz Y, Adan RAH. Microbiota in obesity: interactions with enteroendocrine, immune and central nervous systems. *Obes Rev.* (2018) 19:435–51. doi: 10.1111/obr.12661
12. Strasser B, Berger K, Fuchs D. Effects of a caloric restriction weight loss diet on tryptophan metabolism and inflammatory biomarkers in overweight adults. *Eur J Nutr.* (2015) 54:101–7. doi: 10.1007/s00394-014-0690-3
13. Wang Q, Liu D, Song P, Zou MH. Tryptophan-kynurenine pathway is dysregulated in inflammation, and immune activation. *Front Biosci.* (2015) 20:1116–43. doi: 10.2741/4363
14. Le Floc'h N, Otten W, Merlot E. Tryptophan metabolism, from nutrition to potential therapeutic applications. *Amino Acids.* (2011) 41:1195–205. doi: 10.1007/s00726-010-0752-7
15. Heyes MP, Saito K, Crowley JS, Davis LE, Demitrack MA, Der M, et al. Quinolic acid and kynurenine pathway metabolism in inflammatory and non-inflammatory neurological disease. *Brain.* (1992) 115:1249–73. doi: 10.1093/brain/115.5.1249
16. Oxenkrug GF. Metabolic syndrome, age-associated neuroendocrine disorders, and dysregulation of tryptophan—kynurenine metabolism. *Ann N Y Acad Sci.* (2010) 1199:1–14. doi: 10.1111/j.1749-6632.2009.05356.x
17. Mangge H, Summers KL, Meinitzer A, Zelzer S, Almer G, Prassl R, et al. Obesity-related dysregulation of the Tryptophan–Kynurenine metabolism: Role of age and parameters of the metabolic syndrome. *Obesity.* (2014) 22:195–201. doi: 10.1002/oby.20491
18. Reininghaus EZ, McIntyre RS, Reininghaus B, Geisler S, Bengesser SA, Lackner N, et al. Tryptophan breakdown is increased in euthymic overweight individuals with bipolar disorder: a preliminary report. *Bipolar Disord.* (2014) 16:432–40. doi: 10.1111/bdi.12166
19. Favennec M, Hennart B, Caiazzo R, Leloire A, Yengo L, Verbanck M, et al. The kynurenine pathway is activated in human obesity and shifted toward kynurenine monooxygenase activation. *Obesity.* (2015) 23:2066–74. doi: 10.1002/oby.21199
20. Duncan SH, Lobley GE, Holtrop G, Ince J, Johnstone AM, Louis P, et al. Human colonic microbiota associated with diet, obesity and weight loss. *Int J Obes.* (2008) 32:1720–4. doi: 10.1038/ijo.2008.155
21. Zhang H, DiBaise JK, Zuccolo A, Kudrna D, Braidotti M, Yu Y, et al. Human gut microbiota in obesity and after gastric bypass. *Proc Natl Acad Sci USA.* (2009) 106:2365–70. doi: 10.1073/pnas.0812600106
22. Ridaura VK, Faith JJ, Rey FE, Cheng J, Duncan AE, Kau AL, et al. Gut microbiota from twins discordant for obesity modulate metabolism in mice. *Science.* (2013) 341:1241214. doi: 10.1126/science.1241214
23. Agus A, Planchais J, Sokol H. Gut microbiota regulation of tryptophan metabolism in health and disease. *Cell Host Microbe.* (2018) 23:716–24. doi: 10.1016/j.chom.2018.05.003
24. Roager HM, Licht TR. Microbial tryptophan catabolites in health and disease. *Nat Commun.* (2018) 9:3294. doi: 10.1038/s41467-018-05470-4
25. Rosas HD, Doros G, Bhasin S, Thomas B, Gevorkian S, Malarick K, et al. A systems-level misunderstanding: the plasma metabolome in Huntington's disease. *Ann Clin Transl Neurol.* (2015) 2:756–68. doi: 10.1002/acn3.214
26. Pavlova T, Vidova V, Bienertova-Vasku J, Janku P, Almasi M, Klanova J, et al. Urinary intermediates of tryptophan as indicators of the gut microbial metabolism. *Anal Chim Acta.* (2017) 987:72–80. doi: 10.1016/j.aca.2017.08.022
27. Alexeev EE, Lanis JM, Kao DJ, Campbell EL, Kelly CJ, Battista KD, et al. Microbiota-derived indole metabolites promote human and murine intestinal homeostasis through regulation of interleukin-10 receptor. *Am J Pathol.* (2018) 188:1183–94. doi: 10.1016/j.ajpath.2018.01.011
28. Esser C, Rannug A, Stockinger B. The aryl hydrocarbon receptor in immunity. *Trends Immunol.* (2009) 30:447–54. doi: 10.1016/j.it.2009.06.005
29. Stockinger B, Hirota K, Duarte J, Veldhoen M. External influences on the immune system via activation of the aryl hydrocarbon receptor. *Semin Immunol.* (2011) 23:99–105. doi: 10.1016/j.smim.2011.01.008
30. Zelante T, Iannitti RG, Cunha C, De Luca A, Giovannini G, Pieraccini G, et al. Tryptophan catabolites from microbiota engage aryl hydrocarbon receptor and balance mucosal reactivity via interleukin-22. *Immunity.* (2013) 39:372–85. doi: 10.1016/j.immuni.2013.08.003
31. Raison CL, Rutherford RE, Woolwine BJ, Shuo C, Schettler P, Drake DF, et al. A randomized controlled trial of the tumor necrosis factor antagonist infliximab for treatment-resistant depression: the role of baseline inflammatory biomarkers. *JAMA Psychiatry.* (2013) 70:31–41. doi: 10.1001/2013.jamapsychiatry.4

32. Anesi A, Rubert J, Oluwagbemigun K, Orozco-Ruiz X, Nothlings U, Breteler MMB, et al. Metabolic profiling of human plasma and urine, targeting tryptophan, tyrosine and branched chain amino acid pathways. *Metabolites.* (2019) 9:E261. doi: 10.3390/metabo9110261

33. Virtue AT, McCright SJ, Wright JM, Jimenez MT, Mowel WK, Kotzin JJ, et al. The gut microbiota regulates white adipose tissue inflammation and obesity via a family of microRNAs. *Sci Transl Med.* (2019) 11:eaav1892. doi: 10.1126/scitranslmed.aav1892

34. Widner B, Ledochowski M, Fuchs D. Interferon-gamma-induced tryptophan degradation: neuropsychiatric and immunological consequences. *Curr Drug Metab.* (2000) 1:193–204. doi: 10.2174/1389200003339063

35. Bansal T, Alaniz RC, Wood TK, Jayaraman A. The bacterial signal indole increases epithelial-cell tight-junction resistance and attenuates indicators of inflammation. *Proc Natl Acad Sci USA.* (2010) 107:228–33. doi: 10.1073/pnas.0906112107

36. Wlodarska M, Luo C, Kolde R, d'Hennezel E, Annand JW, Heim CE, et al. Indoleacrylic acid produced by commensal peptostreptococcus species suppresses inflammation. *Cell Host Microbe.* (2017) 22:25–37.e6. doi: 10.1016/j.chom.2017.06.007

37. Rodriguez-Hernandez H, Simental-Mendia LE, Rodriguez-Ramirez G, Reyes-Romero MA. Obesity and inflammation: epidemiology, risk factors, and markers of inflammation. *Int J Endocrinol.* (2013) 2013:678159. doi: 10.1155/2013/678159

38. Friedman M. Analysis, nutrition, and health benefits of tryptophan. *Int J Tryptophan Res.* (2018) 11:1178646918802282. doi: 10.1177/1178646918802282

11

Immunomodulatory Effects of Genetic Alterations Affecting the Kynurenine Pathway

Fanni A. Boros[1] *and László Vécsei*[1,2,3*]

[1] Department of Neurology, Faculty of Medicine, Albert Szent-Györgyi Clinical Center, University of Szeged, Szeged, Hungary,
[2] MTA-SZTE Neuroscience Research Group of the Hungarian Academy of Sciences, University of Szeged, Szeged, Hungary,
[3] Department of Neurology, Interdisciplinary Excellence Centre, University of Szeged, Szeged, Hungary

*Correspondence:
László Vécsei
vecsei.laszlo@med.u-szeged.hu

Several enzymes and metabolites of the kynurenine pathway (KP) have immunomodulatory effects. Modulation of the activities and levels of these molecules might be of particular importance under disease conditions when the amelioration of overreacting immune responses is desired. Results obtained by the use of animal and tissue culture models indicate that by eliminating or decreasing activities of key enzymes of the KP, a beneficial shift in disease outcome can be attained. This review summarizes experimental data of models in which IDO, TDO, or KMO activity modulation was achieved by interventions affecting enzyme production at a genomic level. Elimination of IDO activity was found to improve the outcome of sepsis, certain viral infections, chronic inflammation linked to diabetes, obesity, aorta aneurysm formation, and in anti-tumoral processes. Similarly, lack of TDO activity was advantageous in the case of anti-tumoral immunity, while KMO inhibition was found to be beneficial against microorganisms and in the combat against tumors, as well. On the other hand, the complex interplay among KP metabolites and immune function in some cases requires an increase in a particular enzyme activity for the desired immune response modulation, as was shown by the exacerbation of liver fibrosis due to the elimination of IDO activity and the detrimental effects of TDO inhibition in a mouse model of autoimmune gastritis. The relevance of these studies concerning possible human applications are discussed and highlighted. Finally, a brief overview is presented on naturally occurring genetic variants affecting immune functions *via* modulation of KP enzyme activity.

Keywords: kynurenine pathway, IDO, TDO, KMO, immunomodulation, genetic manipulation

INTRODUCTION

The kynurenine pathway (KP) is the main route of Trp metabolism. The enzymes of the pathway generate numerous metabolites, some of which are pro-inflammatory and/or generate free radicals, while others are known to be anti-inflammatory and/or scavenge free-radicals. Strong links between KP function and the immune system are demonstrated by extensive amounts of data on changes in the levels of KP metabolites and enzyme activities in diseases accompanied by alterations in immune function. Also, inflammatory cytokines are known to enhance the expression of a key KP enzyme, indoleamine 2,3-dioxygenase (IDO). Imbalances in the pathway can be detrimental, as excessive production of either pro-, or anti-inflammatory metabolites can contribute to the development of autoimmunity and/or lead to inefficient immune response against pathogens. Therefore, the understanding of how the KP changes in different immunological states, and, the reverse, how KP effects immunological responses, is cardinal both for understanding the true nature of specific diseases and for identification of therapeutic targets. Genetic manipulations leading either to enhancement or inhibition of the expression of KP enzymes might be a feasible way of restoring the imbalance of the pathway in various diseases. Naturally occurring genetic variations in the coding regions in several genes coding for KP enzymes have been identified [for a review see (1)]. In the majority of these, however, a causal relation between a specific gene variant and disease development has not been elucidated.

This review summarizes available data on the effects of expression modification of KP enzyme coding genes with specific attention to immune modulation. Following a brief overview

---

Abbreviations: KP, kynurenine pathway; IDO, indoleamine 2,3-dioxygenase (protein); *IDO*, indoleamine 2,3-dioxygenase (gene in human); *Ido*, indoleamine 2,3-dioxygenase (murine gene); TDO, tryptophan 2,3-dioxygenase (protein); *Tdo*, tryptophan 2,3-dioxygenase (murine gene); *TDO*, tryptophan 2,3-dioxygenase (gene in human); KMO, kynurenine 3-monooxygenase (protein); *KMO*, kynurenine 3-monooxygenase (gene in human); *Kmo*, kynurenine 3-monooxygenase (murine gene); CNS, central nervous system; L-KYN, L-kynurenine; KYNA, kynurenic acid; KATI-IV, kynurenine aminotransferases; NMDAR, N-methyl-D-aspartate receptor; α7nAChRs, nicotinic acetylcholine receptors; KYNU, kynureninase; AA, anthranilic acid; 3-HK, 3-hydroxy kynurenine; XA, xanthurenic acid; 3-HAA, 3-hydroxyanthranilic acid; ACMS, 2-amino-3-carboxymuconate-semialdehyde; 3-HAO, 3-hydroxyanthranilate 3,4-dioxygenase; PIC, picolinic acid; ACMSD, aminocarboxymuconate-semialdehyde-decarboxylase; QUIN, quinolinic acid; ISRE, IFN stimulated response element; GAS, gamma-activated sequences; DRE, dendritic cell response element; NF-κB, nuclear factor kappa-light-chain-enhancer of activated B-cells; TLRs, toll-like receptors; TGFBR, transforming growth factor beta receptor; AHR, aryl hydrocarbon receptor; IFNBR, interferon beta receptor; IFNGR, interferon gamma receptor; TNFR, tumor necrosis factor receptor; SOCS3, suppressor of cytokine signaling 3; DC, dendritic cell; IFN, interferon; LPS, lipopolysaccharide; IL, interleukines; TNF, tumor necrosis factor; mTOR, mammalian target of rapamycin; NPC, nasopharyngeal carcinoma; AML, acute myeloid leukemia; AHR, aryl hydrocarbon receptor; ROS, reactive oxygen species; siRNA, small interfering RNA; IDO$^{-/-}$, *IDO* knockout; UPEC, Uropathogenic *Escherichia coli*; MuLV, murine leukemia virus; NK cell, natural killer cell; pDC, plasmocytoid dendritic cell; WT, wild type; ECMV, encephalomyocarditis virus; sJIA, systemic juvenile idiopathic arthritis; sHLH, secondary hemophagocytic-lymphohistiocytosis; STING, Stimulator of Interferon Genes; DNP, DNA nanoparticle; EAE, experimental autoimmune encephalitis; MS, multiple sclerosis; MOG, myelin oligodendrocyte glycoprotein; c-diGMP, cyclic diguanylate monophosphate; CIA, collagen induced arthritis; RA, rheumatoid arthritis; AdIDO, adenoviral vector-mediated IDO gene delivery; NOD, non-obese diabetic; MRL*lpr/lpr*, Lupus-prone Murphy Roths large mice; SLE, systemic lupus erythematosus; MAS, macrophage activation syndrome; DR, diabetic retinopathy; AngII, angiotensin II; *ApoE*$^{-/-}$, Apolipoprotein E knockout; NAD(P)H, nicotinamide adenine dinucleotide phosphate; AAA, abdominal aortic aneurysm; VSMC, vascular smooth muscle cell; *Ldlr*$^{-/-}$, low density lipoprotein—receptor deficient; HFD, high fat diet; MMP2, matrix metallopeptidase 2; WAT, white adipose tissue; OGTT, oral glucose tolerance test; ITT, insulin tolerance test; IAA, indole-3 acetic acid; CCl4, carbon-tetrachloride; PMN, polymorph nuclear neutrophil; S.t., *Salmonella typhimurium*; shRNA, short hairpin RNA; RT, radiotherapy; BER, base excision repair; MX, methoxyamine; TS, thymidylate synthase; IRI, ischemia-reperfusion injury; AKI, acute kidney injury; CTL, cytolytic T lymphocyte; PD, Parkinson's disease; SSc, systemic sclerosis; CD, Crohn's disease; BM, bacterial meningitis; CSF, cerebro-spinal fluid.

---

of the metabolites and enzymes of the pathway, we summarize observations which indicate links between KP and immune function. This is followed by an overview of findings obtained by the use of models with targeted ablation and up- or down-regulation of KP enzymes. With respect to diseases related to disorders of the immune system, such as infectious diseases, chronic inflammation, autoimmunity and cancer, these models have focused on three KP enzymes: IDO, tryptophan 2,3-dioxygenase (TDO) and kynurenine 3-monooxygenase (KMO) (**Tables 1–5**). These enzymes and, in particular, IDO are also targeted by several pharmacochemical interventions. Discussion of that field is out of the scope of this review, as we focus on gene level interventions. Readers interested in pharmacologic interventions of KP enzymes can find excellent summaries of the field in Ye et al. (45) and Lemos et al. (46). In the final section, we provide a summary of available data on those naturally occurring KP gene variants which are believed to be associated with different human diseases affecting immune function.

KYNURENINE PATHWAY—THE MAIN ROUTE OF TRYPTOPHAN METABOLISM

Disregarding protein synthesis, the KP is the main route of Trp metabolism, both in the peripheral and in the central nervous system (CNS) (**Figure 1**). In the CNS, 95 percent of the resident Trp is metabolized *via* the KP, and only the minority of the amino acid is transformed into serotonin and melatonin. In consecutive steps of the pathway, numerous metabolites possessing immune- and neuromodulatory properties are synthesized (47).

The first and rate limiting step of Trp metabolism is the conversion of the amino acid into N-formyl-L-kynurenine. This step is catalyzed by one of three enzymes: IDO (often referred to as IDO1), IDO2, or TDO. (Prior to the discovery of IDO 2, "IDO" designation was used exclusively. Today IDO and IDO1 are used as synonyms and IDO2 is reserved for the enzyme recognized in 2007. In this review we will use IDO unless we are referring to IDO2). TDO is expressed mainly in the liver, thus plays a cardinal role in regulating the amount of available Trp throughout the body, outside the CNS. IDO is expressed in several human tissues, among them various cell types of the immune system (48). The enzyme plays a key role in reactions leading to the synthesis of immunoactive KP metabolites, consequently its role in immunomodulation is expected. IDO2 expression pattern and function is not known in detail. A strong argument against the role of this enzyme in Trp metabolism is the frequent occurrence of an IDO2 gene variant that gives rise to a non-functioning enzyme (49), and the high Michaelis Constant of the enzyme for Trp, which is 100-fold above the physiological concentrations of the amino acid (50).

N-formyl-L-kynurenine is converted to L-kynurenine (L-KYN) by formamidase. L-KYN is an important branch point of the KP as it can be alternatively metabolized into three different metabolites of which some are neurotoxic, while others possess neuroprotective and antioxidant properties (51, 52). Firstly, L-KYN can be metabolized into kynurenic acid (KYNA) by kynurenine aminotransferases (KATI-IV)

TABLE 1 | Effects of modulation of IDO function by genetic manipulation in *in vivo* and *in vitro* models of systemic inflammation, viral, and bacterial infections.

Gene	Type of genetic modulation	Disease modeled	Study design	Effect of gene modulation	References
IDO	IDO$^{-/-}$	Systemic inflammation	Mouse model of LPS induced sepsis	Restoration of imbalance of pro-and anti-inflammatory cytokines, increased survival rate	(2)
	IDO$^{-/-}$	Viral infection	Murine leukemia virus induced murine AIDS model	Decreased virus replication; increased number of pDCs and increased type I IFN production; increased survival rate following *Toxoplasma gondii* infection	(3)
	IDO$^{-/-}$	Viral infection	ECMV induced mouse model of acute viral myocarditis	Decreased virus replication and myocardium necrosis; higher survival rate	(4)
	IDO$^{-/-}$	Pain hypersensitivity related to viral infection	Pain hypersensitivity induced by Influenza A virus and MuLV infection	Diminished acute and chronic pain sensitivity related to influenza A and MuLV infections, respectively	(5)
	IDO overexpression	Viral infection	HeLa cells transfected with pcDNA3-IDO	Overexpression of IDO prior to viral infection diminished viral replication thus decreasing infection spread to the neighboring cells	(6)
	IDO$^{-/-}$	Viral infection	LP-BPM5 retrovirus infection of mice - a model of murine AIDS	Gene knockout did not have any effect on disease progression and viral load	(7)
	IDO$^{-/-}$	Bacterial infection	Mouse model of *Mycobacterium tuberculosis* infection	*In vitro* findings showed enhanced T cell proliferation after infection, however, *in vivo* no significant difference could be observed in survival rate or in the number of activated T cells	(8)
	IDO$^{-/-}$	Bacterial infection	Murine cystitis model provoked by uropathogen *Escherichia coli* infection	Increased levels of pro-inflammatory cytokines, higher granulocyte accumulation, and local inflammation of the bladder and decreased survival of the extracellular bacteria	(9)
	IDO$^{-/-}$	Bacterial infection	Mouse model of *Rhodococcus equi* infection	Decreased levels of TGFβ and FOXP3 expression in the liver tissue indicating reduced T regulatory cell responses and prolonged liver inflammation	(10)

IDO, Indoleamine 2,3-dioxygenase gene; IDO$^{-/-}$, IDO knockout; pDC, plasmocytoid dendritic cell; IFN, interferon; ECMV, encephalomyocarditis virus; MuLV, murine leukemia virus; TGFβ, transforming growth factor beta; FOXP3, forkhead box P3.

from which KATII plays the most important role in the human CNS (53, 54). Secondly, L-KYN is also a substrate of kynureninase (KYNU), an enzyme responsible for the formation of anthranilic acid (AA). Finally, the third route of L-KYN metabolism is catalyzed by KMO to form 3-hydroxy kynurenine (3-HK) which can be further transformed into xanthurenic acid (XA) by KATs. 3-HK and AA can both be metabolized into 3-hydroxyanthranilic acid (3-HAA), which, alongside with 3-HK, have free-radical generating properties, thus can lead to oxidative stress and neurodegeneration (55). However, depending on the redox properties of the cell, 3-HK and 3-HAA can also serve as antioxidant molecules (56).

Further down the pathway, the unstable 2-amino-3-carboxymuconate-semialdehyde (ACMS) is formed by 3-hydroxyanthranilate 3,4-dioxygenase (3-HAO). ACMS can be transformed either into picolinic acid (PIC) by an aminocarboxymuconate-semialdehyde-decarboxylase (ACMSD) catalyzed reaction, or it can form the NAD+ and NADP+ precursor quinolinic acid (QUIN) *via* a non-enzymatic conversion. QUIN is a key figure in excitotoxicity mediated neurodegeneration (52, 57, 58).

In light of the numerous enzymes participating and metabolites generated, the involvement of the KP in various disorders is not surprising. Indeed, changes in KP enzyme activity and metabolite levels have been detected in inflammatory, autoimmune, neurodegenerative and psychiatric diseases, as well.

In the following sections of this review we will briefly consider observations that point to existing links between KP and immune function. Then we will overview results obtained by models in which the KP was modulated by interventions effecting gene activity. Finally, we list known genetic alterations in genes of KP enzymes that are believed to be associated with changes in immune functions.

TABLE 2 | Effects of modulation of IDO function by genetic manipulation in animal models of allergy and autoimmunity.

Gene	Type of genetic modulation	Disease modeled	Study design	Effect of gene modulation	References
IDO	IDO⁻/⁻	Airway allergy	Mouse model of acute and chronic allergic airway inflammation	Decrease in Th2 response upon exposure to allergen: diminished Th2 cell activation, Th2 cytokine production, decreased airway inflammation, mucus secretion, and airway hyperresponsiveness	(11)
	IDO⁻/⁻	Autoimmunity	Mice models of sJIA, MAS and sHLH	No difference in the symptoms of IDO⁻/⁻ animals compared to WT—possibility of the presence of other Trp metabolizing enzymes restoring the absence of Ido	(12)
	IDO⁻/⁻	Autoimmunity	EAE mouse model of MS	Immunization with MOG, systemic treatment with DNPs or c-diGMP induced STING signaling, thus potent regulatory immune responses could be achieved, leading to restrained EAE severity and delayed disease onset. However, in the case of lack of IDO in hematopoietic cells, no therapeutic response could be observed	(13)
	IDO⁻/⁻	Autoimmunity	EAE mouse model of MS	Exacerbated EAE disease severity, increased encephalitogenic Th1 and Th17 responses and diminished Treg responses in IDO⁻/⁻ animals.	(14)
	IDO⁻/⁻	Autoimmunity	CIA mouse model of RA	More severe disease demonstrated by increased erosion and cellular infiltration of the joints of IDO⁻/⁻ animals, higher production of IFNγ and IL-17 in the lymph nodes and higher Th1 and Th17 cell frequency in paws	(15)
	AdIDO	Autoimmunity	CIA rat model of RA	Significant reduction of bony destruction, soft tissue swelling and synovial hyperplasia, indicating decreased disease severity	(16)
	Transfection with Ido	Autoimmunity	NOD mouse model of T1D	After TGFβ treatment production of pro-inflammatory cytokines (IL-6 and TNFα) was decreased and pancreatic β-cell auto-antigen generation was diminished	(17)
	IDO⁻/⁻	Autoimmunity	MRLlpr/lpr mouse model of SLE	The injection of apoptotic thymocytes in IDO⁻/⁻ MRLlpr/lpr animals caused elevation of autoantibody titers, pro-inflammatory cytokine production and dysregulated T cell responses leading to lethal autoimmunity due to renal failure	(18)

IDO, Indoleamine 2,3-dioxygenase gene; IDO⁻/⁻, IDO knockout; sJIA, systemic juvenile idiopathic arthritis; MAS, macrophage activation syndrome; sHLH, secondary hemophagocytic-lymphohistiocytosis; WT, wild type; Trp, tryptophan; EAE, experimental autoimmune encephalitis; MS, multiple sclerosis; MOG, myelin oligodendrocyte glycoprotein; DNP, DNA nanoparticle; c-diGMP, cyclic diguanylate monophosphate; CIA, collagen induced arthritis; RA, rheumatoid arthritis; IFNγ, interferon gamma; AdIDO, adenoviral vector-mediated IDO gene delivery; NOD, non-obese diabetic; T1D, type 1 diabetes; TGFβ, transforming growth factor beta; MRLlpr/lpr, Lupus-prone Murphy Roths large mice; SLE, systemic lupus erythematosus.

OBSERVATIONS INDICATING LINKS BETWEEN THE KYNURENINE PATHWAY AND IMMUNE FUNCTIONS

Indoleamine 2,3-Dioxygenase

Interplay between several enzymes of the KP and immune function are well-demonstrated. In this respect IDO, a key enzyme of the pathway, deserves particular attention. IDO is believed to exert its effects on immune function both by direct and indirect mechanisms. As an enzyme, IDO plays a role in Trp utilization and through this, in cellular metabolism *via* mTOR and GCN2 linked pathways. By converting Trp to KYN, IDO has a central role in determining concentrations of KP metabolites, many of which are direct or indirect regulators

TABLE 3 | Effects of modulation of IDO function by genetic manipulation in transplant animal models.

Gene	Type of genetic modulation	Disease modeled	Study design	Effect of gene modulation	References
IDO	Adenoviral *Ido* gene transfer	Transplantation	Adenoviral gene transfer into pancreatic islets; transplantation into diabetogenic mice	Prolonged survival of transplanted tissue; depletion of local Trp; inhibition of T cell proliferation	(19)
	EIAV based *Ido* gene transfer	Transplantation	Mouse model of corneal transplant	Prevention of allogeneic T cell responses; prolonged corneal graft survival	(20)
	hIDO gene transfer *via* PEI	Transplantation	Rat model of lung transplant	Blockage of local T cell responses, inhibition of intracellular ROS formation, thus reducing necrosis and apoptosis of lung cells	(21)
	hIDO gene transfer *via* PEI	Transplantation	Rat model of lung transplant	Selective decrease of complex I activity of the electron transport chain, leading to decreased ATP production in the lung infiltrating T cells, causing damage in their cytotoxic properties	(22)
	Sleeping beauty transposon mediated hIDO delivery	Transplantation	Rat model of lung transplant, investigation of lung fibrosis	Diminished collagen deposition in IDO$^{+/+}$ lungs, resulting in a more preserved bronchus-alveolar architecture. *In vitro* findings revealed that IDO$^{+/+}$ lung cells inhibited the TGFβ mediated proliferation of fibroblasts	(23)
	adenoviral *Ido* gene transfer	Transplantation	Rat model of skin transplant	Wounds with IDO expressing fibroblast healed faster than those with IDO$^{-/-}$ fibroblasts due to enhanced capillary formation	(24)
	adenoviral *Ido* gene transfer	Transplantation	Rat model of cardiac allograft survival	Decreased infiltration of the cardiac allograft with monocytes, macrophages and T cells, accompanied by diminished intragraft levels of IFNγ, TNFα, TGFβ, IL-1β, resulting in prolonged graft survival	(25)
	PEI carrier hIDO transfer	Transplantation	Mouse model of lung transplantation	Prolonged graft survival due to inhibited early T cell responses and diminished memory T cell formation. T cell inhibiting properties were found to be due to the impairment of calcium signaling of the cells	(26)

IDO, Indoleamine 2,3-dioxygenase gene; IDO$^{-/-}$, IDO knockout; Trp, tryptophan; EIAV, Equine infectious anemia virus; PEI, polimer polyethilenimine; ROS, reactive oxygen species; TGFβ, transforming growth factor beta; IFNγ, interferon gamma; TNFα, tumor necrosis factor alpha.

of immunofunction. Furthermore, IDO also acts as a signal protein. In concert with TGFβ, it regulates activation through non-canonical NF-κB response elements, thus affecting of its own production as well (45, 46).

IDO production and activity is controlled at different levels, including both transcriptional and post-translational regulation [reviewed in (46, 59)] (**Figure 2**). At the protein level, both its substrate, Trp, and its co-factor, heme, enhance IDO activity (61, 62). NO was found to reversibly inhibit the enzyme by binding to the active site (63, 64). Antioxidants also inhibit enzyme activity, both at transcriptional and post-transcriptional levels (62). Phosphorylation of two tyrosine side chains also can modulate IDO activity and its halflife (65). Decrease in IDO enzyme levels can be the result of ubiquitylation of the protein by the suppressor of cytokine signaling 3 (SOCS3) factor and proteosomal degradation (66).

At the level of transcription several cis-regulatory elements in the *IDO* promoter transmit regulatory signals. These are IFN stimulated response elements (ISRE), palindromic gamma-activated sequences (GAS), dendritic cell response elements (DRE) and non-canonical NF-κB binding sites [see reviews (60, 65)]. A number of transcription factors have been identified so far, which bind to these elements and play roles in the transcriptional regulation of IDO. Among them are IRF-1, IRF-8, Stat1a, NF-κB (67) and aryl hydrocarbon receptor (AHR). Recently, epigenetic regulation of the gene through histone deacetylase activity has also been reported (68). Through these factors various receptor-ligand pathways converge to determine *IDO* gene expression. These transmit regulatory signals from activated toll-like receptors (TLRs), transforming growth factor beta receptors (TGFBRs), AHR, interferon beta and gamma receptors (IFNBR and IFNGR), and members of the tumor

TABLE 4 | Effects of modulation of IDO function by genetic manipulation in *in vitro* and *in vivo* models of chronic inflammation and cancer.

Gene	Type of genetic modulation	Disease modeled	Study design	Effect of gene modulation	References
IDO	IDO$^{-/-}$	Chronic inflammation	Mouse model of DR	Reduced retinal capillary degeneration	(27)
	IDO$^{-/-}$	Chronic inflammation	AngII induced atherosclerosis mouse model	Reduced ROS production; diminished endothelial cell dysfunction and apoptosis	(28)
	IDO$^{-/-}$	Chronic inflammation	Mouse model of AAA: Ldlr$^{-/-}$ mice infused with AngII and fed with HFD	Reduced VSMC apoptosis	(29)
	IDO$^{-/-}$ and siRNA mediated *Kynu* silencing	Chronic inflammation	AngII induced AAA formation in ApoE$^{-/-}$ mice	Protection against AAA formation—decrease in elastic lamina degradation and aortic expansion	(30)
	IDO$^{-/-}$	Chronic inflammation	Mouse model of obesity	Lower body weight and fat mass; increased number of M2 (anti-inflammatory) macrophages in the WAT; protection against the development of liver steatosis and insulin resistance; diminished LPS plasma levels	(31)
	IDO$^{-/-}$	Chronic inflammation	CCl4 induced mouse model of hepatic fibrosis	Aggravation of liver fibrosis: higher TNFα producing macrophages in the liver; higher TNFα and fibrogenic factor expression	(32)
	IDO$^{-/-}$	Intestinal immunity	*Citrobacter rodentium*-induced colitis mouse model	Attenuated intestinal inflammatory response: less edema, cellular infiltration, epithelial damage and reduced intestinal colonization of bacteria	(33)
	IDO silencing *via* siRNA	Tumor immunity	B16F10 melanoma cells *in vitro* and mouse model	Decrease in tumor size; prevention of T cell apoptosis; restoration of host antitumor immunity	(34)
	IDO silencing *via* shIDO-ST	Tumor immunity	B16F10 melanoma mouse model	Tumor growth is attenuated and the number of lung metastases was diminished	(35)
	IDO silencing *via* shRNA	Tumor immunity	SKOV-3 human ovarian cancer cell line and mouse model	Decrease in tumor growth, peritoneal dissemination and ascites formation, increase in the number of tumor infiltrating NK cells *in vivo*; increased sensitivity to NK cells *in vitro*	(36)
	IDO silencing *via* shRNA	Tumor immunity	Genetic downregulation of IDO in A549 human lung adenocarcinoma cells	Enhanced sensitivity of cells to FK866, MX, pemetrexed and gemcitabine therapy	(37)

IDO, Indoleamine 2,3-dioxygenase gene; Ido$^{-/-}$, Ido knockout; Kynu, kynureninase gene; siRNA, small interfering RNA; shIDO-ST, shRNA: short hairpin RNA; DR, diabetic retinopathy; AngII, Angiotensin II; AAA, abdominal aortic aneurysm; Ldlr$^{-/-}$, low density lipoprotein–receptor deficient; HFD, high fat diet; ApoF$^{-/-}$, Apolipoprotein E knockout; CCl4, carbontetrachloride; ROS, reactive oxygen species; VSMC, vascular smooth cell; WAT, white adipose tissue; LPS, lipopolysaccharide; TNFα, tumor necrosis factor alpha; NK cell, natural killer cell; MX, methoxyamine.

necrosis factor receptor superfamily (TNFRs). Activation of any of these receptors by their ligands can trigger signaling pathways that promote or maintain the expression of *IDO*. Consequently, inflammatory signals, such as IFNs, lipopolysaccharides (LPS), interleukins (ILs) (such as IL-1, IL-2, IL-27, IL-10) TNFs, TGFs, and prostaglandins, can induce IDO production (69, 70). Thus, induction of the enzyme can be very complex and cell type specific [reviewed in (71)]. Moreover, some inflammatory markers act synergistically to increase IDO production and the types of cytokines affecting gene expression may differ in various cell types. This might be reflected by seemingly contradictory reports on the roles of particular ligands in IDO induction. According to some data, IFNγ is one of the main inducers of IDO expression (72). On the other hand, results obtained in LPS induced systemic inflammatory rat model did not support the role of IFNγ in IDO induction in the CNS

and a more important role for other inflammatory cytokines, such as TNFα and IL-6, was proposed. Strengthening this conclusion, in LPS-stimulated glial cell cultures an increase of IDO expression was observed, accompanied by elevated levels of TNFα and IL-6, but no IFNγ expression. Based on these observations, it was concluded that IDO induction in the CNS by LPS is not mediated by IFNγ (73). However, recent findings strongly argue for the role of IFNs in the activation of IDO expression. It was found that not IFNγ but IFNα signaling was essential in enhancing IDO expression after B7 ligation of CTL4-Ig (74). *IDO* expression up-regulation *via* CpG oligodeoxynucleotide binding to TLR9 was also IFNα dependent (75). Futhermore, *IDO* expression was found to be upregulated by cytosolic DNA *via* the STING/IFNαβ pathway (76). Thus, it seems firmly established that type I IFNs play a cardinal role in enhanced *IDO* gene expression with inflammatory signals

TABLE 5 | Effects of modulation of TDO and KMO function by genetic manipulation in *in vitro* and *in vivo* models.

Gene	Type of genetic modulation	Disease modeled	Study design	Effect of gene modulation	References
TDO	Lack of *Tdo* expression	Tumor immunity	P815 mouse tumor model	Slower tumor progression, higher number of cytolytic T cells in the tumor microenvironment	(38)
	TDO$^{-/-}$	Autoimmunity	EAE mouse model of MS	Protective effects against neuronal loss in the spinal cord	(39)
	TDO expression	Infection	HeLa T-Rex cells transfected with pcDNA4-*Tdo* vector containing human liver *TDO* cDNA	Antiparasitic, antiviral, and antibacterial effect; suppression of T cell proliferation	(40)
KMO	KMO$^{-/-}$	Viral infection	EMCV induced mouse model of viral myocarditis	Higher survival rate of *Kmo*$^{-/-}$ animals; decrease in the cellular infiltration of marophages and neutrophiles in heart tissue	(41)
	siRNA mediated *Kmo* silencing	Autoimmunity	Mouse model of autoimmune gastritis	Disease exacerbation due to excessive Th17 cell formation	(42)
	KMO$^{-/-}$	Chronic inflammation	Diabetic mouse and zebrafish models	Proteinuria related to the malfunctioning of kidney podocytes (proposedly due to NAD$^+$ depletion)	(43)
	KMO$^{-/-}$	IRI	IRI leading to AKI in a mouse model	Decreased renal tubular necrosis and neutrophil granulocyte infiltration	(44)

TDO, Tryptophan 2,3-dioxygenase gene; TDO-/-, TDO knockout; KMO, Kynurenine 3-monooxygenase gene; KMO-/-, KMO knockout; EAE, experimental autoimmune encephalitis; MS, multiple sclerosis; EMCV, encephalomyocarditis virus; IRI, ischemia-reperfusion injury; AKI, acute kidney injury.

and that *IDO* expression following LPS treatment is induced by type I IFNs.

IDO is expressed by numerous cells of the immune system: monocytes, dendritic cells (DCs), macrophages and microglia (48). It regulates immune responses in various direct and indirect ways (**Figure 3**). On the one hand, by decreasing the amount of available Trp, it causes an increase in free transfer RNA, thus activating the GCN2 stress-kinase pathway leading to T cell anergy and cell cycle arrest (77). On the other hand, a lack of the amino acid leads to the inhibition of the rapamycin (mTOR) pathway followed by a translational block (78). Moreover, *via* the formation of different immunologically active kynurenine metabolites, IDO also contributes to the apoptosis of effector T cells and promotes the formation of regulatory T cells (59, 79).

Another important link between KP and the immune system is manifested by DCs, in particular in their role in inflammatory processes. Sepsis is a systemic inflammatory response syndrome which leads to hemodynamic shock accompanied by multi-organ failure. It is a major cause of mortality and morbidity among hospitalized patients. Sepsis is the consequence of microbial infection, in which Gram-negative bacteria outer-membrane components (LPS) trigger the uncontrolled production of pro-inflammatory cytokines, which leads to the imbalance of pro-and anti-inflammatory factors. DCs seem to play a cardinal role is sepsis development, as they are capable of producing pro- (IL-12) and anti-inflammatory (IL-10) cytokines, the balance of which was found to be altered during infection (80). In DCs, IDO expression is induced by LPS and the enzyme production contributes to the imbalance of anti- and pro-inflammatory cytokines (2).

A growing body of data shows the involvement of IDO in immune responses to tumors [see in (45, 46, 81)]. A pivotal role

of the enzyme is seen in establishing the immunosuppressive microenvironment of tumors by altering the functions of infiltrating T lymphocytes, thus promoting immune escape and progression of cancer cells (82, 83). Upregulated expression of IDO has been reported in the microenvironment of laryngeal and esophageal carcinomas (84–87) and higher plasma enzyme activity was reported in lung-, gynecological-, breast- and colorectal cancers, and melanoma. Both local expression changes and elevated plasma IDO activity was reported in patients with nasopharyngeal carcinoma (NPC) (81). Interestingly, a significant difference in plasma IDO levels could be detected between healthy controls and NPC patients with metastasis, in contrast to patients without metastasis. Plasma IDO activity was also found to have a prognostic value, as patients with higher levels of enzyme activity had significantly lower rates of survival compared to those with lower IDO activity. Higher enzyme activity was shown to result from higher expression levels: Fukuno et al. reported that IDO mRNA expression in patients with acute myeloid leukemia (AML) was associated with a worse disease outcome (88). In light of the role IDO plays in immune responses to cancer, it is no wonder that IDO modulation is a hot topic in cancer research. Many therapeutic approaches are underway for pharmaceutical enzyme inhibition (65). This review will not discuss these in detail since our aim is to give an overview of findings on approaches targeting the KP by gene modulation.

Tryptophan-Dioxygenase

The first step of the KP can also be catalyzed by TDO, a functional ortholog enzyme of IDO. However, while IDO is mainly expressed by various immune cells, thus regulating the amount of locally available Trp, TDO is expressed in the liver, affecting

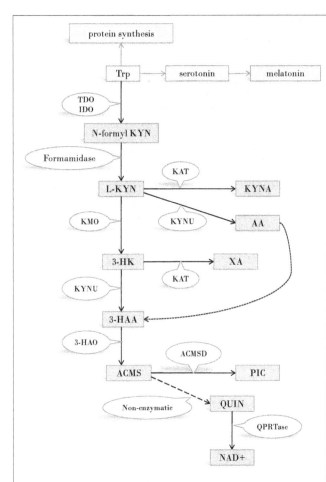

FIGURE 1 | The kynurenine pathway of tryptophan metabolism. Enzymes of the KP metabolise Trp into products possessing immune- and neuromodulatory properties. By the utilization of Trp and generation of NAD coenzyme precursor the KP has profound effects on cellular protein and energy metabolism. Several internal metabolites of the pathway play role on redox regulation and have neuroprotective - or neurotoxic effects. Immune functions are modified by the KP both directly, via immuno modulatory metabolites and indirectly, via changing the metabolism of immune cells by altering amino acid availability, redox status and energy balance. Abbreviations: Trp: tryptophan; TDO:tryptophan 2,3-dioxygenase; IDO:indoleamine 2,3-dioxygenase; N-formyl KYN:N-formyl-kynurenine; L-KYN:L-kynurenine; KAT:kynurenine aminotransferase; KYNA: kynurenic acid; KYNU:kynureninase; AA:anthranilic acid; KMO:kynurenine 3-monooxygenase; 3-HK:3-hydroxy kynurenine; XA: xanthurenic acid; KYNU:kynureninase; 3-HAA: 3-hydroxyanthranilic acid; 3-HAO:3-hydroxyanthranilate 3,4-dioxygenase; ACMS: 2-amino-3-carboxymuconate-semialdehyde; ACMSD: aminocarboxymuconate-semialdehyde-decarboxylase; PIC: picolinic acid; QUIN: quinolinic acid; QPRTase:quinolinate phosphoribosyltransferase; NAD+: nicotinamide adenine dinucleotide; CNS: central nervous system.

the systemic level of the amino acid. The activity of the enzyme can be regulated by various mechanisms. *TDO* transcription is enhanced by glucocorticoids and this is potentiated by glucagon, but inhibited by adrenaline and insulin (89). TDO can also be activated by its cofactor, heme, and its substrate, Trp [reviewed in (61)]. Recent evidence demonstrates TDO presence in rat skin and the CNS of humans (90, 91), thus broadening the

location and raising further questions on the exact role of the enzyme. As Trp stabilizes the TDO enzyme complex (92), and cortisone, a hormone with anti-inflammatory effects, enhances TDO expression (93, 94), one can expect the involvement of the enzyme in immune processes. This was reported first in the early 2000s (95, 96): in 2000, Tatsumi et al. proposed a role for the enzyme in tolerance during embryonic implantation, based on finding upregulated expression of TDO mRNA in murine decidualized stromal cells surrounding the implanted embryo (96). In 2001 Suzuki et al. reported high TDO expression during early murine gestation, preceding the expression of IDO, thus revealing an important role of TDO in fetal tolerance (95). When regarding the immune modulator effects of the KP, research has been mainly focused on IDO, but a growing body of evidence is accumulating on the involvement of TDO as well. It indicates the presence of the enzyme in tumor immune resistance (38, 97) and parasite, viral and microbial infections (98) (**Table 5**). Expression of TDO by several different tumor types—such as melanomas, bladder-, and hepatocarcinomas—drew attention to the possible role of the enzyme in tumor immunity. TDO was found to be constitutively expressed in glioblastomas and excessive production of the AHR agonist KYN was found to contribute to the immune escape, higher motility and survival of tumor cells (38).

Kynurenine Monooxygenase

A third enzyme with assumed immunomodulatory effects of the KP is KMO, which is situated at an important branch point of the pathway. KYN can be catalyzed by KATs into KYNA, representing a neuroprotective and antioxidant branch of the pathway. On the other hand, KMO can convert KYN to 3-HK, which can be further converted into PIC and QUIN. Both of these metabolites are known to have neurotoxic and free radical generating properties. Thus, KMO has a key role in determining the balance between pro- (QUIN, 3-HK, PIC) and anti-inflammatory (KYNA) kynurenine metabolites.

The substrate of the KMO enzyme, KYN, was shown to promote tumor formation and the generation of regulatory T cells *via* AHR (99) and adenylate- and guanylate-cyclase pathway activation (38). However, the mode of action of KYN on AHR raised questions, as the structure of the metabolite does not show the necessary features for high-affinity AHR binding. Recently two KYN condensation products have been identified, which are high affinity AHR ligands, active at low picomolar levels. Thus, KYN seems to be a pro-ligand that spontaneously converts to derivatives possessing AHR agonist properties (100). Theoretically, enhancing the metabolism of KYN *via* KMO upregulation could be protective against the development of tumors. However, upregulation of KMO also leads to the formation of metabolites with reactive oxygen species (ROS) generating properties, such as 3-HK, 3-HAA, and QUIN. QUIN also exerts excitotoxic effects through the activation of NMDARs (38). Pharmacological inhibition of KMO enhances the production of KYNA, a metabolite with neuroprotective effects. Besides its neuroprotective effects (101, 102) KYNA also has an important role in immunomodulation, mainly *via* the activation of GPR35 receptors and AHRs [reviewed: (103)]. KYNA was

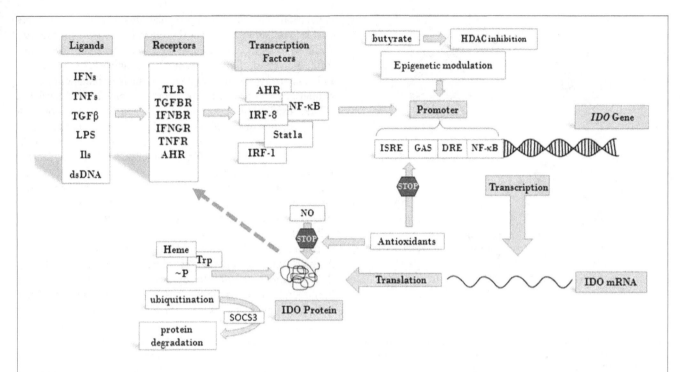

FIGURE 2 | Overview of pathways leading to IDO enzyme production and regulation. IDO activity is regulated at different levels. Its substrate Trp and cofactor heme are positive regulators of the enzyme, whereas antioxidants and NO act as inhibitors. Phosphorylation at tyrosine side chains and ubiquitination modulate IDO activity and half life. At the level of transcription several cis regulatory elements of the IDO promoter collect regulatory signals via binding of transcription factors and epigenetic regulators, which respond to signals arriving from receptors that are activated by cytokines and other immunomodulatory molecules. Extracellular signals produced by other cells or pathogens and intracellular signals, such as cytosolic dsDNA can both induce IDO expression and feed-back regulation of the production has also been described [see text for details and (60)]. Abbreviations: IFN: interferon; TNF: tumor necrosis factor; TGFβ: transforming growth factor beta; LPS: lipopolysaccharide; dsDNA: double strand DNA; TLR: toll-like receptor; TGFBR: transforming growth factor beta receptor; IFNBR: interferon beta receptor; IFNGR: interferon gamma receptor; TNFR: tumor necrosis factor receptor; AHR: aryl hydrocarbon receptor; ISRE: IFN stimulated response element; DRE: dendritic cell response element; GAS: gamma-activated sequences; HDAC: histone deacetylase; ~P: phosphorylation; IDO: indoleamine 2,3-dioxygenase; SOCS3: suppressor of cytokine signaling 3; Trp: tryptophan; NO: nitrogen oxide.

found to attenuate inflammation under inflammatory conditions by several means: by reducing TNF expression in monocytes, IL-4 secretion of T-cell receptor stimulated variant natural killer-like T cells and LPS induced IL-23 formation of DCs [reviewed: (103)]. The expression of KMO was also found to be upregulated in the CNS of rats in LPS induced systemic inflammation, together with a significant increase in pro-inflammatory cytokines such as TNFα and IL-6 (73).

KMO expression and activity have been investigated in autoimmunity related diseases. A link seems to exist through AHRs as these receptors play an important role in the regulation of pro-inflammatory Th17 cell differentiation (42) and Trp metabolites act as agonists of AHRs. KP metabolites play roles in promoting the differentiation of naive T cells into effector Th17 cells (104), which are governors of autoimmune diseases (105). Stephens et al. reported that Th17 cells highly express KMO, and that either the inhibition of the enzyme or the addition of 3-HK augmented the formation of effector T cells (42).

Since these three enzymes of the KP seem to be associated with immune functions, genetic approaches aimed at modifying immune responses are focused on altering their expression. So far, primarily gene knockouts, gene expression regulation by small interfering RNA (siRNA), short hairpin RNA (shRNA)

and different gene delivery techniques into model animals and tissue culture cells have yielded results regarding the immunomodulatory effects of these enzymes. The next section will review these results. We find it important to point out here that with the rapid progress of gene modulatory and gene editing techniques it is expected that the data summarized here will grow in the near future.

IMMUNOMODULATION *VIA* ALTERING THE EXPRESSION OF GENES THAT CODE FOR ENZYMES OF THE KYNURENINE PATHWAY

Indoleamine 2,3-Dioxygenase
Effects of Genetic Modification of Indoleamine 2,3-Dioxygenase Related to Immune Responses in Infection

During the course of sepsis, induction of IDO by bacterial endotoxins plays a pivotal role in the disproportional production of pro- and anti-inflammatory cytokines. Consequently, the detrimental effects of excessive pro-inflammatory stimuli could be lessened by the genetic inhibition of IDO (2). Indeed, in IDO

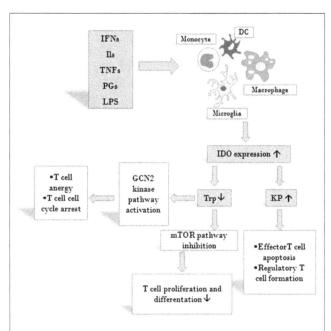

FIGURE 3 | Effects on IDO activity on immune responses. IDO is expressed by various cells of the immune system in response to activation by inflammatory markers such as IFNs, ILs, TNFs, PGs and LPS. By decreasing the amount of available Trp IDO activates the GCN2 stress-kinase pathway leading to T cell anergy and cell cycle arrest, inhibits the mTOR pathway thus diminishing T cell proliferation. By increasing KP metabolite concentrations IDO also contributes to the apoptosis of effector T cells and promotes the formation of T cells of the regulatory subtype. Via these mechanisms IDO might exert profound effects on both systemic and local immune responses. Abbreviations: IFNs: interferons; Ils: interleukins; TNFs: tumor necrosis factors; PGs: prostaglandines; LPS: lipopolysaccharide; DC: dendritic cell; IDO: indoleamine 2,3-dioxygenase; Trp: tryptophan; KP: kynurenine pathway; mTOR: mammalian target of rapamycin.

knockout mice (IDO$^{-/-}$) the balance was shifted toward the production of the anti-inflammatory IL-10. IDO inhibition had beneficial effects on the survival rates as well: overall survival from LPS induced shock was higher among IDO$^{-/-}$ animals compared to wild-type mice (2) (**Table 1**).

In mouse model, Blumenthal et al. found upregulation of *IDO* expression upon *Mycobacterium tuberculosis* infection both *in vitro* and *in vivo*. Though *in vitro* experiments indicated that genetic ablation of the enzyme resulted in enhanced T cell proliferation after infection, such changes were not observed *in vivo*, as there was no significant difference between the numbers of activated T cells in the lungs and lymph nodes of IDO$^{-/-}$ and IDO$^{+/+}$ animals. In accordance with this, the survival rate of *Mycobacterium tuberculosis* infected IDO$^{-/-}$ mice did not differ significantly from that of their IDO expressing counterparts (8). Uropathogenic *Escherichia coli* (UPEC) was also found to elevate IDO expression *in vitro* in human uroepithelial cells and polymorphonuclear leukocytes. In mice *in vivo* genetic ablation of the enzyme (IDO$^{-/-}$) resulted in increased levels of pro-inflammatory cytokines, such as granulocyte-colony stimulating factor, IL-6 and IL-17, leading to an increase in granulocyte accumulation and local inflammation in the bladder of animals and decreased survival of extracellular bacteria as compared to wild type (IDO$^{+/+}$) mice. These observations led to the

conclusion that *via IDO* up-regulation the pathogen reduces host inflammatory responses thus enabling its own survival (9). Similarly to UPEC, infection with *Rhodococcus equi*, a facultative intracellular pathogenic bacterium also enhanced *IDO* expression in DCs and alveolar macrophages. In the liver tissue of *IDO*$^{-/-}$ animals, infection with the pathogen decreased TGFβ level and FOXP3 expression, indicating a reduction in T regulatory cell responses, in parallel with prolonged liver inflammation (10).

The IDO immunomodulatory role was also studied in chronic viral diseases. Infection of mice by LP-BM5 Murine Leukemia Virus (MuLV) resulted in the development of fatal immunodeficiency syndrome, also known as murine AIDS. Similarly to acquired immunodeficiency in humans, murine AIDS is characterized by activation and proliferation of T and B cells with altered functions, a decrease in the number of function of natural killer (NK) cells and abnormal cytokine production. Animals suffering from the disease are more prone to developing B cell lymphoma and to opportunistic infections. Genetic inhibition of IDO was found to evoke protective effects in MuLV infected animals: in IDO$^{-/-}$ mice an increase was observed in the levels of type I IFNs and the number of plasmocytoid dendritic cells (premature type of DCs, pDCs) accompanied by a decrease in virus replication as compared to wild type animals. Interestingly, type I IFN neutralization in IDO deficient animals abolished the decrease in virus replication, suggesting a cardinal role of these IFNs in immune responses against viruses (3). The enhanced production of type I IFNs was attributed to pDCs, which were earlier reported to produce a number of different type I IFNs upon viral infection (106), and are chronically up regulated in HIV patients too (107). According to a further report from the same laboratory, genetic inhibition of IDO expression was also beneficial with the encephalomyocarditis virus (ECMV) murine model of acute viral myocarditis (4). Similarly to the case of MuLV infected mice, IDO$^{-/-}$ animals showed a significantly higher survival rate after ECMV infection compared to WT mice. In knockout animals, ECMV replication was inhibited, as demonstrated by the lower levels of viral genomic RNA in the heart and consequently the decreased levels of myocardial damage. The mechanism of the protective effect in the absence of the enzyme is believed to be the lack of KYN and 3-HK production. These metabolites are proposed to decrease the production of antiviral type I IFNs, key factors in myocardial damage protection. Indeed, treatment of IDO$^{-/-}$ animals with these KP metabolites decreased the otherwise elevated levels of type I IFNs and led to increased myocardial destruction and a prominent reduction in the survival rate. Based on the findings that bone marrow transplantation from IDO$^{-/-}$ animals to IDO$^{+/+}$ mice resulted in significantly higher IFNβ levels than was in the case with IDO$^{-/-}$ animals receiving bone marrow from WT animals, it was proposed that type I IFN production is regulated in the bone marrow. It was concluded that inhibition of antiviral type I IFN production by IDO is the result of multiple mechanisms: on the one hand, the number of activated macrophages is suppressed by the formation of KP metabolites, and on the other hand, local Trp depletion also can contribute to a decrease in type I IFN production (4). In pDCs type I IFN production is regulated by the mTOR pathway (108) that can be antagonized by amino acid starvation (109). Considering that IDO catalyses the metabolism of Trp, one can suppose that the enzyme inhibits mTOR signaling *via* locally depleting Trp (4).

IDO overexpression was also found to be beneficial in the course of West Nile virus infections. Using IDO expressing HeLa cells, it was shown that overexpressing IDO prior to viral infection resulted in a significant decrease in viral replication. Excessive enzyme expression restricted the spread of the infection to the neighboring cells (6).

In contrast with the findings of Hoshi and colleagues, O'Connor et al. reported that IDO deficient LP-BM5 infected mice displayed similar disease severity to their IDO expressing counterparts. These authors detected no differences in retroviral load between IDO$^{-/-}$ and WT animals, thus the lack of enzyme did not seem to affect viral replication or viral spread (7). Similar results were reported by Huang et al., as they found no significant effect of either pharmacological or genetic inhibition of IDO on the outcome and severity of MuLV infection. On the other hand, this study identified IDO as a major factor in pain hypersensitivity related to acute influenza A and MuLV infection. IDO was found to enhance hypersensitivity *via* the production of KYN, and genetic inhibition of IDO resulted in the alleviation of acute and chronic pain related to infection (5).

Effects of Genetic Modification of Indoleamine 2,3-Dioxygenase on Immune Responses in Autoimmune and Allergic Diseases

Besides inflammation related to bacterial and viral infections, the role of IDO in autoimmune and allergic processes has also gained attention (**Table 2**). Studies on the role of IDO in mucosal allergic processes revealed that though the enzyme is not essential for antigen-induced airway immune tolerance, it plays a cardinal role in antigen-induced Th2 mediated immune responses (11). Genetic inhibition of the enzyme in a mouse model of acute allergic airway inflammation led to a decrease in effector T cell formation and in the production of Th2 cytokines, such as IL-4, IL-5, IL-9, and IL-13, which play important roles in asthma and other allergic diseases (110). As a consequence, attenuation in airway inflammation, mucus secretion, airway eosinophilia and hyperresponsiveness was observed in IDO$^{-/-}$ animals when compared to their WT counterparts. Investigation of a chronic asthma model yielded similar results with fewer DCs in the lymph nodes and a decrease in parameters indicating allergic airway inflammation. In accordance with this, IFNγ (a Th1 type cytokine) expression was elevated. In summary, IDO expression of infiltrating DCs seems to be essential in promoting Th2 type immune response upon exposure to airway allergens (11).

In contrast with the above, no effect of knocking out IDO was found in an auto-inflammatory disease, systemic juvenile idiopathic arthritis (sJIA) (12). In a number of sJIA cases secondary hemophagocytic-lymphohistiocytosis (sHLH) develops, a condition characterized by the over-activation of macrophages [macrophage activation syndrome (MAS)], thus leading to a potentially fatal disease state. The development of a cytokine storm—in which IL-1β, IL-6, and IL-18 play cardinal roles—is characteristic of both sJIA and sHLH (111). It has been supposed that both sJIA and sHLH were the consequences of

the lack of effective down regulation of an exaggerated immune response (112, 113). Taking into account the immunomodulatory effects of IDO, assuming the involvement of the enzyme in these disease states seemed well-grounded. However, results of Put et al. did not support this hypothesis. Genetic inhibition of IDO in mice models of sJIA, MAS, and sHLH, did not indicate differences in the symptoms of IDO$^{-/-}$ animals as compared to WT mice. Though neither the level of IDO2 nor TDO was found to be elevated, they hypothesized that the absence of IDO was compensated by other Trp metabolizing enzymes of the KP (12).

According to results reported by Lemos et al., the presence of *IDO* is essential in provoking beneficial immune responses in a mouse model of experimental autoimmune encephalitis (EAE) (13). Cytosolic DNA leads to the activation of the Stimulator of Interferon Genes (STING) adaptor and results in the induction of interferon type I (IFNαβ) production. Continuous activation of STING provokes autoimmunity due to a failure in immune tolerance. In an EAE mouse model of multiple sclerosis (MS), it was found that following immunization with myelin oligodendrocyte glycoprotein (MOG), systemic treatment with DNA nanoparticles (DNPs) or cyclic diguanylate monophosphate (c-diGMP) induced STING signaling. In this way, potent regulatory immune responses could be achieved leading to restrained EAE severity and delayed disease onset. In accordance with this, reduced levels of effector T cell infiltration in the CNS and decreased immune responses to the administered MOG therapy in the spleen were observed. Interestingly, MOG treatment stimulated CNS neurons to express IDO, however, after DNP therapy no IDO expression could be detected in the CNS of immunized mice. The authors concluded that while immunization with MOG led to IDO expression in neurons, DNP induced the enzyme in tissues outside the CNS and paradoxically diminished MOG induced IDO expression in neurons. Based on these findings it was proposed that IDO induction in lymphoid tissues inhibited infiltration of effector immune cells in the CNS and consecutive neuronal IDO expression. In accordance with the above, for therapeutic responses *IDO* gene function was essential only in hematopoietic cells and lack of *IDO* in non-hematopoietic cells did not cause changes in the outcome of DNP therapy. The changes provoked by DNP administration were found to be highly dependent on intact *IDO* and IFNαβ receptor genes, as no therapeutic responses were observed in either STING-KO or IDO$^{-/-}$ animals. It was concluded, that attenuation of immune responses upon DNPs and c-diGMP application was due to the induction of T cell regulatory responses *via* the STING-IFNαβ-IDO pathway. This, accompanied by elevated Trp degradation and changes in the balance of pro-and anti-inflammatory metabolites and cytokines, results in better immune response outcome (13). Earlier reports on diminished Treg responses, exacerbated EAE disease severity and increased encephalitogenic Th1 and Th17 responses in IDO$^{-/-}$ mice supports this notion. Administration of the Trp metabolite 3-HAA, besides inhibiting Th1 and Th17 cells, also enhanced Treg cell responses, thus improving disease outcome. It was concluded that IDO, by promoting the formation of Trp metabolites, such as 3-HAA, enhances Treg differentiation (14).

Investigation of IDO mRNA expression in mice with collagen induced arthritis (CIA), an animal model of rheumatoid arthritis (RA), revealed a significant increase in the level of the transcript in the lymph nodes of affected animals. Enhanced IDO expression was mainly limited to DCs in lymph nodes. By comparing disease progression in IDO deficient to WT mice, it was found that though the severity of the disease was similar at the early stages, in WT animals a plateau was observed 5 days after disease onset, while in $IDO^{-/-}$ mice arthritis progressed further leading to a more severe disease. Increased joint damage, higher production of IFNγ and IL-17 in the lymph nodes and higher Th1 and Th17 cell frequency were observed in paws of IDO deficient animals. These observations led to the conclusion that IDO activation in lymph nodes is essential in reducing the accumulation of Th1 and Th17 cells in joints and thus restraining disease severity and progression in RA animal model (15).

In accordance with the findings of Criado et al., Chen et al. reported that adenoviral vector-mediated intra-articular IDO gene delivery (AdIDO) into ankles of CIA rats ameliorated disease severity. In the ankle joints of CIA animals, a significant reduction was observed in bone destruction, soft tissue swelling and synovial hyperplasia. Furthermore, a significant decrease in CD4+ T cell infiltration accompanied by a higher apoptosis rate and reduced CD68 macrophage infiltration was detected in AdIDO treated CIA animals. Reduced Th17 cell activity was found as well, as was indicated by diminished IL-17, IL-6, IL-1β concentrations and RORγt expression in ankle joints and draining lymph nodes. The authors concluded that IDO gene therapy reduced arthritis via the up-regulation of the Trp degradation pathway, thus increasing kynurenine concentrations, leading to increased CD4+ T cell apoptosis and diminished IL-17 production (16).

Type I diabetes is an autoimmune diseases, in which insulin-producing pancreatic cells are destroyed by activated T lymphoctyes (114). In pDCs IDO expression is triggered by TGFβ via the non-canonical NF-κB pathway. Besides its Trp catabolizing ability, in pDCs IDO acts as a signaling molecule as well: promoting its own and also TGFβ expression, it amplifies immune tolerance and enables the spreading of TGFβ dependent tolerance (115–117).

In a study of non-obese diabetic (NOD) mice, the animal model of autoimmune diabetes, TGFβ failed to activate the non-canonical NF-κB pathway, thus no up-regulation could be achieved in Ido expression. However, after transfection of the Ido gene into NOD pDCs, TGFβ administration led to the activation of the NF-κB pathway. This enhanced IDO expression was accompanied by a decrease in IL-6 and TNFα pro-inflammatory cytokine production and an up-regulation of the anti-inflammatory TGFβ, ensuring a more immune-tolerant setting. Enhanced IDO expression also led to decreased production of pancreatic β-cell auto-antigens. It was concluded, that immunoregulatory functions of TGFβ require a basal expression level of IDO, which could be achieved by the forced expression of the enzyme (17). The observation that enhancement of both the enzymatic and signaling activity of IDO proved to be beneficial in NOD mouse model, might allow us

to expect success from IDO modulation in other, autoimmune diabetes related disorder as well.

A study reported by Ravishankar et al. further strengthens the role of IDO in the course of autoimmune diseases. In a model of Lupus-prone Murphy Roths large (MRLlpr/lpr) mice—an analog of systemic lupus erythematosus (SLE)—significant constitutive IDO expression was observed in the spleen of pre-symptomatic MRLlpr/lpr animals. In contrast, in normal mice little basal IDO activity was present. Treatment of MRLlpr/lpr mice with pharmacological IDO inhibitor, D1MT, yielded significantly elevated autoantibody levels and IgG immune-complex deposition in the skin and kidneys of affected animals, what is a manifestation of loss of self-tolerance. Injecting apoptotic thymocytes in $IDO^{-/-}$ MRLlpr/lpr animals resulted in an increase in autoantibody titers, pro-inflammatory cytokine production, and dysregulated T cell responses culminating in lethal autoimmunity. On the other hand, exposure of $IDO^{+/+}$ MRLlpr/lpr mice to apoptotic cells did not lead to pathogenic autoimmunity, as the response to thymocytes was low and self-limiting. Whether the presence of IDO enables the suppression of T cell responses to the antigens presented or whether it inhibits the antigen presentation itself to potentially autoreactive T cells, needs further elucidation. Nevertheless, the role of IDO in the maintenance of immune homeostasis and in the prevention of autoimmune progression is inevitable (18).

Effects of Genetic Modification of Indoleamine 2,3-Dioxygenase on Transplant Related Immune Responses

Besides studies on the role of IDO in immune responses to infections and autoimmune reactions, its involvement in transplant responses is also a focus of research (**Table 3**). A possible way of treating autoimmune (Type I) diabetes could be the restoration of insulin production via the transplantation of insulin producing pancreas cells (118). However, major concerns are the reappearance of autoimmunity and the rejection of the allograft (119). A study by Alexander et al. yielded promising results with respect of these issues. They found that transplantation of diabetic mice with pancreatic islets expressing IDO via adenoviral gene transfer resulted in prolonged graft survival (19). In vitro experiments revealed a significant depletion of locally available Trp and inhibition of the proliferation of T cells obtained from diabetic animals. The extended in vivo graft survival was proposed to be due to local Trp depletion at the site of transplantation, in accordance with the in vitro findings. These results suggest that transplanted pancreatic cells expressing IDO due to ex vivo genetic editing are capable of inhibiting the proliferation of host diabetic T cells, thus preventing graft rejection (19). These findings open new possible avenues in the treatment of type I diabetes.

Enhanced IDO expression was also found to be beneficial in the case of transplantation of an immune-privileged tissue, the cornea (20). Over expression of IDO in donor corneal endothelial cells prior to the transplant resulted in increased formation of L-KYN in the allograft. As a consequence, the proliferation of allogeneic T cells was locally inhibited, thus permitting the prolonged survival of the graft when compared to no IDO expresser controls. Similarly, enhanced IDO expression prevented lung allograft injury in a rat model. Liu et al. used non-viral gene transfer methods to deliver human IDO gene to enhance IDO expression in the transplanted lungs. They found that both functional and histological properties of IDO overexpressing lungs were significantly improved in comparison to allografts without enhanced gene expression (21, 23). IDO gene delivery blocked local T cell responses, but could not prevent the recruitment of neutrophil granulocytes. Enhanced IDO expression led to the inhibition of intracellular ROS formation, thus reducing ROS induced necrosis and apoptosis of lung cells (21). IDO overexpressing lung allografts displayed more preserved bronchus-alveolar architecture due to significantly less interstitial and peribronchial collagen deposition than controls. In vitro IDO expressing lung cells inhibited the TGFβ mediated proliferation of fibroblasts, however, this could also be prevented by the addition of Trp, suggesting that local Trp depletion due to enhanced IDO expression was the mechanism of fibroblast proliferation prevention (23).

In following studies, Liu et al. found that in transplanted lung allografts IDO overexpression reduced the number of infiltrating CD3+ and CD8+ T cells. CD8+ T cells lost their cytotoxic properties, and a significant reduction was observed in their TNFα and IL-2 production. In vivo findings revealed that IDO overexpression limited ATP production in CD8+ cells. In vitro studies showed that IDO selectively diminished the activity of electron transport chain complex I, which explains the reduced ATP production of infiltrating T cells (22).

Further studies revealed that besides enhanced IDO expression, systemic administration of a KP metabolite, 3-HAA was also capable of prolonging lung allograft survival. Furthermore, IDO overexpression in lung allografts, in addition to TNFα and IL-2, also decreased the level of IFNγ, IL-12, IL-4, IL-5, IL-6, and IL-13. However, there was no reduction in the level of a potential protective cytokine, IL-10. As IL-2, IL-4, IL-12, and IL-6 play important roles in the production of effector memory T cells, it was proposed that IDO overexpression inhibited not only early T cell responses, but also diminished the formation of memory T cells, thus prolonging the survival of the allograft. In vitro findings demonstrated that high IDO environment led to decreases in intracellular calcium levels, phospholipase C-γ1 phosphorylation and mitochondrial mass. These observations offer novel insight into the mechanisms by which IDO exerts T-cell inhibiting properties: namely by impairing T cell receptor activation via decreasing calcium influx, thus impairing calcium signaling (26).

IDO overexpression in fibroblasts diminished CD3+ T cell recruitment at cutaneous wounds as well. The in vitro model showed that wounds receiving IDO expressing human fibroblasts had faster healing rates compared to those grafted with non-treated fibroblasts. This was partly because of the significantly increased vascularisation in wounds prior to receiving IDO expressing fibroblasts as observed in an in vivo rat model. However, the addition of Trp diminished otherwise enhanced angiogenesis, implicating the Trp depleting role of IDO in the course of capillary formation (24).

Overexpression of the enzyme was found to be beneficial regarding cardiac allograft survival as well. Overexpression of IDO in DCs resulted in decreased allogeneic T cell proliferation in vitro. Based on in vivo experiments it was concluded that adenovirus mediated IDO gene transfer in the donor heart led to decreased monocytes, macrophages and T cells infiltrating the organ. This was accompanied by diminished intragraft IFNγ, TNFα, TGFβ, and IL-1β levels and prolonged graft survival (25).

Altogether, these findings underline the feasibility of using IDO gene induction for the purpose of preventing allograft rejection.

Effects of Genetic Modification of Indoleamine 2,3-Dioxygenase on Immune Responses in Disease States Related to Chronic Inflammation and in Intestinal Immunity

In addition to its possible use to modulate immune processes related to infectious diseases, allergy, transplantation, and autoimmunity, the involvement of IDO has also been investigated in diseases accompanied by chronic inflammation, such as diabetes, aorta aneurysm, obesity, and hepatic fibrosis (Table 4).

Hyperglycaemia induced chronic retinal inflammation has a pivotal role in the development of diabetic retinopathy (DR), one of the major causes of visual impairment worldwide (120). In a recent study, Nahomi et al. reported a 50 percent increase of the level of IFNγ in human diabetic retinas accompanied with elevated IDO expression (27). Genetic inhibition of IDO function in diabetic IDO$^{-/-}$ mice was found to reduce retinal capillary degeneration, as acellular capillary formation in knockout mice was alleviated as compared to their WT counterparts (27).

Chronic inflammation has been reported to be a primary feature of atherosclerosis as well (121). The higher angiotensin II (AngII) plasma levels in atherosclerosis suggest hormone involvement in the development of various cardiovascular diseases. This raised the possibility of using the hormone to generate animal models of diseases linked to atherosclerosis. Indeed, infusion of Apolipoprotein E knockout (ApoE$^{-/-}$) mice with AngII led to the development of more severe atherosclerotic lesions in the aorta. In the affected aortic segments, high numbers of lipid-laden macrophages and lymphocytes were observed accompanied by increased macrophage infiltration in the adventitia (122). In a mouse model of atherosclerosis, AngII was found to enhance the expression of IDO in parallel with increased IFNγ expression, indicating a link between the KP and arterial degeneration (28). Inhibition of the enzyme exerted beneficial effects, as in WT mice AngII infusion resulted in increased oxidative stress, dysfunction, and apoptosis of endothelial cells, however, these detrimental effects were all suppressed in IDO$^{-/-}$ animals. AngII infusion also increased plasma kynurenine levels in WT animals, however, such changes were not observed in IDO deficient ones. In vitro studies revealed that upon IFNγ induced Ido activation, 3-HK is formed, which, by increasing nicotinamide adenine dinucleotide phosphate (NAD(P)H) oxidase activity, leads to enhanced ROS production, triggering dysfunction and apoptosis of endothelial cells (28). These results propose a possible therapeutic approach to atherosclerosis linked cardiovascular diseases: genetic inhibition of IDO leading to reduced 3-HK and, consequently, diminished ROS production could be a feasible way of avoiding endothelial cell loss.

Abdominal aortic aneurysm (AAA) is a potentially fatal condition characterized by the abnormal dilatation of the abdominal aorta. The pathomechanism leading to the disease is similar to that seen in atherosclerosis, as it includes the apoptosis of vascular smooth muscle cells (VSMCs), degeneration of the extracellular matrix by a metalloproteinase mediated mechanism, collagen remodeling and chronic inflammation of the aortic wall (123, 124). In a hypercholesterolemic mouse model of AAA, in which low density lipoprotein—receptor deficient ($Ldlr^{-/-}$) mice were infused with AngII and fed with high fat diet (HFD), the absence of IDO was found to be protective against the development of aneurysms (29). In $IDO^{-/-}$ animals infused with AngII, TUNEL assay did not indicate increased levels of apoptosis, but α-actin staining was increased. Both observations suggest the protective effect of IDO exerted *via* the inhibition of apoptosis of VSMC. A comparison of circulating immune cells in $IDO^{+/+}$ and $IDO^{-/-}$ animals revealed no significant difference in the number of neutrophils, monocytes, CD4+ and CD8+ T cells or CD19+ B cells. Similarly, no significant difference was detected in infiltrating macrophages and T lymphocytes in the adventitia and media of the aortic aneurysm. However, IL-17 production was significantly decreased in IDO deficient animals as compared to their IDO expressing counterparts (29). In summary, these findings raise the possibility of a mechanism similar that seen in the development of atherosclerosis. As such, IDO mediated 3-HK formation could be one of the main culprits in arterial wall degeneration (28, 29).

Recently a further kynurenine metabolite and an enzyme of the pathway were identified to take part in the pathomechanism of the disease. According to a study by Wang et al., IDO knockout and siRNA mediated *Kynu* silencing in $ApoE^{-/-}$ mice were protective against AgII induced AAA formation (30). In $ApoE^{-/-}$ mice the genetic inhibition of both IDO and KYNU caused a decrease in elastic lamina degradation and aortic expansion was observed following AngII infusion. The comparison of serum inflammatory markers, such as IFNγ, TNFα, IL-6, and cyclophilin-A, revealed no significant differences between IDO expressing and $IDO^{-/-}$ animals, suggesting another IDO regulated mechanism apart from immune mediation. 3-HAA was identified as a main factor in the pathomechanism of aneurysm development as it was found to upregulate the expression of matrix metallopeptidase 2 (MMP2), which has a central role in the pathophysiology of AAA formation *via* extracellular matrix degeneration (30, 125).

The production of 3-HAA was regulated by both IDO and KYNU. On the one hand, AngII infusion in $IDO^{+/+}$ mice induced the expression of both enzymes, which resulted in the elevation of the level of 3-HAA both in the plasma and aorta of these animals, however, no such changes were observed in the absence of IDO. On the other hand, genetic inhibition of KYNU led to decreased 3-HAA production and diminished MMP2 expression, consequently preventing the formation of AAA (30). The investigation of human AAA samples revealed similar changes in the KP: both IDO and KYNU enzymes were significantly upregulated in human aneurysm samples, accompanied by higher levels of 3-HAA in the affected aortic wall (30). These findings underline the therapeutic potential of interfering in the pathway to prevent vascular degeneration.

Association between obesity, inflammation and the gut microbiome has been intensively investigated in the past decades (31, 126). In a recent study, Laurans et al. reported that $IDO^{-/-}$ mice fed a high fat diet showed lower body weight and fat mass compared to WT animals on the same diet. Knockout animals also had lower liver weights accompanied by less lipid accumulation and decreased macrophage infiltration in the organ, implying the presence of a protective mechanism against steatosis. A decrease in inflammatory processes was also detected in white adipose tissue (WAT) of $IDO^{-/-}$ mice compared to their wild type counterparts. In epididymal and inguinal adipose tissues, lower numbers of infiltrating macrophages were detected and in inguinal WAT the number of M2 type cells was higher, whereas there was no significant change in the number of M1 type cells (31). M2 macrophages are associated with alleviating inflammation, propagating wound healing and are regarded as a "benign" subtype in contrast with the pro-inflammatory, activated M1 type ones (127). In accordance with this, the levels of anti-inflammatory cytokines—such as IL-10, 4, and 5—were significantly higher in animals lacking the enzyme. Besides protection against liver steatosis, genetic inhibition of IDO also proved to be beneficial against the development of insulin resistance, as indicated by lower insulin concentrations measured during oral glucose tolerance tests (OGTT) and better results to insulin tolerance tests (ITT) by $IDO^{-/-}$ animals compared to WT mice. These findings suggest the protective role of IDO inhibition against obesity and obesity related pathological changes in metabolism affecting the liver and glucose homeostasis. Laurans et al. also attempted to identify the causative role of IDO in obesity and related disorders. They found that KYN and KYNA supplementation did not abolish the positive effects of IDO deletion on body weight, thus it is unlikely that the beneficial metabolic changes seen in the case of IDO inhibition are the consequences of the lack of these metabolites (31). Several previous observations on obesity related intestinal dysbiosis and gut derived LPS translocation (128), the demonstration of high IDO expression in the gastrointestinal tract, and that activity of IDO was increased in the intestine of high fat diet animals (129) support the assumption that higher intestinal IDO expression leads to a shift toward kynurenine production instead of the formation of indole derivatives (31). In concert with this assumption, Laurans and colleagues found that in the $IDO^{-/-}$ HFD fed mice higher intestinal levels of indole-3 acetic acid (IAA) were present. In parallel with this, the levels of two cytokines known to be dependent on indole derivatives (130), IL-17 and IL-22 [which both play primary roles in rapid immune response of the host against microbes (131)] were increased, accompanied by the decreased expression of inflammation related genes. These changes in the intestinal tract were accompanied by significantly diminished LPS levels in the plasma of $IDO^{-/-}$ animals on HFD compared to WT HFD animals. All combined, these findings strongly suggest a causative effect of IDO deletion in maintaining an intact intestinal immune barrier in obesity (31).

However, while the absence of IDO can be beneficial, as in most of the cases cited above, the lack of the enzyme can also have detrimental effects in certain cases. The seemingly opposing findings demonstrate the diverse and complex role of the enzyme in the regulation of immune processes. Hepatic fibrosis is a consequence of chronic inflammation which can be triggered by various agents, such as viral infection, drugs, metabolic and autoimmune diseases (32). Elevated expression of IDO has been reported in hepatitis (132), leading to the assumption that the enzyme might be involved in hepatic fibrosis. Based on data of elevated levels of pro-inflammatory cytokines, such as TNFα and IL-6, in a hepatitis model, Ogiso et al. proposed that the induction of IDO by pro-inflammatory agents might play a role in the disease. In a carbon-tetrachloride (CCl4) induced animal model of the disease, the absence of IDO was found to aggravate the progress of fibrosis. The number of macrophages producing TNFα was significantly higher in the liver of IDO knockout animals, leading to a rise in the level of TNFα accompanied by the elevated expression of fibrogenic factors as compared to WT animals. On the grounds that IDO activation leads to a decrease in available Trp with the simultaneous production of kynurenine metabolites and that Trp is cardinal in the activation of NK and T cells, it was proposed that the elimination of IDO activity contributes to liver fibrosis by a dual mechanism: the inhibition of the enzyme results in sufficiently high Trp levels for lymphocyte activation and prevents the formation of kynurenine metabolites that suppress lymphocytes (32).

IDO seems to play an important role in intestinal immunity under normal circumstances as well. Harrington et al. reported a significant elevation of IgA and IgG in the gut and sera of IDO$^{-/-}$ mice as compared to wild type animals (33). Antibiotic treatment of IDO$^{-/-}$ animals led to a decrease in IgA and IgG levels indicating that the increased level of these Igs was a consequence of the lack of IDO modulatory effects on gut microbiota. Based on the observation that the elevated baseline Ig levels of IDO null animals could be corrected by antibiotic treatment, the authors proposed the involvement of IDO in a negative-feedback mechanism, which limits B lymphocyte responses to commensal microorganisms in the intestinal tract. This notion was supported by the finding that infection of IDO$^{-/-}$ mice with a bacterial enteropathogen similar to the human pathogen Escherichia coli, Citrobacter rodentium, resulted in attenuated intestinal inflammatory responses. This was manifested in less oedema, cellular infiltration, epithelial damage and reduced intestinal colonization of the bacteria in IDO null animals as compared to WT (33). These beneficial effects were attributed to the elevated formation of natural secretory IgA, which facilitated the prevention of intestinal colocalization of the pathogen. It was hypothesized that IDO regulated gut microbiota by stimulating Ig production via the formation of cytotoxic kynurenine metabolites, as these kynurenines could inhibit the proliferation of the antibody producing B cells. Another mechanism by which the enzyme can affect B cell responses is by its ability to modulate T cell activity (33).

Effects of Genetic Modification of Indoleamine 2,3-Dioxygenase on Immune Responses to Cancer

A steadily growing body of data shows upregulated states of IDO in various cancer types making it a potent target for therapeutic approaches. To date, several chemical inhibitors of the enzyme have reached clinical trials, however, there are only a handful of those therapeutic approaches which attempt to modulate the enzyme function by genetic means [reviewed in (65)]. Besides post-translational modifications, the activity of the enzyme is also controlled at the transcriptional level (65), and in most interventions a decrease in the enzyme activity is desired, so genetic modulation seems feasible and exploring ways to achieve it is highly warranted. As upregulated IDO expression has been reported in various tumors (81), silencing the IDO gene could be an effective way for interfering immune escape in malignancies (**Table 4**). Report that IDO silencing by siRNA technology in cultured B16F10 melanoma cells diminished Trp catabolism and prevented apoptosis of T cells supports this notion. Transplantation of IDO inhibited tumor cells into mice resulted in the formation of smaller tumors. Moreover, in vivo IDO-siRNA treatment enabled the recovery of T cell responses, thus restoring host antitumor immunity, and silencing the gene also caused a delay in tumor onset (34). In melanoma mouse model, silencing injection of IDO specific shRNA, expressed from a plasmid in Salmonella typhimurium, attenuated tumor growth and led to a significant decrease in the number of lung metastases. In Ido-silenced animals massive tumor cell death was observed accompanied by polymorph nuclear neutrophil (PMN) infiltration in tumors. The production of excessive amounts of ROS led to the apoptosis of cancerous cells. Though it is likely that cytotoxic PMN recruitment is primarily to clear off S.t. cells, the production of ROS generates a microenvironment that is disadvantageous for tumor growth (35, 133). IDO silencing has been demonstrated to be effective in ovarian cancer as well (36). Injection of SKOV-3 human ovarian cancer cells with short hairpin RNA (shRNA) silenced IDO (SKOV-3/shIDO) into mice resulted in reduced tumor growth when compared to animals receiving IDO expressing cells. Simultaneously, peritoneal dissemination and ascites formation was inhibited and NK cell accumulation in the tumors was increased in SKOV-3/shIDO cell injected mice compared to those injected with tumor cells without IDO inhibition. In vitro studies revealed that in co-culture with NK cells, SKOV-3/shIDO cells displayed significantly decreased survival rates compared to those of non-IDO inhibited SKOV-3 cells, suggesting that IDO inhibition increases cancer cell sensitivity to NK cells (36).

In a recent study Wang et al. reported that radiotherapy (RT) treatment of patients with non-small cell lung carcinoma caused a decrease in KYN/Trp ratio, indicating diminished IDO activity, which was restored post-RT. They also reported a significant correlation between IDO activity and the clinical outcome of patients receiving RT. Those patients who had a higher KYN/Trp ratio prior to RT treatment showed significantly poorer survival than those with a lower KYN/Trp ratio. Similarly, there was correlation between greater KYN levels pre- and post-RT treatment and modest survival. These data suggested that

RT induced favorable immune activity changes and IDO activity depended on the dose of implemented RT therapy. The authors hypothesized that defining the optimal dose of therapy is crucial in the modulation of IDO function, as a low dose would not be able to cause satisfactory immunomodulatory changes, whereas overdose can lead to detrimental impairment of the immune system (134).

The potential of enhancing cancer treatment efficacy by IDO function modulation was also demonstrated by Vareki et al. Anti-IDO shRNA transfected A549 human lung adenocarcinoma cells exhibit enhanced sensitivity to anti-cancer treatment. Genetic depletion of IDO sensitized the cells to the NAD+ inhibitor FK866, base excision repair (BER) inhibitor methoxyamine (MX), the folate anti-metabolite pemetrexed and the nucleoside analog gemcitabine—the latter two are already approved anticancer drugs. Simultaneous downregulation of IDO and thymidylate synthase (TS), a rate-limiting and key enzyme of DNA repair, led to the sensitization of the cells to 5FUdR as well. These results demonstrate the potential of genetic inhibition of IDO in combination with chemotherapy in cancer treatment (37).

Thus far, IDO targeting in cancer research and in therapeutic approaches involves mainly pharmaceutical enzyme inhibition. However, the use of IDO inhibitors has limitations [reviewed in (135)], underpinning the importance of genetic interventions, both alone and in combination therapy. Most of the known IDO inhibitors are analogs of the enzyme's natural substrate and act as competitive inhibitors of the enzyme. Thus, in order to exert the desired effect, these molecules either need to be used in concentrations at which they can compete with Trp in the target site, or need to show higher affinity for the enzyme than its own substrate. Trp analogs can also interfere with amino acid supply, thus misleading the cell, which in turn cannot give competent responses to changes in nutrient levels. A further limitation is that several of the applied drugs, such as 1-MT, Epacadostat, Norharmane, and Navoximod are AHR activators. This calls for specific attention, since there are data on AHR ligands possessing pro-carcinogenic effects [reviewed in (135)], though results are conflicting in regard of this question and further investigation is needed in order to clarify this issue. On the other hand, it must be emphasized here that similarly to the disadvantages and concerns regarding pharmaceutical enzyme inhibition, genetic modifications also carry dangers and raise several questions [reviewed in (136)]. There are concerns regarding the use of both viral and non-viral vectors and the off-target effects. Integration of the transfected genetic material into unwanted sites might evoke unwanted, potentially fatal immune responses for the host. While choosing sides between the two therapeutic approaches at present is hardly possible, in light of the progress of drug design and gene delivery techniques, it is likely that IDO targeting in either way or in combination will enter into the regiment of treatments of important malignancies.

Tryptophan-Dioxygenase

Similarly to IDO, the effect of the functional ortholog enzyme, TDO, expression was studied on the immune response to tumors in animal models. Pilotte compared tumor rejection rate observed upon injecting TDO expressing and TDO non-expressing P815 tumor cells into the peritoneal cavity of mice (38). Though both cell lines produced tumors, the growth of tumors resulting from cells not expressing TDO was slower than those originating from cells which expressed TDO. TDO expression led to a decrease in T lymphocyte proliferation in the tumor microenvironment, indicated by the fewer cytolytic T lymphocytes (CTL) detected in the peritoneal cavity of animals. They concluded that TDO inhibition promotes tumor rejection. Furthermore, they concluded that inhibition of IDO and TDO might have synergestic effects in improving host response to tumors. Interestingly, pharmacological inhibition of TDO potentiated tumor-rejecting ability (38). These findings raise the possibility of targeting the TDO enzyme in an anti-tumor therapy.

While inhibition of T lymphocytes resulting from TDO expression can be detrimental for anti-tumor activity, the activity of the enzyme can be beneficial in the fight against infectious diseases. TDO expressing HeLa cells were found to exert antiparasitic, antiviral and antibacterial effects, as these cells were found to be able to inhibit the growth of *Toxoplasma gondii*, *Herpes simplex virus* and *Staphylococcus aureus* after tetracycline stimulation. Similarly to the finding of diminished T lymphocyte proliferation in the tumor microenvironment upon TDO expression, the presence of the enzyme resulted in the restriction of T cell proliferation in cells pre-treated with anti-CD3 mitogenic antibody. Furthermore, supernatant obtained from TDO expressing cells was capable of inhibiting allogeneic T cell responses. Both the antimicrobial and T cell proliferation inhibitory effects of TDO expressing cells were blocked by administering exogenous Trp, suggesting that the mechanism by which these effects are achieved is due to the decreased level of Trp available because of its metabolization by TDO (40).

A recent study of Elbers et al. revealed that hypoxia significantly impaired both antibacterial, antiparasitic and immunoregulatory properties of TDO. Investigation of TDO expression and enzymatic activity in HeLa cells engineered to express the enzyme and murine liver homogenates revealed that under low oxygen conditions, though the expression was not affected, the enzymatic activity of the protein was significantly reduced. In line with this, under hypoxic conditions, the growth of *Enterococcus faecalis* and *Staphylococcus aureus* was no longer inhibited, and T cell proliferation was restricted. Considering that hypoxia can often be observed in tumoral tissues and that infected tissues often exhibit low oxygen levels, the loss of normoxia could be a key factor in the loss of appropriate immune responses against pathogens and tumors (137).

Genetic inhibition of TDO was also investigated in EAE model of MS. Though TDO deficiency had no impact on leukocyte infiltration in the CNS, nor on the rate of demyelination, disease activity or degradation of the optic nerve, it had protective effects against neuronal loss in the spinal cord. This discrepancy could be explained either by the different sensitivities of these areas and/or by the diverse expression of TDO in separate brain areas (39).

As TDO is expressed in the liver, and some corticoids which are widely used in immunosuppressive therapy following transplant induce its expression (93, 138), it follows that TDO modulation might be exploited in allogeneic liver transplant protection. Reduction of locally available Trp in the liver can diminish T cell responses (40), while simultaneous production of kynurenines can promote the development of suppressive, rather than effector dendritic cells, thus further inhibiting T cell responses (138). At present, however, there is no available data on findings on the effects of the genetic modulation of TDO on liver transplantation. Taking into account the reasons mentioned above and the positive effects of IDO modulation on allograft rejection, investigating the possibility of TDO use in this respect seems warranted.

Kynurenine 3-Monooxygenase

The third enzyme of the KP which has been subject to studies concerning its immunomodulatory roles is KMO. In light of the position of KMO in the hierarchy of KP enzymes, and that the induction of KMO is likely to shift the balance toward the production of neurotoxic and pro-inflammatory metabolites, targeting enzyme inhibition is a tempting approach for interfering in excessive inflammatory processes. Indeed, modulation of KYNA production by KMO inhibition has gained interest in the past decades and is a promising therapeutic approach for disease states linked to neurodegeneration, major depression, cancer, and immunological abnormalities (139). Besides utilizing specific KMO inhibitors, Kmo knockout animals are also efficient tools for investigating the effects of the lack of the enzyme (**Table 5**).

Giorgini et al. generated $Kmo^{-/-}$ mice and investigated the levels of different KP metabolites in the brain, liver, and plasma of the animals. The levels of Trp and NAD^+ tended to be only slightly decreased in these tissues. The marginal decrease in Trp level suggests that KMO inhibition has only a slight influence on upstream KP enzymes such as IDO and TDO. The findings that practically no difference in NAD^+ levels was found supports the assumption that alternative NAD generating mechanisms are able to produce the necessary amount of metabolite when the KP is inhibited. The levels of KYN, AA, and KYNA were elevated, with a more striking increase in the level of the latter in the periphery than in the brain. Interestingly, though the levels of the product of the enzyme, 3-HK, were significantly decreased both in the periphery and the brain, the metabolite was still detectable. This observation suggests that in $KMO^{-/-}$ animals other enzyme isoform(s) are capable of producing the metabolite in small quantities (139). Noteworthy was the difference between levels of QUIN in the periphery and in the CNS of Kmo null animals. A significant decrease in the level of this excitotoxic metabolite was detected both in the liver and plasma of $KMO^{-/-}$ animals, but there was only a moderate decrease in the brain. Based on these findings the authors concluded that peripheral inhibition of KMO might be sufficient for neuroprotection, as targeted inhibition of KMO in the CNS would not result in a more prominent decrease in the levels

of QUIN (139). Though the decrease in the amount of 3-HK and QUIN accompanied by the increase of KYNA levels in the CNS could shift neurotoxicity toward neuroprotection, excessive elevation of KYNA holds plenty of danger (140). There is a growing body of evidence on the association of exaggerated KYNA levels and impairment in cognitive functions (101, 141–143).

Genetic modulation of KMO activity as a possible therapeutic approach for intervening infections was investigated by Kubo et al. in an EMCV induced mice model of viral myocarditis (41). They found that the survival rate of $KMO^{-/-}$ mice was significantly higher compared to WT animals. This was accompanied by a significant decrease in the cellular infiltration of macrophages and neutrophils in the heart tissue of knockout animals. Moreover, the number of EMCV infected cells was significantly reduced in $KMO^{-/-}$ specimens in parallel with lower levels of EMCV genomic RNA. Viral infection upregulated the expression of Kmo as significantly higher Kmo mRNA levels were detected in $KMO^{+/+}$ animals after EMCV infection. These findings support the notion that links upregulated enzyme expression to higher mortality upon viral infection. Differences between WT and knockout animals were detected not only in the heart tissue but also in the periphery. In the serum of $KMO^{-/-}$ mice lower chemokine and cytokine levels, while higher levels of KYN and KYNA were detectable compared to WT animals (41). KYN has been shown to inhibit T and NK cell proliferation, and, via the generation of ROS, induces the apoptosis of NK cells (144–146). KYNA also exerts immune modulating effects by restricting TNF production of macrophages via G protein-coupled receptor GPR35 activation (147). Based on the anti-inflammatory effects of KYN and KYNA, elevated levels of these metabolites are proposed to be key factors in decreased inflammatory responses seen in $KMO^{-/-}$ animals. Thus, genetic inhibition of the enzyme is expected to exert beneficial effects by preventing excessive cytokine and chemokine production and decreasing the recruitment of cells of the immune system (41).

In a mouse model of autoimmune gastritis, siRNA mediated gene silencing of Kmo led to the exacerbation of the disease. A self-regulatory mechanism was proposed, whereby the expression of Kmo ensures kynurenine catabolism, therefore reducing the amount of available AHR agonist kynurenine, thus lessening the formation of Th17 cells and pro-inflammatory IL-17 production. Accordingly, the inhibition of the enzyme exacerbated inflammatory processes via promoting the formation of Th17 cells (42).

Changes in KMO function have been reported in diseases linked to chronic inflammation as well. The expression of KMO in podocytes was found to be decreased in a diabetic environment, both in human and mouse kidneys (43). Genetic inhibition of the enzyme under diabetic conditions in mice and zebrafish resulted in proteinuria, a condition often related to diabetes. Serum kynurenine metabolite levels in these animals were changed showing an increase in the levels of KYNA and KYN parallel with a decrease in the level of AA, suggesting a shift in the KP. Depletion of NAD^+ was found to have a negative effect on insulin sensitivity and also on the proper functioning of podocytes. Based on these findings, decreased expression and/or genetic inhibition of KMO leading to decreased production of NAD$^+$ was proposed to contribute to diabetes related proteinuria (43).

In a recent study of Zheng et al., genetic deletion of KMO was found to be protective against ischemia-reperfusion injury (IRI) induced acute kidney injury (AKI). KMO$^{-/-}$ mice showed better kidney function and significantly diminished tubular necrosis in the kidney tissue than KMO$^{+/+}$ animals. Similarly, significantly less neutrophil granulocyte infiltration was measured in the renal tissue upon KMO deficiency. Following IRI, the levels of Trp were significantly decreased in both KMO$^{-/-}$ and KMO$^{+/+}$ groups compared to animals without IRI. IRI also led to increased levels of the protective KYNA in KMO$^{-/-}$ mice. The plasma level of 3-HK was elevated followed by IRI in KMO expressing animals, however, such changes were not observed in KMO deficient animals. Considering the ROS generating, thus potentially pro-apoptotic properties of 3-HK, it could be concluded that genetic ablation of KMO, followed by decreased production of 3-HK, carry potential for preventing AKI after IRI (44).

Despite that these findings suggest promising results upon *KMO* ablation, inhibition of the enzyme might hold disadvantages as well. Recently Badawy has proposed, that QUIN is the most potent immunosuppressant KP metabolite, and it plays antagonistic role with the anti-inflammatory KNYA (148). Though downregulation of KMO might be beneficial in regards to elevated anti-inflammatory KYNA production, this would be accompanied by a diminished amount of the immunosuppressant QUIN. This situation clearly represents the complexity and delicate balance of the pathway and its metabolites, and raises further difficulties to be overcome.

ASSOCIATIONS BETWEEN GENE VARIATIONS LEADING TO CHANGES IN KP ENZYME FUNCTION AND HUMAN DISEASES

With the advent of new generation sequencing, a growing body of data is accumulating on polymorphisms in the human genome. It is, however, a great challenge to establish causality between genomic changes and the appearance and/or progression of specific diseases, and associations between genetic variants with disease states remain mostly obscure. Variants of genes encoding KP enzymes have been found to occur in frequencies differing between patient groups of specific diseases and samples of healthy population (1). Association of *IDO* variants have been suggested with depression (48, 149, 150) and autoimmune diseases such as systemic sclerosis (151) and Crohn's disease (152). *TDO* variants are believed to be associated with hypertryptophanemia (153) and psychiatric disorders such as Tourette syndrome (154) and autism (155). *KMO* mutations were found to be related to psychiatric diseases such as schizophrenia (156–161), bipolar disorder (162), and postpartum depression (163), and also in multiple sclerosis (164). Variations of the *AADAT* gene encoding the KATII enzyme were found to be associated with bacterial meningitis (165–167), changes in *KYNU* are believed to be

related to essential hypertension (168, 169) and xanthurenic aciduria (170). An SNP in the *HAAO* gene encoding 3-HAO was found to be associated to hypospadiasis by a so far unknown mechanism (171), and changes in *ACMSD* were proposed to be linked with Parkinson's disease (PD) (172).

Despite the numerous findings pointing to possible associations of specific SNPs with specific diseases, only in very few cases are known where a change in a gene sequence results in a change in the activity of an enzyme connected to the disease, thus indicating direct causal link between gene variant(s) and disorder(s). In the following part of this section we summarize findings of those naturally occurring variations in KP genes that disturb the activity of the encoded enzyme and thus are proposedly linked to human diseases in which immune functions are altered.

Several *IDO* gene variants -present in the population with differing frequencies-have been shown to impact enzyme function (173). Nonetheless, there are only a very limited number of studies on these variants, despite the great clinical relevance they might have in a better understanding the pathomechanisms of specific diseases.

Systemic sclerosis (SSc), a connective tissue disease of which a hallmark is autoimmunity, is indicated by the infiltration of circulating antibodies and activated T cells in the affected tissues (151). Underlying the role of altered immune response in the disease are findings of disequilibrium of the pro-inflammatory Th17 and regulatory T cell functions in patients with SSc (174). Considering the T cell modulatory effects of IDO, one can easily foresee the involvement of the enzyme in the disease. Tardito and colleagues investigated the occurrence of five *IDO* SNPs in SSc (151). Three of these nucleotide alterations are located in the coding region of the *IDO* gene, which all result in amino acid changes, the other two are in the intronic regions. The frequency of the 5 SNPs in the worldwide population vary between 1 and 22 percent, and each occur both in homo- and heterozygous forms (based on data of www.ensembl.org). In the case of four out of the five SNPs involved in this study there were no observable frequency differences in their appearance among groups of SSc and control samples.

A comparison of the frequency of SNP rs7820268 between a group of SSc patients and a matching control group of healthy controls revealed significant difference (151). Rs7820268 is a change of a C to T within intron 5 of the *IDO* gene. The minor allele is present in 22 percent of the population worldwide with 37 percent as the highest population minor allele frequency (based on data of www.ensembl.org). The frequency of T allele was significantly higher among patients compared to healthy controls, and similarly higher were the frequencies of both genotypes carrying the T allele (TT and TC). By comparing the suppression activity of T regulatory cells of patients with at least one T allele to those homozygous for the C allele, it was shown that CD8+ Treg suppression activity was impaired in individuals carrying the minor (T) allele. The authors concluded that the rs7820268 *IDO* SNP possibly affects *IDO* expression and/or activity in a certain type of immune cells, e.g., DCs, which, *via* cell-to-cell crosstalk affect the suppressive function of

CD8+ Treg cells leading to the evolution of autoimmune processes (151).

Association of *IDO* gene variants with another autoimmune disease, Crohn's disease (CD), has been reported by Lee et al. (152). CD is a chronic inflammatory bowel disease, which includes the involvement of the gastrointestinal tract and often several extraintestinal manifestations, further worsening the phenotype. In CD the expression of *IDO1* was found to be upregulated, and the activity of the enzyme was found to be in positive correlation with disease severity and inflammatory markers such as erythrocyte sedimentation rate and C-reactive protein (175). A comparison of the frequencies of 6 different *IDO1* variants among CD patients and healthy controls did not reveal significant differences, nevertheless the higher frequencies of three of the investigated variants were found to be associated with the severity of the disease (152). Both rs35059413 and rs35099072 are a C to T nucleotide change (indicated in reverse orientation) resulting in a Ala to Thr and Arg to His amino acid change in the 4th and 77th amino acid position of the protein, respectively (based on data of www.ensembl.org). The third variant is a C to A nucleotide change in exon 7. Patients carrying any of these three coding *IDO1* gene variants were more likely to show extraintestinal manifestations such as arthritis, uveitis, and perianal disease, indicators of CD severity. Serum KYN/Trp ratio, that is an indicator of *IDO* activity, revealed a decrease in enzyme activity in patients possessing *IDO1* SNPs. These findings strongly support the existence of an association between a more severe disease phenotype and a decrease in IDO1 activity which is likely to originate from mutations of the *IDO* gene (152).

Investigation of genetic variants of another KP gene, *AADAT*, that encodes KATII, revealed that in a SNP (rs1480544), a C to T change in the intronic region of the gene might be associated with bacterial meningitis (BM) (165). The minor allele was found to be more frequent among patients suffering from the disease than in healthy volunteers. The TT genotype was found to be accompanied by a decrease in several inflammatory markers in the blood, such as TNFα, IL1β, and IL6, and a diminished immune cell number in the cerebrospinal fluid (CSF) (165). These findings led to the hypothesis that this genetic variant could affect the course of the infection by influencing the recruitment of immune cells at the site of infection and the production of inflammation-related cytokines. Further studies focusing on this genetic variant revealed that in individuals with the TT genotype an increased level of KYNA and an elevation in the level of an anti-inflammatory cytokine, IL-10, were observed compared to those carrying the CC genotype (166). This led to the conclusion that BM patients bearing this *AADAT* SNP might expect a better disease outcome due to a less excessive inflammatory response. As the SNP is located in a putative exonic silencer, it is hypothesized that it leads to enhanced *AADAT* mRNA production and consequently to an increase in the amount of protein produced (166, 176). As a consequence, production of the neuroprotective and antioxidant KYNA is increased in carriers of the SNP, further alleviating neuronal damage caused by infection (166).

CONCLUSIONS

In light of the large number of metabolites that are able to evoke neurotoxic vs. neuroprotectant, ROS generating vs. antioxidant, pro- vs. anti-inflammatory effects, it is no wonder that alterations of the KP have been linked to disease states. Indeed, altered kynurenine production has been shown in several neurodegenerative (177–179), psychiatric (180), and inflammatory diseases (181). Several of these ailments are characterized by altered immune functions, primarily as the result of altered levels of specific metabolites resulting from a change in the activity of key enzymes of the pathway such as IDO, TDO, or KMO. Interfering in the pathway in order to restore the imbalances of kynurenine metabolites could be a feasible way of ameliorating symptoms and reducing the progression of disease states. Results obtained using animal models indicate that frequently, though not exclusively, specific enzyme activity at either normal or increased levels could be the culprit behind unwanted immune reactions. On the other hand, this might offer possibilities to restore normal function by downregulating specific genes. The emerging technique of genetic therapy is a promising therapeutic approach that has been or is currently attempted in a regimen of diseases: e.g., neurological disorders such as Huntington's disease [IONIS-HTTRx; ClinicalTrials.govidentifier: NCT02519036; (182)] and spinal muscular atrophy (SMA) (140), immunological diseases as severe combined immune deficiency due to adenosine-deaminase deficiency [ADA-SCID; (183)], cardiovascular diseases (184) and malignant diseases like acute lymphoblastic leukemia (185) or non-Hodgkin lymphoma (186). In most cases genetic therapy is viewed as a technology by which entire genes or gene segments are inserted or removed to/from the genome. However, an effective genetic approach could be selective inhibition of the expression of a specific gene at a given tissue type and/or in a specific time frame. Results from animal models suggest that this could be a possibility in the cases of several diseases in which an overreaction of the immune response might be ameliorated by inhibiting KP enzyme activity locally and temporarily.

Regarding the modulation of immune function *via* the KP by genetic interventions, the first and rate limiting enzyme, IDO has been in the focus of research. Most of these studies use animal models, primarily mice knockouts. Several studies, on the other hand, were performed by modifying KP enzyme expression in animal or human cells in tissue culture. Inhibition of the enzyme at a genetic level was found to be beneficial in animal models of bacterial (2) and viral (3, 4) infections, immune modulation following organ transplant (19, 20) and diseases in which chronic inflammation plays a crucial role, such as DR (27), atherosclerosis (28), AAA (29, 30) and metabolic changes linked to obesity (31). Inhibition of the enzyme is also a promising way of interfering in tumor mediated immunological changes, thus restoring anti-tumor immunity (33, 34, 36, 45, 46). Genetic inhibition of a functional ortholog of the enzyme, TDO, was also found to be beneficial in the combat against tumors (38). On the other hand, cell culture studies also revealed antimicrobial effects of enhanced expression of the enzyme (40). Genetic modulation of another KP enzyme, KMO has also proven to be two sided: inhibition was found to be protective against EMCV infection in a mouse model of viral myocarditis (41), however, lack of KMO was reported to lead to autoimmune disease exacerbation (42) and also caused malfunction of podocytes in the kidney and consequent proteinuria (43).

Genome wide association studies have proposed several genetic variants of genes encoding KP enzymes to be associated with human diseases. However, there are only a handful of studies on the effects of these genetic changes on enzyme function. Thus, establishing cause-case relations between specific SNPs and disease development requires a great amount of further work. Nonetheless, findings obtained from genetically modified animal studies suggest that intervention in the KP by genetic modulation might be a promising therapeutic approach. Thus, research aimed at uncovering the effects of naturally occurring gene variations on the expression and function of the encoded enzymes is highly warranted, as results of these studies combined with preclinical findings can help in the identification of novel therapeutic targets and in the development of suitable therapeutic approaches.

AUTHOR CONTRIBUTIONS

LV and FB contributed conception and design of the manuscript. FB did data collection and wrote the manuscript in consultation with LV. LV contributed to manuscript revision and to the refinement of the final manuscript. All authors read and approved the submitted version.

FUNDING

This work was supported by GINOP-2.3.2-15-2016-00034, Hungarian Brain Research Program—Grant No. 2017-1.2.1-NKP-2017-00002 NAP VI/4, Ministry of Human Capacities, Hungary grant 20391-3/2018/FEKUSTRAT, the MTA-SZTE Neuroscience Research Group of the Hungarian Academy of Sciences and the University of Szeged and the University of Szeged Open Access Fund—Grant No. 4238.

ACKNOWLEDGMENTS

We would like to thank Jennifer Tusz (Edmonton, Canada) for the careful linguistic revision of the manuscript.

REFERENCES

1. Boros FA, Bohár Z, Vécsei L. Genetic alterations affecting the genes encoding the enzymes of the kynurenine pathway and their association with human diseases. *Mutat Res Mutat Res.* (2018) 776:32–45. doi: 10.1016/j.mrrev.2018.03.001

2. Jung ID, Lee M, Chang JH, Lee JS, Jeong Y, Lee C-M, et al. Blockade of indoleamine 2,3-dioxygenase protects mice against lipopolysaccharide-induced endotoxin shock. *J Immunol.* (2009) 182:3146–54. doi: 10.4049/jimmunol.0803104

3. Hoshi M, Saito K, Hara A, Taguchi A, Ohtaki H, Tanaka R, et al. The absence of IDO upregulates type I IFN production, resulting in suppression of viral replication in the retrovirus-infected mouse. *J Immunol.* (2010) 185:3305–12. doi: 10.4049/jimmunol.0901150

4. Hoshi M, Matsumoto K, Ito H, Ohtaki H, Arioka Y, Osawa Y, et al. l-tryptophan–kynurenine pathway metabolites regulate type I IFNs of acute viral myocarditis in mice. *J Immunol.* (2012) 188:3980–7. doi: 10.4049/jimmunol.1100997

5. Huang L, Ou R, Rabelo de Souza G, Cunha TM, Lemos H, Mohamed E, et al. Virus infections incite pain hypersensitivity by inducing indoleamine 2,3 dioxygenase. *PLoS Pathog.* (2016) 12:e100561. doi: 10.1371/journal.ppat.1005615

6. Yeung AWS, Wu W, Freewan M, Stocker R, King NJC, Thomas SR. Flavivirus infection induces indoleamine 2,3-dioxygenase in human monocyte-derived macrophages via tumor necrosis factor and NF-κB. *J Leukoc Biol.* (2012) 91:657–66. doi: 10.1189/jlb.1011532

7. O'Connor MA, Green WR. The role of indoleamine 2,3-dioxygenase in LP-BPM5 murine retroviral disease progression. *Virol J.* (2013) 10:1–10. doi: 10.1186/1743-422X-10-154

8. Blumenthal A, Nagalingam G, Huch JH, Walker L, Guillemin GJ, Smythe GA, et al. *M. tuberculosis* induces potent activation of IDO-1, but this is not essential for the immunological control of infection. *PLoS ONE.* (2012) 7:e37314. doi: 10.1371/journal.pone.0037314

9. Loughman JA, Hunstad DA. Induction of indoleamine 2,3-dioxygenase by uropathogenic bacteria attenuates innate responses to epithelial infection. *J Infect Dis.* (2012) 205:1830–39. doi: 10.1093/infdis/jis280

10. Heller MC, Drew CP, Jackson KA, Griffey S, Watson JL. A potential role for indoleamine 2,3-dioxygenase (IDO) in Rhodococcus equi infection. *Vet Immunol Immunopathol.* (2010) 138:174–82. doi: 10.1016/j.vetimm.2010.07.013

11. Xu H, Oriss TB, Fei M, Henry AC, Melgert BN, Chen L, et al. Indoleamine 2,3-dioxygenase in lung dendritic cells promotes Th2 responses and allergic inflammation. *Proc Natl Acad Sci USA.* (2008) 105:6690–5. doi: 10.1073/pnas.0708809105

12. Put K, Brisse E, Avau A, Imbrechts M, Mitera T, Janssens R, et al. IDO1 deficiency does not affect disease in mouse models of systemic juvenile idiopathic arthritis and secondary hemophagocytic lymphohistiocytosis. *PLoS ONE.* (2016) 11:e0150075. doi: 10.1371/journal.pone.0150075

13. Lemos H, Huang L, Chandler PR, Mohamed E, Souza GR, Li L, et al. Activation of the Stimulator of Interferon Genes (STING) adaptor attenuates experimental autoimmune encephalitis. *J Immunol.* (2014) 192:5571–8. doi: 10.4049/jimmunol.1303258

14. Yan Y, Zhang G-X, Gran B, Fallarino F, Yu S, Li H, et al. IDO upregulates regulatory T cells via tryptophan catabolite and suppresses encephalitogenic T cell responses in experimental autoimmune encephalomyelitis. *J Immunol.* (2010) 185:5953–61. doi: 10.4049/jimmunol.1001628

15. Criado G, Šimelyte E, Inglis JJ, Essex D, Williams RO. Indoleamine 2,3 dioxygenase-mediated tryptophan catabolism regulates accumulation of Th1/Th17 cells in the joint in collagen-induced arthritis. *Arthritis Rheum.* (2009) 60:1342–51. doi: 10.1002/art.24446

16. Chen S-Y, Wu C-L, Lai M-D, Lin C-C, Yo Y-T, Jou I-M, et al. Amelioration of rat collagen-induced arthritis through CD4+ T cells apoptosis and synovial interleukin-17 reduction by indoleamine 2,3-dioxygenase gene therapy. *Hum Gene Ther.* (2011) 22:145–54. doi: 10.1089/hum.2009.217

17. Pallotta MT, Orabona C, Bianchi R, Vacca C, Fallarino F, Belladonna ML, et al. Forced IDO1 expression in dendritic cells restores immunoregulatory signalling in autoimmune diabetes. *J Cell Mol Med.* (2014) 18:2082–91. doi: 10.1111/jcmm.12360

18. Ravishankar B, Liu H, Shinde R, Chandler P, Baban B, Tanaka M, et al. Tolerance to apoptotic cells is regulated by indoleamine 2,3-dioxygenase. *Proc Natl Acad Sci USA.* (2012) 109:3909–14. doi: 10.1073/pnas.1117736109

19. Alexander AM, Crawford M, Bertera S, Rudert WA, Takikawa O, Robbins PD, et al. Indoleamine 2,3-dioxygenase expression in transplanted NOD Islets prolongs graft survival after adoptive transfer of diabetogenic splenocytes. *Diabetes.* (2002) 51:356–65. doi: 10.2337/diabetes.51.2.356

20. Beutelspacher SC, Pillai R, Watson MP, Tan PH, Tsang J, McClure MO, et al. Function of indoleamine 2,3-dioxygenase in corneal allograft rejection and prolongation of allograft survival by over-expression. *Eur J Immunol.* (2006) 36:690–700. doi: 10.1002/eji.200535238

21. Liu H, Liu L, Fletcher BS, Visner GA. Novel action of indoleamine 2,3-dioxygenase attenuating acute lung allograft injury. *Am J Respir Crit Care Med.* (2006) 173:566–72. doi: 10.1164/rccm.200509-1413OC

22. Liu H, Liu L, Liu K, Bizargity P, Hancock WW, Visner GA. Reduced cytotoxic function of effector CD8+ T cells is responsible for indoleamine 2,3-dioxygenase-dependent immune suppression. *J Immunol.* (2009) 183:1022–31. doi: 10.4049/jimmunol.0900408

23. Liu H, Liu L, Fletcher BS, Visner GA. Sleeping Beauty-based gene therapy with indoleamine 2,3-dioxygenase inhibits lung allograft fibrosis. *FASEB J.* (2006) 20:2384–6. doi: 10.1096/fj.06-6228fje

24. Li Y, Tredget EE, Ghaffari A, Lin X, Kilani RT, Ghahary A. Local expression of indoleamine 2,3-dioxygenase protects engraftment of xenogeneic skin substitute. *J Invest Dermatol.* (2006) 126:128–36. doi: 10.1038/sj.jid.5700022

25. Li J, Meinhardt A, Roehrich ME, Golshayan D, Dudler J, Pagnotta M, et al. Indoleamine 2,3-dioxygenase gene transfer prolongs cardiac allograft survival. *Am J Physiol Heart Circ Physiol.* (2007) 293:3415–23. doi: 10.1152/ajpheart.00532.2007

26. Iken K, Liu K, Liu H, Bizargity P, Wang L, Hancock WW, et al. Indoleamine 2,3-dioxygenaseand metabolites protect murine lung allografts and impair the calcium mobilization of T cells. *Am J Respir Cell Mol Biol.* (2012) 47:405–16. doi: 10.1165/rcmb.2011-0438OC

27. Nahomi RB, Sampathkumar S, Myers AM, Elghazi L, Smith DG, Tang J, et al. The absence of indoleamine 2,3-dioxygenase inhibits retinal capillary degeneration in diabetic mice. *Invest Ophthalmol Vis Sci.* (2018) 59:2042–53. doi: 10.1167/iovs.17-22702

28. Wang Q, Zhang M, Ding Y, Wang Q, Zhang W, Song P, et al. Activation of NAD(P)H oxidase by tryptophan-derived 3-hydroxykynurenine accelerates endothelial apoptosis and dysfunction *in vivo*. *Circ Res.* (2014) 114:480–92. doi: 10.1161/CIRCRESAHA.114.302113

29. Metghalchi S, Vandestienne M, Haddad Y, Esposito B, Dairou J, Tedgui A, et al. Indoleamine 2 3-dioxygenase knockout limits angiotensin II-induced aneurysm in low density lipoprotein receptor-deficient mice fed with high fat diet. *PLoS ONE.* (2018) 13:e0193737. doi: 10.1371/journal.pone.0193737

30. Wang Q, Ding Y, Song P, Zhu H, Okon I, Ding N-Y, et al. Tryptophan-derived 3-hydroxyanthranilic acid contributes to angiotensin II-induced abdominal aortic aneurysm formation in mice *in vivo*. *Circulation.* (2017) 136:2271–83. doi: 10.1161/CIRCULATIONAHA.117.030972

31. Laurans L, Venteclef N, Haddad Y, Chajadine M, Alzaid F, Metghalchi S, et al. Genetic deficiency of indoleamine 2,3-dioxygenase promotes gut microbiota-mediated metabolic health. *Nat Med.* (2018) 24:1113–23. doi: 10.1038/s41591-018-0060-4

32. Ogiso H, Ito H, Ando T, Arioka Y, Kanbe A, Ando K, et al. The deficiency of indoleamine 2,3-dioxygenase aggravates the CCl4-induced liver fibrosis in mice. *PLoS ONE.* (2016) 11:e0162183. doi: 10.1371/journal.pone.0162183

33. Harrington L, Srikanth CV, Antony R, Rhee SJ, Mellor AL, Shi HN, et al. Deficiency of indoleamine 2,3-dioxygenase enhances commensal-induced antibody responsesand protects against Citrobacter rodentium-induced colitis. *Infect Immun.* (2008) 76:3045–53. doi: 10.1128/IAI.00193-08

34. Zheng X, Koropatnick J, Li M, Zhang X, Ling F, Ren X, et al. Reinstalling antitumor immunity by inhibiting tumor-derived immunosuppressive molecule IDO through RNA interference. *J Histochem Cytochem.* (2006) 177:5639–46. doi: 10.4049/jimmunol.177.8.5639

35. Blache CA, Manuel ER, Kaltcheva TI, Wong AN, Ellenhorn JDI, Blazar BR, et al. Systemic delivery of *Salmonella typhimurium* transformed with IDO shRNA enhances intratumoral vector colonization and suppresses tumor growth. *Cancer Res.* (2013) 72:6447–56. doi: 10.1158/0008-5472.CAN-12-0193

36. Wang D, Saga Y, Mizukami H, Sato N, Nonaka H, Fujiwara H, et al. Indoleamine-2,3-dioxygenase, an immunosuppressive enzyme that inhibits natural killer cell function, as a useful target for ovarian cancer therapy. *Int J Oncol.* (2012) 40:929–34. doi: 10.3892/ijo.2011.1295

37. Vareki SM, Chen D, Di Cresce C, Ferguson PJ, Figueredo R, Pampillo M, et al. IDO downregulation induces sensitivity to pemetrexed, gemcitabine, FK866,

38. and methoxyamine in human cancer cells. *PLoS ONE.* (2015) 10:e0143435. doi: 10.1371/journal.pone.0143435

38. Pilotte L, Larrieu P, Stroobant V, Colau D, Dolusic E, Frédérick R, et al. Reversal of tumoral immune resistance by inhibition of tryptophan 2,3-dioxygenase. *Proc Natl Acad Sci USA.* (2012) 109:2497–502. doi: 10.1073/pnas.1113873109

39. Lanz TV, Williams SK, Stojic A, Iwantscheff S, Sonner JK, Grabitz C, et al. Tryptophan-2,3-dioxygenase (TDO) deficiency is associated with subclinical neuroprotection in a mouse model of multiple sclerosis. *Nat Sci Rep.* (2017) 7:1–13. doi: 10.1038/srep41271

40. Schmidt SK, Müller A, Heseler K, Woite C, Spekker K, Mackenzie CR, et al. Antimicrobial and immunoregulatory properties of human tryptophan 2,3-dioxygenase. *Eur J Immunol.* (2009) 39:2755–64. doi: 10.1002/eji.200939535

41. Kubo H, Hoshi M, Mouri A, Tashita C, Yamamoto Y, Nabeshima T, et al. Absence of kynurenine 3-monooxygenase reduces mortality of acute viral myocarditis in mice. *Immunol Lett.* (2016) 181:94–100. doi: 10.1016/j.imlet.2016.11.012

42. Stephens GL, Wang Q, Swerdlow B, Bhat G, Kolbeck R, Fung M. Kynurenine 3-monooxygenase mediates inhibition of Th17 differentiation via catabolism of endogenous aryl hydrocarbon receptor ligands. *Eur J Immunol.* (2013) 43:1727–34. doi: 10.1002/eji.201242779

43. Korstanje R, Deutsch K, Bolanos-Palmieri P, Hanke N, Schroder P, Staggs L, et al. Loss of kynurenine 3-mono-oxygenase causes proteinuria. *J Am Soc Nephrol.* (2016) 27:3271–7. doi: 10.1681/ASN.2015070835

44. Zheng X, Zhang A, Binnie M, McGuire K, Webster SP, Hughes J, et al. Kynurenine 3-monooxygenase is a critical regulator of renal ischemia–reperfusion injury. *Exp Mol Med.* (2019) 51:1–14. doi: 10.1038/s12276-019-0210-x

45. Ye Z, Yue L, Shi J, Shao M, Wu T. Role of IDO and TDO in cancers and related diseases and the therapeutic implications. *J Cancer.* (2019) 10:2771–82. doi: 10.7150/jca.31727

46. Lemos H, Huang L, Prendergast GC, Mellor AL. Immune control by amino acid catabolism during tumorigenesis and therapy. *Nat Rev Cancer.* (2019) 19:162–75. doi: 10.1038/s41568-019-0106-z

47. Vecsei L, Szalardy L, Fulop F, Toldi J. Kynurenines in the CNS: recent advances and new questions. *Nat Rev Drug Discov.* (2013) 12:64–82. doi: 10.1038/nrd3793

48. Smith AK, Simon J, Gustafson E, Noviello S, Cubells J, Epstein M, et al. Association of a polymorphism in the indoleamine-2,3- dioxygenase gene and interferon-α-induced depression in patients with chronic hepatitis C. *Mol Psychiatry.* (2012) 17:781–9. doi: 10.1038/mp.2011.67

49. Metz R, DuHadaway JB, Kamasani U, Laury-Kleintop L, Muller AJ, Prendergast GC. Novel tryptophan catabolic enzyme IDO2 is the preferred biochemical target of the antitumor indoleamine 2,3-dioxygenase inhibitory compound D-1-methyl-tryptophan. *Cancer Res.* (2007) 67:7082–7. doi: 10.1158/0008-5472.CAN-07-1872

50. Yuasa HJ, Ball HJ, Fern Y, Austin CJD, Whittington CM, Belov K, et al. Characterization and evolution of vertebrate indoleamine 2,3-dioxygenases IDOs from monotremes and marsupials. *Comp Biochem Physiol Part B.* (2009) 153:137–44. doi: 10.1016/j.cbpb.2009.02.002

51. Sas K, Szabó E, Vécsei L. Mitochondria, oxidative stress and the kynurenine system, with a focus on ageing and neuroprotection. *Molecules.* (2018) 23:E191. doi: 10.3390/molecules23010191

52. Németh H, Toldi J, Vécsei L. Role of kynurenines in the central and peripheral nervous systems. *Curr Neurovasc Res.* (2005) 2:249–60. doi: 10.2174/1567202054368326

53. Han Q, Cai T, Tagle DA, Li J. Structure, expression and function of kynurenine aminotransferases in human and rodent brains. *Cell Mol Life Sci.* (2010) 67:353–68. doi: 10.1007/s00018-009-0166-4

54. Okuno E, Nakamura M, Schwarcz R. Two kynurenine aminotransferases in human brain. *Brain Res.* (1991) 542:307–12. doi: 10.1016/0006-8993(91)91583-M

55. Shoki O, Nobuyoshi N, Hiroshi S, Hiroshi K. 3-Hydroxykynurenine, an endogenous oxidative stress generator, causes neuronal cell death with apoptotic features and region selectivity. *J Neurochem.* (1998) 70:299–307. doi: 10.1046/j.1471-4159.1998.70010299.x

56. Zhuravlev AV, Zakharov GA, Shchegolev BF, Savvateeva-Popova EV. Antioxidant properties of kynurenines: density functional

theory calculations. *PLOS Comput Biol.* (2016) 12:e1005213. doi: 10.1371/journal.pcbi.1005213

57. Guillemin GJ. Quinolinic acid, the inescapable neurotoxin. *FEBS J.* (2012) 279:1356–65. doi: 10.1111/j.1742-4658.2012.08485.x

58. Bohár Z, Toldi J, Fülöp F, Vécsei L. Changing the face of kynurenines and neurotoxicity: therapeutic considerations. *Int J Mol Sci.* (2015) 16:9772–93. doi: 10.3390/ijms16059772

59. Munn DH, Mellor AL. Indoleamine 2,3 dioxygenase and metabolic control of immune responses. *Trends Immunol.* (2013) 34:137–43. doi: 10.1016/j.it.2012.10.001

60. Mbongue JC, Nicholas DA, Torrez TW, Kim NS, Firek AF, Langridge WHR. The role of indoleamine 2,3-dioxygenase in immune suppression and autoimmunity. *Vaccines.* (2015) 3:703–29. doi: 10.3390/vaccines3030703

61. Badawy AA-B. Tryptophan availability for kynurenine pathway metabolism across the life span: control mechanisms and focus on aging, exercise, diet and nutritional supplements. *Neuropharmacology.* (2017) 112:248–63. doi: 10.1016/j.neuropharm.2015.11.015

62. Thomas SR, Salahifar H, Mashima R, Hunt NH, Richardson DR, Stocker R. Antioxidants inhibit indoleamine 2,3-dioxygenase in IFN-γ-activated human macrophages: posttranslational regulation by pyrrolidine dithiocarbamate. *J Immunol.* (2001) 166:6332–40. doi: 10.4049/jimmunol.166.10.6332

63. Thomas SR, Mohr D, Stocker R. Nitric oxide inhibits indoleamine 2,3-dioxygenase activity in interferon-y primed mononuclear phagocytes. *J Biol Chem.* (1994) 269:14457–64.

64. Thomas SR, Terentis AC, Cai H, Takikawa O, Levina A, Lay PA, et al. Post-translational regulation of human indoleamine 2,3-dioxygenase activity by nitric oxide. *J Biol Chem.* (2007) 282:23778–87. doi: 10.1074/jbc.M700669200

65. Hornyák L, Dobos N, Koncz G, Karányi Z, Páll D, Szabó Z, et al. The role of indoleamine-2, 3- dioxygenase in cancer development, diagnostics, and therapy. *Front Immunol.* (2018) 9:151. doi: 10.3389/fimmu.2018.00151

66. Orabona C, Pallotta MT, Volpi C, Fallarino F, Vacca C, Bianchi R, et al. SOCS3 drives proteasomal degradation of indoleamine 2,3-dioxygenase (IDO) and antagonizes IDO-dependent tolerogenesis. *PNAS.* (2008) 105:20828–33. doi: 10.1073/pnas.0810278105

67. Du MX, Sotero-Esteva WD, Taylor MW. Analysis of transcription factors regulating induction of indoleamine 2,3-dioxygenase by IFN-γ. *J Interf Cytokine Res.* (2000) 20:133–42. doi: 10.1089/107999000312531

68. Martin-Gallausiaux C, Larraufie P, Jarry A, Béguet-Crespel F, Marinelli L, Ledue F, et al. Butyrate produced by commensal bacteria down-regulates indolamine 2,3-dioxygenase 1 (IDO-1) expression via a dual mechanism in human intestinal epithelial cells. *Front Immunol.* (2018) 9:2838. doi: 10.3389/fimmu.2018.02838

69. Carbotti G, Barisione G, Airoldi I, Mezzanzanica D, Bagnoli M, Ferrero S, et al. IL-27 induces the expression of IDO and PD-L1 in human cancer cells. *Oncotarget.* (2015) 6:43267–80. doi: 10.18632/oncotarget.6530

70. Yanagawa Y, Iwabuchi K, Onoé K. Co-operative action of interleukin-10 and interferon-γ to regulate dendritic cell functions. *Immunology.* (2009) 127:345–53. doi: 10.1111/j.1365-2567.2008.02986.x

71. Mellor AL, Munn DH. IDO expression by dendritic cells: tolerance and tryptophan catabolism. *Nat Rev Immunol.* (2004) 4:762–74. doi: 10.1038/nri1457

72. Mándi Y, Vécsei L. The kynurenine system and immunoregulation. *J Neural Transm.* (2012) 119:197–209. doi: 10.1007/s00702-011-0681-y

73. Connor TJ, Starr N, O'Sullivan JB, Harkin A. Induction of indolamine 2,3-dioxygenase and kynurenine 3-monooxygenase in rat brain following a systemic inflammatory challenge: a role for IFN-γ? *Neurosci Lett.* (2008) 441:29–34. doi: 10.1016/j.neulet.2008.06.007

74. Baban B, Hansen AM, Chandler PR, Manlapat A, Bingaman A, Kahler DJ, et al. A minor population of splenic dendritic cells expressing CD19 mediates IDO-dependent T cell suppression via type I IFN signaling following B7 ligation. *Int Immunol.* (2005) 17:909–19. doi: 10.1093/intimm/dxh271

75. Mellor AL, Baban B, Chandler PR, Manlapat A, Kahler DJ, Munn DH. Cutting edge: CpG oligonucleotides induce splenic CD19+ dendritic cells to acquire potent indoleamine 2,3-dioxygenase-dependent T cell regulatory functions via IFN Type 1 signaling. *J Immunol.* (2005) 175:5601–5. doi: 10.4049/jimmunol.175.9.5601

76. Lemos H, Mohamed E, Huang L, Ou R, Pacholczyk G, Arbab AS, et al. STING promotes the growth of tumors characterized by low antigenicity via IDO activation Henrique. *Cancer Res.* (2017) 76:2076–81. doi: 10.1158/0008-5472.CAN-15-1456

77. Munn DH, Sharma MD, Baban B, Harding HP, Zhang Y, Ron D, et al. GCN2 kinase in T cells mediates proliferative arrest and anergy induction in response to indoleamine 2,3-dioxygenase. *Immunity.* (2005) 22:633–42. doi: 10.1016/j.immuni.2005.03.013

78. Cobbold SP, Adams E, Farquhar CA, Nolan KF, Howie D, Lui KO, et al. Infectious tolerance via the consumption of essential amino acids and mTOR signaling. *Proc Natl Acad Sci USA.* (2009) 106:12055–60. doi: 10.1073/pnas.0903919106

79. Mezrich JD, Fechner JH, Zhang X, Johnson BP, William JB, Bradfield CA. An interaction between kynurenine and the aryl hydrocarbon receptor can generate regulatory T cells. *J Immunol.* (2010) 185:3190–8. doi: 10.4049/jimmunol.0903670

80. Wen H, Hogaboam CM, Gauldie J, Kunkel SL. Severe sepsis exacerbates cell-mediated immunity in the lung due to an altered dendritic cell cytokine profile. *Am J Pathol.* (2006) 168:1940–50. doi: 10.2353/ajpath.2006.051155

81. Ben-haj-ayed A, Moussa A, Ghedira R, Gabbouj S, Miled S, Bouzid N, et al. Prognostic value of indoleamine 2,3-dioxygenase activity and expression in nasopharyngeal carcinoma. *Immunol Lett.* (2016) 169:23–32. doi: 10.1016/j.imlet.2015.11.012

82. Munn DH, Mellor AL. IDO in the tumor microenvironment: inflammation, counter-regulation, and tolerance. *Trends Immunol.* (2016) 37:193–207. doi: 10.1016/j.it.2016.01.002

83. Uyttenhove C, Pilotte L, Théate I, Stroobant V, Colau D, Parmentier N, et al. Evidence for a tumoral immune resistance mechanism based on tryptophan degradation by indoleamine 2,3-dioxygenase. *Nat Med.* (2003) 9:1269–74. doi: 10.1038/nm934

84. Liu J, Lu G, Tang F, Liu Y, Cui G. Localization of indoleamine 2,3-dioxygenase in human esophageal squamous cell carcinomas. *Virchows Arch.* (2009) 455:441–8. doi: 10.1007/s00428-009-0846-3

85. Milano F, Jorritsma T, Rygiel AM, Bergman JJ, Sondermeijer C, Brinke A, et al. Expression pattern of immune suppressive cytokines and growth factors in oesophageal adenocarcinoma reveal a tumour immune escape-promoting microenvironment. *Scand J Immunol.* (2008) 68:616–23. doi: 10.1111/j.1365-3083.2008.02183.x

86. Ye J, Liu H, Hu Y, Li P, Zhang G, Li Y. Tumoral indoleamine 2,3-dioxygenase expression predicts poor outcome in laryngeal squamous cell carcinoma. *Virchows Arch.* (2013) 462:73–81. doi: 10.1007/s00428-012-1340-x

87. Zhang G, Liu W-L, Zhang L, Wang J, Kuang M-H, Liu P, et al. Involvement of indoleamine 2,3-dioxygenase in impairing tumor-infiltrating CD8 T-cell functions in esophageal squamous cell carcinoma. *Clin Dev Immunol.* (2011) 2011:384726. doi: 10.1155/2011/384726

88. Fukuno K, Hara T, Tsurumi H, Shibata Y, Mabuchi R, Nakamura N, et al. Expression of indoleamine 2,3-dioxygenase in leukemic cells indicates an unfavorable prognosis in acute myeloid leukemia patients with intermediate-risk cytogenetics. *Leuk Lymphoma.* (2015) 56:1398–405. doi: 10.3109/10428194.2014.953150

89. Nakamura T, Niimi S, Nawa K, Noda C, Ichihara A, Takagi Y, et al. Multihormonal regulation of transcription of the tryptophan 2,3-dioxygenase gene in primary cultures of adult rat hepatocytes with special reference to the presence of a transcriptional protein mediating the action of glucocorticoids. *J Biol Chem.* (1987) 262:727–33.

90. Miller CL, Llenos IC, Dulay JR, Weis S. Upregulation of the initiating step of the kynurenine pathway in postmortem anterior cingulate cortex from individuals with schizophrenia and bipolar disorder. *Brain Res.* (2006) 1073–1074:25–37. doi: 10.1016/j.brainres.2005.12.056

91. Ishiguro I, Naito J, Saito K, Nagamurac Y. Skin L-tryptophan-2,3-dioxygenase and rat hair growth. *FEBS Lett.* (1993) 329:178–82. doi: 10.1016/0014-5793(93)80217-I

92. Nakamura T, Shinno H, Ichihara A. Insulin and glucagon as a new regulator system for tryptophan oxygenase activity demonstrated in primary cultured rat hepatocytes. *J Biol Chem.* (1980) 255:7533–5.

93. Rubin RT. Adrenal cortical activity changes in manic-depressive illness. Influence on intermediary metabolism of tryptophan. *Arch*

Gen Psychiatry. (1967) 17:671–9. doi: 10.1001/archpsyc.1967.01730300031006

94. Oxenburg GF. Tryptophan kynurenine metabolism as a common mediator of genetic and environmental impacts in major depressive disorder: the serotonin hypothesis revisited 40 years later. *Isr J Psychiatry Relat Sci.* (2010) 47:56–63. doi: 10.3410/f.13356987.14726252

95. Suzuki S, Toné S, Takikawa O, Kubo T, Kohno I, Minatogawa Y. Expression of indoleamine 2,3-dioxygenase and tryptophan 2,3-dioxygenase in early concepti. *Biochem J.* (2001) 355:425–9. doi: 10.1042/bj3550425

96. Tatsumi K, Higuchi T, Fujiwara H, Nakayama T, Egawa H, Itoh K, et al. Induction of tryptophan 2, 3-dioxygenase in the mouse endometrium during implantation. *Biochem Biophys Res Commun.* (2000) 274:166–70. doi: 10.1006/bbrc.2000.3115

97. Opitz CA, Litzenburger UM, Sahm F, Ott M, Tritschler I, Trump S, et al. An endogenous ligand of the human aryl hydrocarbon receptor promotes tumor formation. *Nature.* (2011) 478:197–203. doi: 10.1038/nature10491

98. Schmidt SK, Ebel S, Keil E, Woite C, Ernst JF, Benzin AE, et al. Regulation of IDO activity by oxygen supply: inhibitory effects on antimicrobial and immunoregulatory functions. *PLoS ONE.* (2013) 8:e63301. doi: 10.1371/journal.pone.0063301

99. Nguyen NT, Nakahama T, Le DH, Van Son L, Chu HH, Kishimoto T. Aryl hydrocarbon receptor and kynurenine: recent advances in autoimmune disease research. *Front Immunol.* (2014) 5:551. doi: 10.3389/fimmu.2014.00551

100. Seok SH, Ma ZX, Feltenberger JB, Chen H, Chen H, Scarlett C, et al. Trace derivatives of kynurenine potently activate the aryl hydrocarbon receptor (AHR). *J Biol Chem.* (2018) 293:1994–2005. doi: 10.1074/jbc.RA117.000631

101. Foster AC, Vezzani A, French ED, Schwarcz R. Kynurenic acid blocks neurotoxicity and seizures induced in rats by the related brain metabolite quinolonoc acid. *Neurosci Lett.* (1984) 48:273–8. doi: 10.1016/0304-3940(84)90050-8

102. Andiné P, Lehmann A, Ellrén K, Wennberg E, Kjellmer I, Nielsen T, et al. The excitatory amino acid antagonist kynurenic acid administered after hypoxic-ischemia in neonatal rats offers neuroprotection. *Neurosci Lett.* (1988) 90:208–12. doi: 10.1016/0304-3940(88)90813-0

103. Wirthgen E, Hoeflich A, Rebl A, Günther J. Kynurenic acid: the Janus-faced role of an immunomodulatory tryptophan metabolite and its link to pathological conditions. *Front Immunol.* (2017) 8:1957. doi: 10.3389/fimmu.2017.01957

104. Veldhoen M, Hirota K, Christensen J, O'Garra A, Stockinger B. Natural agonists for aryl hydrocarbon receptor in culture medium are essential for optimal differentiation of Th17 T cells. *J Exp Med.* (2009) 206:43–9. doi: 10.1084/jem.20081438

105. Hu Y, Shen F, Crellin NK, Ouyang W. The IL-17 pathway as a major therapeutic target in autoimmune diseases. *Ann N Y Acad Sci.* (2011) 1217:60–76. doi: 10.1111/j.1749-6632.2010.05825.x

106. Kadowaki N, Antonenko S, Lau JY, Liu Y. Natural interferon alpha/beta-producing cells link innate and adaptive immunity. *J Exp Med.* (2000) 192:219–26. doi: 10.1084/jem.192.2.219

107. Tilton JC, Manion MM, Luskin MR, Johnson AJ, Patamawenu AA, Hallahan CW, et al. Human immunodeficiency virus viremia induces plasmacytoid dendritic cell activation *in vivo* and diminished alpha interferon production *in vitro.* *J Virol.* (2008) 82:3997–4006. doi: 10.1128/JVI.01545-07

108. Costa-Mattioli M, Sonenberg N. RAPping production of type I interferon in pDCs through mTOR. *Nat Immunol.* (2008) 9:1097–9. doi: 10.1038/ni1008-1097

109. Gao X, Zhang Y, Arrazola P, Hino O, Kobayashi T, Yeung RS, et al. Tsc tumour suppressor proteins antagonize amino-acid–TOR signalling. *Nat Cell Biol.* (2002) 4:699–704. doi: 10.1038/ncb847

110. Barnes PJ. Th2 cytokines and asthma: an introduction. *Respir Res.* (2001) 2:64–5. doi: 10.1186/rr39

111. Canna SW, Behrens EM. Making sense of the cytokine storm: a conceptual framework for understanding, diagnosing, and treating hemophagocytic syndromes. *Pediatr Clin North Am.* (2012) 59:329–44. doi: 10.1016/j.pcl.2012.03.002

112. Mellins ED, Macaubas C, Grom AA. Pathogenesis of systemic juvenile idiopathic arthritis: some answers, more questions. *Nat Rev Rheumatol.* (2014) 7:416–26. doi: 10.1038/nrrheum.2011.68

113. Janka G, zur Stadt U. Familial and acquired hemophagocytic lymphohistiocytosis. *Hematol Am Soc Hematol Educ Progr.* (2005) 2005:82–8. doi: 10.1182/asheducation-2005.1.82

114. Bach JF. Insulin-dependent diabetes mellitus as an autoimmune disease. *Endocr Rev.* (1994) 15:516–42. doi: 10.1210/edrv-15-4-516

115. Pallotta MT, Orabona C, Volpi C, Vacca C, Belladonna ML, Bianchi R, et al. Indoleamine 2,3-dioxygenase is a signaling protein in long-term tolerance by dendritic cells. *Nat Immunol.* (2011) 12:870–8. doi: 10.1038/ni.2077

116. Orabona C, Pallotta MT, Grohmann U. Different partners, opposite outcomes: a new perspective of the immunobiology of indoleamine 2,3-dioxygenase. *Mol Med.* (2012) 18:834–42. doi: 10.2119/molmed.2012.00029

117. Belladonna ML, Orabona C, Grohmann U, Puccetti P. TGF-β and kynurenines as the key to infectious tolerance. *Trends Mol Med.* (2009) 15:41–9. doi: 10.1016/j.molmed.2008.11.006

118. Samuel T, Cockwell P. Islet cell transplantation. *J R Soc Med.* (2002) 95:31–3. doi: 10.1177/014107680209500109

119. ShapiroAM, Lakey JR, Ryan EA, Korbutt GS, Toth E, Warnock GL, et al. Islet transplantation in seven patients with type 1 diabetes mellitus using a glucocorticoid-free immunosuppressive regimen. *N Engl J Med.* (2000) 343:230–8. doi: 10.1056/NEJM200007273430401

120. Tarr JM, Kaul K, Chopra M, Kohner EM, Chibber R. Pathophysiology of diabetic retinopathy. *ISRN Ophthalmol.* (2013) 2013:343560. doi: 10.1155/2013/343560

121. Conti P, Shaik-Dasthagirisaeb Y. Atherosclerosis: a chronic inflammatory disease mediated by mast cells. *Cent Eur J Immunol.* (2015) 40:380–6. doi: 10.5114/ceji.2015.54603

122. Daugherty A, Manning MW, Cassis LA. Angiotensin II promotes atherosclerotic lesions and aneurysms in apolipoprotein E – deficient mice. *J Clin Invest.* (2000) 105:1605–12. doi: 10.1172/JCI7818

123. Lu H, Daugherty A. Aortic Aneurysms. *Arterioscler Thromb Vasc Biol.* (2017) 37:59–66. doi: 10.1161/ATVBAHA.117.309578

124. Hellmann DB, Grand DJ, Freischlag JA. Inflammatory abdominal aortic aneurysm. *JAMA.* (2007) 297:395–400. doi: 10.1001/jama.297.4.395

125. Hellenthal FA, Buurman WA, Wodzig WK, Schurink GW. Biomarkers of AAA progression. Part 1: extracellular matrix degeneration. *Nat Rev Cardiol.* (2009) 6:464–74. doi: 10.1038/nrcardio.2009.80

126. Dandona P, Aljada A, Bandyopadhyay A. Inflammation: the link between insulin resistance, obesity and diabetes. *Trends Immunol.* (2004) 25:4–7. doi: 10.1016/j.it.2003.10.013

127. Roszer T. Understanding the mysterious M2 macrophage through activation markers and effector mechanisms. *Mediat Inflamm.* (2015) 2015:1–16. doi: 10.1155/2015/816460

128. Cani PD, Amar J, Iglesias MA, Poggi M, Knauf C, Bastelica D, et al. Metabolic endotoxemia initiates obesity and insulin resistance. *Diabetes.* (2007) 56:1761–72. doi: 10.2337/db06-1491

129. Cherayil BJ. Indoleamine 2,3-dioxygenase in intestinal immunity and inflammation. *Inflamm Bowel Dis.* (2009) 15:1391–6. doi: 10.1002/ibd.20910

130. Lamas B, Richard ML, Leducq V, Pham H-P, Michel M-L, Da Costa G, et al. CARD9 impacts colitis by altering gut microbiota metabolism of tryptophan into aryl hydrocarbon receptor ligands. *Nat Med.* (2016) 22:598–605. doi: 10.1038/nm.4102

131. Valeri M, Raffatellu M. Cytokines IL-17 and IL-22 in the host response to infection. *Pathog Dis.* (2016) 74:1–65. doi: 10.1093/femspd/ftw111

132. Iwamoto N, Ito H, Ando K, Ishikawa T, Hara A, Taguchi A, et al. Upregulation of indoleamine 2,3-dioxygenase in hepatocyte during acute hepatitis caused by hepatitis B virus-specic cytotoxic T lymphocytes *in vivo.* *Liver Int.* (2009) 22:277–83. doi: 10.1111/j.1478-3231.2008.01748.x

133. Manuel ER, Diamond DJ. A road less traveled paved by IDO silencing. Harnessing the antitumor activity of neutrophils. *Oncoimmunology.* (2013) 2:e23322. doi: 10.4161/onci.23322

134. Wang W, Huang L, Jin J-Y, Jolly S, Zang Y, Wu H, et al. IDO immune status after chemoradiation may predict survival in lung cancer patients. *Cancer Res.* (2018) 78:809–16. doi: 10.1158/0008-5472.CAN-17-2995

135. Günther J, Däbritz J, Wirthgen E. Limitations and off-target effects of tryptophan-related IDO inhibitors in cancer treatment. *Front Immunol.* (2019) 10:1801. doi: 10.3389/fimmu.2019.01801

136. Goswami R, Subramanian G, Silayeva L, Newkirk I, Doctor D, Chawla K, et al. Gene therapy leaves a vicious cycle. *Front Oncol.* (2019) 9:297. doi: 10.3389/fonc.2019.00297

137. Elbers F, Woite C, Antoni V, Stein S, Funakoshi H, Nakamura T, et al. Negative impact of hypoxia on tryptophan 2,3-dioxygenase function. *Mediat Inflamm.* (2016) 2016:1638916. doi: 10.1155/2016/1638916

138. Benseler V, Mccaughan GW, Schlitt HJ, Bishop GA, Bowen DG, Bertolino P. The liver: a special case in transplantation tolerance. *Semin Liver Dis.* (2007) 27:194–213. doi: 10.1055/s-2007-979471

139. Giorgini F, Huang SY, Sathyasaikumar KV, Notarangelo FM, Thomas MAR, Tararina M, et al. Targeted deletion of kynurenine 3-monooxygenyse in mice a new tool for studying kynurenine pathway metabolism in periphery and brain. *J Biol Chem.* (2013) 288:36554–66. doi: 10.1074/jbc.M113.503813

140. Rózsa É, Hermina R, Vécsei L, Toldi J. The Janus-face kynurenic acid. *J Neural Transm.* (2008) 115:1087–91. doi: 10.1007/s00702-008-0052-5

141. Chess AC, Simoni MK, Alling TE, Bucci DJ. Elevations of endogenous kynurenic acid produce spatial working memory deficits. *Schizophr Bull.* (2007) 33:797–804. doi: 10.1093/schbul/sbl033

142. Erhardt S, Schwieler L, Emanuelsson C, Geyer M. Endogenous kynurenic acid disrupts prepulse inhibition. *Biol Psychiatry.* (2004) 56:255–60. doi: 10.1016/j.biopsych.2004.06.006

143. Chess AC, Landers AM, Bucci DJ. L-kynurenine treatment alters contextual fear conditioning and context discrimination but not cue-specific fear conditioning. *Behav Brain Res.* (2009) 201:325–31. doi: 10.1016/j.bbr.2009.03.013

144. Frumento G, Rotondo R, Tonetti M, Damonte G, Benatti U, Ferrara GB. Tryptophan-derived catabolites are responsible for inhibition of T and natural killer cell proliferation induced by indoleamine 2,3-dioxygenase. *J Exp Med.* (2002) 196:459–68. doi: 10.1084/jem.20020121

145. Terness P, Bauer TM, Röse L, Dufter C, Watzlik A, Simon H, et al. Inhibition of allogeneic T cell proliferation by indoleamine 2,3-dioxygenase – expressing dendritic cells: mediation of suppression by tryptophan metabolites. *J Exp Med.* (2002) 196:447–57. doi: 10.1084/jem.20020052

146. Song H, Park H, Kim Y, Kim DK, Lee H-K, Cho D-H, et al. L- Kynurenine-induced apoptosis in human NK cells is mediated by reactive oxygen species. *Int Immunopharmacol.* (2011) 11:932–8. doi: 10.1016/j.intimp.2011.02.005

147. Wang J, Simonavicius N, Wu X, Swaminath G, Reagan J, Tian H, et al. Kynurenic acid as a ligand for orphan G protein-coupled receptor GPR35. *J Biol Chem.* (2006) 281:22021–8. doi: 10.1074/jbc.M603503200

148. Badawy AAB. Hypothesis kynurenic and quinolinic acids: the main players of the kynurenine pathway and opponents in inflammatory disease. *Med Hypotheses.* (2018) 118:129–38. doi: 10.1016/j.mehy.2018.06.021

149. Galvão-de Almeida A, Quarantini LC, Sampaio AS, Lyra AC, Parise CL, Paraná R, et al. Lack of association of indoleamine 2,3-dioxygenase polymorphisms with interferon-alpha-related depression in hepatitis C. *Brain Behav Immun.* (2011) 25:1491–7. doi: 10.1016/j.bbi.2011.06.001

150. Cutler JA, Rush AJ, McMahon FJ, Laje G. Common genetic variation in the indoleamine-2,3-dioxygenase genes and antidepressant treatment outcome in major depressive disorder. *J Psychopharmacol.* (2012) 26:360–7. doi: 10.1177/0269881111434622

151. Tardito S, Negrini S, Conteduca G, Ferrera F, Parodi A, Battaglia F, et al. Indoleamine 2,3 dioxygenase gene polymorphisms correlate with CD8+ Treg impairment in systemic sclerosis. *Hum Immunol.* (2013) 74:166–9. doi: 10.1016/j.humimm.2012.11.008

152. Lee A, Kanuri N, Zhang Y, Sayuk GS, Li E, Ciorba MA. IDO1 and IDO2 non-synonymous gene variants: correlation with Crohn's disease risk and clinical phenotype. *PLoS ONE.* (2014) 9:e115848. doi: 10.1371/journal.pone.0115848

153. Ferreira P, Shin I, Sosova I, Dornevil K, Jain S, Dewey D, et al. Hypertryptophanemia due to tryptophan 2,3-dioxygenase deficiency. *Mol Genet Metab.* (2017) 120:317–24. doi: 10.1016/j.ymgme.2017.02.009

154. Comings D. Blood serotonin and tryptophan in tourette syndrome. *Am J Med Genet.* (1990) 36:418–30. doi: 10.1002/ajmg.1320360410

155. Nabi R, Serajee FJ, Chugani DC, Zhong H, Hug AH. Association of tryptophan 2,3 dioxygenase gene polymorphism with autism. *Am J Med Genet B Neuropsychiatr Genet.* (2004) 125B:63–8. doi: 10.1002/ajmg.b.20147

156. Wonodi I, Stine O, Sathyasaikumar K, Roberts R, Mitchell B, Hong L, et al. Downregulated kynurenine 3-monooxygenase gene expression and enzyme activity in schizophrenia and genetic association with schizophrenia endophenotypes. *Arch Gen Psychiatry.* (2011) 68:665–74. doi: 10.1001/archgenpsychiatry.2011.71

157. Holtze M, Saetre P, Erhardt S, Schwieler L, Werge T, Hansen T, et al. Kynurenine 3-monooxygenase (KMO) polymorphisms in schizophrenia: an association study. *Schizophr Res.* (2011) 127:270–2. doi: 10.1016/j.schres.2010.10.002

158. Aoyama N, Takahashi N, Saito S, Maeno N, Ishihara R, Ji X, et al. Association study between kynurenine 3-monooxygenase gene and schizophrenia in the Japanese population. *Genes Brain Behav.* (2006) 5:364–8. doi: 10.1111/j.1601-183X.2006.00231.x

159. Golimbet VE, Lezheiko TV, Alfimova MV, Abramova LI, Kondrat'ev NV. Association of kynurenine-3-monooxygenase gene with schizophrenia. *Russ J Genet.* (2014) 50:634–7. doi: 10.1134/S1022795414060039

160. Wonodi I, McMahon RP, Krishna N, Mitchell BD, Liu J, Glassman M, et al. Influence of kynurenine 3-monooxygenase (KMO) gene polymorphism on cognitive function in schizophrenia. *Schizophr Res.* (2014) 160:80–7. doi: 10.1016/j.schres.2014.10.026

161. Holtze M, Saetre P, Engberg G, Schwieler L, Werge T, Andreassen OA, et al. Kynurenine 3-monooxygenase polymorphisms: relevance for kynurenic acid synthesis in patients with schizophrenia and healthy controls. *J Psychiatry Neurosci.* (2012) 37:53–7. doi: 10.1503/jpn.100175

162. Lavebratt C, Olsson S, Backlund L, Frisén L, Sellgren C, Priebe L, et al. The KMO allele encoding Arg452 is associated with psychotic features in bipolar disorder type 1, and increased CSF KYNA level and reduced KMO expression. *Mol Psychiatry.* (2014) 19:334–41. doi: 10.1038/mp.2013.11

163. Wang S-Y, Duan K-M, Tan X-F, Yin J-Y, Mao X-Y, Zheng W, et al. Genetic variants of the kynurenine-3-monooxygenase and postpartum depressive symptoms after cesarean section in Chinese women. *J Affect Disord.* (2017) 215:94–101. doi: 10.1016/j.jad.2017.03.023

164. McCauley J, Zuvich R, Bradford Y, Kenealy S, Schnetz-Boutaud N, Gregory S, et al. Follow-up examination of linkage and association to chromosome 1q43 in multiple sclerosis. *Genes Immun.* (2009) 10:624–30. doi: 10.1038/gene.2009.53

165. de Souza FRS, Fontes FL, da Silva TA, Coutinho LG, Leib SL, Agnez-Lima LF. Association of kynurenine aminotransferase II gene C401T polymorphism with immune response in patients with meningitis. *BMC Med Genet.* (2011) 12:51. doi: 10.1186/1471-2350-12-51

166. Coutinho LG, Christen S, Bellac CL, Fontes FL, de Souza FRS, Grandgirard D, et al. The kynurenine pathway is involved in bacterial meningitis. *J Neuroinflamm.* (2014) 11:169. doi: 10.1186/s12974-014-0169-4

167. Fontes FL, de Araújo LF, Coutinho LG, Leib SL, Agnez-Lima LF. Genetic polymorphisms associated with the inflammatory response in bacterial meningitis. *BMC Med Genet.* (2015) 16:70. doi: 10.1186/s12881-015-0218-6

168. Zhang Y, Zhang K, He X, Yuan W, Wang G, Mao S, et al. A polymorphism of kynureninase gene in a hypertensive candidate chromosomal region is associated with essential hypertension. *Chinese J Cardiol.* (2005) 33:588–91. doi: 10.3760/j:issn:0253-3758.2005.07.002

169. Zhang Y, Shen J, He X, Zhang K, Wu S, Xiao B, et al. A rare variant at the KYNU gene is associated with kynureninase activity and essential hypertension in the Han Chinese population. *Circ Cardiovasc Genet.* (2011) 4:687–94. doi: 10.1161/CIRCGENETICS.110.959064

170. Christensen M, Duno M, Lund AM, Skovby F, Christensen E. Xanthurenic aciduria due to a mutation in KYNU encoding kynureninase. *J Inherit Metab Dis.* (2007) 30:248–55. doi: 10.1007/s10545-007-0396-2

171. Geller F, Feenstra B, Carstensen L, Pers TH, van Rooij IALM, Körberg IB, et al. Genome-wide association analyses identify variants in developmental genes associated with hypospadias. *Nat Genet.* (2014) 46:957–63. doi: 10.1038/ng.3063

172. Nalls MA, Plagnol V, Hernandez DG, Sharma M, Sheerin UM, Saad M, et al. Imputation of sequence variants for identification of genetic risks for Parkinson's disease: a meta-analysis of genome-wide association studies. *Lancet.* (2011) 377:641–9. doi: 10.1016/S0140-6736(10)6 2345-8

173. Arefayene M, Philips S, Cao D, Mamidipalli S, Desta Z, Flockhart DA, et al. Identification of genetic variants in the human indoleamine 2,3-dioxygenase (IDO1) gene,which have altered enzyme activity. *Pharmacogenet Genomics.* (2009) 19:464–76. doi: 10.1097/FPC.0b013e32832 c005a

174. Fenoglio D, Battaglia F, Parodi A, Stringara S, Negrini S, Panico N, et al. Alteration of Th17 and Treg cell subpopulations co-exist in patients affected with systemic sclerosis. *Clin Immunol.* (2011) 139:249–57. doi: 10.1016/j.clim.2011.01.013

175. Gupta NK, Thaker AI, Kanuri N, Riehl TE, Rowley CW, Stenson WF, et al. Serum analysis of tryptophan catabolism pathway: correlation with Crohn's disease activity. *Inflamm Bowel Dis.* (2012) 18:1214–20. doi: 10.1002/ibd.21849

176. Královičová J, Vorechovský I. Global control of aberrant splice-site activation by auxiliary splicing sequences: evidence for a gradient in exon and intron definition. *Nucleic Acids Res.* (2007) 35:6399–413. doi: 10.1093/nar/gkm680

177. Guillemin GJ, Williams KR, Smith DG, Smythe GA, Croitoru-Lamoury J, Brew BJ. Quinolinic acid in the pathogenesis of Alzheimer's disease. *Adv Exp Med Biol.* (2003) 527:167–76. doi: 10.1007/978-1-4615-0135-0_19

178. Beal MF, Matson WR, Storey E, Milbury P, Ryan EA, Ogawa T, et al. Kynurenic acid concentrations are reduced in Huntington's disease cerebral cortex. *J Neurol Sci.* (1992) 108:80–7. doi: 10.1016/0022-510X(92)90191-M

179. Németh H, Toldi J, Vécsei L. Kynurenines, Parkinson's disease and other neurodegenerative disorders: preclinical and clinical studies. *J Neural Transm.* (2006) 70:285–304. doi: 10.1007/978-3-211-45295-0_45

180. Myint AM, Kim KY, Verkerk R, Scharpé S, Steinbusch H, Leonard B. Kynurenine pathway in major depression: evidence of impaired neuroprotection. *J Affect Disord.* (2007) 98:143–51. doi: 10.1016/j.jad.2006.07.013

181. Cribbs AP, Williams RO. Role of the kynurenine pathway in immune-mediated inflammation. In: Mittal S, editor. *Targeting the Broadly Pathogenic Kynurenine Pathway.* Cham: Springer International Publishing (2015). p. 93–107.

182. Wurster CD, Ludolph AC. Antisense oligonucleotides in neurological disorders. *Ther Adv Neurol Disord.* (2018) 11:1–19. doi: 10.1177/1756286418776932

183. Blaese RM, Culver KW, Miller AD, Carter CS, Fleisher T, Clericij M, et al. T lymphocyte-directed gene therapy for ADA- SCID: initial trial results after 4 years. *Science.* (1995) 270:475–80. doi: 10.1126/science.270.5235.475

184. Deev RV, Bozo IY, Mzhavanadze ND, Voronov DA, Gavrilenko AV, Chervyakov YV, et al. pCMV- vegf165 intramuscular gene transfer is an effective method of treatment for patients with chronic lower limb ischemia. *J Cardiovasc Pharmacol Ther.* (2015) 20:473–82. doi: 10.1177/1074248415574336

185. Maude SL, Laetsch TW, Buechner J, Rives S, Boyer M, Bittencourt H, et al. Tisagenlecleucel in children and young adults with B-cell lymphoblastic leukemia. *N Engl J Med.* (2018) 378:439–48. doi: 10.1056/NEJMoa1709866

186. Roberts ZJ, Better M, Bot A, Roberts MR, Ribas A. Axicabtagene ciloleucel, a first-in-class CAR T cell therapy for aggressive NHL. *Leuk Lymph.* (2018) 59:1785–96. doi: 10.1080/10428194.2017.1387905

Limitations and Off-Target Effects of Tryptophan-Related IDO Inhibitors in Cancer Treatment

Juliane Günther[1†], Jan Däbritz[2] and Elisa Wirthgen[2†]*

[1] Research Group Epigenetics, Metabolism and Longevity, Leibniz Institute for Farm Animal Biology, Dummerstorf, Germany,
[2] Department of Pediatrics, Rostock University Medical Center, Rostock, Germany

Correspondence:
Elisa Wirthgen
elisa.wirthgen@med.uni-rostock.de

[†] *These authors have contributed equally to this work*

Immunooncology is still a growing area in cancer therapy. Drugs within this therapeutic approach do not directly target/attack the tumor but interfere with immune checkpoints and target or reprogram key metabolic pathways critical for anti-cancer immune defense. Indolamine 2,3-dioxygenase 1 (IDO1) and the tryptophan (TRP)-kynurenine pathway were identified as critical mechanisms in cancer immune escape and their inhibition as an approach with promising therapeutic potential. Particularly, a multitude of IDO1 inhibiting tryptophan analogs are widely applied in several clinical trials. However, this therapy results in a variety of implications for the patient's physiology. This is not only due to the inhibition of an enzyme important in almost every organ and tissue in the body but also because of the general nature of the inhibitor as an analog of a proteinogenic amino acid as well as the initiation of cellular detoxification known to affect inflammatory pathways. In this review we provide a deeper insight into the physiological consequences of an IDO1 inhibiting therapy based on TRP related molecules. We discuss potential side and off-target effects that contribute to the interpretation of unexpected positive as well as negative results of ongoing or discontinued clinical studies while we also highlight the potential of these inhibitors independent of the IDO1 signaling pathway.

Keywords: IDO inhibitors, immunooncology, arylhydrocarbon receptor, TRP mimetics, pharmakokinetics

INTRODUCTION

The degradation of tryptophan (TRP) along the kynurenine pathway (KP) plays a crucial role in the regulation of the immune response, notably as a counter-regulatory mechanism in the context of inflammation (1, 2). Three rate limiting enzymes of KP have been described thus far, tryptophan 2,3-dioxygenase (TDO2), and indolamine 2,3-dioxygenase (IDO) 1 and 2, which are regulated by both nutritional and inflammatory pathways (3). In cancers, it has been shown that an increased IDO1 activity promotes the development of an immunosuppressive microenvironment that can inhibit effective anti-tumor immune responses (4). Besides cancer cells, the tumor microenvironment included heterogeneous cell types, including endothelial cells, immune cells, and mesenchymal stromal cells (MSCs) (5). There are indications that especially MSCs contribute to a solid tumor environment by IDO-mediated immunosuppressive effects such as reducing both tumor-infiltrating T-cells as well as B-cells (6). Furthermore, studies of the microenvironment in acute myeloid leukemia demonstrate a positive correlation between increased IDO expression in MSC and elevated level of immunosuppressive regulatory T-cells (7).

Therefore, the inhibition of IDO1 activity is of special interest as a target for anti-cancer therapy in order to restore tumor immunity.

In consequence, several IDO1-inhibitors are currently tested *in vitro* as well as in clinical trials (8). Many of these inhibitors such as 1-methyltryptophan (1-MT, Indoximod), INCB024360 (Epacadostat), NLG919 (Navoximod), or Norharmane are structurally related to TRP, the natural IDO substrate. These inhibitors bind to the IDO enzyme; however, they are not catabolized to N-formyl kynurenine. Frequently used IDO inhibitors in cancer therapy are Indoximod and Epacadostat which are currently under investigation in several clinical trials (https://clinicaltrials.gov). The application of IDO inhibitors should prevent both the depletion of TRP and the production of immunomodulatory TRP metabolites such as kynurenine (KYN) or kynurenic acid (KYNA) contributing to a suppression of IDO-induced immune escape of cancer cells. Although some promising results were described *in vitro* and in rodent models (9–15), however, controversy results regarding the efficiency of IDO-inhibitors were reported (16–18). This may be the result of pharmacokinetic or off-target effects such as the activation of detoxification pathways or the pretense of a nutritional signal due to TRP mimicry. This should be considered for application of TRP-related molecules *in vivo* since these effects can negatively affect the outcome of cancer treatments.

PHARMACOKINETIC ASPECTS AFFECTING EFFICACY OF IDO INHIBITORS

The effective inhibition of IDO1 activity is anticipated to result in a reduced catalytic degradation of TRP to KYN and an altered metabolite profile along the KP in response to inflammatory stimuli. Most IDO1 inhibitors are synthetic TRP analogs acting as competitive inhibitors of the enzyme. To function as potent inhibitors it is necessary to reach similar or higher levels than TRP in the target tissue or to have a higher affinity to IDO than the natural substrate TRP which has a Michaelis constant (K_m) of $\sim 7\,\mu M$ (19). Regarding the reported K_i or IC_{50} values shown in **Figure 1** it is assumed that the TRP analogs D- and L-1-MT (21) as well as the TRP derivate Norharmane (22) act on micromolar levels while BMS-986205 (23), Epacadostat (21), and Navoximod (24) exert inhibitory effects on nanomolar levels.

Indoximod

During last years, two stereoisomers, 1-methyl-D-tryptophan (D-1-MT = Indoximod) and 1-methyl-L-tryptophan (L-1-MT) were scrutinized as IDO inhibitors. Indoximod, which is under investigation in several clinical trials, showed therapeutic effects in murine tumor models reversing the suppression of T-cell proliferation and inducing retardation, but no total arrest of tumor growth (9, 10, 13). Unexpectedly, in an IDO1 positive ovarian cancer cell line, Indoximod triggered an increased IFNγ-induced release of the TRP metabolite KYN concurrent with an increase of IDO1 mRNA (25) indicating an activation of KP instead of anticipated inhibition. An acceleration of TRP

degradation was also reported in mice and pigs after oral or subcutaneous applications of L-1-MT, which is not applied in clinical trials but used as IDO inhibitor in preclinical studies (14, 17). However, in these studies, KYNA, a stable end product of KP was increased in plasma rather than KYN, which is an intermediate metabolite of KP. However, IDO expression on mRNA or protein levels was not further investigated in these studies. Nevertheless, these results indicate that 1-MT induce an increase of TRP degradation via the KP instead of a downregulation by IDO inhibition.

One reason for the lack of effective IDO1 inhibition could be that the concentration of 1-MT was too low to inhibit IDO1 activity *in vivo*. A phase I trial of tumor patients using Indoximod as an IDO1 inhibitor has shown that doses higher than 1,200 mg 1-MT in a patient do not increase peak serum levels over $\sim 16\,\mu M$ (26), indicating a limited accumulation of the applied inhibitor. This finding is in accordance with previous findings in pigs showing that a steady-state 1-MT concentration is already reached after the second 1-MT injection of 1,000 mg/animal/day (27), increasing 1-MT to plasma levels similar to those of TRP ($\sim 30\,\mu M$). In studies using a recombinant IDO1 enzyme in cell-free assay systems determined that the L-isomer of 1-MT inhibits 50% of IDO1 activity at concentrations of $19\,\mu M$ whereas the D-isomer was not effective (13). Interestingly, in mature human dendritic cells, L-1-MT only diminished IFNγ-induced increase of KYN at concentrations of 1 mM, whereas $200\,\mu M$ showed no effect (28). This indicates that 1-MT was unable to prevent the production of KYN under physiological conditions in these cells which might be due to a low affinity of the inhibitor to the enzyme. Thereby, the half maximal inhibitory concentration (IC_{50}) of L-1-MT and D-1-MT was $120\,\mu M$ and more than 2.5 mM, respectively. As shown for 1-MT, it should be considered that K_i values from cell-free assays may not reflect the inhibitory effect *in vivo* resulting in inefficient inhibition at physiological concentrations. According to the reported IC_{50} values in HeLa cells it is assumed that both L- and D-1-MT are *in vivo* relatively ineffective IDO inhibitors. Nevertheless, significant effects of these drugs on immune response and KP reveal off-target modes of actions. The ineffective IDO inhibition by 1-MT *in vivo* should be considered for the interpretation of published studies using 1-MT.

Navoximod

Navoximod is a dual specific inhibitor that inhibits IDO1 and TDO, but with only 20-fold ($EC_{50} = 1.5\,\mu M$) selectivity against the later enzyme (24). Navoximod is very potent in the inhibition of IDO1 and was recently used in a phase 1 trial in combination with Azolizumab against solid tumors (29). According to the pharmacokinetics data published for orally administered doses in this study (600 or 1,000 mg), the plasma concentration of the drug should be sufficient to achieve EC_{50} inhibition of TDO. This may explain some of the effects and side effects of the treatment. The question to what extent a combined IDO1 and TDO inhibition is advantageous or disadvantageous is currently still under debate. A recently published article demonstrates the quickly absorption and moderate bioavailability of Navoximod and shows that this drug is extensively metabolized mainly by

Natural IDO substrate		K_m
L-tryptophan (TRP)	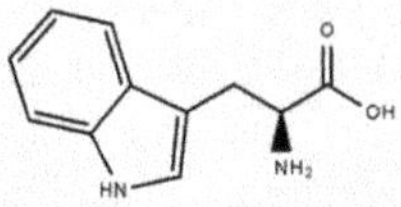	rhIDO 7.0 ± 0.8 μM [19]

TRP-analogues	Structure	In clinical trials	K_i / IC_{50}
1-Methyl-D-tryptophan (Indoximod)	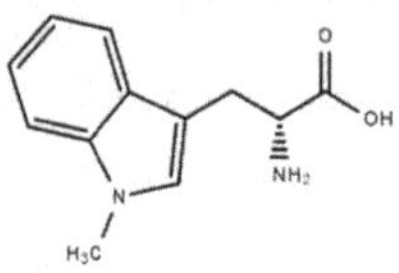	**Yes**: alone and in combination with different biologicals or drugs in advanced cancers in phase 1 and 2 trials (18 studies)	K_i > 100 μM HeLa IC_{50} 2.5 mM [20]
1-Methyl-L-tryptophan	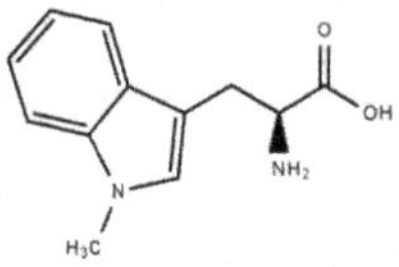	**No**	K_i 19 μM HeLa IC_{50} 120 μM [20]
BMS-986205	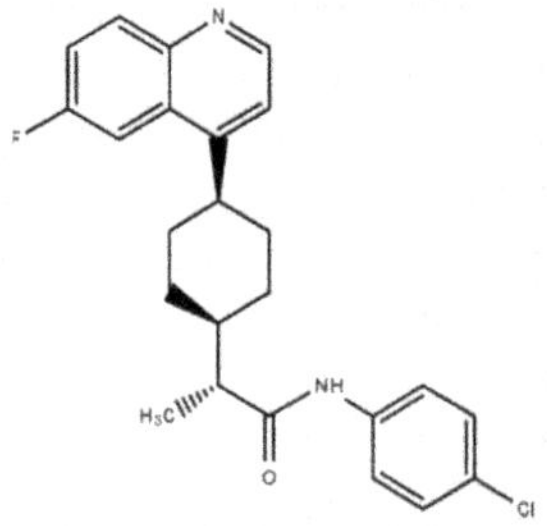	**Yes**: alone and in combination with different biologicals or drugs in advanced cancer diseases in phase 1 and 2 trials (21 studies)	HeLa IC_{50} 1.7 nM [22]
INCB024360 (Epacadostat)	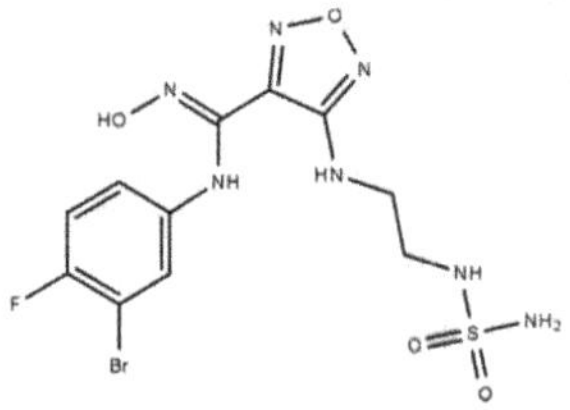	**Yes**: alone and in combination with different biologicals or drugs in several cancer diseases in phase 1 and 2 studies (57 studies)	IDO1 IC_{50} 73 nM HeLa IC_{50} 7.4 nM [20]
NLG919 (GDC-0919, Navoximod)	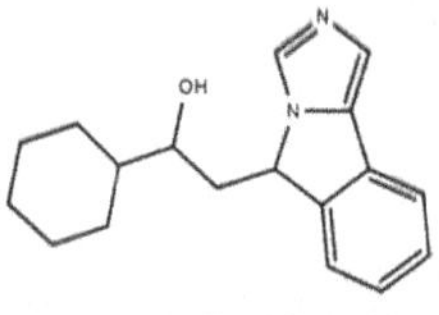	**Yes**: alone and in combination with Atezolizumab in patients with solid tumors in phase 1 studies (2 studies)	K_i 7 nM HeLa IC_{50} 28 nM [23]
Norharmane	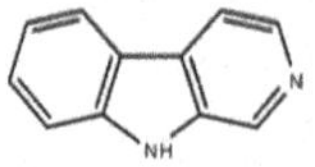	**No**	K_i 176 μM [21]

FIGURE 1 | Overview of TRP-related IDO-inhibitors currently under investigation for cancer therapy in preclinical studies or clinical trials (according to their matches under https://clinicaltrials.gov, date of access: 2019-04-03). For L-TRP, one natural IDO substrate, the Michaelis constant (K_m) is presented (defined as the substrate concentration at 1/2 the maximum velocity). The values K_i or the IC_{50} concentration are presented to compare the relative potency of IDO-Inhibitors. The IC_{50} value quantifies the concentration at which 50% inhibition is observed and describes the functional strength of the inhibitor under specified assay conditions (20). In contrast, K_i denotes the equilibrium constant of the dissociation of the inhibitor-bound enzyme complex reflecting the binding affinity of the inhibitor. It is assumed that lower values of IC_{50} or K_i denote a better inhibition or a tighter binding, respectively. TRP, tryptophan; IDO, indolamine 2,3-dioxygenase; K_i, inhibitory constant.

UDP-glucuronosyltransferases (UGT) (30). It would be advisable to also check the bioactivity of the resulting metabolites.

Epacadostat

Epacadostat is described as highly potent and selective IDO1 inhibitor with moderate oral bioavailability (31). *In vitro* studies reveal that Epacadostat decreases the proliferation of regulatory T-cells concurrent with an increase of activity of cytotoxic T-lymphocytes (32). The *in vivo* IC_{50} after multiple dosing of Epacadostat is ~70 nM (33) suggesting a more potent inhibitory activity on IDO than 1-MT (21). After 100 mg oral Epacadostat application twice daily a maximum plasma concentration of 0.8 μM on day 1 and 0.9 μM on day 8 can be reached (34). It was shown that after oral application Epacadostat is metabolized in the body to IDO inactive plasma metabolites (35). The main metabolic route is glucuronidation via UGT enzymes. Another negligible primary metabolite is produced by reductive metabolism of intestinal microbiota. Further conversion of this metabolite can occur in the liver via cytochrome P450 (CYP) metabolism after absorption of this metabolite in the gut. However, data on the bioactivity of these metabolites are still missing.

In vivo IDO inhibition could be demonstrated in a phase I study in patients with advanced solid malignancies describing an effective normalization of serum KYN levels after oral application of Epacadostat, however, objective responses to the treatment were not observed (36). According to the promising findings that Epacadostat improves the anti-tumor response in combination with other drugs such as Nivolumab or Pembrolizumab (34, 37) the efficacy of Epacadostat in combination with various drug partners was investigated in ECHO 301–310 trials (8). However, the negative results of the phase III trial ECHO 301 in melanoma patients revealed no improvement of progression-free or overall survival by Epacadostat compared to the single treatment with the checkpoint inhibitor Pembrolizumab, which is an antibody against the programmed cell death ligand 1 (PD-L1) (38). These results raise fundamental questions about the benefits of IDO inhibition in cancer treatment. Analysis in endothelial cells of patients with advanced melanoma showed that only 17 out of 43 patients have an increased IDO expression and only 2 of 43 patients were IDO1 and PD-L1 double positive (39) revealing that IDO is not an appropriate target for the majority of melanoma patients. In this context it might be helpful to identify patients with specific immune marker phenotypes in order to develop a personalized / tailored immunotherapy.

BMS-986205

Preclinical data reveal the potent and selective IDO1 inhibitory properties of BMS-986205 (IC$_{50}$ = 1.7 nM in HeLa cells). Preliminary results of a clinical phase 1/2a trail with BMS-986205 alone or in combination with Nivolumab demonstrate that an IC$_{90}$ can be reliably achieved with 200 mg daily oral application with this IDO inhibitor (23). Furthermore, it could be shown that the intratumoral KYN concentrations can be reduced by 90%. Unfortunately, there are no published data regarding the metabolization of the BMS-986205.

POTENTIAL "OFF-TARGET" EFFECTS OF IDO INHIBITORS

Activation of Arylhydrocarbon Receptor

There is evidence that IDO inhibitors including 1-MT (both isomers), Epacadostat, Navoximod, and Norharmane activate the ubiquitously expressed promiscuous ligand-operated arylhydrocarbon receptor (AhR) (18, 40). This is supported by the fact that Epacadostat and Navoximod are extensively metabolized by enzymes (UGT, CYP) controlled by AhR indicating that these drugs activate this signaling pathway. AhR is a ubiquitously expressed promiscuous ligand-operated receptor which mediates pleiotropic effects on the regulation of the immune response (41). As natural ligands of AhR the

tryptophan metabolites, L-KYN (42), 6-formylindolcarbazole (FICZ, a photoproduct of TRP) (43) and KYNA (44), are described. After ligand-binding, AhR dimerizes with the AhR nuclear translocator (ARNT) and acts as a transcription factor, which mediates crucial effects on the pro- and anti-inflammatory regulation of the immune response (41). In this context, there is evidence that the direction of ligand-activated AhR signaling depends on the specific AhR ligand and the microenvironment (homeostatic or inflammatory) (45). In addition to transcriptional regulation, it has been suggested that AhR activation by tryptophan metabolites mediates non-enzymatic functions of IDO1. Thereby, IDO1 act as a signaling protein that contributes to TGF-β-driven tolerance in inflammatory and non-inflammatory context (42, 46). Furthermore, it is assumed that in cancer cells the AhR-mediated transcription of IL6 leads to the autocrine activation of IDO expression via STAT3 (AhR-IL6-STAT3 loop), which is associated with a poor prognosis in lung cancer (47).

The activation of AhR by IDO inhibitors may be detrimental to the assumed treatment concept of downregulating the KP by IDO inhibition. This supports several studies describing pro-carcinogenic effects of AhR ligands in several human cancers including prostate, lung, breast, pancreatic and gastric cancer (45). In transgenic mice, a constitutively active AhR induces stomach tumors (48) demonstrating an oncogenic potential of the AhR. On the other hand, there are also several reports suggesting that AhR ligands have anti-carcinogenic properties. In human colon cancer cell lines the treatment with AhR ligands such as methylcholanthrene or 3,3′diindolylmethane was able to inhibit cell proliferation and stimulate apoptosis (45). Currently, effects of prolonged AhR activation by IDO inhibitors on cancer progression are hard to predict. AhR is expressed by many cell types, including immune cells, which are important in anti-tumor response.

TRP Mimetics in Somatic Cells

An important off-target mode of action of TRP-related IDO inhibitors is that they mimic TRP even in the context as fake nutritional signals. They may target the mammalian target of rapamycin (mTOR) signaling which is the central pathway in amino acid sensing and signaling (49). Activation of mTOR via amino acids leads to initiation of a range of cellular processes including cell growth, proliferation, differentiation, and metabolic alterations. High amounts of TRP analogs may feign an amino acid oversupply. This could potentially be dangerous because cells cannot react adequately to the amount of nutrients actually available. However, it is known that 1-MT can reactivate the mTOR activity inhibited by TRP depletion in cancer microenvironment (50). This has beneficial effects for subsequent chemotherapeutic intervention and may be the most important cause of antitumor effects of this inhibitor (16) (**Figure 2**). Most cytotoxic drugs used in anti-cancer therapy target highly proliferative cells. Therefore, an enhanced mTOR activity, especially in otherwise "cold" tumors, may boost the efficacy of these cytotoxic therapies. Furthermore, T-cells are important players of the host immune system against cancer. These immune cells depend on mTOR signaling to integrate

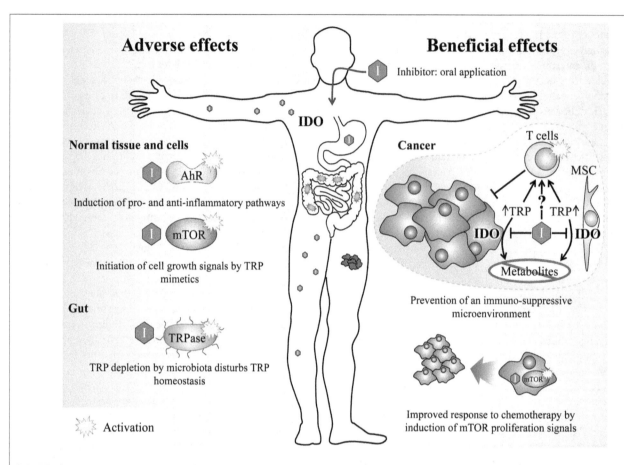

FIGURE 2 | Overview of beneficial and potential adverse effects after treatment with IDO inhibitors. Beneficial effects: IDO inhibitors can break the tumour's immune escape mechanisms (immunosuppressive microenvironment) by inhibiting the TRP depletion either by inhibiting the IDO enzyme in cancer cells as well as in surrounding mesenchymal stroma cells (MSC) and thus reducing the TRP conversion or by acting as TRP mimetics. Both mechanisms can reactivate an adequate T-cell response previously suppressed by the tumor. On the other hand, the inhibition of IDO leads to a reduction of anti-inflammatory TRP metabolites, which also counteracts the formation of an immunosuppressive microenvironment. Furthermore, the activation of mTOR by TRP mimetics induces proliferation signals in the tumor. This may beneficially complement a cytotoxic anti-cancer therapy, which is most effective on proliferating cells. Adverse effects: The unspecific activation of AhR or mTOR by IDO inhibitors may induce inflammatory signaling pathways or growth signals. In the gut, TRP analogs maybe sensed by microbiota as amino acid and induce an enhanced TRP depletion by activation of the TRPase operon. TRP, tryptophan; IDO, indolamine 2,3-dioxygenase; mTOR, mammalian target of rapamycin; AhR, arylhydrocarbon receptor, TRPase, tryptophanase.

danger signals for their proper activation (51). Therefore, the TRP depleted microenvironment typical for a range of tumors impairs T-cell proliferation and function. Reactivation of T-cell function via activation of mTOR may overcome the tumor immune escape and beneficially complement an anti-cancer therapy.

TRP Mimetics in Microbiota

It has been shown *in vitro* that the 1-MT-induced increase in TRP may impede the antimicrobial and immunoregulatory functions of LPS-induced TRP depletion (52), facilitating chronic infections due to impaired pathogen growth arrest (53). During cancer therapy, this might increase the risk of chronic uncontrolled infections due to an insufficient host immune response. A problem of oral TRP mimetic application is furthermore, that subsets of enteric bacteria express TRP degrading enzymes (54). Tryptophanase is one of these bacterial enzymes which are known to be induced by TRP in the gut (55). Most TRP analogs like 1-MT are no substrate of this enzyme (56). However, they are sensed by the bacteria as amino acid and therefore equally effective induce the tryptophanase operon necessary for high enzyme expression (56). This may lead to enhanced TRP depletion in the gut by microbiota. Although, the physiological consequences of the described effects remain unknown, it can be concluded that the systemic application of TRP analogs disturbs the homeostasis of TRP metabolism which might affect cell metabolism, immune response, and growth of potential enteric bacteria. The TRP mimetic properties were extensively investigated only for 1-MT. However, it cannot be excluded that other TRP-related inhibitors may also mimic TRP and interfere with the described metabolic pathways.

CONCLUSION

Several IDO1-inhibitors are currently tested *in vitro* as well as in clinical trials. However, there are controversial results regarding the efficacy of IDO inhibitors for IDO inhibition and cancer treatment. It should be considered that some competitive inhibitors such as 1-MT or Norharmane can hardly induce effective *in vivo* IDO inhibition due to their low *in vitro* potency and the fact that they reach plasma concentrations similar to those of the IDO substrate TRP. Therefore, the immunomodulatory effect of these inhibitors in the body is most likely related to off-target effects such as AhR activation or fake nutritional signaling rather than IDO inhibition. This should be considered when interpreting the significance of IDO in *in vitro* and *in vivo* studies with these inhibitors. In contrast to 1-MT and Norharmane, more potent inhibitors such as Epacadostat or Navoximod inhibit IDO on nanomolar levels resulting in decreased KYN production *in vitro* and *in vivo*. Nevertheless, the failure of a large phase III clinical trial with Epacadostat in melanoma patients indicates that IDO, at least in this type of cancer, is not a suitable target to improve the efficacy of drugs such as Pembrolizumab. In this context, it might be beneficial, for example, to use a molecular diagnostic approach such as biomarker profiles to clarify in advance to what extent IDO inhibition can be beneficial for the respective cancer treatment strategy. Furthermore, the pro- and anti-carcinogenic effects of mTOR and/or AhR activation may be a double-edged sword depending on the type of cancer, the tumor environment and the concurrent anticancer treatment. These side effects, which have so far not been considered sufficiently, should definitely be taken into account in the development of beneficial synergistic drug combinations in cancer therapy. In this context, computational approaches and bioinformatic modeling could become increasingly important in the future.

AUTHOR CONTRIBUTIONS

EW and JG wrote the first draft of the manuscript. JD critically revised the manuscript for important intellectual content. Each author has approved the final version of the manuscript before publication.

FUNDING

This work was supported by the German Research Foundation (DFG, GU 1487/1-1) and by the Rostock University Medical Center (UMR, FORUN 889021). The publication of this article was funded by the Open Access Fund of the University of Rostock.

REFERENCES

1. Wirthgen E, Hoeflich A. Endotoxin-induced tryptophan degradation along the kynurenine pathway: the role of indolamine 2, 3-dioxygenase and aryl hydrocarbon receptor-mediated immunosuppressive effects in endotoxin tolerance and cancer and its implications for immunoparalysis. *J Amino Acids.* (2015) 2015:973548. doi: 10.1155/2015/973548
2. Wirthgen E, Hoeflich A, Rebl A, Günther J. Kynurenic acid: the janus-faced role of an immunomodulatory tryptophan metabolite and its link to pathological conditions. *Front Immunol.* (2018) 8:1957. doi: 10.3389/fimmu.2017.01957
3. Mándi Y, Vécsei L. The kynurenine system and immunoregulation. *J Neural Transm.* (2012) 119:197–209. doi: 10.1007/s00702-011-0681-y
4. Liu X, Newton RC, Friedman SM, Scherle PA. Indoleamine 2, 3-dioxygenase, an emerging target for anti-cancer therapy. *Curr Cancer Drug Targets.* (2009) 9:938–52. doi: 10.2174/156800909790192374
5. Poggi A, Varesano S, Zocchi MR. How to hit mesenchymal stromal cells and make the tumor microenvironment immunostimulant rather than immunosuppressive. *Front Immunol.* (2018) 9:262. doi: 10.3389/fimmu.2018.01342
6. Ling W, Zhang J, Yuan Z, Ren G, Zhang L, Chen X, et al. Mesenchymal stem cells use IDO to regulate immunity in tumor microenvironment. *Cancer Res.* (2014) 74:1576–87. doi: 10.1158/0008-5472.CAN-13-1656
7. Mansour I, Zayed RA, Said F, Latif LA. Indoleamine 2,3-dioxygenase and regulatory T cells in acute myeloid leukemia. *Hematology.* (2016) 21:447–53. doi: 10.1080/10245332.2015.1106814
8. Komiya T, Huang CH. Updates in the clinical development of epacadostat and other indoleamine 2,3-dioxygenase 1 inhibitors (IDO1) for human cancers. *Front Oncol.* (2018) 8:423. doi: 10.3389/fonc.2018.00423
9. Uyttenhove C, Pilotte L, Théate I, Stroobant V, Colau D, Parmentier N, et al. Evidence for a tumoral immune resistance mechanism based on tryptophan degradation by indoleamine 2, 3-dioxygenase. *Nat Med.* (2003) 9:1269–74. doi: 10.1038/nm934
10. Muller AJ, DuHadaway JB, Donover PS, Sutanto-Ward E, Prendergast GC. Inhibition of indoleamine 2, 3-dioxygenase, an immunoregulatory target of the cancer suppression gene Bin1, potentiates cancer chemotherapy. *Nat Med.* (2005) 11:312–9. doi: 10.1038/nm1196
11. Yang H-J, Yen M-C, Lin C-C, Lin C-M, Chen Y-L, Weng T-Y, et al. A combination of the metabolic enzyme inhibitor APO866 and the immune adjuvant L-1-methyl tryptophan induces additive antitumor activity. *Exp Biol Med.* (2010) 235:869–76. doi: 10.1258/ebm.2010.010001
12. Okamoto T, Toné S, Kanouchi H, Miyawaki C, Ono S, Minatogawa Y. Transcriptional regulation of indoleamine 2, 3-dioxygenase (IDO) by tryptophan and its analogue. *Cytotechnology.* (2007) 54:107–13. doi: 10.1007/s10616-007-9081-4
13. Hou DY, Muller AJ, Sharma MD, DuHadaway J, Banerjee T, Johnson M, et al. Inhibition of indoleamine 2,3-dioxygenase in dendritic cells by stereoisomers of 1-methyl-tryptophan correlates with antitumor responses. *Cancer Res.* (2007) 67:792–801. doi: 10.1158/0008-5472.CAN-06-2925
14. Kiank C, Zeden J-P, Drude S, Domanska G, Fusch G, Otten W, et al. Psychological stress-induced, IDO1-dependent tryptophan catabolism: implications on immunosuppression in mice and humans. *PLoS ONE.* (2010) 5:e11825. doi: 10.1371/journal.pone.0011825
15. Qian F, Villella J, Wallace PK, Mhawech-Fauceglia P, Tario JD, Andrews C, et al. Efficacy of levo-1-methyl tryptophan and dextro-1-methyl tryptophan in reversing indoleamine-2, 3-dioxygenase–mediated arrest of T-Cell proliferation in human epithelial ovarian cancer. *Cancer Res.* (2009) 69:5498–504. doi: 10.1158/0008-5472.CAN-08-2106
16. Prendergast GC, Malachowski WP, DuHadaway JB, Muller AJ. Discovery of IDO1 inhibitors: from bench to bedside. *Cancer Res.* (2017) 77:6795–811. doi: 10.1158/0008-5472.CAN-17-2285
17. Wirthgen E, Otten W, Tuchscherer M, Tuchscherer A, Domanska G, Brenmoehl J, et al. Effects of 1-methyltryptophan on immune responses and the kynurenine pathway after lipopolysaccharide challenge in pigs. *Int J Mol Sci.* (2018) 19:3009. doi: 10.3390/ijms19103009
18. Moyer BJ, Rojas IY, Murray IA, Lee S, Hazlett HF, Perdew GH, et al. Indoleamine 2, 3-dioxygenase 1 (IDO1) inhibitors activate the aryl hydrocarbon receptor. *Toxicol Appl Pharmacol.* (2017) 323:74–80. doi: 10.1016/j.taap.2017.03.012

19. Basran J, Rafice SA, Chauhan N, Efimov I, Cheesman MR, Ghamsari L, et al. A kinetic, spectroscopic, and redox study of human tryptophan 2, 3-dioxygenase. *Biochemistry.* (2008) 47:4752–60. doi: 10.1021/bi702393b

20. Cheng Y-C. Relationship between the inhibition constant (Ki) and the concentration of inhibition, which causes 50% inhibition (IC50) of an enzymatic reaction. *Biochem Pharmacol.* (1973) 22:3099–108. doi: 10.1016/0006-2952(73)90196-2

21. Liu X, Shin N, Koblish HK, Yang G, Wang Q, Wang K, et al. Selective inhibition of IDO1 effectively regulates mediators of antitumor immunity. *Blood.* (2010) 115:3520–30. doi: 10.1182/blood-2009-09-246124

22. Kudo Y, Boyd CAR. Human placental indoleamine 2,3-dioxygenase: cellular localization and characterization of an enzyme preventing fetal rejection. *Biochim Biophys Acta.* (2000) 1500:119–24. doi: 10.1016/S0925-4439(99)00096-4

23. Siu LL, Gelmon K, Chu Q, Pachynski R, Alese O, Basciano P, et al. Abstract CT116: BMS-986205, an optimized indoleamine 2,3-dioxygenase 1 (IDO1) inhibitor, is well tolerated with potent pharmacodynamic (PD) activity, alone and in combination with nivolumab (nivo) in advanced cancers in a phase 1/2a trial. *Cancer Res.* (2017) 77(13 Suppl.):CT116-CT. doi: 10.1158/1538-7445.AM2017-CT116

24. Mautino MR, Jaipuri FA, Waldo J, Kumar S, Adams J, Van Allen C, et al. Abstract 491: NLG919, a novel indoleamine-2,3-dioxygenase (IDO)-pathway inhibitor drug candidate for cancer therapy. *Cancer Res.* (2013) 73(8 Suppl.):491. doi: 10.1158/1538-7445.AM2013-491

25. Opitz CA, Litzenburger UM, Opitz U, Sahm F, Ochs K, Lutz C, et al. The indoleamine-2, 3-dioxygenase (IDO) inhibitor 1-methyl-D-tryptophan upregulates IDO1 in human cancer cells. *PLoS ONE.* (2011) 6:e19823. doi: 10.1371/journal.pone.0019823

26. Soliman HH, Jackson E, Neuger T, Dees EC, Harvey RD, Han H, et al. A first in man phase I trial of the oral immunomodulator, indoximod, combined with docetaxel in patients with metastatic solid tumors. *Oncotarget.* (2014) 5:8136–46. doi: 10.18632/oncotarget.2357

27. Wirthgen E, Kanitz E, Tuchscherer M, Tuchscherer A, Domanska G, Weitschies W, et al. Pharmacokinetics of 1-methyl-L-tryptophan after single and repeated subcutaneous application in a porcine model. *Exp Anim.* (2016) 65:147–55. doi: 10.1538/expanim.15-0096

28. Löb S, Konigsrainer A, Schafer R, Rammensee H-G, Opelz G, Terness P. Levo-but not dextro-1-methyl tryptophan abrogates the IDO activity of human dendritic cells. *Blood.* (2008) 111:2152–4. doi: 10.1182/blood-2007-10-116111

29. Jung KH, LoRusso PM, Burris HA, Gordon MS, Bang Y-J, Hellmann MD, et al. Phase I study of the indoleamine 2,3-dioxygenase 1 (IDO1) inhibitor navoximod (GDC-0919) administered with PD-L1 inhibitor (atezolizumab) in advanced solid tumors. *Clin Cancer Res.* (2019) 25:3220–8. doi: 10.1158/1078-0432.CCR-18-2740

30. Ma S, Suchomel J, Yanez E, Yost E, Liang X, Zhu R, et al. Investigation of the absolute bioavailability and human mass balance of navoximod, a novel IDO1 inhibitor. *Br J Clin Pharmacol.* (2019). 85:1751–60. doi: 10.1111/bcp.13961

31. Yue EW, Sparks R, Polam P, Modi D, Douty B, Wayland B, et al. INCB24360 (Epacadostat), a Highly Potent and Selective Indoleamine-2,3-dioxygenase 1 (IDO1) Inhibitor for Immuno-oncology. *ACS Med Chem Lett.* (2017) 8:486–91. doi: 10.1021/acsmedchemlett.6b00391

32. Jochems C, Fantini M, Fernando RI, Kwilas AR, Donahue RN, Lepone LM, et al. The IDO1 selective inhibitor epacadostat enhances dendritic cell immunogenicity and lytic ability of tumor antigen-specific T cells. *Oncotarget.* (2016) 7:37762–72. doi: 10.18632/oncotarget.9326

33. Shi JG, Bowman KJ, Chen X, Maleski J, Leopold L, Yeleswaram S. Population pharmacokinetic and pharmacodynamic modeling of epacadostat in patients with advanced solid malignancies. *J Clin Pharmacol.* (2017) 57:720–9. doi: 10.1002/jcph.855

34. Mitchell TC, Hamid O, Smith DC, Bauer TM, Wasser JS, Olszanski AJ, et al. Epacadostat plus pembrolizumab in patients with advanced solid tumors: phase I results from a multicenter, open-label phase I/II trial (ECHO-202/KEYNOTE-037). *J Clin Oncol.* (2018) 36:3223–30. doi: 10.1200/JCO.2018.78.9602

35. Boer J, Young-Sciame R, Lee F, Bowman KJ, Yang X, Shi JG, et al. Roles of UGT, P450, and gut microbiota in the metabolism of epacadostat in humans. *Drug Metab Dispos.* (2016) 44:1668–74. doi: 10.1124/dmd.116.070680

36. Beatty GL, O'Dwyer PJ, Clark J, Shi JG, Bowman KJ, Scherle PA, et al. First-in-human phase I study of the oral inhibitor of indoleamine 2,3-dioxygenase-1 epacadostat (INCB024360) in patients with advanced solid malignancies. *Clin Cancer Res.* (2017) 23:3269–76. doi: 10.1158/1078-0432.CCR-16-2272

37. Perez RP, Riese MJ, Lewis KD, Saleh MN, Daud A, Berlin J, et al. Epacadostat plus nivolumab in patients with advanced solid tumors: preliminary phase I/II results of ECHO-204. *J Clin Oncol.* (2017) 35(15_Suppl.):3003. doi: 10.1200/JCO.2017.35.15_suppl.3003

38. Long GV, Dummer R, Hamid O, Gajewski TF, Caglevic C, Dalle S, et al. Epacadostat plus pembrolizumab versus placebo plus pembrolizumab in patients with unresectable or metastatic melanoma (ECHO-301/KEYNOTE-252): a phase 3, randomised, double-blind study. *Lancet Oncol.* (2019). doi: 10.1016/S1470-2045(19)30274-8. [Epub ahead of print]

39. Krähenbühl L, Goldinger SM, Mangana J, Kerl K, Chevolet I, Brochez L, et al. A longitudinal analysis of IDO and PDL1 expression during immune- or targeted therapy in advanced melanoma. *Neoplasia.* (2018) 20:218–25. doi: 10.1016/j.neo.2017.12.002

40. Lewis HC, Chinnadurai R, Bosinger SE, Galipeau J. The IDO inhibitor 1-methyl tryptophan activates the aryl hydrocarbon receptor response in mesenchymal stromal cells. *Oncotarget.* (2017) 8:91914. doi: 10.18632/oncotarget.20166

41. Nguyen NT, Nakahama T, Le DH, Van Son L, Chu HH, Kishimoto T. Aryl hydrocarbon receptor and kynurenine: recent advances in autoimmune disease research. *Front Immunol.* (2014) 5:551. doi: 10.3389/fimmu.2014.00551

42. Bessede A, Gargaro M, Pallotta MT, Matino D, Servillo G, Brunacci C, et al. Aryl hydrocarbon receptor control of a disease tolerance defence pathway. *Nature.* (2014) 511:184–90. doi: 10.1038/nature13323

43. Bunaciu RP, Yen A. 6-Formylindolo (3, 2-b) carbazole (FICZ) enhances retinoic acid (RA)-induced differentiation of HL-60 myeloblastic leukemia cells. *Mol Cancer.* (2013) 12:39. doi: 10.1186/1476-4598-12-39

44. DiNatale BC, Murray IA, Schroeder JC, Flaveny CA, Lahoti TS, Laurenzana EM, et al. Kynurenic acid is a potent endogenous aryl hydrocarbon receptor ligand that synergistically induces interleukin-6 in the presence of inflammatory signaling. *Toxicol Sci.* (2010) 115:89–97. doi: 10.1093/toxsci/kfq024

45. Lamas B, Natividad JM, Sokol H. Aryl hydrocarbon receptor and intestinal immunity. *Mucosal Immunol.* (2018) 11:1024–38. doi: 10.1038/s41385-018-0019-2

46. Pallotta MT, Orabona C, Volpi C, Vacca C, Belladonna ML, Bianchi R, et al. Indoleamine 2, 3-dioxygenase is a signaling protein in long-term tolerance by dendritic cells. *Nat Immunol.* (2011) 12:870–8. doi: 10.1038/ni.2077

47. Litzenburger UM, Opitz CA, Sahm F, Rauschenbach KJ, Trump S, Winter M, et al. Constitutive IDO expression in human cancer is sustained by an autocrine signaling loop involving IL-6, STAT3 and the AHR. *Oncotarget.* (2014) 5:1038–51. doi: 10.18632/oncotarget.1637

48. Anderson G, Maes M. Interactions of tryptophan and its catabolites with melatonin and the alpha 7 nicotinic receptor in central nervous system and psychiatric disorders: role of the aryl hydrocarbon receptor and direct mitochondria regulation. *Int J Tryptophan Res.* (2017) 10:1178646917691738. doi: 10.1177/1178646917691738

49. Yoon MS, Choi CS. The role of amino acid-induced mammalian target of rapamycin complex 1(mTORC1) signaling in insulin resistance. *Exp mol Med.* (2016) 48:e201. doi: 10.1038/emm.2015.93

50. Metz R, Rust S, Duhadaway JB, Mautino MR, Munn DH, Vahanian NN, et al. IDO inhibits a tryptophan sufficiency signal that stimulates mTOR: a novel IDO effector pathway targeted by D-1-methyl-tryptophan. *Oncoimmunology.* (2012) 1:1460–8. doi: 10.4161/onci.21716

51. Chi H. Regulation and function of mTOR signalling in T cell fate decisions. *Nat Rev Immunol.* (2012) 12:325–38. doi: 10.1038/nri3198

52. Schmidt SK, Siepmann S, Kuhlmann K, Meyer HE, Metzger S, Pudelko S, et al. Influence of tryptophan contained in 1-Methyl-Tryptophan on antimicrobial and immunoregulatory functions of indoleamine 2,3-dioxygenase. *PLoS ONE.* (2012) 7:e44797. doi: 10.1371/journal.pone.0044797

53. Greco FA, Coletti A, Camaioni E, Carotti A, Marinozzi M, Gioiello A, et al. The Janus-faced nature of IDO1 in infectious diseases: challenges and therapeutic opportunities. *Future med Chem.* (2016) 8:39–54. doi: 10.4155/fmc.15.165

54. Gao J, Xu K, Liu H, Liu G, Bai M, Peng C, et al. Impact of the gut microbiota on intestinal immunity mediated by tryptophan metabolism. *Front Cell Infect Microbiol.* (2018) 8:13. doi: 10.3389/fcimb.2018.00013

55. Wikoff WR, Anfora AT, Liu J, Schultz PG, Lesley SA, Peters EC, et al. Metabolomics analysis reveals large effects of gut microflora on mammalian blood metabolites. *Proc Natl Acad Sci USA.* (2009) 106:3698–703. doi: 10.1073/pnas.0812874106

56. Yanofsky C, Horn V, Gollnick P. Physiological studies of tryptophan transport and tryptophanase operon induction in *Escherichia coli.* *J Bacteriol.* (1991) 173:6009–17. doi: 10.1128/jb.173.19.6009-6017. 1991

13

IDO and Kynurenine Metabolites in Peripheral and CNS Disorders

Yi-Shu Huang, Joy Ogbechi, Felix I. Clanchy, Richard O. Williams and Trevor W. Stone*

The Kennedy Institute of Rheumatology, NDORMS, University of Oxford, Oxford, United Kingdom

*Correspondence:
Trevor W. Stone
trevor.stone@kennedy.ox.ac.uk

The importance of the kynurenine pathway in normal immune system function has led to an appreciation of its possible contribution to autoimmune disorders such as rheumatoid arthritis. Indoleamine-2,3-dioxygenase (IDO) activity exerts a protective function, limiting the severity of experimental arthritis, whereas deletion or inhibition exacerbates the symptoms. Other chronic disorder with an inflammatory component, such as atherosclerosis, are also suppressed by IDO activity. It is suggested that this overall anti-inflammatory activity is mediated by a change in the relative production or activity of Th17 and regulatory T cell populations. Kynurenines may play an anti-inflammatory role also in CNS disorders such as Huntington's disease, Alzheimer's disease and multiple sclerosis, in which signs of inflammation and neurodegeneration are involved. The possibility is discussed that in Huntington's disease kynurenines interact with other anti-inflammatory molecules such as Human Lymphocyte Antigen-G which may be relevant in other disorders. Kynurenine involvement may account for the protection afforded to animals with cerebral malaria and trypanosomiasis when they are treated with an inhibitor of kynurenine-3-monoxygenase (KMO). There is some evidence that changes in IL-10 may contribute to this protection and the relationship between kynurenines and IL-10 in arthritis and other inflammatory conditions should be explored. In addition, metabolites of kynurenine downstream of KMO, such as anthranilic acid and 3-hydroxy-anthranilic acid can influence inflammation, and the ratio of these compounds is a valuable biomarker of inflammatory status although the underlying molecular mechanisms of the changes require clarification. Hence it is essential that more effort be expended to identify their sites of action as potential targets for drug development. Finally, we discuss increasing awareness of the epigenetic regulation of IDO, for example by DNA methylation, a phenomenon which may explain differences between individuals in their susceptibility to arthritis and other inflammatory disorders.

Keywords: kynurenine, arthritis, lymphocyte antigens, 3-hydroxyanthranilic acid, Huntington's disease, T-cells

INTRODUCTION

Widespread interest in the kynurenine pathway (**Figure 1**) and its roles in the nervous and immune systems developed in parallel from the discoveries of indoleamine-2,3-dioxygenase (IDO) activation by interferon-γ (1) and the subsequent discovery of a major functional role in placental immunity (2, 3) and the observation that catabolites of the IDO product, kynurenine, had modulatory effects on neuronal function (4–6) (**Figure 2**). It is now recognized that similar mechanisms may be involved at the molecular level of neuronal and non-neuronal processes and that activity along the kynurenine pathway is fundamental to the development of some central and peripheral disorders. Examples of these will be presented in this review, with the initial emphasis on disorders of primarily peripheral origin, including arthritis and atherosclerosis. A later section will emphasize the important links between peripheral and central inflammation by noting the roles of kynurenines and immune function in Alzheimer's disease, multiple sclerosis and Huntington's disease, where a relationship has been described between IDO and Human Lymphocyte Antigen-G. Those interactions may contribute to the roles of immune system activity in physiology and disease pathogenesis, with potentially common targets of therapeutic intervention for central and peripheral disorders.

KYNURENINES AND PERIPHERAL INFLAMMATORY DISORDERS

Rheumatoid Arthritis

The interface between tissue and immune system cells is seen clearly in peripheral inflammatory disorders such as rheumatoid arthritis (RA). In this condition, local tissue trauma and degeneration are accompanied by leukocyte infiltration and pannus formation which diminishes the volume of the joint space. This cellular infiltration and cytokine production eventually results in tissue damage and a positive feedback cycle in which the joint damage exacerbates the inflammatory response which in turn produces further bone and joint erosion.

Much work on the kynurenine metabolites in this condition has centered on the first enzymes of the pathway (IDO and tryptophan-2,3-dioxygenase, TDO), the isoforms of which have been discussed in depth (7). Where the identity of an isoform is known, it will be indicated in this review. The indeterminate form "IDO" implies that no distinction was made in the original literature. In general TDO, found mainly in the liver, exhibits greater selectivity for tryptophan whereas IDO, which occurs or can be induced in several tissues, acts on a wider range of indole-based substrates. As the enzyme most highly activated by interferon-γ (IFN-γ), IDO has often been the primary target used to explore disease mechanisms. In the case of RA, we have demonstrated that the inhibition of IDO (by 1-methyl-DL-tryptophan) or deletion of IDO1 increased the severity of arthritic symptoms in the collagen-induced model of arthritis (CIA) (8). The symptoms were, however, reduced significantly by the administration of kynurenine indicating that it was probably the loss of kynurenine or its downstream catabolites which were responsible for enhancing the arthritic symptoms and histopathology. Importantly, the effects of IDO inhibition included an increase in the numbers of IFN-γ- and interleukin-17- (IL-17)- producing T lymphocytes, particularly in the joints (8), suggesting a normally restraining influence of IDO. This is entirely consistent with the concept that RA is characterized by pathogenic T cells, including Th1 and Th17 cells.

In order to assess whether these observations might be relevant to RA in human patients, we considered mechanisms by which IDO or its activation processes might be affected in human subjects. One important mechanism for the regulation of IDO1 results from interaction between the B7 complex on dendritic cells (DCs) with Cytotoxic T-lymphocyte Antigen-4 (CTLA-4) expressed in the membranes of regulatory T cells. This ligation induces and activates IDO1 in the DCs and is maintained by Transforming Growth Factor-β (TGF-β) and inflammatory mediators via non-canonical actions of Nuclear Factor-κB (NFκB). This route is one of the major processes by which immune tolerance is maintained in a stable, long-term manner (9) and is an important link between arthritic damage and the kynurenine pathway. Subsequently we were able to demonstrate that in patients with RA there was a defect of IDO1 induction in the immune system involving the B7 / CTLA-4 interaction. The mechanism of this defect proved to be aberrant DNA methylation at the CTLA-4 promoter, leading to a loss of Treg cells and increased symptoms in the patients (10). The genetically impaired IDO1 activation thus reproduced the effect of arthritis exacerbation in IDO1-/- mice. The full cycle of events which explains the development, progression and remission of RA remains to be defined, but it is clear that IDO in DCs plays a significant role in that cycle. Since the simple procedure of administering kynurenine can reduce the degree of tissue damage and disability (8), this might represent a potential avenue for novel treatments.

It is perhaps unfortunate that IDO is such a clear and easily reproducible feature of inflammation since many studies have focussed almost exclusively on this enzyme and have interpreted the findings in terms of the full kynurenine pathway. The ratio of kynurenine to tryptophan concentrations in the blood or tissues has become a widely accepted marker of immune system activation, without a full appreciation of changes in the levels and relative amounts of metabolites downstream of kynurenine-3-mono-oxygenase (KMO). It is now clear that the effects of IDO activation are mediated not only via the reduced availability of tryptophan, but also by those downstream metabolites. These compounds have direct effects on the immune system that regulate the initiation, progression and termination of immune responses to infection or tissue damage.

Examples of these effects include the ability of kynurenine or kynurenic acid to activate the Aryl Hydrocarbon Receptor (AHR) which in turn induces an increased expression of IDO and TDO, providing a positive feedback circuit (11–14). The progressively increasing levels of kynurenine have two critical actions: induction of the transcription factor Forkhead Box-P3 (FoxP3) (15–17) and suppression of the transcription factor Retinoic Acid Receptor-related Orphan Receptor-γt (RORγt) (18, 19). FoxP3 promotes the differentiation of CD4+ T cells to CD4+CD25+FoxP3+ regulatory T helper cells (Tregs) which are able to inhibit other CD4+ cells and the cytotoxic effector T cells such as CD8+ T cells and Natural Killer (NK) cells. The inhibition of RORγt expression prevents the differentiation of CD4+ T cells into generally pro-inflammatory Th17 cells. Since the work described above had indicated a role for Th17 and Treg cells in CIA, involvement of the AHR and its feed-forward generation of IDO/TDO might be relevant.

Activation of AHRs by their classic agonist hydrocarbon molecules such as benzo[a]pyrene and 2, 3, 7, 8-tetrachlorodibenzo-p-dioxin (TCDD) could potentially account

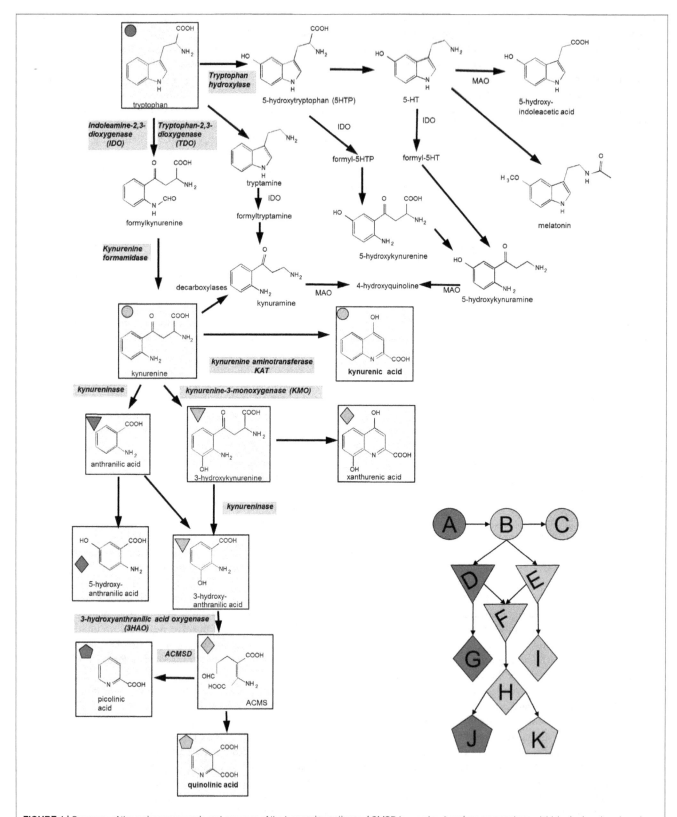

FIGURE 1 | Summary of the major compounds and enzymes of the kynurenine pathway. ACMSD is α-amino-β-carboxymuconate semialdehyde decarboxylase. In cells lacking this enzyme the molecule in parentheses (ACMS) rearranges spontaneously (non-enzymatically) to quinolinic acid. When present, ACMSD converts ACMS to picolinic acid. Key metabolites include (A) Tryptophan, (B) Kynurenine, (C) Kynurenic acid, (D) Anthranilic acid, (E) 3-hydroxy-kynurenine, (F) 3-hydroxy-anthranilic acid, (G) 5-hydroxy-anthranilic acid, (H) ACMS, (I) xanthurenic acid, (J) picolinic acid, and (K) quinolinic acid.

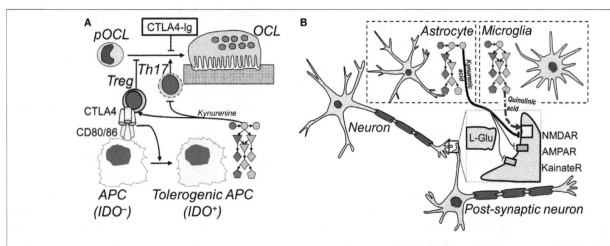

FIGURE 2 | Cell-specific IDO pathways in inflammation. **(A)** In the immune system, APCs upregulate expression of the complete IDO pathway when activated. Tolerogenic APCs promote the differentiation of Tregs and inhibit Th17 differentiation. Tregs inhibit APC activation via CTLA-4, which also inhibits differentiation of pre-osteoclasts (pOCL) to osteoclasts (OCL); soluble CTLA4-Ig (ipilimumab) also inhibits OCL differentiation. Conversely, Th17 promote osteoclastogenesis. **(B)** In the CNS, microglia express low levels of kynurenine aminotransferase, pushing the IDO pathway to the production of excitatory and potentially neurotoxic quinolinic acid (dashed arrow). Astrocytes express low levels of KMO which leads to the accumulation of the NMDA receptor blocker and neuroprotective kynurenic acid (full arrows). See **Figure 1** for legend to IDO pathway metabolites.

for the exacerbation of RA in cigarette smokers (20–22). Indeed, activation of AHRs by the constituents of cigarette smoke can potentiate the induction of NFkB by Tumor Necrosis Factor-α (TNF-α), leading not only to increased inflammatory activity but also reducing the efficacy of anti-TNF-α medications and possibly explaining both the apparent resistance of some patients to these drugs but also the high rate of non-compliance or discontinuation (23). The mechanism of AHR in these cases is likely to involve changes in the number and activity of Th17 cells (21) consistent with the evidence noted above. The exacerbation of symptoms in models of arthritis such as CIA and antigen-induced arthritis (AIA) is prevented by deletion of either AHRs or of IL-17 receptors (21) supporting the view that AHR activation can drive Th17 differentiation.

Helping to understand the mechanisms underlying RA, osteoarthritis (OA) and osteoporosis (OP) is the finding that the effects of AHR activation are potentiated by Human Leucocyte Antigen-DRB1, a significant risk factor for the development of arthritis (24). The synergism is sufficient to increase osteoclast generation and thus bone damage but, even more relevant systemically, the combination increases Th17 cell differentiation with high IL-17 levels noted in arthritic joints and draining lymph nodes.

Conversely the activation of AHRs by compounds with known anti-arthritic potential, such as sinomenine and norisoboldine, promote the differentiation of Treg cells (25, 26). Since the AHR is known to respond differentially to various compounds and to produce effects that depend qualitatively on the agonist, it will be of interest to determine whether these effects reflect a known or novel target site on the AHR complex which might be amenable to new drug development. An unrelated compound, tetrandrine, combines both these actions and normalizes the Th17: Treg ratio by a mechanism which involved the AHR (27). However, it is

unclear whether the compound acts on two distinct target sites on the AHR, or whether the result of acting at a single site drives two different responses in Th17/Treg precursor cells. It is possible, for example, that tetrandrine has different sites of action in the two populations or that it induces different responses when acting on AHRs in cells destined to become Th17 and Treg precursors. These uncertainties would be important matters to clarify as they could lead to more selective molecules with a single mechanism of action which might be devoid of unwanted effects on other cell populations.

In addition to these promoters of AHR activity, several routes are now known by which AHR activity can be down-regulated. The microRNA molecule miR-223 for example suppresses AHR activity by interfering with the AHR Nuclear Translocator (ARNT) (28). Of particular interest was the observation that this interaction occurred in macrophages, but was less prominent in patients with RA than those with osteoarthritis, supporting proposals that these cells play an important role in the etiology of RA. However, these results are difficult to reconcile with the report that AHR deletion from thymocytes reduced arthritic parameters in mice with CIA, whereas deletion selectively from macrophages had no effect (13).

Since AHR expression is seen in most cell types, it is important to consider that immune system cells may be the dominant population involved in the regulation of arthritic inflammation. Nevertheless, it has been reported that the fibroblast-like synovial cells, which exhibit a high rate of proliferation and migration within the joints of patients with RA, also express AHRs. Activation of the receptors comprehensively inhibits the synovial cells, reducing proliferation, migration and invasion of surrounding tissue (29). A role for IDO in these phenomena has not been studied in depth but would be predicted as a significant feature of AHR activation elsewhere.

Although there is continuing controversy about the relative importance of tryptophan depletion and kynurenine metabolite activity in immune system regulation (30, 31), it is likely that both mechanisms are relevant to some extent. While kynurenine and its metabolites are the primary biologically active compounds in the kynurenine pathway, the changes of their concentrations in blood or CSF are often small, as is the reduction in tryptophan concentration resulting from its oxidation (to kynurenine) by IDO or TDO. Much of the behavioral work in experimental animals, or clinical work in humans, includes the measurement of the kynurenine: tryptophan (K/T) ratio, which provides a larger and statistically more useful parameter. The effects of tryptophan depletion are likely to be mediated by activation of the Generalized Controller Non-derepressible-2 Kinase (GCN2) (16, 32, 33), a sensor of cellular amino acid levels. A reduction in the concentration of tryptophan, for example, results in increased numbers of free tryptophanyl-tRNA molecules which induce GCN2 activation. Cells expressing IDO, such as plasmacytoid DCs, therefore, can induce T cell anergy by reduced proliferation and induced apoptosis (32, 34). Although GCN2 is usually considered to be necessary for linking tryptophan deficiency to the inhibition of cell cycling, it is possible that this relationship operates differently in CD4+ and CD8+ T cells (35). The effect of tryptophan depletion is potentiated by tryptophan catabolites in the kynurenine pathway (16).

Osteoporosis

Osteoporosis is another musculo-skeletal disorder in which inflammation is thought to play a significant role although the involvement of kynurenines remains poorly understood. When quantifying the levels of kynurenines in patients newly diagnosed with osteoporosis (and therefore receiving no relevant medication at the time), it was found that the serum content of 3-hydroxy-anthranilic acid (3HAA) was substantially *lower* (around 10-fold) than that in a parallel cohort of normal control subjects. Moreover, there was a comparably *increased* concentration of anthranilic acid (AA), generating an overall difference in concentration between these compounds of approximately 100:1. After treatment with the standard drugs - bisphosphonates or Selective Estrogen Receptor Modulators (SERMs) for 2 years, these values had returned to the levels determined in control subjects, accompanied by a significant improvement in measurements of bone density (36).

Both the mechanism and the pathological significance of this remain unclear. There have been suggestions of enzymic conversion of AA to 3HAA (37) which, potentially, might be inhibited during the course of inflammation resulting in a higher AA: 3HAA ratio. It is not known, however, whether these changes in the kynurenine pathway are primary or secondary contributory factors in the development of osteoporosis. 3HAA exerts inhibitory control of Th1 cells, changing the important ratio between inflammatory, IFN-γ-secreting Th1 cells and anti-inflammatory IL-10 secreting Th2 cells with a resulting anti-inflammatory polarization of immune system function (38). A loss of 3HAA should therefore result in a pro-inflammatory environment and could account for the emergence of a disorder

such as osteoporosis in which the immune system is likely to be involved (39–41).

But what could generate the loss of 3HAA? Could it simply be a defective enzyme converting anthranilate to AA to 3HAA? Or might there be a reduced oxidation by KMO of kynurenine to 3-hydroxy-kynurenine (3HK), with kynureninase catabolising the excess kynurenine to AA? Why then is there no comparable increase in the conversion of kynurenine to kynurenic acid via kynurenine aminotransferase (KAT)? Do therapeutic agents affect the kynurenine pathway directly, in which case those effects might drive the AA:3HAA ratio and determine the initiation and time course of inflammation, or are all the kynurenine pathway changes a result of altered levels of a crucial factor such as a regulatory cytokine, chemokine or growth factor? Certainly 3HAA is less stable than AA in aqueous media, as discussed previously (42), largely because it is a reactive compound which auto-oxidizes to a form which dimerises spontaneously to cinnabarinic acid (43, 44). However, this molecular difference does not readily account for the differences in concentrations observed between two populations of patients, since the chemical and redox environment should not differ greatly between the groups.

The importance of these questions lies not simply in an understanding of osteoporosis, but also in accounting for similar changes in a wide range of disorders in which an underlying inflammation appears to be involved. Thus, similar, though not as dramatic, changes in AA: 3HAA ratio have been reported in a range of disorders [see (30, 31, 42)] where they can change progressively with the development of disease symptoms (45).

In attempting to explain some of these phenomena, several groups have turned to vitamins and the possible relevance of a deficiency in their availability. One plausible view is that disturbances to the kynurenine pathway may result from a deficiency of pyridoxal phosphate, one form of vitamin B6 which is a crucial co-factor for several kynurenine pathway enzymes such as kynureninase and kynurenine aminotransferase. Although not previously considered, riboflavin (vitamin B2) is also required, along with pyridoxal phosphate, for the activation of KMO (46, 47). Infections and inflammation are associated with increased turnover of this cofactor (48), lowering cytosolic concentrations, a relationship consistent with the ability of riboflavin to inhibit the production of inflammatory cytokines (49), to potentiate the effects of anti-inflammatory drugs (49, 50) and to enhance host resistance (51, 52). Conversely, reduced riboflavin availability is associated with greater inflammatory activity in arthritis (53). Thus, the lowering of riboflavin content associated with the onset of inflammation, in turn producing suppressed KMO activity and the preferential metabolism of kynurenine to AA, could account for the high AA: 3HAA ratio observed in osteoporosis (36). As noted above, a similar elevation in this ratio has been reported in patients with arthritis (54) and other chronic disorders involving tissue inflammation (42).

As in RA, the AHRs seem to play a significant role in the regulation of bone turnover and fragility. Activation of AHRs enhances osteoblast production with corresponding increases in bone formation and strength (55). Similarly, Michalowska et al. (56) reported that kynurenine promotes osteoblast formation, possibly resulting from its inhibition of myeloid mesenchymal stem cell proliferation and the consequent loss of osteoblast precursors. On the other hand, there is evidence that the renal deficiency which results from kidney damage or loss increases the expression of AHRs in osteocytes and elevates plasma levels of a range of metabolites including kynurenine and 3-hydroxykynurenine (3HK) (57). These changes are associated with increased numbers of osteoclasts, with kynurenine levels inversely related to several parameters of bone formation. Overall it was suggested that the AHR-mediated production of kynurenines mediated the osteoclast generation. In addition, while AHR generation of kynurenines promotes bone formation, the activation by AHR of the Cytochrome P450 enzymes promotes osteoclast activity so reducing osteogenesis, whereas AHR deletion was reported to increase bone development and density (58). It is clearly important not only to establish the reasons for the differing conclusions on kynurenine activity but also whether the various effects of AHR activation are mediated by kynurenine metabolites, cytochrome enzymes or other routes, and how those different routes interact with each other and with overall tissue function.

Also introducing an element of confusion is evidence that the presence of inflammation may alter the actions of AHRs. Thus, increased expression of AHRs was demonstrated in mesenchymal stem cells from mice with CIA (59) and this was associated with reduced production of osteoblasts. Treating the animals with AHR agonists further reduced bone formation, potentially representing a contributory mechanism in osteoporosis (55). Clearly it is essential to know whether the behavior of cells and receptors differs significantly between a normal physiological state and that of the pathological, diseased state since it would impact on the approach needed for therapeutic developments.

These various factors may also be complicated by dietary considerations. Increasing attention is being devoted to dietary regulation of metabolism, with directly acting AHR agonists such as 3,3'-diindolylmethane being of special interest. This and related compounds occur in several *Brassica* species of vegetables and have been found to inhibit osteoclast numbers and activity, resulting in enhanced bone formation (60). Again, it will be valuable to establish whether the kynurenine pathway is involved in this, and how it interacts with, and possibly modifies, the other consequences of AHR activation.

The importance of kynurenines on bone formation is dependent not only on AHR expression but also on activity in the CTLA-4 and B7-mediated interactions between T cells and DCs. CTLA-4 inhibits T cell activation by blocking the interaction between the T cell receptor co-activator CD28 and the B7 (CD80/CD86) complex. This results in increased generation of Wnt-10b which promotes bone formation (61).

The activation of IDO in DCs is also regulated by the B7 complex, with activation by CTLA-4 expressed on Tregs producing a tolerogenic profile in the DCs. The loss of bone tissue which follows the menopause or ovariectomy has been associated with increased activity in DCs, but preventing CTLA-4 activity preserves bone tissue (62), suggesting a potential use of the stable, synthetic construct CTLA-4Ig in reducing osteoporosis. As with several other instances of IDO and kynurenine involvement in

pathology, it remains uncertain whether the modulation of DC activity is via local changes in tryptophan concentration or the generation of pro-apoptotic compounds such as 3HK and 3HAA.

In addition, CTLA-4 acts directly on the CD80/86 proteins on monocytes to inhibit their differentiation to osteoclasts, resulting in reduced bone destruction (63–66). Clearly, with such a range of sites of action for CTLA-4 and CTLA-4Ig, some of which influence bone formation and destruction, it is uncertain how important the regulation of kynurenine and its catabolites is to the overall control of bone formation in health or disease. In particular, it is not known whether changes in the concentration of any components of the kynurenine pathway are able to modulate any of the interactions between CD28, CD80, CD86, and CTLA-4. In view of the growing use of CTLA-4Ig in RA, and of the CTLA-4 blocking antibody ipilimumab in melanomas, however, these questions might be worthy of investigation. It is tempting to speculate on the range of studies that, while not specifically examining the actions of kynurenine and its metabolites, nonetheless have generated results which might contribute to understanding the full extent of tryptophan metabolite involvement. Thus, while the anabolic steroid dehydroepiandrosterone increased osteoblastogenesis and bone formation, it also increased the numbers of FoxP3+ Treg cells, an effect that might be generated via kynurenine pathway activation (67).

Finally it is interesting to note that bone formation may be affected indirectly by changes in vitamin D metabolism. Benzo[a]pyrene, for example promotes the catabolism of the vitamin and would thus hinder calcium absorption and bone formation (68). This would certainly be an important consideration for individuals concerned about osteoporosis following many years of cigarette use. It would be of great interest to determine whether these effects are the result of benzo[a]pyrene activation of AHRs and the subsequent activation of IDO or TDO.

Atherosclerosis

The overall anti-inflammatory effect of kynurenine in arthritis is reflected in similar properties in several other peripheral disorders. Atherosclerosis is characterized by vascular endothelial deposits known as plaques in which accumulated leukocytes are tightly enmeshed with a calcified complex of fatty materials, blood cells and platelets. These plaques reduce the effective diameter of the vascular lumen, restricting blood flow and affecting blood pressure and tissue viability as a result (69). Atherosclerosis is a major risk factor for disability and mortality and a full understanding of the underlying causative factors remains uncertain. Although the regulation of cholesterol metabolism by apoenzyme-E (ApoE) is believed to play a prominent role in the disorder, rodents specifically lacking ApoE exhibit little vascular abnormality. When ApoE deficiency is combined with the deletion or inhibition of IDO1, however, there is a marked exacerbation of the pathology, as noted above in arthritis, with the deposition of atherosclerotic plaques comparable to the natural disorder in humans (69, 70). The importance of IDO activation has been demonstrated by reports that the promotion of Treg differentiation by IDO-expression tolerogenic DCs produces a reduction in atherosclerotic plaque deposition (71, 72).

Consistent with the studies on trypanosomiasis described below (section Psychiatric Disorders), in which kynurenine levels were positively correlated with IL-10, down-regulation of IDO1 in the atherosclerosis model resulted in a diminished expression of IL-10 in most lymphoid tissues including peripheral blood, spleen and lymph node B cells (69). However, there is not a simple cause-and-effect relationship between these compounds since IL-10 expression was not induced or elevated by kynurenine administration *in vivo*. On the other hand, kynurenine did increase IL-10 production by B cells *in vitro* (69).

Not only are these results interesting in terms of understanding the importance of IDO activity in maintaining immune tolerance and thus restraining the extent of disease, but they support the possible explanation of some apparently conflicting results noted above. If the kynurenine induction or promotion of IL-10 expression is specifically exerted on B cells, the overall relationship between the two compounds will depend on the relative involvement of T cells, B cells and probably other leukocyte populations, as stated earlier.

CENTRAL NEURO-INFLAMMATION

Understanding the role of kynurenines in the Central Nervous System (CNS) has involved work in two areas of tissue function which are more problematic in this region than elsewhere. The first is the question of pathway localization at the cellular level. Detailed histological studies on the presence and distribution of the various enzymes along the kynurenine pathway revealed a differential localization in cell types. For example, KMO was absent from astrocytes (73, 74), so that these cells are only able to generate the glutamate antagonist and neuroprotective kynurenic acid. In contrast, microglia express all components of the pathway, so that their activation by inflammatory mediators could result in increased levels of quinolinic acid. This is consistent with the phenotypic resemblance of microglial cells to that of resident phagocytes in other organs, as macrophages also convert tryptophan to all components of the kynurenine pathway including quinolinic acid (74–76). The ability to generate quinolinic acid and other damaging kynurenines such as 3HK, explains why the inflammatory activation of microglia could cause local cellular damage or death. As IDO1 was constitutively active in most glial cells (74, 77), it had not been clear why the generation of quinolinic acid would not produce a significant ongoing loss of cells. That could now be understood as the result of kynurenine and kynurenic acid production by astrocytes which—in the absence of KMO and downstream enzymes— could accumulate these compounds to a level at which they could antagonize glutamate and quinolinic acid to prevent neural over-excitation and excitotoxicity (73, 77). Kynurenine crosses cell membranes readily and kynurenic acid, despite its poor membrane permeability, also enters the extracellular space (78, 79). Whether this is simply the result of slow diffusion, a facilitated transfer by pinocytosis or the excretion of kynurenate in exosomes, remains unclear.

There remains significant debate on this hypothesis, as quinolinic acid synthesis by activated microglia may exceed kynurenate production, resulting in local cell damage. In such an inflammatory situation, IDO will also be activated in astrocytes and the increased production of kynurenine—in view of its higher membrane permeability—could well diffuse into the activated microglia much more rapidly than would kynurenic acid. The result could be a potentiation of microglial kynurenine metabolism with even greater levels of quinolinic acid being produced.

Interestingly, the expression of KAT can also vary between cell types in the CNS. Microglia express lower levels of the more active KAT2 relative to KAT1 (73) so that the conversion of kynurenine to quinolinic acid in these cells will be further enhanced relative to cells expressing more of this enzyme. Subtle differences such as these between cell types may be critical in regulating the relative production of different kynurenine metabolites depending on the balance of neural and glial cell activity under any given functional circumstances such as different cytokine profiles.

Huntington's Disease

The term "central neuro-inflammation" encompasses several disorders in which the initiating defect involves neurons or glial cells but which results in abnormal functioning of the nervous system as a whole. One such disorder is Huntington's disease which can now be understood in terms of newly recognized interactions between kynurenines and aspects of immune function and which may contribute to their roles in physiology and disease pathogenesis.

In the CNS many of the pathological effects of kynurenine pathway activity may result from a balance between the concentrations of quinolinic acid, an agonist at glutamate receptors sensitive to N-methyl-D-aspartate (NMDA) (4, 6, 80) and kynurenic acid, an antagonist at glutamate receptors but with greatest efficacy blocking NMDA receptors (5, 81, 82). An excess of the former may result in excessive depolarization, calcium influx and neurotoxicity (83), leading to the speculation that an over-production or suppressed removal of quinolinate might be a factor in neurodegenerative disorders such as Huntington's disease with a possibly similar role in Alzheimer's disease and other central disorders (84, 85).

In addition, over-activation of NMDA receptors is accompanied by increased microglial proliferation and activation together with cytokine production. This indicates that an inflammatory environment has been induced in which the levels of potentially pathogenic cytokines are likely to cause, or contribute to the induction of neuronal damage or death (86, 87). Consistent with this idea, the levels of quinolinic acid in the CNS are increased by at least two orders of magnitude during and following viral infection (88, 89), or following exposure of experimental animals to Toll-Like Receptor agonists such as bacterial lipopolysaccharides (LPS) or viral-RNA-mimetic poly(I:C). These phenomena recall the induction and activation of the kynurenine pathway by IFN-γ (1) and the importance of these phenomena in host responses to infection, the protection of allogeneic embryos or the maintenance of tissue grafts resulting from the depletion of tryptophan and generation of kynurenine catabolites (2, 3, 90–92).

It is now clear that there are also major changes in the immune system associated with some central disorders, of which Huntington's disease represents a good example. Huntington's disease is a genetic, inherited disorder in which the early degeneration of striatal regions produces progressive motor disorders and later cortical involvement leading to cognitive dysfunction. It is one of few conditions in which involvement of the kynurenine pathway has been implicated on the basis of studies on prokaryotes, *in vitro* and *in vivo* mammalian models and human patients (93–95) and for which the kynurenine pathway has been considered as a therapeutic target (96–98). Increasingly, evidence indicates parallel disturbances in the immune system (94, 99–102). Central microglia are activated and peripheral monocytes of patients with Huntington's disease are hyper-sensitive to immunogenic stimuli (103). A variety of changes in cytokine expression have been reported in the disorder (100, 104) and it is claimed that immunosuppressant treatment can produce significant amelioration of Huntington's disease symptoms and progression (105).

Particularly intriguing is the finding that soluble Human Leucocyte Antigen-G (sHLA-G) levels in the serum of patients show a clear trend of correlation with symptom severity, and a statistically significant effect in the most severely affected patients (100). HLA-G has been associated primarily with materno-fetal tolerance (106) but elevated HLA-G expression has been noted in several CNS disorders in which its effects are largely immune-suppressant (107, 108). The full importance of this was not appreciated at the time of the original study, but the molecule is of great interest since it is a secreted protein with the ability to inhibit T cell and cytotoxic cell activity (109).

sHLA-G also promotes the differentiation of Treg cells (110), the effect of which is to enhance the progression and metastasis of tumors. IDO expression is greater in tumors than normal tissue so that these two molecules—IDO and sHLA-G—might act synergistically as tumor promoters. Such synergism might explain the poor performance of selective IDO1 inhibitors in clinical oncogenic trials (111–113). Since IDO1 and sHLA-G are not restricted to the cell membrane or cytoplasm, but can be released into the extracellular medium, their immunosuppressant activity will be exerted around a wider cellular environment than would otherwise be the case with corresponding implications for generalized inflammation and tumor surveillance.

Importantly, it has been proposed that under some circumstances, especially in the presence of high concentrations of IFN-γ, the major immunosuppressive activity of activated DCs may be mediated to a greater extent by the expression and release of sHLA-G than by IDO (114). The inhibition of cytotoxic CD8+ T cells is largely prevented by antibody blockade of sHLA-G rather than by IDO inhibition. The relationship between high levels of IFN-γ and HLA-G is quite specific since antigen induction is around 20-fold greater than other HLA antigens and neither IL-6 nor IL-10 mediate the effects of interferons on HLA-G expression. It has been suggested that the relative potencies of IDO and HLA-G-mediated immunosuppression might contribute to the dual nature of interferon activity, this being a major Th1 cytokine inducing inflammatory mediators in the early phase of immune responses to stimuli, but exerting an auto-limiting suppression of inflammation in the later phases (115). High concentrations of IFN-γ induce HLA-G expression in DCs which are then responsible for cytotoxic T-lymphocyte inhibition. HLA-G also acts on macrophages (116) to promote their differentiation into the M2 phenotype which is characterized by increased CD163 and reduced CD86 expression. Placental and decidual M2 cells are involved in fetal protection against maternal T cell attack *in utero* (117–119) with increased activity of IDO1, a known contributor to fetal protection. Overall, therefore, the parallel changes in Huntington's disease severity and sHLA-G expression and their correlation with the genetic mutation (100) may reflect a significant relevance of immune function in the progression of the disorder.

Questions also remain about these relationships, especially that between immune system function in the peripheral and CNS, given that markers of inflammation have been widely reported in the blood and peripheral organs and tissues of patients with Huntington's disease. A version of the mutated huntingtin protein—which is believed to the primary cause of neurodegeneration in Huntington's disease—also induces disturbances to immune function (99) and there are marked similarities in the altered profile of gene expression in the blood cells and neurons of Huntington's disease patients (104). Do these changes arise simultaneously from an undefined factor, or does one act as a trigger for changes in the other? What would happen in patients treated with an anti-inflammatory agent which was confined to the blood and peripheral tissues? Would such a drug break the degeneration-inflammation cycle sufficiently to reduce the symptoms of Huntington's disease or, possibly, halt its progression? Highly relevant to these considerations are reports that the treatment of patients with Huntington's disease using an immune-modulating drug such as glatiramer acetate showed significant beneficial effects (105), emphasizing the need to understand the neuro-immune interactions at the heart of the disorder.

Alzheimer's Disease and Multiple Sclerosis

In addition to its activation of NMDA receptors, quinolinic can induce the expression of immunologically active molecules in astrocytes including IL-8, Chemokine Ligand-5 (CCL5) and Macrophage Inflammatory Protein-1 (MIP-1) as well as several chemokine receptors such as CXCR4, CXCR6, CCR3, and CCR5 which promote leukocyte attraction across the blood-brain barrier (120, 121). Several of these proteins are increased in the brains of patients with Alzheimer's disease, so the similarity of this activity to the action of β-amyloid fragments has prompted the suggestion that the kynurenine pathway may be involved in the etiology of this disorder, an idea consistent with the demonstration that amyloid-β induces IDO expression (122, 123). It is possible that quinolinic acid could initiate a positive feedback cycle of cell activation, further quinolinic acid generation, mediator induction and further activation, from which it may be difficult for cells to escape. Stimulation of NMDA receptors by quinolinic acid stimulates glial proliferation, further enhancing these events (120, 124).

The increased kynurenine pathway activity in Alzheimer's disease (74, 77, 125, 126) has been linked with β-amyloid production and tau hyperphosphorylation which can be induced by quinolinic acid (74, 77, 122, 124, 127, 128). There is also good evidence that the kynurenines plays a role in the formation of neurofibrillary tangles and senile plaques (126). IDO1 inhibition suppresses plaque development, neuronal death and cognitive dysfunction (60).

Neurons express ACMSD (**Figure 1**) and can therefore divert the conversion of 3HAA from quinolinic acid to picolinic which also regulates inflammatory mediator release (129–131). It also prevents some of the deleterious actions of quinolinic acid including its toxicity on cholinergic and dopaminergic neurons (132–134). It has been suggested that this component of the kynurenine pathway is important in the production of suicidal ideation and behavior (135).

Some of these considerations are especially important in multiple sclerosis (MS) where the underlying problem is inflammatory and the products of kynurenine pathway activation, primarily quinolinic acid, are toxic not only to neurons but also to oligodendrocytes, thus contributing to the loss of central myelination. Kynurenine pathway activity is abnormal in patients with MS, suggesting cell activation (136–139). In patients with MS or in the animal model of this disorder (experimental autoimmune encephalomyelitis, EAE), IDO1 and KMO are increased (85, 137, 140) possibly as a result of the high levels of TNF-α and IFN-γ. IDO inhibition exacerbates EAE severity in mice (141, 142). MS appears to be a disorder in which the beneficial effects of kynurenine pathway activation (induction of T cell tolerance) is in competition with the generation of potentially damaging levels of quinolinic acid (76, 143).

The question of membrane permeability by kynurenine is also important in the relationship between kynurenine pathway activity in the peripheral circulation or tissues and the CNS. The stimulation of immune system cells activates several enzymes in the kynurenine pathway which are relevant to the control of leukocyte populations and the balance between pro- and anti-inflammatory cells and their products. At least two of these—quinolinic acid and kynurenic acid, as noted above—can regulate neuronal excitability and plasticity. It could be life-threatening if the delicate CNS control of bodily functions—somatic and autonomic—were to be influenced significantly by the variety of infective, traumatic, allergic or inflammatory changes that involve the peripheral immune system. The brain is protected from these, however, by the blood-brain barrier, across which kynurenine and 3HK can cross quite readily, but quinolinic acid and kynurenic acid cross very slowly. Indeed, the clinical consequences of intense or chronically elevated levels of peripheral immune system activation appears to be a major factor in several psychiatric disorders such as depression (144) and schizophrenia (145–147) resulting from the altered balance between kynurenic acid and glutamate receptor agonists, including quinolinic acid. Some of these issues have been discussed in detail elsewhere (148). It has been shown that the cerebrovascular cells intimately involved in blood-brain barrier function express elements of the kynurenine pathway. On activation, the vascular endothelial cells and pericytes produce kynurenine which is released from basolateral sites providing a short path to diffuse across into the brain parenchyma. They also synthesize kynurenic acid which, with picolinic acid, are protective by their abilities to block glutamate receptors and to suppress the secretion of inflammatory mediators, respectively. It has been pointed out that these properties of the blood-brain barrier may be critical factors in HIV-Associated Neurocognitive Disorder (HAND) since the kynurenine produced from barrier cells by systemic inflammatory mediators can enter the CNS rapidly in large amounts, being then converted by microglia to quinolinic acid at a rate sufficient to overwhelm kynurenate production or entry. The resulting excitotoxic loss of neurons may than contribute significantly to the emergence of dementia (148).

Quite apart from the neuroimmunological activity of quinolinic acid, it can increase the permeability of the blood-brain barrier (149–152), an effect intriguingly opposed by kynurenic acid (153). Not only would this allow inflammatory mediators easier access to the CNS cells but it would also facilitate passage of leukocytes directly into the brain parenchyma.

Psychiatric Disorders

The kynurenine pathway may be involved in several psychiatric disorders, several of which have been reviewed in detail (144–146, 154–157). Perhaps the strongest evidence is for a role in schizophrenia (145, 146). One issue which has aroused controversy in this area is a claim that the role of kynurenic acid in schizophrenia could involve the block of nicotinic receptors in addition to NMDA receptors. While the levels of kynurenic acid are increased in the CNS and probably contribute to the symptoms of schizophrenia (146) and other CNS disorders involving defective cognition, that claim has not been substantiated and cannot be replicated [see (158)]. Any apparent effect of kynurenic acid on nicotinic receptors appears to be secondary to the effects of nicotinic receptors on the release of glutamate and other neuroactive compounds (158).

There is also very good evidence that activation of the kynurenine pathway is a major factor in the production of depression and related illnesses. Certainly the K/T ratio correlates well with the induction and severity of depressive symptoms following the administration of IDO inducers such as interferon-β or exposure to stress (144, 154–157). The levels of kynurenines are also closely associated with severe depression and the development of suicidal thoughts and behavior (135).

There has been less interest in the role of kynurenines in anxiety disorders, probably because of the difficulties of interpretation in studies of a psychological process which is hard to translate from experimental animals to humans. Nevertheless, there is increasing evidence that the kynurenine pathway is involved in anxiety behaviors, especially related to primary events in the immune system, such as inflammation (159).

Malaria and Trypanosomiasis

Infective, rather than genetic examples of neuroinflammation are the parasitic infestations of cerebral malaria and trypanosomiasis. Approximately 20% of people who contract malaria will proceed to develop cerebral malaria, a condition which causes serious somatic and psychiatric changes in patients and, in most cases, results in death. Infection of C57BL/6J mice with the strain *Plasmodium berghei ANKA* generates an animal model in which the cerebrovascular histology and functional involvement closely reproduce these phenomena in humans (160). When treated with *P. berghei ANKA* almost all the tested mice died within 7 days, but animals treated simultaneously with Ro61-8048 (an inhibitor of KMO) survived up to the end of the study at 21 days (160). KMO inhibition increased the endogenous levels of kynurenine and kynurenic acid as reported in other studies (161–164) and seen in KMO-deficient animals (165, 166). The blockade of neuronal glutamate receptors by kynurenate was probably the main factor accounting for the protective inhibition of neurotoxicity and animal survival. Although this initial study did not take account of changes in the immune system, the results were sufficiently clear that a similar study was performed subsequently in trypanosomiasis. Here, an animal model was used to assess the infiltration of brain parenchyma and vascular or ventricular endothelia by reactive leukocytes (167). The results indicated that KMO inhibition was able to reduce significantly the extent of leukocyte infiltration into the brain as well as the histological assessment of neuronal death.

To follow up these results in human patients, levels of kynurenine and its catabolites were measured in the cerebrospinal fluid of patients suffering from trypanosomiasis and the samples were also examined for levels of IL-6 and IL-10. There was a close and highly significant correlation between levels of kynurenine and IL-6, supporting the view that an inflammatory response had been initiated within the CNS. However, there was also a strongly positive correlation between kynurenine and IL-10, a largely immunosuppressive cytokine secreted primarily by anti-inflammatory leukocytes which suppress DC activation and IDO expression. It is not obvious why there should be an increase in IL-10 production associated with tryptophan metabolism, but several other groups have also reported positive relationships between the kynurenine pathway and IL-10 (168–171). In a cohort of healthy young individuals a clear positive association was seen between IL-10 levels and those of kynurenine, the kynurenine: tryptophan ratio, 3HK and 3HAA levels (172). A reduction of TNF-α and IL-17 expression by mesenchymal stem cells has been associated with increased IL-10 and kynurenine levels (170), although LPS produces parallel increases in TNF-α, IL-10, and IDO activity (173).

In other cases kynurenine and IL-10 behave differently. Subjects responding to BCG vaccinations and patients with inflammatory bowel disease have increased kynurenine and IFN-γ levels but reduced IL-10 as expected of an immune response (174, 175). IDO1 activity has been shown to increase IL-10 production in B cells, whereas *in vitro* kynurenine did not do so, implying that another IDO1 product might be involved. A correlation was reported between pro-inflammatory TNF-α and kynurenine levels, whereas the neuroprotective kynurenic acid was correlated with IL-10 levels (176). Indeed kynurenic acid has been reported to increase IL-10 production (177) so whether kynurenine production is positively or negatively related to IL-10 may depend on the balance of B cell, T cell and monocyte activity

in addition to being dependent on activity in different parts of the kynurenine pathway (**Figures 1, 2**).

Administration of the statin group of drugs reduces IL-6 production but increases IL-10 and kynurenine (178). This expected opposite movement of IL-10 and IL-6 has been observed in IDO1-deficient DCs in which there is the anticipated loss of AHR activity and reduced levels of IL-10, but increased IL-6 and TNF-α production (179); conversely both IL-6 and IL-10 were increased after surgery (180). Kynurenine itself suppresses IL-6 release but kynurenic acid has been reported to increase it. Since both compounds increase IL-10 production, the ratio between kynurenine and kynurenic acid may be a particularly important factor in determining the inflammatory cytokine balance (181).

Nevertheless, despite their opposite immune system bias, IL-6 and IL-10 have been shown to change in parallel in patients with depression, in which inflammatory drive (IFN-γ, TNF-α, CRP) is reduced. In this same condition IDO activation increases kynurenine concentrations, producing a negative correlation with the cytokines (182). Parallel increases in IL-6 and IL-10 were observed in patients with obsessive-compulsive disorder (183) and chronic hepatitis where the correlation between levels of these proteins was particularly high ($P = 0.005$) (184). Those changes were not accompanied by any change in IFN-γ levels, perhaps indicating a critical role of IDO metabolites and the IL-6:IL-10 balance in the regulation of IFN-γ. It may be relevant that expression of the IL-10 receptor is also affected by tryptophan catabolites, since it is increased by IFN-γ stimulation and activation of AHRs by kynurenine regulates activity of the promoter region of the IL-10 receptor α-subunit to increase receptor expression (185).

Increasing evidence indicates that IDO activation and IL-10 production can be induced by the same stimuli, leading to the view that the anti-inflammatory and tolerogenic actions of both proteins may be at least complementary and potentially synergistic (186, 187). Functionally, IDO and IL-10 show important interactions with some degree of mutual redundancy. Thus, amniotic fluid stem cells which are closely related to mesenchymal stem cells and possess the same profile of molecular markers, powerfully suppress the proliferation of peripheral blood mononuclear cells induced by phorbol-12-myristate-13-acetate (PMA). This inhibition is mediated by the combination of IDO and IL-10 production by the amniotic cells, with both being required for maximal suppression of proliferation (188).

The relationship between IDO and IL-10 may be particularly relevant in the presence of microbial invasion since some bacteria can induce DCs to facilitate IL-10 production by subpopulations of T cells such as the FoxP3-negative Tr1-like cells. This is achieved by the microbial induction of appropriate T cell polarizing molecules including IDO1 (189). Consistent with the overall anti-inflammatory balance which this generates, the production of IDO1 and IL-10 is accompanied by a reduction in the secretion of pro-inflammatory TNF-α and IL-12 components. The simultaneous presence of IDO1 and IL-10 can also influence non-infective inflammation such as that associated with tumor development. For many tumors, it is recognized that compounds with characteristics of Damage-Associated Molecular Patterns in the local microenvironment promote tolerogenic dendritic and mesenchymal stem cells which in turn induce the stable co-expression of IDO and IL-10 to further suppress lymphocyte aggression (190). Among the compounds able to initiate this activity are uric acid and the S100A4 protein, both of which have been linked to a variety of inflammatory states in peripheral and central tissues.

ENVIRONMENTAL FACTORS AND THE KYNURENINE PATHWAY: DEVELOPMENT AND EPIGENETICS

It is a common experience that the existence and severity of arthritic symptoms can vary substantially throughout life, at different times of day, with changes in affective status (mood, stress, anxiety etc.) or with changes in dietary habits. It is important to recognize, therefore, that many such factors do impact directly on the kynurenine pathway and could modulate inflammatory symptoms, peripheral, or central. Exposure to stressful conditions activates the hypothalamo-pituitary-adrenal axis leading to the secretion of corticosteroids which are potent inducers of TDO and will therefore increase kynurenine pathway activity. Cruciferous vegetables in particular contain alkaloids such as brassinins which inhibit IDO1 (191) and a variety of indole-derived compounds such as indole-3-carbinol and di-indolyl-methane which are agonists at AHRs (192, 193), thus regulating the IDO/TDO-kynurenine-AHR feedback cycle described above and giving the compounds significant anti-inflammatory properties (194, 195). The influence of such factors may be of paramount importance in determining the occurrence and severity of arthritis and related disorders, since we have demonstrated a role of the kynurenine pathway in tissue development of the embryo, and the methylation state of IDO1 appears to determine the magnitude of induced arthritis.

Embryonic Development

The normal, physiological roles of the kynurenine pathway have received less attention than their potential pathological relevance but recent reports have indicated the probability of important functions in early development of the embryo. The treatment of pregnant rats in late gestation with an inhibitor of KMO (**Figure 1**), results in an accumulation of kynurenine as well as promoting its transamination to kynurenic acid. These changes resulted in significant molecular, structural, immunocytochemical and functional (electrophysiological) changes in neonates produced by the treated dams and changes in all these parameters persisted into adulthood (161–164). Similar results were obtained by the administration of kynurenine itself to pregnant animals (196–199), and in animals lacking KMO by genetic manipulation (165, 166).

These results indicate that the kynurenine pathway is playing a significant role in early development and the initial hypothesis to explain these effects was based on the known importance of glutamate and its receptors in the early formation of the brain. In particular, the NMDA-sensitive subtype of receptors are involved in neurogenesis, progenitor cell migration, axon and dendrite growth and guidance as well as spine and synapse formation.

The activity of these NMDA receptors—and therefore brain development—would be dependent on the ratio of the NMDA receptor agonist quinolinic acid and the antagonist kynurenic acid. The occurrence and long-term maintenance of altered brain structure and function might contribute to the development of neurological and psychiatric disorders in adult life. The most established examples of such "neurodevelopmental" disorders are schizophrenia (145–147, 197, 199, 200) and major depression (154, 155) including suicide vulnerability (135).

If these changes in CNS development are mirrored in the actions of kynurenines on the immune system, they could contribute significantly to immune system responses and to the susceptibility of offspring to a range of immunological problems including autoimmune diseases such as RA. Thus, in the brain development studies there may have been changes in immune function mediated by the altered levels of kynurenines, such as abnormal cytokine or chemokine levels in the pregnant dam or embryonic brain, changes to microglial activation, or modifications to peripheral leukocyte function and their infiltration into the pre- or postnatal brain. Any effects of prenatal interference with the kynurenine pathway on immune function would represent a highly important area of investigation, especially in the light of evidence that some leukocyte populations express NMDA receptors and other targets of kynurenine and its catabolites such as AHRs and the G-protein coupled receptor GPR35 (82).

While there is a growing literature on the effects of prenatal inflammatory stimuli on CNS development and function in the adult offspring (161–164, 201–204), few studies have yet addressed the immunological consequences of such maternal factors. In one such study, however, it is clear that prenatal activation of the maternal immune system using bacterial LPS or the viral mimetic poly(inosinic:cytidylic) acid (poly[I:C], PIC) can affect the concentrations of several cytokines in the offspring in parallel with changes in expression of IDO (205). The most interesting result of this study was that a repeat immunological challenge in adulthood produced less change in the test animals than controls, indicating a long-lasting and possibly permanent depression of immune system function which could have significant implications for the development of autoimmune disease. However, a previous study reached the opposite conclusion, that prenatal immune activation induced increased adaptive immune responses in the offspring (206) raising the possibility that subtle differences in experimental animals or procedures may have a major influence on the outcome.

While these factors do not fall under the classification of "epigenetic" they will clearly interact with epigenetic processes described below in determining the final, overall activity and effectiveness of the kynurenine pathway in neurological and immunological function in postnatal life.

Epigenetics of IDO

If the kynurenine pathway is as widely and fundamentally important as the above discussions imply, any modifications to the various components of the pathway would carry substantial implications for a variety of disorders. Relevant changes could include genetic mutations or epigenetic changes. The latter do not involve changes directly to the genetic machinery or nucleotide sequence, but consist of minor changes to the gene or related segments of the chromosome such as promoter sequences, which alter the functionality of that gene. This may change the extent to which a section of gene is transcribed, or the properties of the transcribed protein. Epigenetic changes are often the result of environmental factors (diet, stress, disease) which affect the activity of key enzymes such as acetyl- or methyl-donors, altering their activity on the genome. Epigenetic changes are often reversible but, if they affect the germ-line cells, they may be inherited.

Several of the disorders discussed above may be susceptible to epigenetic influences. The brains of patients with Huntington's disease exhibit evidence of alterations in methylation status (207, 208) or acetylation status (209) and inhibition of a histone deacetylase may prevent the development of cognitive deficits as well as huntingtin expansion (210). Such changes may contribute significantly to the course of the disorder and its heritability, especially since DNA methylation has been shown to produce extension of the mutant CAG repeat sequence (211).

RA may involve defects in acetylation (212), reflected in the beneficial activity of a histone deacetylase inhibitor in CIA (213). It is also likely that there are changes in DNA methylation (214–217) as has been noted in regulatory T cells (218) and synovial fibroblasts (219). The methylation pattern has been claimed to reflect therapeutic efficacy of the TNF-α inhibitor etanercept (220) and so may be relevant to explaining the non-responsiveness to this drug of some patients.

The aberrant methylation of Treg cells, affecting the *FOXP3* and *CTLA4* genes, reduces their immunosuppressant activity. We have found that the DNA-demethylating compound decitabine reduces this suppression and restores immunosuppression associated with increased expression of Treg markers. In the CIA model of arthritis decitabine increased the suppression function of Treg cells along with a decrease in pro-inflammatory Th1 and Th17 cells and their infiltration into arthritic paws. Of major relevance to the kynurenine pathway, these effects of demethylation were associated with increased expression of IDO1 which is normally an important aspect of the immunosuppressant behavior of Treg cells mediated by the CTLA-4 ligation of B7 proteins, and further differentiation of Treg cells by the promotion of FoxP3 expression.

When CIA was induced in IDO1-deficient mice on a C57/BL6N.Q (H-2^q) background), decitabine administration reduced both the early symptoms and pathology of the disorder but also reduced the expression of transcription factors characterizing pro-inflammatory cells (IFNγ+ and Tbet$^+$ in Th1; IL17+ and RoRγt$^+$ in Th17 cells). In contrast, symptoms were exacerbated in the later stages of disease in parallel with a loss of FoxP3$^+$ Tregs and an increased number of Tbet$^+$ Th1 and RoRγt$^+$ Th17 cells. This time course would be consistent with the concept that IDO1 activity is a critical feature of the interactions needed to maintain long-term Treg-mediated immune tolerance. Decitabine also increased the number of IDO1-positive monocytes while a combination of

ADC/decitabine and IFN-γ allowed myeloid DCs to increase their IDO1 expression.

Overall, because of its critical, central role in immune function and tolerogenesis, the methylation of IDO1 appears to be an important factor in determining its activity. If these factors affect germline DNA, as noted above, they may significantly affect the immunological competence of offspring and their susceptibility to a range of disorders.

CLINICAL POTENTIAL

This review has introduced a few of the many disorders afflicting peripheral tissues or the CNS in which inflammation is implicated, but that is enough to recognize the therapeutic potential of influencing the kynurenine pathway by pharmacological interference. Many academic and commercial laboratories have demonstrated the promise of analogs or derivatives of kynurenine and its catabolites to act as receptor agonists, antagonists or enzyme inhibitors (138, 221, 222).

In the CNS work has been concentrated on inhibitors of KMO to reduce quinolinic acid synthesis and thereby reduce neural activity and excitotoxicity in neurodegenerative disorders as well as in the suppression of peripheral inflammation, especially in the pancreas (223–226). A different approach is in the development of KAT inhibitors intended to reduce kynurenic acid formation in psychiatric disorders such as schizophrenia (227–230). Of course these two approaches, being essentially contrary in their objectives, raise concerns that schizoid symptoms might be induced in response to KMO inhibition, or that KAT inhibition could divert more kynurenine via KMO to quinolinic acid.

In a similar vein, there has been a major effort to develop inhibitors of IDO1 to prevent the immune-suppressant activity of this enzyme and thus to drive tumor cell death or to facilitate the effects of anti-tumor drugs (231–235). In principle, this approach might lead to the initiation or exacerbation of clinical inflammatory and autoimmune disorders described above. While this would remain a problem which would need careful monitoring, clinical trials with IDO1 inhibitors have recently been found to be less effective anti-cancer agents than anticipated (111–113), raising doubts about the continuation of this strategy.

Despite these concerns, major advances are being made in kynurenine-related treatments for Huntington's disease and schizophrenia, and the range of conditions potentially amenable to kynurenine-related therapy continues to escalate. The factors which can recruit kynurenine pathway involvement such as infection, inflammation, dietary changes, various forms of stress and others make it highly likely that the kynurenine pathway will prove to be a valuable source of new therapeutic agents in the near future.

SUMMARY AND CONCLUSIONS

Some of the inter-relationships between IDO or its kynurenine-derived catabolites and aspects of the immune system have been discussed, focusing on several examples of disorders affecting peripheral tissues or the CNS. In many cases there are important questions to be resolved, such as which components of the kynurenine pathway are responsible for different elements of immune regulation. It seems likely that a fuller appreciation of these issues will not only help to understand the molecular basis of some disorders, but will further the development of increasingly sophisticated and targeted therapies (236). This will be especially important if methods can be identified to modify or prevent epigenetic changes which alter the expression or functional capacity of relevant enzymes, receptors or transduction systems. Finally, more detailed investigation of the immunological consequences of stress, infection and immune system activation during pregnancy—all of which involve activity in the kynurenine pathway—may be highly relevant to understanding postnatal susceptibility to autoimmune disorders and cancer, much as recent work has shown lasting effects on the nervous system. With growing interest in the importance of neuroimmune interactions for disease development and resolution, a combined knowledge of both these areas might yield synergistic advances in medicine and therapeutics.

AUTHOR CONTRIBUTIONS

All authors contributed to the writing and proof-reading of this manuscript.

ACKNOWLEDGMENTS

The authors acknowledge personal support from the Ministry of Science and Technology (Taiwan)(Y-SH) and Cancer Research UK (FC); JO was a vs. Arthritis Postdoctoral Research Fellow. TS is an Honorary Senior Research Fellow.

REFERENCES

1. Yoshida R, Imanishi J, Oku T, Kishida T, Hayaishi O. Induction of pulmonary indoleamine 2,3-dioxygenase by interferon. *Proc Nat Acad Sci USA.* (1981) 78:129–32. doi: 10.1073/pnas.78.1.129

2. Munn DH, Zhou M, Attwood JT, Bondarev I, Conway SJ, Marshall B, et al. Prevention of allogeneic fetal rejection by tryptophan catabolism. *Science.* (1998) 281:1191–3. doi: 10.1126/science.281.538 0.1191

3. Mellor AL, Munn DH. Immunology at the maternal-fetal interface: lessons for T cell tolerance and suppression. *Ann Rev Immunol.* (2000) 18:367–91. doi: 10.1146/annurev.immunol.18.1.367

4. Stone TW, Perkins MN. Quinolinic acid: a potent endogenous excitant at amino acid receptors in CNS. *Eur J Pharmacol.* (1981) 72:411–2. doi: 10.1016/0014-2999(81)90587-2

5. Perkins MN, Stone TW. An iontophoretic investigation of the actions of convulsant kynurenines and their interaction with the endogenous excitant quinolinic acid. *Brain Res.* (1982) 247:184–7. doi: 10.1016/0006-8993(82)91048-4

6. Perkins MN, Stone TW. Pharmacology and regional variations of quinolinic acid-evoked excitations in the rat central nervous system. *J Pharmacol Exp Ther.* (1983) 226:551–7.

7. Fatokun AA, Hunt NH, Ball HJ. Indoleamine 2,3-dioxygenase 2 (IDO2) and the kynurenine pathway: characteristics and potential roles in health and disease. *Amino Acids.* (2013) 45:1319–29. doi: 10.1007/s00726-013-1602-1

8. Criado G, Simelyte E, Inglis JJ, Essex D, Williams RO. Indoleamine 2,3 dioxygenase-mediated tryptophan catabolism regulates accumulation of Th1/Th17 Cells in the joint in collagen-induced arthritis. *Arthritis Rheum.* (2009) 60:1342–51. doi: 10.1002/art.24446

9. Onodera T, Jang MH, Guo ZJ, Yamasaki M, Hirata T, Bai ZB, et al. Constitutive expression of IDO by dendritic cells of mesenteric lymph nodes: functional involvement of the CTLA-4/B7 and CCL22/CCR4 interactions. *J Immunol.* (2009) 183:5608–14. doi: 10.4049/jimmunol.0804116

10. Cribbs AP, Kennedy A, Penn H, Read JE, Amjadi P, Green P, et al. Treg cell function in rheumatoid arthritis is compromised by CTLA-4 promoter methylation resulting in a failure to activate the indoleamine 2,3-dioxygenase pathway. *Arthritis Rheumatol.* (2014) 66:2344–54. doi: 10.1002/art.38715

11. DiNatale BC, Murray IA, Schroeder JC, Flaveny CA, Lahoti TS, Laurenzana EM, et al. Kynurenic acid is a potent endogenous aryl hydrocarbon receptor ligand that synergistically induces interleukin-6 in the presence of inflammatory signaling. *Toxicol Sci.* (2010) 115:89–97. doi: 10.1093/toxsci/kfq024

12. Nguyen NT, Kimura A, Nakahama T, Chinen I, Masuda K, Nohara K, et al. Aryl hydrocarbon receptor negatively regulates dendritic cell immunogenicity via a kynurenine-dependent mechanism. *Proc Nat Acad Sci USA.* (2010) 107:19961–6. doi: 10.1073/pnas.1014465107

13. Nakahama T, Kimura A, Nguyen NT, Chinen I, Hanieh H, Nohara K, et al. Aryl hydrocarbon receptor deficiency in T cells suppresses the development of collagen-induced arthritis. *Proc Nat Acad Sci USA.* (2011) 108:14222–7. doi: 10.1073/pnas.1111786108

14. Li Q, Harden JL, Anderson CD, Egilmez NK. Tolerogenic phenotype of IFN-g–induced IDO+ dendritic cells is maintained via an autocrine IDO–kynurenine/ AhR–IDO loop. *J Immunol.* (2016) 197:962–70. doi: 10.4049/jimmunol.1502615

15. Xie FT, Cao JS, Zhao J, Yu Y, Qi F, Dai XC. IDO expressing dendritic cells suppress allograft rejection of small bowel transplantation in mice by expansion of Foxp3(+) regulatory T cells. *Transpl Immunol.* (2015) 33:69–77. doi: 10.1016/j.trim.2015.05.003

16. Fallarino F, Grohmann U, You S, McGrath BC, Cavener DR, Vacca C, et al. The combined effects of tryptophan starvation and tryptophan catabolites down-regulate T cell receptor zeta-chain and induce a regulatory phenotype in naive T cells. *J Immunol.* (2006) 176:6752–61. doi: 10.4049/jimmunol.176.11.6752

17. Fallarino F, Grohmann U. Using an ancient tool for igniting and propagating immune tolerance: IDO as an inducer and amplifier of regulatory T cell functions. *Curr Med Chem.* (2011) 18:2215–21. doi: 10.2174/092986711795656027

18. Romani L, Fallarino F, de Luca A, Montagnoli C, D'Angelo C, Zelante T, et al. Defective tryptophan catabolism underlies inflammation in mouse chronic granulomatous disease. *Nature.* (2008) 451:211–5. doi: 10.1038/nature06471

19. Romani L, Zelante T, de Luca A, Fallarino F, Puccetti P. IL-17 and therapeutic kynurenines in pathogenic inflammation to fungi. *J Immunol.* (2008) 180:5157–62 doi: 10.4049/jimmunol.180.8.5157

20. Cheng L, Qian L, Xu ZZ, Tan Y, Luo CY. Aromatic hydrocarbon receptor provides a link between smoking and rheumatoid arthritis in peripheral blood mononuclear cells. *Clin Exp Rheumatol.* (2019) 37:445–9.

21. Talbot J, Peres RS, Pinto LG, Oliveira RDR, Lima KA, Donate PB, et al. Smoking-induced aggravation of experimental arthritis is dependent of aryl hydrocarbon receptor activation in Th17 cells. *Arthritis Res Ther.* (2018) 20:119. doi: 10.1186/s13075-018-1609-9

22. Nguyen NT, Nakahama T, Kishimoto T. Aryl hydrocarbon receptor and experimental autoimmune arthritis. *Semin Immunopathol.* (2013) 35:637–44. doi: 10.1007/s00281-013-0392-6

23. Nii T, Kuzuya K, Kabata D, Matsui T, Murata A, Ohya T, et al. Crosstalk between tumor necrosis factor-alpha signaling and aryl hydrocarbon receptor signaling in nuclear factor -kappa B activation: a possible molecular mechanism underlying the reduced efficacy of TNF-inhibitors

in rheumatoid arthritis by smoking. *J Autoimmun.* (2019) 98:95–102. doi: 10.1016/j.jaut.2018.12.004

24. Fu J, Nogueira SV, van Drongelen V, Coit P, Ling S, Rosloniec EF, et al. Shared epitope-aryl hydrocarbon receptor crosstalk underlies the mechanism of gene-environment interaction in autoimmune arthritis. *Proc Nat Acad Sci USA.* (2018) 115:4755–60. doi: 10.1073/pnas.1722124115

25. Tong B, Yuan X, Dou Y, Wu X, Wang Y, Xia Y, et al. Sinomenine induces the generation of intestinal Treg cells and attenuates arthritis via activation of aryl hydrocarbon receptor. *Lab Invest.* (2016) 96:1076–86. doi: 10.1038/labinvest.2016.86

26. Tong B, Yuan X, Dou Y, Wu X, Chou G, Wang Z, et al. Norisoboldine, an isoquinoline alkaloid, acts as an aryl hydrocarbon receptor ligand to induce intestinal Treg cells and thereby attenuate arthritis. *Int J Biochem Cell Biol.* (2016) 75:63–73. doi: 10.1016/j.biocel.2016.03.014

27. Yuan X, Tong B, Dou Y, Wu X, Wei Z, Dai Y. Tetrandrine ameliorates collagen-induced arthritis in mice by restoring the balance between Th17 and Treg cells via the aryl hydrocarbon receptor. *Biochem Pharmacol.* (2016) 101:87–99. doi: 10.1016/j.bcp.2015.11.025

28. Ogando J, Tardaguila M, Diaz-Alderete A, Usategui A, Miranda-Ramos V, Jorge Martinez-Herrera D, et al. Notch-regulated miR-223 targets the aryl hydrocarbon receptor pathway and increases cytokine production in macrophages from rheumatoid arthritis patients. *Sci Rep.* (2016) 6:20223. doi: 10.1038/srep20223

29. Lahoti TS, Hughes JM, Kusnadi A, John K, Zhu B, Murray IA, et al. Aryl hydrocarbon receptor antagonism attenuates growth factor expression, proliferation, and migration in fibroblast-like synoviocytes from patients with rheumatoid arthritis. *J Pharmacol Exp Ther.* (2014) 348:236–45. doi: 10.1124/jpet.113.209726

30. Badawy AA. Kynurenine pathway of tryptophan metabolism: regulatory and functional aspects. *Int J Tryptophan Res.* (2017) 10:1178646917691938. doi: 10.1177/1178646917691938

31. Badawy AA. Hypothesis kynurenic and quinolinic acids: the main players of the kynurenine pathway and opponents in inflammatory disease. *Med Hypoth.* (2018) 118:129–38. doi: 10.1016/j.mehy.2018.06.021

32. Munn DH, Sharma MD, Baban B, Harding HP, Zhang YH, Ron D, et al. GCN2 kinase in T cells mediates proliferative arrest and anergy induction in response to indoleamine 2,3-dioxygenase. *Immunity.* (2005) 22:633–42. doi: 10.1016/j.immuni.2005.03.013

33. Yan Y, Zhang G-X, Gran B, Fallarino F, Yu S, Li H, et al. IDO upregulates regulatory T cells via tryptophan catabolite and suppresses encephalitogenic T cell responses in experimental autoimmune encephalomyelitis. *J Immunol.* (2010) 185:5953–61. doi: 10.4049/jimmunol.1001628

34. Ravindran R, Khan N, Nakaya HI, Li SZ, Loebbermann J, Maddur MS, et al. Vaccine activation of the nutrient sensor GCN2 in dendritic cells enhances antigen presentation. *Science.* (2014) 343:313–7. doi: 10.1126/science.1246829

35. van de Velde LA, Guo XZJ, Barbaric L, Smith AM, Oguin TH, Thomas PG, et al. Stress kinase GCN2 controls the proliferative fitness and trafficking of cytotoxic T cells independent of environmental amino acid sensing. *Cell Rep.* (2016) 17:2247–58. doi: 10.1016/j.celrep.2016.10.079

36. Forrest CM, Mackay GM, Oxford L, Stoy N, Stone TW, Darlington LG. Kynurenine pathway metabolism in patients with osteoporosis after two years of drug treatment. *Clin Exp Pharmacol Physiol.* (2006) 33:1078–87. doi: 10.1111/j.1440-1681.2006.04490.x

37. Baran H, Schwarcz R. Presence of 3-hydroxyanthranilic acid in rat-tissues and evidence for its production from anthranilic acid in the brain. *J Neurochem.* (1990) 55:738–44. doi: 10.1111/j.1471-4159.1990.tb04553.x

38. Fallarino I, Grohmann U, Vacca C, Bianchi R, Orabona C, Spreca A, et al. T cell apoptosis by tryptophan catabolism. *Cell Death Differ.* (2002) 9:1069–77. doi: 10.1038/sj.cdd.4401073

39. Pietschmann P, Mechtcheriakova D, Meshcheryakova A, Föger-Samwald U, Ellinger I. Immunology of osteoporosis: a mini-review. *Gerontology.* (2016) 62:128–37. doi: 10.1159/000431091

40. Iseme RA, Mcevoy M, Kelly B, Agnew L, Walker FR, Attia J. Is osteoporosis an autoimmune mediated disorder? *Bone Rep.* (2017) 7:121–31. doi: 10.1016/j.bonr.2017.10.003

41. Caetano-Lopes J, Canhão H, Fonseca JE. Osteoimmunology–the hidden immune regulation of bone. *Autoimmun Rev.* (2009) 8:250–55. doi: 10.1016/j.autrev.2008.07.038

42. Darlington LG, Forrest CM, Mackay GM, Smith RA, Smith AJ, Stoy N, et al. On the biological importance of the 3-hydroxyanthranilic acid: anthranilic acid ratio. *Int J Tryptophan Res.* (2010) 3:51–9. doi: 10.4137/IJTR.S4282

43. Dykens JA, Sullivan SG, Stern A. Oxidative reactivity of the tryptophan metabolites 3-hydroxyanthranilate, quinolinate and picolinate. *Biochem Pharmacol.* (1987) 36:211–7.

44. Ishii T, Iwahashi H, Sugata R, Kido R, Fridovich I. Superoxide disumutases enhance the rat of autoxidation of 3-hydroxyanthranilic acid. *Arch Biochem Biophys.* (1990) 276:248–50. doi: 10.1016/0003-9861(90)90034-V

45. Sternberg JM, Forrest CM, Dalton RN, Turner C, Rodgers J, Stone TW, et al. Kynurenine pathway activation in human african trypanosomiasis. *J Infect Dis.* (2017) 215:806–12. doi: 10.1093/infdis/jiw623

46. Charconnet-Harding F, Dalgliesh CE, Neuberger A. The relation between riboflavin and tryptophan metabolism, studied in the rat. *Biochem J.* (1953) 53:513–21. doi: 10.1042/bj0530513

47. Stevens CO, Henderson LM. Riboflavin and hepatic kynurenine hydroxylase. *J Biol Chem.* (1959) 234:1191–4.

48. Brijal S, Lakshmi AV. Tissue distribution and turnover of [3H]riboflavin during respiratory infection in mice. *Metabolism.* (1999) 48:1608–11. doi: 10.1016/S0026-0495(99)90253-6

49. Menezes RR, Godin AM, Rodrigues FF, Coura GME, Melo ISF, Brito A, et al. Thiamine and riboflavin inhibit production of cytokines and increase the anti-inflammatory activity of a corticosteroid in a chronic model of inflammation induced by complete freund's adjuvant. *Pharmacol Rep.* (2017) 69:1036–43. doi: 10.1016/j.pharep.2017.04.011

50. Dey S, Bishayi B. Riboflavin along with antibiotics balances reactive oxygen species and inflammatory cytokines and controls *Staphylococcus aureus* infection by boosting murine macrophage function and regulates inflammation. *J Inflamm.* (2016) 13:36. doi: 10.1186/s12950-016-0145-0

51. Pinkerton H, Bessey OA. The loss of resistance to murine typhus infection resulting from riboflavin deficiency in rats. *Science.* (1939) 89:368–70. doi: 10.1126/science.89.2312.368

52. Verdrengh M, Tarkowski A. Riboflavin in innate and acquired immune responses. *Inflamm Res.* (2005) 54:390–3. doi: 10.1007/s00011-005-1372-7

53. Mulherin DM, Thurnham DI, Situnayake RD. Glutathione reductase activity, riboflavin status, and disease activity in rheumatoid arthritis. *Ann Rheum Dis.* (1996) 55:837–40. doi: 10.1136/ard.55.11.837

54. Igari T, Tsuchizawa M, Shimamura T. Alteration of tryptophan-metabolism in the synovial-fluid of patients with rheumatoid-arthritis and osteoarthritis. *Tohoku J Exp Med.* (1987) 153:79–86. doi: 10.1620/tjem.153.79

55. Ge L, Cui Y, Cheng K, Han J. Isopsoralen enhanced osteogenesis by targeting AhR/ERα. *Molecules.* (2018) 23:2600. doi: 10.3390/molecules23102600

56. Michalowska M, Znorko B, Kaminski T, Oksztulska-Kolanek E, Pawlak D. New insights into tryptophan and its metabolites in the regulation of bone metabolism. *J Physiol Pharmacol.* (2015) 66:779–91.

57. Kalaska B, Pawlak K, Domaniewski T, Oksztulska-Kolanek E, Znorko B, Roszczenko A, et al. Elevated levels of peripheral kynurenine decrease bone strength in rats with chronic kidney disease. *Front Physiol.* (2017) 8:836. doi: 10.3389/fphys.2017.00836

58. Iqbal J, Sun L, Cao J, Yuen T, Lu P, Bab I, et al. Smoke carcinogens cause bone loss through the aryl hydrocarbon receptor and induction of Cyp1 enzymes. *Proc Nat Acad Sci USA.* (2013) 110:11115–20. doi: 10.1073/pnas.1220919110

59. Tong Y, Niu M, Du Y, Mei W, Cao W, Dou Y, et al. Aryl hydrocarbon receptor suppresses the osteogenesis of mesenchymal stem cells in collagen-induced arthritic mice through the inhibition of beta-catenin. *Exp Cell Res.* (2017) 350:349–57. doi: 10.1016/j.yexcr.2016.12.009

60. Yu TY, Pang WJ, Yang GS. 3,3 '-Diindolylmethane increases bone mass by suppressing osteoclastic bone resorption in mice. *J Pharmacol Sci.* (2015) 127:75–82. doi: 10.1016/j.jphs.2014.11.006

61. Roser-Page S, Vikulina T, Zayzafoon M, Weitzmann MN. CTLA-4Ig-Induced T cell anergy promotes Wnt-10b production and bone formation in a mouse *model. Arthritis Rheumatol.* (2014) 66:990–9. doi: 10.1002/art.38319

62. Grassi F, Tell G, Robbie-Ryan M, Gao Y, Terauchi M, Yang X, et al. Oxidative stress causes bone loss in estrogen-deficient mice through enhanced bone

marrow dendritic cell activation. *Proc Nat Acad Sci USA.* (2007) 104:15087–92. doi: 10.1073/pnas.0703610104

63. Axmann R, Herman S, Zaiss M, Franz S, Polzer K, Zwerina J, et al. CTLA-4 directly inhibits osteoclast formation. *Ann Rheum Dis.* (2008) 67:1603–9. doi: 10.1136/ard.2007.080713

64. Dubrovsky AM, Lim MJ, Lane NE. Osteoporosis in rheumatic diseases: anti-rheumatic drugs and the skeleton. *Calcif Tissue Int.* (2018) 102:607–18. doi: 10.1007/s00223-018-0401-9

65. Bozec A, Zaiss MM, Kagwiria R, Voll R, Rauh M, Chen Z, et al. T cell costimulation molecules CD80/86 inhibit osteoclast differentiation by inducing the IDO/Tryptophan pathway. *Sci Transl Med.* (2014) 6:235ra60. doi: 10.1126/scitranslmed.3007764

66. Bozec A, Zaiss MM. T regulatory cells in bone remodelling. *Curr Osteoporos Rep.* (2017) 15:121–5. doi: 10.1007/s11914-017-0356-1

67. Qiu X, Gui Y, Xu Y, Li D, Wang L. DHEA promotes osteoblast differentiation by regulating the expression of osteoblast-related genes and Foxp(3+) regulatory T cells. *Biosci Trends.* (2015) 9:307–14. doi: 10.5582/bst.2015.01073

68. Matsunawa M, Amano Y, Endo K, Uno S, Sakaki T, Yamada S, et al. The Aryl hydrocarbon receptor activator benzo[a]pyrene enhances vitamin D-3 catabolism in macrophages. *Toxicol Sci.* (2009) 109:50–8. doi: 10.1093/toxsci/kfp044

69. Cole JE, Astola N, Cribbs AP, Goddard ME, Park I, Green P, et al. Indoleamine 2,3-dioxygenase-1 is protective in atherosclerosis and its metabolites provide new opportunities for drug development. *Proc Nat Acad Sci USA.* (2015) 112:13033–8. doi: 10.1073/pnas.1517820112

70. Polyzos KA, Ovchinnikova O, Berg M, Baumgartner R, Agardh H, Pirault J, et al. Inhibition of indoleamine-2,3-dioxygenase promotes vascular inflammation and increases atherosclerosis in apoE-/- mice. *Cardiovasc Res.* (2015) 106:295–302. doi: 10.1093/cvr/cvv100

71. Forteza MJ, Polyzos KA, Baumgartner R, Suur BE, Mussbacher M, Johansson DK, et al. Activation of the regulatory T-cell/indoleamine-2,3-dioxygenase axis reduces vascular inflammation and atherosclerosis in hypoerlipidemic mice. *Front Immunol.* (2018) 9:950. doi: 10.3389/fimmu.2018.00950

72. Yun TJ, Lee JS, Machmach K, Shim D, Choi J, Wi YJ, et al. Indoleamine-2,3-dioxygenase-expressing plasmacytoid dendritic cells protect against atherosclerosis by induction of regulatory T cells. *Cell Metab.* (2016) 23:852–66. doi: 10.1016/j.cmet.2016.04.010

73. GuilleminGJ, Kerr SJ, Smythe GA, Smith DG, Kapoor V, ArmatiPJ, et al. Kynurenine pathway metabolism in human astrocytes: a paradox for neuronal protection. *J Neurochem.* (2001) 78:842–53. doi: 10.1046/j.1471-4159.2001.00498.x

74. Guillemin GJ, Brew BJ, Noonan CE, Takikawa O, Cullen KM. Indoleamine 2,3 dioxygenase and quinolinic acid immunoreactivity in Alzheimer's disease hippocampus. *Neuropathol Appl Neurobiol.* (2005) 31:395–404. doi: 10.1111/j.1365-2990.2005.00655.x

75. Chiarugi A, Calvani M, Meli E, Traggiai E, Moroni F. Synthesis and release of neurotoxic kynurenine metabolites by human monocyte-derived macrophages. *J Neuroimmunol.* (2001) 120:190–8. doi: 10.1016/S0165-5728(01)00418-0

76. Heyes MP, Saito K, Markey SP. Human macrophages convert L-tryptophan into the neurotoxin quinolinic acid. *Biochem J.* (1992) 283:633–5. doi: 10.1042/bj2830633

77. Guillemin GJ, Smythe G, Takikawa O, Brew BJ. Expression of indoleamine 2,3-dioxygenase and production of quinolinic acid by human microglia, astrocytes, and neurons. *Glia.* (2005) 49:15–23. doi: 10.1002/glia.20090

78. Notarangelo FM, Beggiato S, Schwarcz R. Assessment of prenatal kynurenine metabolism using tissue slices: focus on the neosynthesis of kynurenic acid in mice. *Dev Neurosci.* (2019) 41:102–11. doi: 10.1159/000499736

79. Heredi J, Cseh EK, Berko A, Magyarine A, Veres G, Zadori D, et al. Investigating kynurenic acid production and kynurenergic manipulation on acute mouse brain slice preparations. *Brain Res Bull.* (2019) 146:185–91. doi: 10.1016/j.brainresbull.2018.12.014

80. Stone TW. The neuropharmacology of quinolinic and kynurenic acids. *Pharmacol Rev.* (1993) 45:309–79.

81. Stone TW, Darlington LG. Endogenous kynurenines as targets for drug discovery and development. *Nat Rev Drug Discov.* (2002) 1:609–20. doi: 10.1038/nrd870

82. Stone TW, Stoy N, Darlington LG. An expanding range of targets for kynurenine metabolites of tryptophan. *Trends Pharmacol Sci.* (2013) 34:136–43. doi: 10.1016/j.tips.2012.09.006

83. Schwarcz R, Whetsell WO, Mangano RM. Quinolinic acid - an endogenous metabolite that produces axon-sparing lesions in rat brain. *Science.* (1983) 219:316–8. doi: 10.1126/science.6849138

84. Ting KK, Brew BJ, Guillemin GJ. Effect of quinolinic acid on human astrocytes morphology and functions: implications in Alzheimer's disease. *J Neuroinflammation.* (2009) 6:36. doi: 10.1186/1742-2094-6-36

85. Lovelace MD, Varney B, Sundaram G, Lennon MJ, Lim CK, Jacobs K, et al. Recent evidence for an expanded role of the kynurenine pathway of tryptophan metabolism in neurological diseases. *Neuropharmacology.* (2017) 112:373–88. doi: 10.1016/j.neuropharm.2016.03.024

86. Samuelsson AM, Jennische E, Hansson HA, Holmang A. Prenatal exposure to interleukin-6 results in inflammatory neurodegeneration in hippocampus with NMDA / GABA(A) dysregulation and impaired spatial learning. *Am J Physiol Regul Integr Comp Physiol.* (2006) 290:R1345–56. doi: 10.1152/ajpregu.00268.2005

87. Zou J, Crews FT. Glutamate/NMDA excitoxicity and HMGB1/TLR4 neuroimmune toxicity converge as components of neurodegeneration. *AIMS Mol Sci.* (2015) 2:77–100. doi: 10.3934/molsci.2015.2.77

88. Heyes MP, Mefford IN, Quearry BJ, Dedhia M, Lackner A. Increased ratio of quinolinic acid to kynurenic acid in cerebrospinal-fluid of d-retrovirus-infected rhesus macaques - relationship to clinical and viral status. *Ann Neurol.* (1990) 27:666–75. doi: 10.1002/ana.410270614

89. Heyes MP, Jordan EK, Lee K, Saito K, Frank JA, Snoy PJ, et al. Relationship of neurologic status in macaques infected with the simian immunodeficiency virus to cerebrospinal-fluid quinolinic acid and kynurenic acid. *Brain Res.* (1992) 570:237–50. doi: 10.1016/0006-8993(92)90587-Y

90. Pfefferkorn ER. Interferon-gamma blocks the growth of *toxoplasma-gondii* in human-fibroblasts by inducing the host-cells to degrade tryptophan. *Proc Nat Acad Sci USA.* (1984) 81:908–12. doi: 10.1073/pnas.81.3.908

91. Terness P, Bauer TM, Rose L, Dufter C, Watzlik A, Simon H, et al. Inhibition of allogeneic T cell proliferation by indoleamine 2,3-dioxygenase-expressing dendritic cells: mediation of suppression by tryptophan metabolites. *J Exp Med.* (2002) 196:447–57. doi: 10.1084/jem.20020052

92. Terness P, Chuang JJ, Opelz G. The immunoregulatory role of IDO-producing human dendritic cells revisited. *Trends Immunol.* (2006) 27:68–73. doi: 10.1016/j.it.2005.12.006

93. Giorgini F, Guidetti P, Nguyen QV, Bennett SC, Muchowski PJ. A genomic screen in yeast implicates kynurenine 3-monooxygenase as a therapeutic target for Huntington disease. *Nat Genet.* (2005) 37:526–31. doi: 10.1038/ng1542

94. Schwarcz R, Guidetti P, Sathyasaikumar KV, Muchowski PJ. Of mice, rats and men: revisiting the quinolinic acid hypothesis of Huntington's disease. *Prog Neurobiol.* (2010) 90:230–45. doi: 10.1016/j.pneurobio.2009.04.005

95. Stoy N, Mackay GM, Forrest CM, Christofides J, Egerton M, Stone TW, et al. Tryptophan metabolism and oxidative stress in patients with Huntington's disease. *J Neurochem.* (2005) 93:611–23. doi: 10.1111/j.1471-4159.2005.03070.x

96. Boros FA, Klivenyi P, Toldi J, Vecsei L. Indoleamine-2,3-dioxygenase as a novel therapeutic target for Huntington's disease. *Exp Opin Ther Targets.* (2019) 23:39–51. doi: 10.1080/14728222.2019.1549231

97. Stone TW, Forrest CM, Darlington LG. Kynurenine pathway inhibition as a therapeutic strategy for neuroprotection. *FEBS J.* (2012) 279:1386–97. doi: 10.1111/j.1742-4658.2012.08487.x

98. Stone TW, Forrest CM, Stoy N, Darlington LG. Involvement of kynurenines in Huntington's disease and stroke-induced brain damage. *J Neural Transm.* (2012) 119:261–74. doi: 10.1007/s00702-011-0676-8

99. Andre R, Carty L, Tabrizi SJ. Disruption of immune cell function by mutant huntingtin in Huntington's disease pathogenesis. *Curr Opin Pharmacol.* (2016) 26:33–8. doi: 10.1016/j.coph.2015.09.008

100. Forrest CM, Mackay GM, Stoy N, Spiden SL, Taylor R, Stone TW, et al. Blood levels of kynurenines, interleukin-23 and soluble human leucocyte antigen-G at different stages of Huntington's disease. *J Neurochem.* (2010) 112:112–22. doi: 10.1111/j.1471-4159.2009.06442.x

101. Ellrichmann G, Reick C, Saft C, Linker RA. The role of the immune system in Huntington's disease. *Clin. Dev. Immunol.* (2013) 2013:541259. doi: 10.1155/2013/541259

102. Sathyasaikumar KV, Stachowski EK, Amori L, Guidetti P, Muchowski PJ, Schwarcz R. Dysfunctional kynurenine pathway metabolism in the R6/2 mouse model of Huntington's disease. *J Neurochem.* (2010) 113:1416–25. doi: 10.1111/j.1471-4159.2010.06675.x

103. Crotti A, Glass CK. The choreography of neuroinflammation in Huntington's disease. *Trends Immunol.* (2015) 36:364–73. doi: 10.1016/j.it.2015.04.007

104. Moss DJH, Flower MD, Lo KK, Miller JRC, van Ommen GJB, 't Hoen PA, et al. Huntington's disease blood and brain show a common gene expression pattern and share an immune signature with Alzheimer's disease. *Sci Rep.* (2017) 7:44849. doi: 10.1038/srep44849

105. Corey-Bloom J, Aikin AM, Gutierrez AM, Nadhem JS, Howell TL, Thomas EA. Beneficial effects of glatiramer acetate in Huntington's disease mouse models: evidence for BDNF-elevating and immunomodulatory mechanisms. *Brain Res.* (2017) 1673:102–10. doi: 10.1016/j.brainres.2017.08.013

106. Kostlin N, Ostermeir AL, Spring B, Schwarz J, Marme A, Walter CB, et al. HLA-G promotes myeloid-derived suppressor cell accumulation and suppressive activity during human pregnancy through engagement of the receptor ILT4. *Eur J Immunol.* (2017) 47:374–84. doi: 10.1002/eji.201646564

107. Wiendl H, Feger U, Mittelbronn M, Jack C, Schreiner B, Stadelmann C, et al. Expression of the immune-tolerogenic major histocompatibility molecule HLA-G in multiple sclerosis: implications for CNS immunity. *Brain.* (2005) 128:2689–704. doi: 10.1093/brain/awh609

108. Fainardi E, Rizzo R, Melchiorri L, Castellazzi M, Paolino E, Tola MR, et al. Intrathecal synthesis of soluble HLA-G and HLA-I molecules are reciprocally associated to clinical and MRI activity in patients with multiple sclerosis. *Mult Scler.* (2006) 12:2–12. doi: 10.1191/1352458506ms1241oa

109. Abumaree M, Al Jumah M, Pace RA, Kalionis B. Immunosuppressive properties of mesenchymal stem cells. *Stem Cell Rev Rep.* (2012) 8:375–92. doi: 10.1007/s12015-011-9312-0

110. Nasef A, Mathieu N, Chapel A, Frick J, Francois S, Mazurier C, et al. Immuno-suppressive effects of mesenchymal stem cells: involvement of HLA-G. *Transplantation.* (2007) 84:231–7. doi: 10.1097/01.tp.0000267918.07906.08

111. Long GV, Dummer R, Humid O, Gajewski TF, Caglevic C, Dalle S, et al. Epacadostat plus pembrolizumab versus placebo plus pembrolizumab in patients with unresectable or metastatic melanoma (ECHO-301/KEYNOTE-252): a phase 3, randomised, double-blind study. *Lancet Oncol.* (2019) 20:1083–97. doi: 10.1016/S1470-2045(19)30274-8

112. Guenther J, Daebritz J, Wirthgen E. Limitations and off-target effects of tryptophan-related IDO inhibitors in cancer treatment. *Front Immunol.* (2019) 10:1801. doi: 10.3389/fimmu.2019.01801

113. Komiya T, Huang CH. Updates in the clinical development of epacadostat and other indoleamine 2,3-dioxygenase 1 inhibitors (IDO1) for human cancers. *Front Oncol.* (2018) 8:423. doi: 10.3389/fonc.2018.00423

114. Svajger U, Obermajer N, Jeras M. IFN-γ-rich environment programs dendritic cells toward silencing of cytotoxic immune responses. *J Leukoc Biol.* (2014) 95:33–46. doi: 10.1189/jlb.1112589

115. Feuerer M, Eulenburg K, Loddenkemper C, Hamann A, Huehn J. Self-limitation of Th1-mediated inflammation by IFN-gamma. *J Immunol.* (2006) 176:2857–86. doi: 10.4049/jimmunol.176.5.2857

116. Lee CL, Guo Y, So KH, Vijayan M, Guo Y, Wong VHH, et al. Soluble human leukocyte antigen G5 polarizes differentiation of macrophages toward a decidual macrophage-like phenotype. *Hum Reprod.* (2015) 30:2263–74. doi: 10.1093/humrep/dev196

117. Leidi M, Gotti E, Bologna L, Miranda E, Rimoldi M, Sica A, et al. M2 macrophages phagocytose rituximab-opsonized leukemic targets more efficiently than M1 Cells In vitro. *J Immunol.* (2009) 182:4415–22. doi: 10.4049/jimmunol.0713732r

118. Tsai YC, Tseng JT, Wang CY, Su MT, Huang JY, Kuo PL. Medroxyprogesterone acetate drives M2 macrophage differentiation toward a phenotype of decidual macrophage. *Mol Cell Endocrinol.* (2017) 452:74–83. doi: 10.1016/j.mce.2017.05.015

119. Wheeler KC, Jena MK, Pradhan BS, Nayak N, Das S, Hsu CD, et al. VEGF may contribute to macrophage recruitment and M2 polarization in the decidua. *PLoS ONE.* (2018) 13:e0191040. doi: 10.1371/journal.pone.0191040

120. Guillemin GJ, Croitoru-Lamoury J, Dormont D, Armati PJ, Brew BJ. Quinolinic acid upregulates chemokine production and chemokine receptor expression in astrocytes. *Glia.* (2003) 41:371–81. doi: 10.1007/978-1-4615-0135-0_4

121. Fiala M, Zhang L, Gan XH, Sherry B, Taub D, Graves MC, et al. Amyloid-beta induces chemokine secretion and monocyte migration across a human blood-brain barrier model. *Mol Med.* (1998) 4:480–9. doi: 10.1007/BF03401753

122. Guillemin GJ, Smythe GA, Veas LA, Takikawa O, Brew BJ. A beta 1-42 induces production of quinolinic acid by human macrophages and microglia. *Neuroreport.* (2003) 14:2311–5. doi: 10.1097/00001756-200312190-00005

123. Guillemin GJ, Williams KR, Smith DG, Smythe GA, Croitoru-Lamoury J, Brew BJ. Quinolinic acid in the pathogenesis of Alzheimer's disease. *Adv Exp Med Biol.* (2003) 527:167.e176. doi: 10.1007/978-1-4615-0135-0_19

124. Ting KK, Brew B, Guillemin G. The involvement of astrocytes and kynurenine pathway in Alzheimer's disease. *Neurotox Res.* (2007) 12:247–62. doi: 10.1007/BF03033908

125. Widner B, Leblhuber F, Walli J, Tilz GP, Demel U, Fuchs D. Tryptophan degradation and immune activation in Alzheimer's disease. *J Neural Transm.* (2000) 107:343–53. doi: 10.1007/s007020050029

126. Wu W, Nicolazzo JA, Wen L, Chung R, Stankovic R, Bao SS, et al. Expression of tryptophan 2,3-dioxygenase and production of kynurenine pathway metabolites in triple transgenic mice and human Alzheimer's disease brain. *PLoS ONE.* (2013) 8:e59749. doi: 10.1371/journal.pone.0059749

127. Guillemin GJ, Wang L, Brew BJ. Quinolinic acid selectively induces apoptosis of human astrocytes: potential role in AIDS dementia complex. *J Neuroinflammation.* (2005) 2:16. doi: 10.1186/1742-2094-2-16

128. Rahman A, Ting K, Cullen KM, Braidy N, Brew BJ, Guillemin GJ. The excitotoxin quinolinic acid induces tau phosphorylation in human neurons. *PLoS ONE.* (2009) 4:e6344. doi: 10.1371/journal.pone.0006344

129. Bosco MC, Rapisarda A, Massazza S, Melillo G, Young H, Varesio L. The tryptophan catabolite picolinic acid selectively induces the chemokines macrophage inflammatory protein-1 alpha and-1 beta in macrophages. *J Immunol.* (2000) 164:3283–91. doi: 10.4049/jimmunol.164.6.3283

130. Melillo G, Cox GW, Radzioch D, Varesio L. Picolinic-acid, a catabolite of l-tryptophan, a costimulus for the induction of reactive nitrogen intermediate production in murine macrophages. *J Immunol.* (1993) 150:4031–40.

131. Guillemin GJ, Cullen KM, Lim CK, Smythe GA, Garner B, Kapoor V, et al. Characterization of the kynurenine pathway in human neurons. *J Neurosci.* (2007) 27:12884–92.doi: 10.1523/JNEUROSCI.4101-07.2007

132. Jhamandas K, Boegman RJ, Beninger RJ, Bialik M. Quinolinate-induced cortical cholinergic damage - modulation by tryptophan-metabolites. *Brain Res.* (1990) 529:185–91. doi: 10.1016/0006-8993(90)90826-W

133. Vrooman L, Jhamandas K, Boegman RJ, Beninger RJ. Picolinic-acid modulates kainic acid-evoked glutamate release from the striatum in-vitro. *Brain Res.* (1993) 627:193–8. doi: 10.1016/0006-8993(93)90320-M

134. Beninger RJ, Colton AM, Ingles JL, Jhamandas K, Boegman, RJ. Picolinic-acid blocks the neurotoxic but not the neuroexcitant properties of quinolinic acid in the rat-brain - evidence from turning behavior and tyrosine-hydroxylase immunohistochemistry. *Neuroscience.* (1994) 61:603–12. doi: 10.1016/0306-4522(94)90438-3

135. Bryleva EY, Brundin L. Kynurenine pathway metabolites and suicidality. *Neuropharmacology.* (2017) 112:324–30. doi: 10.1016/j.neuropharm.2016.01.034

136. Mancuso R, Hernis A, Agostini S, Rovaris M, Caputo D, Fuchs D, et al. Indoleamine 2,3 dioxygenase (IDO) expression and activity in relapsing-remitting multiple sclerosis. *PLoS ONE.* (2015) 10:e0130715. doi: 10.1371/journal.pone.0130715

137. Lim CK, Brew BJ, Sundaram G, Guillemin GJ. Understanding the roles of the kynurenine pathway in multiple sclerosis progression. *Int J Tryptophan Res.* (2010) 3:157–67. doi: 10.4137/IJTR.S4294

138. Platten M, Ho PP, Youssef S, Fontoura P, Garren H, Hur EM, et al. Treatment of autoimmune neuroinflammation with a synthetic tryptophan metabolite. *Science.* (2005) 310:850–5. doi: 10.1126/science.1117634

139. Hartai Z, Klivenyi P, Janaky T, Penke B, Dux L, Vecsei L. Kynurenine metabolism in multiple sclerosis. *Acta Neurol Scand.* (2005) 112:93–6. doi: 10.1111/j.1600-0404.2005.00442.x

140. Chiarugi A, Cozzi A, Ballerini C, Massacesi L, Moroni F. Kynurenine 3-mono-oxygenase activity and neurotoxic kynurenine metabolites increase in the spinal cord of rats with experimental allergic encephalomyelitis. *Neuroscience.* (2001) 102:687–95. doi: 10.1016/S0306-4522(00)00504-2

141. Sakurai K, Zou JP, Tschetter JR, Ward JM, Shearer GM. Effect of indoleamine 2,3-dioxygenase on induction of experimental autoimmune encephalomyelitis. *J Neuroimmunol.* (2002) 129:186–96. doi: 10.1016/S0165-5728(02)00176-5

142. Kwidzinski E, Bunse J, Aktas O, Richter D, Mutlu L, Zipp F, et al. Indolamine 2,3-dioxygenase is expressed in the CNS and down-regulates autoimmune inflammation. *FASEB J.* (2005) 19:1347–9. doi: 10.1096/fj.04-3228fje

143. Kwidzinski E, Bechmann I. IDO expression in the brain: a double-edged sword. *J Mol Med.* (2007) 85:1351–9. doi: 10.1007/s00109-007-0229-7

144. Savitz J, Dantzer R, Meier TB, Wurfel BE, Victor TA, McIntosh SA, et al. Activation of the kynurenine pathway is associated with striatal volume in major depressive disorder. *Psychoneuroendocrinology.* (2015) 62:54–8. doi: 10.1016/j.psyneuen.2015.07.609

145. Stone TW, Darlington LG. The kynurenine pathway as a therapeutic target in cognitive and neurodegenerative disorders. *Br J Pharmacol.* (2013) 169:1211–27. doi: 10.1111/bph.12230s

146. Erhardt S, Schwieler L, Imbeault S, Engberg G. The kynurenine pathway in schizophrenia and bipolar disorder. *Neuropharmacology.* (2017) 112:297–306. doi: 10.1016/j.neuropharm.2016.05.020

147. Wonodi I, Stine OC, Sathyasaikumar KV, Robers RC, Mitchell BD, Hong LE, et al. Downregulated kynurenine 3-monooxygenase gene expression and enzyme activity in schizophrenia and genetic association with schizophrenia endophenotypes. *Arch Gen Psychiatry.* (2011) 68:665–74. doi: 10.1001/archgenpsychiatry.2011.71.

148. Owe-Young R, Webster NL, Mukhtar M, Pomerantz RJ, Smythe G, Walker D, et al. Kynurenine pathway metabolism in human blood-brain-barrier cells: implications for immune tolerance and neurotoxicity. *J Neurochem.* (2008) 105:1346–57. doi: 10.1111/j.1471-4159.2008.05241.x

149. Steiner J, Bogerts B, Sarnyai Z, Walter M, Gos T, Bernstein HG, et al. Bridging the gap between the immune and glutamate hypotheses of schizophrenia and major depression: potential role of glial NMDA receptor modulators and impaired blood-brain barrier integrity. *World J Biol Chem.* (2012) 13:482–92. doi: 10.3109/15622975.2011.583941

150. Guillemin GJ. Quinolinic acid, the inescapable neurotoxin. *FEBS J.* (2012) 79:1356–65. doi: 10.1111/j.1742-4658.2012.08485.x

151. St'astný F, Skultétyová I, Pliss L, Jezová D. Quinolinic acid enhances permeability of rat brain microvessels to plasma albumin. *Brain Res Bull.* (2000) 53:415–20. doi: 10.1016/S0361-9230(00)00368-3

152. Baranyi A, Amouzadeh-Ghadikolai O, vone Lewinski D, Breitenecker RJ, Stojakovic T, Maerz W, et al. Beta-trace protein as a new noninvasive immunological marker for quinolinic acid-induced blood-brain barrier integrity. *Sci Rep.* (2017) 7:43642. doi: 10.1038/srep43642

153. Olah G, Heredi J, Menyhart A, Czinege Z, Nagy D, Fuzik J, et al. Unexpected effects of peripherally administered kynurenic acid on cortical spreading depression and related blood-brain barrier permeability. *Drug Des Dev Ther.* (2013) 7:981–7. doi: 10.2147/DDDT.S44496

154. Maes M, Yirmiya R, Noraberg J, Brene S, Hibbeln J, Perini G, et al. The inflammatory and neurodegenerative hypothesis of depression: leads for future research and new drug developments in depression. *Metab Brain Dis.* (2009) 24:27–53. doi: 10.1007/s11011-008-9118-1

155. Dantzer R, O'Connor JC, Lawson MA, Kelley KW. (2011). Inflammation-associated depression: from serotonin to kynurenine. *Psychoneuroendocrinology.* 36:426–436. doi: 10.1016/j.psyneuen.2010.09.012

156. Reus GZ, Jansen K, Titus S, Carvalho AF, Gabbay V, Quevedo J. Kynurenine pathway dysfunction in the pathophysiology and treatment of depression: evidences from animal and human studies. *J Psychiat Res.* (2015) 68:316–28. doi: 10.1016/j.jpsychires.2015.05.007

157. Sforzini L, Nettis MA, Mondelli V, Pariante CM. Inflammation in cancer and depression: a starring role for the kynurenine pathway. *Psychopharmacology.* (2019) 236:2997–3011. doi: 10.1007/s00213-019-05200-8

158. Stone TW. Does kynurenic acid act on nicotinic receptors? *An assessment of the evidence. J. Neurochem.* (in press). doi: 10.1111/jnc.14907

159. Miller AH, Haroon E, Raison CL, Felger JC. Cytokine targets in the brain: impact on neurotransmitters and neurocircuits. *Depress Anxiety.* (2013) 30:297–306. doi: 10.1002/da.22084

160. Clark CJ, Mackay GM, Smythe GA, Bustamante S, Stone TW, Phillips RS. Prolonged survival of a murine model of cerebral malaria by kynurenine pathway inhibition. *Infect Immun.* (2005) 73:5249–51. doi: 10.1128/IAI.73.8.5249-5251.2005

161. Forrest CM, Khalil OS, Pisar M, Darlington LG, Stone TW. Prenatal inhibition of the tryptophan - kynurenine pathway alters synaptic plasticity and protein expression in the rat hippocampus. *Brain Res.* (2013) 1504:1–15. doi: 10.1016/j.brainres.2013.01.031

162. Forrest CM, Khalil OS, Pisar M, McNair K, Kornisiuk E, Snitcofsky M, et al. Changes in synaptic transmission and protein expression in the brains of adult offspring after prenatal inhibition of the kynurenine pathway. *Neuroscience.* (2013) 254:241–59. doi: 10.1016/j.neuroscience.2013.09.034

163. Khalil OS, Pisar M, Forrest CM, Vincenten MCJ, Darlington LG, Stone TW. Prenatal inhibition of the kynurenine pathway leads to structural changes in the hippocampus of adult rat offspring. *Euro J Neurosci.* (2014) 39:1558–71. doi: 10.1111/ejn.12535

164. Pisar M, Forrest CM, Khalil OS, McNair K, Vincenten MCJ, Qasem S, et al. Modified neocortical and cerebellar protein expression and morphology following prenatal inhibition of the kynurenine pathway. *Brain Res.* (2014) 1576:1–17. doi: 10.1016/j.brainres.2014.06.016

165. Forrest CM, McNair K, Pisar M, Khalil OS, Darlington LG, Stone TW. Altered hippocampal plasticity by prenatal kynurenine administration, kynurenine-3-monoxygenase (KMO) deletion or galantamine. *Neuroscience.* (2015) 310:91–105. doi: 10.1016/j.neuroscience.2015.09.022

166. Giorgini F, Huang SY, Sathyasaikumar KV, Notarangelo FM, Thomas MAR, Tararina M, et al. Targeted deletion of kynurenine 3-monooxygenase in mice: a new tool for studying kynurenine pathway metabolism in periphery and brain. *J Biol Chem.* (2013) 288:36554–66. doi: 10.1074/jbc.M113.503813

167. Rodgers J, Stone TW, Barrett MP, Bradley B, Kennedy PGE. Kynurenine pathway inhibition reduces central nervous system inflammation in a model of human African trypanosomiasis. *Brain.* (2009) 132:1259–67. doi: 10.1093/brain/awp074

168. Milosavljevic N, Gazdic M, Markovic BS, Arsenijevic A, Nurkovic J, Dolicanin Z, et al. Mesenchymal stem cells attenuate liver fibrosis by suppressing Th17 cells - an experimental study. *Transpl Int.* (2018) 31:102–15. doi: 10.1111/tri.13023

169. Markovic BS, Gazdic M, Arsenijevic A, Jovicic N, Jeremic J, Djonov V, et al. Mesenchymal stem cells attenuate cisplatin-induced nephrotoxicity in iNOS-dependent manner. *Stem Cells Int.* (2017) 2017:1315378. doi: 10.1155/2017/1315378

170. Gazdic M, Markovic BS, Jovicic N, Misirkic-Marjanovic M, Djonov V, Jakovljevic V, et al. Mesenchymal stem cells promote metastasis of lung cancer cells by downregulating systemic antitumor immune response. *Stem Cells Int.* (2017) 2017:6294717. doi: 10.1155/2017/6294717

171. Mariuzzi L, Domenis R, Orsaria M, Marzinotto S, Londero AP, Bulfoni M, et al. Functional expression of aryl hydrocarbon receptor on mast cells populating human endometriotic tissues. *Lab Invest.* (2016) 96:959–71. doi: 10.1038/labinvest.2016.74

172. Deac OM, Mills JL, Gardiner CM, Shane B, Quinn L, Midttun O, et al. Serum immune system biomarkers neopterin and interleukin-10 are strongly related to tryptophan metabolism in healthy young adults. *J Nutr.* (2016) 146:1801–6. doi: 10.3945/jn.116.230698

173. Wirthgen E, Otten W, Tuchscherer M, Tuchscherer A, Domanska G, Brenmoehl J, et al. Effects of 1-methyltryptophan on immune responses and the kynurenine pathway after lipopolysaccharide challenge in pigs. *Int J Mol Sci.* (2018) 19:3009. doi: 10.3390/ijms19103009

174. Farup PG, Ueland T, Rudi K, Lydersen S, Hestad K. Functional bowel disorders are associated with a central immune activation. *Gastroenterol Res Pract.* (2017) 2017:1642912. doi: 10.1155/2017/1642912

175. Pichler R, Gruenbacher G, Culig Z, Brunner A, Fuchs D, Fritz J, et al. Intratumoral Th2 predisposition combines with an increased Th1 functional phenotype in clinical response to intravesical BCG in bladder cancer. *Cancer Immunol Immunother.* (2017) 66:427–40. doi: 10.1007/s00262-016-1945-z

176. Coutinho LG, Christen S, Bellac CL, Fontes FL, Soares de Souza FR, Grandgirard D, et al. The kynurenine pathway is involved in bacterial meningitis. *J Neuroinflamm.* (2014) 11:169.doi: 10.1186/s12974-014-0169-4

177. Metghalchi S, Ponnuswamy P, Simon T, Haddad Y, Laurans L, Clement M, et al. Indoleamine 2,3-dioxygenase fine-tunes immune homeostasis in atherosclerosis and colitis through repression of interleukin-10 production. *Cell Metab.* (2015) 22:460–71. doi: 10.1016/j.cmet.2015.07.004

178. Maneechotesuwan K, Kasetsinsombat K, Wamanuttajinda V, Wongkajornsilp A, Barnes PJ. Statins enhance the effects of corticosteroids on the balance between regulatory T cells and Th17 cells. *Clin Exp Allergy.* (2013) 43:212–22. doi: 10.1111/cea.12067

179. de Araujo EF, Feriotti C, de Lima Galdino NA, Preite NW, Garcia CVL, Loures FV. The IDO-AHR axis controls Th17/treg immunity in a pulmonary model of fungal infection. *Front Immunol.* (2017) 8:880. doi: 10.3389/fimmu.2017.00880

180. Zheng S, Shao S, Qiao Z, Chen X, Piao C, Yu Y, et al. Clinical parameters and gut microbiome changes before and after surgery in thoracic aortic dissection in patients with gastrointestinal complications. *Sci Rep.* (2017) 7:15228. doi: 10.1038/s41598-017-15079-0

181. Matysik-Wozniak A, Paduch R, Turski WA, Maciejewski R, Juenemann AG, Rejdak R. Effects of tryptophan, kynurenine and kynurenic acid exerted on human reconstructed corneal epithelium *in vitro. Pharmacol Rep.* (2017) 69:722–9. doi: 10.1016/j.pharep.2017.02.020

182. Wiedlocha M, Marcinowicz P, Krupa R, Janoska-Jazdzik M, Janus M, Debowska W, et al. Effect of antidepressant treatment on peripheral inflammation markers - a meta-analysis. *Progr Neuropsychopharmacol Biol Psychiatry.* (2018) 80:217–26. doi: 10.1016/j.pnpbp.2017.04.026

183. Rao NP, Venkatasubramanian G, Ravi V, Kalmady S, Cherian A, Reddy J. Plasma cytokine abnormalities in drug-naive, comorbidity-free obsessive-compulsive disorder. *Psychiatry Res.* (2015) 229:949–52. doi: 10.1016/j.psychres.2015.07.009

184. Yang RN, Gao N, Chang Q, Meng XC, Wang WH. The role of IDO, IL-10 and TGF-β in the HCV-associated chronic hepatitis, liver cirrhosis and hepatocellular carcinoma. *J Med Virol.* (2019) 91:265–71. doi: 10.1002/jmv.25083

185. Lanis JM, Alexeev EE, Curtis VF, Kitzenberg DA, Kao DJ, Battista KD, et al. Tryptophan metabolite activation of the aryl hydrocarbon receptor regulates IL-10 receptor expression on intestinal epithelia. *Mucosal Immunol.* (2017) 10:1133–44. doi: 10.1038/mi.2016.133

186. Kim NS, Torrez T, Langridge W. LPS enhances CTB-insulin induction of IDO1 and IL-10 synthesis in human dendritic cells. *Cell Immunol.* (2019) 338:32–42. doi: 10.1016/j.cellimm.2019.03.003

187. Coquerelle C, Oldenhove G, Acolty V, Denoeud J, Vansanten G, Verdebout JM, et al. Anti-CTLA-4 treatment induces IL-10-producing ICOS+ regulatory T cells displaying IDO-dependent anti-inflammatory properties in a mouse model of colitis. *Gut.* (2009) 58:1363–73. doi: 10.1136/gut.2008.162842

188. Luo CF, Jia WW, Wang K, Chi FL, Gu YQ, Yan XL, et al. Human amniotic fluid stem cells suppress PBMC proliferation through IDO and IL-10-dependent pathways. *Curr Stem Cell Res Ther.* (2014) 9:36–45. doi: 10.2174/1574888X113086660067

189. Alameddine J, Godefroy E, Papargyris L, Sarrabayrouse G, Tabiasco J, Bridonneau C, et al. *Faecalibacterium prausnitzii* skews human DC to prime IL10-producing T cells through TLR2/6/JNK signalling and IL-10, IL-27, CD39 and IDO-1 induction. *Front Immunol.* (2019) 10:143. doi: 10.3389/fimmu.2019.00143

190. Eisenbacher JL, Schrezenmeier H, Jahrsdorfer B, Kaltenmeier C, Rojewski MT, Yildiz T, et al. S100A4 and uric acid promote mesenchymal stromal cell induction of IL-10(+)/IDO+ lymphocytes. *J Immunol.* (2014) 192:6102–10. doi: 10.4049/jimmunol.1303144

191. Banerjee T, DuHadaway JB, Gaspari P, Sutanto-Ward E, Munn DH, Mellor AL, et al. A key *in vivo* antitumor mechanism of action of natural product-based brassinins is inhibition of indoleamine-2,3-dioxygenase. *Oncogene.* (2008) 27:2851–7. doi: 10.1038/sj.onc.1210939

192. Miller CA. Expression of the human aryl hydrocarbon receptor complex in yeast. Activation of transcription by indole compounds. *J Biol Chem.* (1997) 272:32824–9. doi: 10.1074/jbc.272.52. 32824

193. Guengerich PF, Martin MV, McCormick WA, Nguyen LP, Glover E, Bradfield CA. Aryl hydrocarbon receptor response to indigoids *in vitro* and *in vivo. Arch Biochem Biophys.* (2004) 423:309–16. doi: 10.1016/j.abb.2004.01.002

194. Benson JM, Shepherd DM. Aryl hydrocarbon receptor activation by tcdd reduces inflammation associated with Crohn's Disease. *Toxicol Sci.* (2011) 120:68–78. doi: 10.1093/toxsci/kfq360

195. Benson JM, Shepherd DM. Dietary ligands of the aryl hydrocarbon receptor induce anti-inflammatory and immunoregulatory effects on murine dendritic cells. *Toxicol Sci.* (2011) 124:327–38. doi: 10.1093/toxsci/kfr249

196. Notarangelo FM, Pocivavsek A. Elevated kynurenine pathway metabolism during neurodevelopment: Implications for brain and behaviour. *Neuropharmacology.* (2017) 112:275–85. doi: 10.1016/j.neuropharm.2016.03.001

197. Pocivavsek A, Thomas MAR, Elmer GI, Bruno JP, Schwarcz R. Continuous kynurenine administration during the prenatal period, but not during adolescence, causes learning and memory deficits in adult rats. *Psychopharmacology.* (2014) 231:2799–809. doi: 10.1007/s00213-014-3452-2

198. Pocivavsek A, Elmer GI, Schwarcz R. Inhibition of kynurenine aminotransferase II attenuates hippocampus-dependent memory deficit in adult rats treated prenatally with kynurenine. *Hippocampus.* (2019) 29:73–7. doi: 10.1002/hipo.23040

199. Hahn B, Reneski CH, Pocivavsek A, Schwarcz R. Prenatal kynurenine treatment in rats causes schizophrenia-like broad monitoring deficits in adulthood. *Psychopharmacology.* (2018) 235:651–61.doi: 10.1007/s00213-017-4780-9

200. Schwieler L, Larsson MK, Skogh E, Kegel ME, Orhan F, Abdelmoaty S, et al. Increased levels of IL-6 in the cerebrospinal fluid of patients with chronic schizophrenia - significance for activation of the kynurenine pathway. *J Psychiat Neurosci.* (2015) 40:126–33. doi: 10.1503/jpn.140126

201. Anderson G, Maes M. Schizophrenia: linking prenatal infection to cytokines, the tryptophan catabolite (TRYCAT) pathway, NMDA receptor hypofunction, neuro-development and neuroprogression. *Progr Neuropsychopharmacol Biol Psychiatry.* (2013) 42:5–19. doi: 10.1016/j.pnpbp.2012.06.014

202. Vorhees CV, Graham DL, Braun AA, Schaefer TL, Skelton MR, Richtand NM, et al. Prenatal immune challenge in rats: Effects of polyinosinic-polycytidylic acid on spatial learning, prepulse inhibition, conditioned fear, and responses to MK-801 and amphetamine. *Neurotoxicol Teratol.* (2015) 47:54–65. doi: 10.1016/j.ntt.2014.10.007

203. Meehan C, Harms L, Frost JD, Barreto R, Todd J, Schall U, et al. Effects of immune activation during early or late gestation on schizophrenia-related behaviour in adult rat offspring. *Brain Behav Immun.* (2017) 63:8–20. doi: 10.1016/j.bbi.2016.07.144

204. Mueller N. Inflammation in schizophrenia: pathogenetic aspects and therapeutic considerations. *Schizophrenia Bull.* (2018) 44:973–82. doi: 10.1093/schbul/sby024

205. Clark SM, Notarangelo FM, Li X, Chen S, Schwarcz R, Tonelli LH. Maternal immune activation in rats blunts brain cytokine and kynurenine pathway responses to a second immune challenge in early adulthood. *Prog Neuropsychopharmacol Biol Psychiatry.* (2019) 89:286–94. doi: 10.1016/j.pnpbp.2018.09.011

206. Zager A, Pinheiro ML, Ferraz-de-Paula V, Ribeiro A, Palermo-Neto J. Increased cell-mediated immunity in male mice offspring exposed to maternal immune activation during late gestation. *Int Immunopharmcol.* (2013) 17:633–637. doi: 10.1016/j.intimp.2013.08.007

207. Song W, Zsindely N, Farago A, Marsh JL, Bodai L. Systematic genetic interaction studies identify histone demethylase UTX as potential target for ameliorating Huntington's disease. *Hum Mol Genet.* (2018) 27:649–66. doi: 10.1093/hmg/ddx432

208. Thomas EA. DNA methylation in Huntington's disease: implications for trans-generational effects. *Neurosci Lett.* (2016) 625:34–9. doi: 10.1016/j.neulet.2015.10.060

209. Yeh HH, Young D, Gelovani JG, Robinson A, Davidson Y, Herholz K, et al. Histone deacetylase class II and acetylated core histone immune-histochemistry in human brains with Huntington's disease. *Brain Res.* (2013) 1504:16–24. doi: 10.1016/j.brainres.2013.02.012

210. Suelves N, Kirkham-McCarthy L, Lahue RS, Gines S. A selective inhibitor of histone deacetylase 3 prevents cognitive deficits and suppresses striatal

CAG repeat expansions in Huntington's disease mice. *Sci Rep.* (2017) 7:6082. doi: 10.1038/s41598-017-05125-2

211. Mollica PA, Reid JA, Ogle RC, Sachs PC, Bruno RD. DNA Methylation leads to DNA repair gene down-regulation and trinucleotide repeat expansion in patient-derived Huntington disease cells. *Am J Pathol.* (2016) 186:1967–76. doi: 10.1016/j.ajpath.2016.03.014

212. Angiolilli C, Kabala PA, Grabiec AM, Van Baarsen IM, Ferguson BS, Garcia S, et al. Histone deacetylase 3 regulates the inflammatory gene expression programme of rheumatoid arthritis fibroblast-like synoviocytes. *Ann Rheum Dis.* (2017) 76:277–85. doi: 10.1136/annrheumdis-2015-209064

213. Oh BR, Suh DH, Bae D, Ha N, Choi Y, Yoo HJ, et al. Therapeutic effect of a novel histone deacetylase 6 inhibitor, CKD-L, on collagen-induced arthritis *in vivo* and regulatory T cells in rheumatoid arthritis *in vitro. Arthritis Res Ther.* (2017) 19:154. doi: 10.1186/s13075-017-1357-2

214. Ai R, Hammaker D, Boyle DL, Morgan R, Walsh AM, Fan S, et al. Joint-specific DNA methylation and transcriptome signatures in rheumatoid arthritis identify distinct pathogenic processes. *Nat Comm.* (2016) 7:11849. doi: 10.1038/ncomms11849

215. Lin Y, Luo Z. Aberrant methylation patterns affect the molecular pathogenesis of rheumatoid arthritis. *Int Immunopharmacol.* (2017) 46:141–5. doi: 10.1016/j.intimp.2017.02.008

216. Glossop JR, Nixon NB, Emes RD, Sim J, Packham JC, Mattey DL, et al. DNA methylation at diagnosis is associated with response to disease-modifying drugs in early rheumatoid arthritis. *Epigenomics.* (2017) 9:419–28. doi: 10.2217/epi-2016-0042

217. Fang G, Zhang QH, Tang Q, Jiang Z, Xing S, Li J, et al. Comprehensive analysis of gene expression and DNA methylation datasets identify valuable biomarkers for rheumatoid arthritis progression. *Oncotarget.* (2018) 9:2977–83. doi: 10.18632/oncotarget.22918

218. Zafari P, Yari K, Mostafaei S, Iranshahi N, Assar S, Fekri A, et al. Analysis of Helios gene expression and Foxp3 TSDR methylation in the newly diagnosed rheumatoid arthritis patients. *Immunol Invest.* (2018) 47:632–42. doi: 10.1080/08820139.2018.1480029

219. Araki Y, Aizaki Y, Sato K, Oda H, Kurokawa R, Mimura T. Altered gene expression profiles of histone lysine methyltransferases and demethylases in rheumatoid arthritis synovial fibroblasts. *Clin Exp Rheumatol.* (2018) 36:314–6.

220. Plant D, Webster A, Nair N, Oliver J, Smith SL, Eyre S, et al. Differential methylation as a biomarker of response to etanercept in patients with rheumatoid arthritis. *Arthritis Rheumatol.* (2016) 68:1353–60. doi: 10.1002/art.39590

221. Jacobs KR, Castellano-Gonzalez G, Guillemin GJ, Lovejoy DB. Major developments in the design of inhibitors along the kynurenine pathway. *Curr Med Chem.* (2017) 24:2471–95. doi: 10.2174/0929867324666170502123114

222. Dounay AB, Tuttle JB, Verhoestt PR. Challenges and opportunities in the discovery of new therapeutics targeting the kynurenine pathway. *J Med Chem.* (2015) 26:8762–82. doi: 10.1021/acs.jmedchem.5b00461

223. Phillips RS, Iradukunda EC, Hughes T, Bowen JP. Modulation of Enzyme Activity in the Kynurenine Pathway by Kynurenine Monooxygenase Inhibition. *Front Molec Biosci.* (2019) 6:3. doi: 10.3389/fmolb.2019.00003

224. Hutchinson JP, Rowland P, Taylor MRD, Christodoulou EM, Haslam C, Hobbs CI, et al. Structural and mechanistic basis of differentiated inhibitors of the acute pancreatitis target kynurenine-3-monooxygenase. *Nature Commun.* (2017) 8:15827. doi: 10.1038/ncomms15827

225. Walker AL, Ancellin N, Beaufils B, Bergeal M, Binnie M, Bouillot A et al. Development of a series of kynurenine 3-monooxygenase inhibitors leading to a clinical candidate for the treatment of acute pancreatitis. *J Med Chem.* (2017) 60:3383–04. doi: 10.1021/acs.jmedchem.7b00055

226. Amin SA, Adhikari N, Jha, T, Gayen S. First molecular modeling report on novel arylpyrimidine kynurenine monooxygenase inhibitors through multi-QSAR analysis against Huntington's disease: A proposal to chemists! *Bioorg Med Chem Lett.* (2016) 26:5712–18. doi: 10.1016/j.bmcl.2016.10.058

227. Rossi F, Miggiano R, Ferraris DM, Rizzi M. The synthesis of kynurenic acid in mammals: an updated kynurenine aminotransferase structural katalogue. *Front Molec Biosci.* (2019) 6:7. doi: 10.3389/fmolb.2019.00007

228. Nematollahi A, Sun GC, Jayawickrama GS, Hanrahan JR, Church WB. Study of the activity and possible mechanism of action of a reversible inhibitor of recombinant human KAT-2: a promising lead in neurodegenerative and cognitive disorders. *Molecules.* (2016) 21:856. doi: 10.3390/molecules21070856

229. Pellicciari R, Liscio P, Giacche N, De Franco F, Carotti A, Robertson J. et al. Alpha-Amino-beta-carboxymuconate-epsilon-semialdehyde Decarboxylase (ACMSD) inhibitors as novel modulators of de novo nicotinamide adenine dinucleotide (NAD(+)) biosynthesis. *J Med Chem.* (2018) 61:745–59. doi: 10.1021/acs.jmedchem.7b01254

230. Yoshida Y, Fujigaki H, Kato K, Yamazaki K, Fujigaki S, Kunisawa K, et al. Selective and competitive inhibition of kynurenine aminotransferase 2 by glycyrrhizic acid and its analogues. *Sci Rept.* (2019) 9:10243. doi: 10.1038/s41598-019-46666-y

231. Hu H, Li M, Wu D, Li ZW, Miao RF, Liu Y, et al. Design, synthesis and biological evaluation of novel aryl-acrylic derivatives as novel indoleamine-2,3-dioxygenase 1 (IDO1) inhibitors. *Bioorg Med Chem.* (2019) 27:3135–44. doi: 10.1016/j.bmc.2019.05.048

232. Yang R, Chen Y, Pan LK, Yang YY, Zheng Q, Hu Y, et al. Design, synthesis and structure-activity relationship study of novel naphthoindolizine and indolizinoquinoline-5,12-dione derivatives as IDO1 inhibitors. *Bioorg Med Chem.* (2018) 26:4886–97. doi: 10.1016/j.bmc.2018.08.028

233. Pan LK, Zheng Q, Chen Y, Yang R, Yang YY, Li ZJ, et al. Design, synthesis and biological evaluation of novel naphthoquinone derivatives as IDO1 inhibitors. *Europ J Med Chem.* (2018) 157:423–36. doi: 10.1016/j.ejmech.2018.08.013

234. Zou Y, Wang F, Wang Y, Sun QR, Hu Y, Li YZ, et al. Discovery of imidazoleisoindole derivatives as potent IDO1 inhibitors: Design, synthesis, biological evaluation and computational studies. *Europ J Med Chem.* (2017) 140:293–304. doi: 10.1016/j.ejmech.2017.09.025

235. Gao DD, Li YX. Identification and preliminary structure-activity relationships of 1-Indanone derivatives as novel indoleamine-2,3-dioxygenase 1 (IDO1) inhibitors. *Bioorg Med Chem.* (2017) 25:3780–91. doi: 10.1016/j.bmc.2017.05.017

236. Schwarcz R, Stone TW. The kynurenine pathway and the brain: challenges, controversies and promises. *Neuropharmacology.* (2017) 112:237–47. doi: 10.1016/j.neuropharm.2016.08.003

14

The Opposite Effects of Kynurenic Acid and Different Kynurenic Acid Analogs on Tumor Necrosis Factor-α (TNF-α) Production and Tumor Necrosis Factor-Stimulated Gene-6 (TSG-6) Expression

Yvette Mándi[1]*, Valéria Endrész[1], Timea Mosolygó[1], Katalin Burián[1], Ildikó Lantos[1], Ferenc Fülöp[2], István Szatmári[2], Bálint Lőrinczi[2], Attila Balog[3] and László Vécsei[4]

[1] Department of Medical Microbiology and Immunobiology, University of Szeged, Szeged, Hungary, [2] Institute of Pharmaceutical Chemistry and Research Group for Stereochemistry, Hungarian Academy of Sciences, University of Szeged, Szeged, Hungary, [3] Department of Rheumatology and Immunology, University of Szeged, Szeged, Hungary, [4] Department of Neurology, University of Szeged, Szeged, Hungary

*Correspondence:
Yvette Mándi
mandi.yvette@med.u-szeged.hu

Purpose: The investigation of anti-inflammatory and immunosuppressive functions of Kynurenic acid (KYNA) is now in focus. There is also substantial evidence that TSG-6 has an anti-inflammatory activity. Therefore, in the present study, we compared the effects of newly synthetized KYNA analogs on the TNF-α production in U-937 monocytic cells in correlation with the effects on the TSG-6 expression.

Methods: TNF-α production was measured by ELISA, the TSG-6 expression was determined by RTqPCR method. As cytokine inducers *Staphylococcus aureus* and *Chlamydia pneumoniae* were used.

Results: KYNA and KYNA analogs attenuated TNF-α production and increased TSG-6 mRNA expression in U-937 cells stimulated by heat inactivated *Staphylococcus aureus*. In contrast, KYNA and some of the KYNA analogs increased the TNF-α production of *C. pneumoniae* infected U-937 cells; however, the newly synthetized analogs (SZR104, SZR 105, and SZR 109) exerted significant inhibitory effects on the TNF-α synthesis. The inhibitory and stimulatory effects correlated inversely with the TSG-6 expression.

Conclusions: TSG-6 expression following activation with bacterial components could participate in the suppression of inflammatory cytokines, such as TNF-α, We suppose that the elevation of the TSG-6 expression by KYNA and especially by new KYNA analogs might be one of the mechanisms that are responsible for their suppressive effect on TNF-α production as a feedback mechanism. KYNA and KYNA analogs have an important role in influencing TSG-6 expression, and there is a possible benefit of targeting TSG-6 expression by kynurenines in inflammatory conditions following infections.

Keywords: kynurenic acid, TNF-α, TSG-6, U-937, *Staphylococcus, Chlamydia pneumoniae*

INTRODUCTION

There is an increasing interest in the role of kynurenines in the immune function. The kynurenine pathway is a regulator of both innate and adaptive immune responses, and the tryptophan metabolism kynurenine and production reflect a crucial interface between the immune and nervous systems (1, 2). Kynurenic acid (KYNA) is one of the products of the kynurenine pathway of tryptophan metabolism (3–5). KYNA as an antagonist of ionotropic glutamate receptors N-methyl-D-aspartate (NMDA) and the α7 nicotinic acetylcholine receptor (α7nAchR) exert neuroprotective effects (2, 4–10). KYNA acts both as a blocker of the glycine co-agonistic site of the NMDA receptor and as a non-competitive inhibitor of the α7 nicotinic acetylcholine receptor (11). The investigation of anti-inflammatory and immunosuppressive functions of KYNA is now in focus. It has been proved that these immunomodulatory properties are based on the signaling by G-protein-coupled receptor 35 (GP35) and aryl hydrocarbon receptor (AHR)-mediated pathways ys (2, 12–14).

Several studies have revealed that KYNA can attenuate inflammation induced by different stimuli (2, 15, 16). Previously, we demonstrated that KYNA and a KYNA analog reduced the TNF-α secretion from human mononuclear cells (17). In the present study, we compared the effects of newly synthetized KYNA analogs on the α TNF-α production in U-937 monocytic cell line. We focused on the potential correlation between the effects on the TSG-6 (TNFα- stimulated gene 6) expression and the influence, i.e., the suppression, of TNF-α production by different KYNA analogs.

Tumor necrosis factor -stimulated gene-6 (TSG-6) product is an 35-kDa hyaluronan(HA)-binding protein (18, 19) that is secreted by a wide range of cell types in response to inflammatory mediators. TSG-6 expression has been shown to be induced in fibroblasts, chondrocytes, monocytes, mesenchymal stem cells, vascular smooth muscle cells upon stimulation by proinflammatory signals (20). Moreover, TSG-6 is expressed by astrocytes in the brain (21). A substantial number of studies have shown that TSG-6 has anti-inflammatory activity (18, 20, 22–27).

TSG-6 has been reported to inhibit the association of TLR4 with MyD88, thereby suppressing NF-κB activation (26). TSG-6 has also prevented the expression of proinflammatory proteins (iNOS, IL-6, TNFα, IL-1β). TSG-6 functions by converting macrophages from a proinflammatory to an anti-inflammatory phenotype by suppression of TLR4/NF-κB signaling and STAT1 and STAT3 activation (26).The inhibition of the TLR2 pathway has also been reported (28).

Therefore, the aim of the present study is to evaluate a possible connection between the capacity of KYNA and KYNA analogs on the TSG-6 expression and the inhibition of TNF-α production first of all in U-937 monocytic cells. Our hypothesis was that activation of TSG-6 expression might be at least partially responsible for the TNF-α inhibitory effect of KYNA. TNF-α induction in U-937 cells was performed with heat killed *Staphylococcus aureus*, and the effects were compared with *Chlamydia pneumoniae (C. pneumoniae)*. *Staphylococcus aureus* is a Gram-positive pyogenic coccus and a good inducer of TNF in mononuclear cells, and it mimics natural conditions (29, 30). *Chlamydia pneumoniae* is a Gram-negative bacterium, growing intracellularly, and it is responsible for different inflammatry conditions, especially in the lungs and in atherosclerosis. *Chlamydia pneumoniae* attach monocytes and multiply in them (31).The main question was, whether the production of TNF-α, and TSG-6 could be induced by these criteriae in U-937 cells. It was demonstrated in a previous study, that *C.pneumoniae* upregulated. numerous inflammatory genes in U-937 cells (32).

MATERIALS AND METHODS

Reagents

KYNA (Kynurenic acid) was purchased from Sigma-Aldrich (Steinheim, Germany). Compounds SZR-72, SZR-73, and SZR-81 were synthesized by direct amidation of KYNA (33). In case of SZR-104, SZR-105, and SZR-109, the syntheses were achieved starting from the corresponding amides followed by C-3 aminoalkylation with morpholine or with diethylamine in the presence of formaldehyde (34, 35) (**Table 1**). KYNA and the analogs were dissolved in phosphate buffered saline (PBS) and added in increasing concentration in the μM range to the cell cultures.

Cell Lines and Infection

U-937 cells were grown in RPMI 1640 medium supplemented with 10% heat-inactivated FBS (Biowest, Nuaille, France), 2 mmol/L L-glutamine, 1x nonessential amino acids, HEPES 4 mmol/L, 25 μg/mL gentamicin, and 0.5 μg/mL fungizone. HEp-2 cells were maintained in minimal essential medium (MEM) with Earle's salts completed with 10% FBS, 2 mmol/L L-glutamine, 1x nonessential amino acids, 25 μg/mL gentamicin, and 0.5 μg/mL fungizone. All reagents were purchased from SIGMA, St. Louis, MO, USA, unless otherwise indicated. The cell lines were purchased from ATCC. For TNF-α and TSG-6 induction, 5 × 10^5 U-937 cells/mL were infected with 10^7 heat inactivated *Staphylococcus aureus (S.aureus)*, or with 5 MOI (multiplicity of infection) *Chlamydia pneumoniae*. Cell supernatants were tested for TNF-α content by ELISA and cell lysates for TSG-6 mRNA by RT qPCR.

Bacterial Strains

Staphylococcus aureus (S. aureus, SA1) 10^8 /mL, were heat inactivated (29) and were used as a TNF-α inducer (30).

Chlamydia pneumoniae (C. pneumoniae) CWL029 strain from American Types Culture Collection (ATCC) was propagated in HEp-2 cells. Infective chlamydiae were quantitated by indirect immunofluorescent method applying anti-Chlamydia lipopolysaccharide (cLPS) monoclonal antibody (AbD Serotec, Oxford, United Kingdom) and FITC-labeled anti-mouse IgG (Sigma-Aldrich, St. Louis, MO). The concentration of infective elementary bodies (EB)-s was expressed as inclusion forming units/mL (IFU/mL).

TABLE 1 | KYNA and KYNA analogs used in the experiments.

Code	Structure	Chemical name	Empirical formula and Mw
KYNA		4-hydroxyquinolin-2-carboxylic acid	$C_{10}H_7NO_3$ 189.17
SzR-72		N-(2-(dimethylamino)ethyl)-4-hydroxyquinoline-2-carboxamide hydrochloride	$C_{14}H_{18}ClN_3O_2$ 295.76
SzR-73		N-(3-(dimethylamino)propyl)-4-hydroxyquinoline-2-carboxamide hydrochloride	$C_{15}H_{20}ClN_3O_2$ 309.79
SzR-81		N-(2-(pyrrolidin-1-yl)ethyl)-4-hydroxyquinoline-2-carboxamide hydrochloride	$C_{16}H_{20}ClN_3O_2$ 321.80
SzR-104		N-(2-(dimethylamino)ethyl)-3-(morpholinomethyl)-4-hydroxyquinoline-2-carboxamide	$C_{19}H_{26}N_4O_3$ 358.43
SzR-105		N-(2-(pyrrolidin-1-yl)ethyl)-3-(morpholinomethyl)-4-hydroxyquinoline-2-carboxamide	$C_{21}H_{28}N_4O_3$ 384.47
SzR-109		N-(2-(pyrrolidin-1-yl)ethyl)-3-((diethylamino)methyl)-4-hydroxyquinoline-2-carboxamide	$C_{21}H_{30}N_4O_2$ 370.49

Stimulation of U 937 Cells by Bacteria Infection

(a) U-937 cells (5 × 10^5 cells/mL) were stimulated with 10^7 heat inactivated *S. aureus* (29) as a TNF inducer (30) and were incubated for 24 h in CO_2 incubator at 37°C in complete RPMI. In parallel experiments, the cell cultures were pretreated for 30 min with KYNA and KYNA analoques at a concentration of 250–500 μM. In our prevous experiments (17), these concentrations proved to be optimal in reducing cytokine production. Cell supernatants were tested for TNF-α and TSG-6 content by ELISA and cell lysates for TSG-6 mRNA by RT qPCR.

(b) U-937 cells were seeded in 24-well plates (5 × 10^5 cells/well), and the cells were then infected with *C. pneumoniae* at a multiplicity of infection (MOI) of 5 in complete RPMI with 0.5% glucose and centrifuged at 800 × g for 1 h RT. The growth medium was replaced in the wells with a medium containing KYNA analogs at a concentration of 250–500 μM. The culture plates were incubated for 24 h in CO_2 incubator at 37°C. Cell supernatants were tested for TNF-α and TSG-6 content by ELISA and cell lysates for TSG-6 mRNA by RT qPCR.

Chlamydial DNA Quantitation

For the quantitative assessment of chlamydial replication, a direct DNA quantitation method was used (36). The cells in the 96-well plates were infected with *C. pneumoniae* at a multiplicity of infection (MOI) of 5. After 24 and 48 h, the infected cells in 3 parallel wells were washed in the plates twice with 200 μL/well phosphate buffered saline (PBS). Then 100 μL Milli-Q water was added to the wells, and the plates were stored at −80°C. In order to free the DNA from the cells, two freeze-thaw cycles were applied. Thoroughly mixed lysates were used as templates directly for quantitative PCR (qPCR) using SsoFast™ EvaGreen® Supermix (BioRad). For the detection of *C. pneumoniae* DNA, the following primers were used: *ompA* F: 5′ TGCGACGCTATTAGCTTACGT 3′ and *ompA* R: 5′ TAGTTTGCAGCAGCGGATCCA 3′. A BLAST search was performed to check the specificity of the product target sequence of the primer sets. The primers were synthetized by Integrated DNA Technologies Inc. (Montreal, Quebec, Canada). During qPCR reaction, after the 10 min at 95°C polymerase activation step, 40 PCR cycles of 20 s at 95°C, and 1 min at 64°C were performed. The fluorescence intensity was measured at the end of the annealing–extension step. The specificity of amplification was confirmed by the melting curve analysis. For each PCR, the cycle threshold (Ct) corresponding to the cycle, where the amplification curve crossed the base line, was determined. The difference in Ct values detected in the samples incubated with KYNA and the analogs at a concentration of 250 and 500 μM compared to that of the untreated samples was calculated.

TNF-α ELISA

The TNF-α concentrations in the supernatants were quantified by using the TNF-α ELISA kit (Legend Max BioLegend San Diego) according to the instructions of the manufacturer.

TSG-6 ELISA

The TSG-6 concentrations in the supernatants were quantified by using the TSG-6 ELISA kit (SIGMA U.S.A. St. Louis) according to the instructions of the manufacturer.

TSG-6 mRNA Quantification by Reverse Transcription Quantitative PCR (RT qPCR)

Total RNA was extracted from the samples by using TRI Reagent (Sigma-Aldrich, St. Louis, MO, USA) according to the manufacturer's protocol. The quality and the quantity of the extracted RNA were assessed by a NanoDrop Lite spectrophotometer (Thermo Scientific, Waltham, MA, USA). First-strand cDNA was synthesized by using 2 μg of total RNA with High-Capacity cDNA Reverse Transcription Kit (Applied Biosystems, Foster City, CA, USA) strictly adhering to the manufacturer's recommendations. The qPCR was conducted with cDNA, 1 μL of primers (10 μM) and SensiFast SYBR® No-ROX Mix (Bioline GmbH, Luckenwalde, Germany) in a total volume of 10 μL. The primers used in the assay were the following: TSG-6 sense 5′- ACT CAA GTA TGG TCA GCG TAT TC−3′, TSG-6 antisense 5′- GCC ATG GAC ATC ATC GTA ACT−3′; β-actin sense 5′- TTC TAC AAT GAG CTG CGT GTG GCT−3′, and β-actin antisense 5′- TAG CAC AGC CTG GAT AGC AAC GTA−3′. All primers were synthetized by Integrated DNA Technologies Inc. (Montreal, Quebec, Canada). The RT-qPCR was performed in a CFX96 Touch PCR detection system (Bio-Rad, Hercules, CA, USA). Thermal cycling was initiated with a denaturation step of 2 min at 95 °C followed by 40 cycles each of 10 s at 95°C and 1 min at 60°C. The fluorescence intensity was detected at the end of the annealing–extension steps. The specificity of amplification was confirmed by carrying out a melting curve analysis. The cycle threshold (C$_t$) corresponding to the cycle, where the amplification curve crossed the base line, was determined. The Ct of target transcripts was compared with that of β-actin, the difference being referred to as ΔC$_t$. The relative expression level was given as $2^{-(\Delta\Delta Ct)}$, where $\Delta\Delta C_t = \Delta C_t$ for the experimental sample minus ΔC$_t$ for the control sample. Increases in transcripts >2-fold compared to the control samples were considered to be significant. Uninfected cells were used as controls. All of the measurements were performed in duplicate from 3 biological repetitions.

Human Blood Samples

EDTA-anticoagulated peripheral blood samples from 10 healthy volunteers were obtained.

Samples (1 mL each) were incubated in the presence of heat inactivated S, aureus for 18 hr. Parallel blood samples were pretreated for 30 min with KYNA and KYNA analogs at a concentration of 500 μM. Following the incubation period, the blood samples were centrifuged at 300 × g, and the supernatants were tested for TNF-α and TSG-6 content by ELISA.

For the experiments performed with the human blood we have the approval of the ethics commitee of the Medical Faculty of the University. of Szeged (ETT-TUKEB 905/PI/09). This study was conducted in full accordance with the tenets of Declaration of Helsinki (1964).

Statistical Analysis

Data are expressed as means ± SD. Differences between group means were determined by the unpaired Student *t*-test. *p*-values <0.05 were considered significant. Data of box and whiskers analysis were evaluated by Mann-Whitney test. The correlation between the TNF-α production and expression of TSG-6 was evaluated by correlation analysis. All statistical calculations were performed with the Graph-Pad Prism 5 statistical program (GraphPad Software Inc., San Diego, CA, USA).

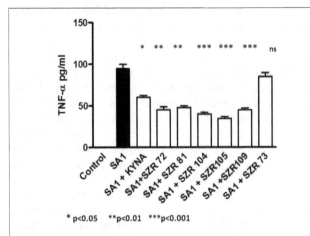

FIGURE 1 | KYNA and KYNA analogs attenuate TNF-α levels in SA1 stimulated U-937 cells. U-937 cells (5 × 10⁵/ml) were stimulated with heat inactivated SA (107/ml) alone, (filled bar), or incubated together with KYNA or KYNA analogs at a concentration of 500 μM, which were added for 30 min prior to the addition of SA1 (open bars). The TNF-α levels in the supernatants were determined after 24 h by ELISA. Each concentration was tested in duplicate. Data are shown as means ± SD of three experiments. *$p < 0.01$; **$p < 0.001$ vs. the samples induced only with SA1 determined by the Student t-test.

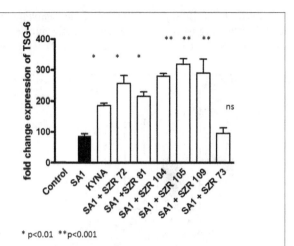

FIGURE 2 | Effect of 500 μM of KYNA and KYNA analogs on TSG-6 mRNA levels in U-937 monocytic cells stimulated with SA1. TSG-6 expressions were normalized to reference gene of β-actin by using quantitative real-time PCR. Relative expression was calculated by using the $2^{-(\Delta\Delta Ct)}$ method and is given as a ratio between the target and the reference gene. Control: TSG-6 mRNA expression without stimulation, Filled bar: TSG-6 mRNA expression in SA1-stimulated cells without KYNA or KYNA analoques, open bars: TSG-6 mRNA expression in SA1-stimulated cells in the presence of 500 μM KYNA or KYNA analogs. Data are shown as means ± SD of the results of three independent experiments. *$p < 0.01$ vs. SA1 induced cells without chemicals, **$p < 0.001$ vs. SA1 induced cells without chemicals, determined by the Student t-test.

RESULTS

KYNA and KYNA Analogs Attenuate TNF-α Production in U-937 Human Monocytic Cells Stimulated by Heat Inactivated *Staphylococcus aureus*

The maximum TNF-α concentrations in the supernatants in SA1-induced cultures of U-937 cells without pretreatment of KYNA and derivates were 95. ± 8.5 pg/mL. At a concentration of 500 μM, all KYNA analogs suppressed the TNF-α level significantly, except SZR 73 (**Figure 1**). The new analogs SZR 104, 105, and 109 exerted the most potent inhibitory effects ($p < 0.001$) in equimolar (500 μM) concentration. Results obtained with 500 μM of the chemicals are demonstrated in **Figure 1**. In our previous experiments (17), 25 μM KYNA and SZR72 proved to be ineffective. At increasing concentrations (125, 250, and 500 μM), KYNA and SZR72 exhibited increasing inhibitory effects on TNF-α production. Similar results were obtained in the present experiments (data not shown), but only the result with the most effective concentration (500 μM) is demonstrated in this paper (**Figure 1**).

KYNA and KYNA Analogs Increase TSG-6 mRNA Expression in U-937 Cells

To gain further insight into the connection between the inhibition of TNF-α production and the induction of TSG-6 expression exerted by KYNA analoques, we determined the effects of KYNA analoques on TSG-6 mRNA expression. Both KYNA and KYNA analogs increased the TSG-6 relative expression at equimolar concentrations of 500 μM (**Figure 2**) significantly. SZR 73 was not effective in this respect, similarly

as it was observed in the experiments with TNF-α production. Thus, we suspect that there is a connection between the attenuation of SA1-induced TNF protein synthesis and the TSG-6 gene transcription, which is elevated by KYNA and KYNA analoques.

KYNA and the KYNA Analogs Differently Influence TNF-α Production Induced by *C. pneumoniae* in U-937 Human Monocytic Cells

We wanted to compare the effects of KYNA and KYNA derivates on TNF-α production when the inducer is a Gram-negative, intracellular bacterium, i.e., *Chlamydia pneumoniae (C. pneumoniae)*. Our results were unexpected; instead of having inhibitory effects, KYNA and some of the KYNA analoques increased the TNF-α production of *C. pneumoniae* infected U-937 cells. In contrast, the newly synthetized analogs (SZR104, SZR 105, and SZR 109) exerted a significant inhibitory effect on the cytokine synthesis (**Figure 3**).

KYNA and KYNA Analogs Differently Influence TSG-6 mRNA Expression in U-937 Cells Infected With *Chlamydia pneumoniae*

C. pneumoniae induced a considerable TSG-6 expression in U-937 cells. KYNA, SZR72, and SZR81 inhibited the rate of expression (**Figure 4A**). Interestingly, the same chemicals enhanced the TNF-α production of *C. pneumoniae*-induced U-937 cells (**Figure 3**). On the other hand, further KYNA analoques (SZR 104, SZR 105, and SZR 109) with different

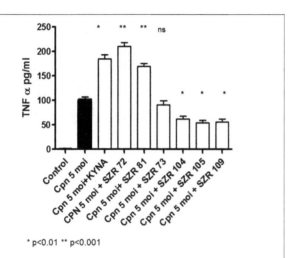

*p<0.01 **p<0.001

FIGURE 3 | Effect of KYNA and KYNA analogs on TNF-α production in U-937 human monocytic cells stimulated by *Chlamydia pneumonia*. U-937 cells were pretreated for 30 min with KYNA or KYNA analogs and thereafter incubated for 24 h with 5 MOI of *Chlamydia pneumoniae*. U-937 cells (5 × 10⁵/mL) were infected with 5 MOI of *Chlamydia pneumoniae* alone (filled bar), or incubated together with KYNA or KYNA analogs at a concentration of 500 μM, which were added for 30 min prior to the addition of the bacteria (open bars). The TNF-α levels in the supernatants were determined after 24 h. Each concentration was tested in duplicate. Data are shown as means ± SD of three experiments. *$p < 0.01$; **$p < 0.001$ vs. the samples induced only with *C. pneumoniae* determined by the Student *t*-test.

chemical structure (see **Table 1**) stimulated TSG-6 expression (**Figure 4B**). It is also noteworthy that only these analoques inhibited significantly the TNF-α production of *C. pneumoniae*-induced U-937 cells (**Figure 3**). Considering the variable effects of KYNA analogs on the TSG-6 expression and also on the TNF-α production, we checked the correlation between the two effects. As it was expected, a significant inverse correlation was found between the effects on the TNF-α secretion and the TSG-6 expression exerted by different KYNA analogs (**Figure 5**). KYNA, SZR72, and SZR81 induced higher TNF-α secretion by U-937 cells after *C. pneumoniae* infection, but they decreased the TSG-6 expression compared to the cells that were infected only with *C. peumomiae*, without any of the compounds (i.e., Cpn in **Figure 5**). In contrast, in the case of the highest rate of TSG-6 expression (SZR 105), a maximal rate of inhibition of TNF-α production was observed. Therefore, we suppose that the different effects of KYNA analoques on the TSG-6 expression in *C. pneumoniae* infected cells might explain the difference in their effects on the secretion of TNF-α.

Altogether, from these data, it seems that inhibition of TNF-α is not only in correlation with the antiinflammatory effect of TSG-6, but in this situations, KYNA analogs are able to increase or even decrease the expression of TSG-6.

Effects of KYNA Analoques on the Quantity of *C. pneumoniae*

To ascertain that the effects of KYNA analoques on the TNF-α or TSG-6 induction is not simply due to their effects on the replication of *C. pneumoniae*, we performed experiments for quantitative assessment of chlamydial replication by a direct

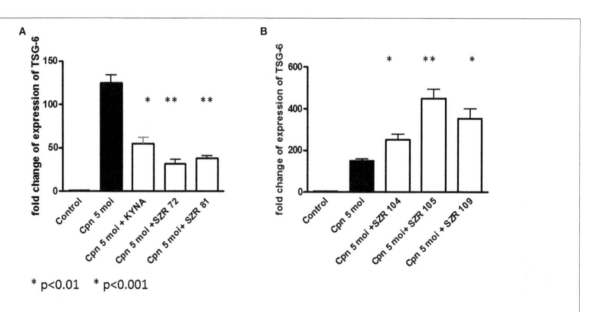

* p<0.01   * p<0.001

FIGURE 4 | Effect of 500 μM of KYNA and KYNA analogs on TSG-6 mRNA levels in U-937 monocytic cells stimulated with *Chlamydia pneumoniae* at a MOI 5. TSG-6 expressions were normalized to the reference gene of β-actin by using quantitative real-time PCR. Relative expression was calculated by using the $2^{-(\Delta\Delta Ct)}$ method and is given as a ratio between the target and the reference gene. Control: TSG-6 mRNA expression without stimulation, Filled bar: TSG-6 mRNA expression in *C. pneumoniae*-stimulated cells without KYNA or KYNA analoques, open bars: TSG-6 mRNA expression in *C. pneumoniae*-stimulated cells in the presence of 500 μM KYNA or KYNA analoques. Data are shown as means ± SD of the results of three independent experiments. *$p < 0.01$ vs. *C. pneumoniae*- induced cells without chemicals, **$p < 0.001$ vs. *C. pneumoniae*-induced cells without chemicals, determined by the Student *t*-test. **(A)** Decreasing, **(B)** Increasing effects.

quantitative PCR method (36). *C. pneumoniae* ompA gene was detected in the lysate of U-937 cells infected with *C. pneumoniae* at a MOI of 5 in the presence or absence of KYNA analoques at a concentration of 250 or 500 μM, respectively. Direct detection of *C. pneumoniae* DNA in the lysate of infected cells was done at 24 and 48 h postinfection. There was no significant inhibition or even elevation in the quantity of chlamydial DNA in the presence of different KYNA analoques after the 24 h (open bars) or 48 h (filled bars) incubation period. The results of the samples tested at 24 and 48 h of incubation are presented in **Figure 6**. Therefore,

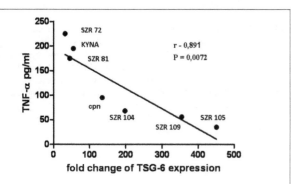

FIGURE 5 | Correlation between the TSG-6 expression and TNF-α production by U-937 cells infected with *C. pneumoniae* at a MOI 5 in the presence of KYNA or the analogs. U-937 cells were pretreated for 30 min with KYNA or KYNA analogs at a concentration of 500 μM, and thereafter incubated for 24 h with 5 MOI of *Chlamydia pneumoniae*. The TNF-α levels in the supernatants were determined with ELISA assay, and the TSG-6 expression by RT qPCR reactions. The significance of correlation was calculated by correlation analysis with the Graph-Pad Prism 5 statistical program. Symbols and numbers represent the data obtained with KYNA or KYNA analogs. Cpn: incubation only with *Chlamydia pneumoniae* without compounds. The correlation coefficient, r value is-0.891, the p-value = 0.0072, the 95% confidence interval is −0.9838 to −0,4174.

we assume that KYNA analoques do not influence the replication or the quantity of *C. pneumoniae*.

Effects of KYNA Analogs on TGS-6 Protein Production in U-937 Human Monocytic Cells Stimulated With Heat Inactivated *S. aureus* or by *Chlamydia pneumoniae*

To ascertain whether the effects of KYNA and analogs on the TSG-6 expression influence parallelly the protein level, the TSG-6 concentrations in the supernatants of U-937 cells were determined.

At a concentration of 500 μM, KYNA and KYNA analogs increased the TGF-6 level significantly, except SZR 73 in SA1 induced cells (**Figure 7A**). The new analogs SZR 104, 105, and 109 exerted the most potent stimulatory effects (*p* < 0.001) in equimolar (500 μM) concentration. *C. pneumoniae* induced also TSG-6 production in U-937 cells, but KYNA, SZR72, and SZR81 decreased the level of TSG-6 protein expression (**Figure 7B**). On the other hand, further KYNA analoques (SZR 104, SZR 105, and SZR 109) increased the TSG-6 concentration in the supernatants (7b). These experiments obtained with 500 μM of KYNA and KYNA analogs support the results obtained with RT PCR data demonstrating the effects of the chemicals on the TSG-6 RNA expression.

KYNA Analogs SZR 72 and SZR 105 Attenuate TNF-α Production and Increase TSG-6 Secretion in Human Whole Blood Cells Stimulated by Heat Inactivated *Staphylococcus aureus*

Some of the results obtained by *in vitro* experiments with U-937 monocytic cells were repeated by "*ex vivo*" experimets

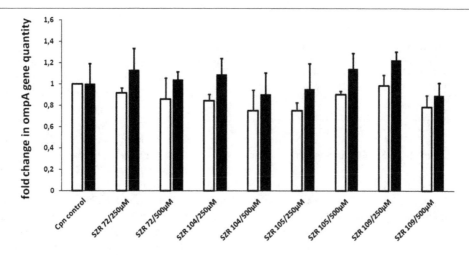

FIGURE 6 | Analysis of the effect of kynurenic acid derivates on *C. pneumoniae* growth in U-937 cells based on quantitation of chlamydial DNA by qPCR. The cells were infected in 96-well plates at a MOI of 5 in a medium containing kinurenic acid derivates. Direct detection of *C. pneumoniae* ompA gene in the lysate of infected cells was performed at 24 (open bars) and 48 h (filled bars) postinfection. Fold change in the quantity of chlamydial DNA in kinurenic acid derivate treated cultures compared to the quantities detected in non-treated cultures was calculated. The mean of fold change in 3 parallel cultures and SD are shown. The differences are not significant.

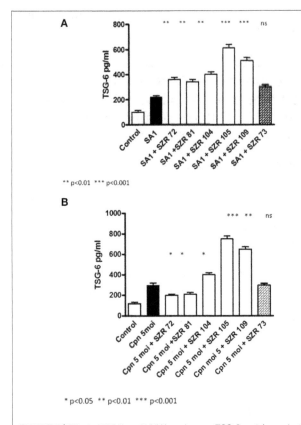

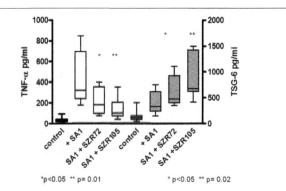

FIGURE 8 | Effect of KYNA analogs SZR 72 and SZR 105 on the TNF-α production and TSG-6 secretion in human whole blood cells stimulated by heat inactivated *Staphylococcus aureus*. EDTA-anticoagulated blood samples 1–1 mL each of 10 donors were incubated with SZR72 or SZR105 at a concentration of 500 μM for 30 min prior to the addition of heat inactivated *Staphylococcus aureus* (10^7/ml) The concentrations of TNF-α and that of TSG-6 in the plasma were determined after 18 h incubation period by TNF-α and TSG-6 ELISA plotted on the left and right Y axis, respectively. The data are depicted as box and whiskers plots, where the lines inside the boxes denote medians, and the boxes mark the interval between 25 and 75 percentile, and the whiskers the maximum and minimum. Significance were determined by the Mann-Whitney test.

FIGURE 7 | Effect of KYNA and KYNA analogs on TGS-6 protein production in U-937 human monocytic cells stimulated with heat inactivated *S. aureus* (SA1) **(A)** or by *Chlamydia pneumoniae* **(B)**. **(A)** U-937 cells (5×10^5/ml) were stimulated with heat inactivated SA1 (10^7/ml) alone, (filled bar), or incubated together with KYNA or KYNA analogs at a concentration of 500 μM, which were added for 30 min prior to the addition of SA1 (open bars). The TSG-6 levels in the supernatants were determined after 24 h by ELISA. Each concentration was tested in duplicate. Data are shown as means ± SD of three experiments. *$p < 0.01$; **$p < 0.001$ vs. the samples induced only with SA1 determined by the Student *t*-test. **(B)** U-937 cells were pretreated for 30 min with KYNA or KYNA analogs and thereafter incubated for 24 h with 5 MOI of *Chlamydia pneumoniae*. U-937 cells (5×10^5/mL) were infected with 5 MOI of *Chlamydia pneumoniae* alone (filled bar), or incubated together with KYNA or KYNA analogs at a concentration of 500 μM, which were added for 30 min prior to the addition of the bacteria (open bars). The TSG-6 levels in the supernatants were determined after 24 h. Each concentration was tested in duplicate. Data are shown as means ±SD of three experiments. *$p < 0.01$; **$p < 0.001$ vs. the samples induced only with *C. pneumoniae* determined by the Student *t*-test.

investigating the effects of two KYNA analogs in human peripheral blood.

There was big individual differences in the TNF-α concentrations and in TSG-6 concentrations in the supernatants in SA1-induced blood cultures (**Figure 8**), between 179 pg/ml and 850 pg/ml, and between 150 and 750 pg/ml, respectively. At a concentration of 500 μM, both SZR 72 and SZR 105 suppressed the TNF-α level significantly in the S. aureus induced blood cultures. Again, the new analog SZR 105 exerted more potent inhibitory effect ($p = 0.001$) in equimolar (500 μM) concentration. Similarly to the effects on U-937 cells, the KYNA analogs SZR72 and SZR 105 significantly

increased the TSG-6 concentrations in SA1 induced blood samples (**Figure 8**).

DISCUSSION

In our experiments, KYNA and different KYNA derivates inhibited the TNF-α production of U-937 cells stimulated with heat inactivated *Staphylococcus aureus*. The rate of the inhibition was variable according the structure of the analoques (**Figure 1**). The effect of the analogs were compared in equimolar concentration on the TNF-α production when the inducer was *Chlamydia pneumoniae*, a Gram negative, intracellular bacterium. In these experiments, however, not all KYNA derivates inhibited TNF-α production by U-937 monocytic cells; moreover, KYNA itself, and SZR72 and SZR81 increased it (**Figure 3**). We hypothesized that the difference in the influence on the TNF-α production might be connected with the difference in the TSG-6 expression (**Figure 4**).

The production of TNF-α in *C. pneumoniae* infected cells was inhibited only by the KYNA derivates (SZR 104, SZR105, SZR109) that upregulated the expression of TSG-6 (**Figures 4, 5**).

It is noteworthy, that TSG-6 itself does not only exert an antiinflammatory effect (20, 26, 27), but its expression might be under the influence of KYNA (37). It has been published that kynurenic acid controls TSG-6-mediated immunosuppression of the human mesenchymal stem cells (MSCs). In elegant experiments, it has been demonstrated that KYNA specifically regulates TSG-6 production by activating aryl hydrocarbon receptor (AHR). KYNA activates AHR, which directly binds to the TSG-6 promoter to enhance TSG-6 expression. Moreover, KYNA-pretreated MSCs can further boost TSG-6 production, and thus enhance the therapeutic capacity of human

MSCs against lipopolysaccharide (LPS)-induced acute lung injury (37).

We found that in most experiments, TSG-6 expression was up-regulated in U-937 monocytic cells stimulated with bacterial components, and KYNA and KYNA analogs were able to influence the rate of expression of TSG-6. The elevation of the TSG-6 expression might be one of the mechanisms that are responsible for the suppression of TNF-α production as a feedback effect. This effect was clearly demonstrated in our experiments using heat inactivated *S. aureus* as a cytokine inducer. In the case of *C. pneumoniae* infection, however, KYNA and KYNA analoques did not exert this effect uniformly. Some of them increased TSG-6 expression with a concomitant inhibition of the production of TNF-α, but several compounds (KYNA, SZR72, and SZR 81) rather decreased the expression of TSG-6, and it is very likely that this could lead to an elevated TNF-α production compared to the TNF-α production of U-937 cells infected with *C. pneumoniae* without any KYNA analoque. We hypothesized that the explanation of the difference in the results might be due to the different chemical structure of the analoques (see **Table 1**). The examined substrates (SZR-72, SZR-73 SZR-81, SZR-104, SZR-105, and SZR-109) can be classified into two classes of compounds: the first are amide derivatives (SZR-72, SZR-73, SZR-81) containing cationic center at the amide side chain. The second class of compounds (SZR-104, SZR-105, and SZR-109) are the C-3 aminoalkylated amides, therefore they can be interpreted as derivatives with dual cationic centers.

They could differently influence the binding of *C. pneumoniae* to the Toll-like receptor 2 (TLR2), and especially, differently activate AHR in the presence of *C. pneumoniae*. It has to be highlighted that the newly synthetized analogs, SZR 105 and SZR 109, were the most potent inducers of TSG-6 expression, and the highest inhibitors of TNF-α production in both types of bacterial inducers. The study of the exact effect of *Chlamydia pneumoniae* on the interaction between AHR and some KYNA analogs needs to be further investigated and proved.

Whatever the explanation is, our results indicate that there is a close connection between TNF production and TSG-6 expression, and there is an inverse correlation between the TSG-6 expression and TNF-α production in the presence of KYNA and KYNA analogs.

This negative correlation was further demonstrated at the protein level of TSG-6 measured in the supernatants of U-937 cells. and also in unseparated human peripheral blood samples

The stimulation of TSG-6 expression by KYNA and KYNA derivates might be one of the mechanisms that have an important role in their suppressive effect on TNF-α production. TSG-6 expression following activation with bacterial components could participate in the suppression of inflammatory cytokines, such as TNF-α, and it is noteworthy that KYNA and especially KYNA analogs are able to enhance this effect. Further studies are required to elucidate the different effects of KYNA derivates in the case of different bacterial inducers and the possible benefits of targeting TSG-6 expression by kynurenines in inflammatory conditions following infections.

AUTHOR CONTRIBUTIONS

YM designed research and wrote the manuscript. VE, KB, and IL conducted experiments with *Chlamydia*. TM performed experiments with RT-PCR. FF, IS, and BL contributed new reagents. AB provided the blood samples, YM and VE analyzed data. LV organized research for neurological project. All authors read and approved the manuscript.

FUNDING

This work was supported by GINOP 2.3.2-2015-16-00034 and Ministry of Human Capacities, Hungary Grant, 20391-3/2018/FEKUSTRAT.

REFERENCES

1. Mándi Y, Vécsei L. The kynurenine system and immunoregulation. *J Neural Transm Vienna Austr.* (2012) 119:197–209. doi: 10.1007/s00702-011-0681-y

2. Wirthgen E, Hoeflich A, Rebl A, Günther J. Kynurenic Acid: the janus-faced role of an immunomodulatory tryptophan metabolite and its link to pathological conditions. *Front Immunol.* (2017) 8:1957. doi: 10.3389/fimmu.2017.01957

3. Swartz KJ, During MJ, Freese A, Beal MF. Cerebral synthesis and release of kynurenic acid: an endogenous antagonist of excitatory amino acid receptors. *J Neurosci Off J Soc Neurosci.* (1990) 10:2965–73.

4. Stone TW. Development and therapeutic potential of kynurenic acid and kynurenine derivatives for neuroprotection. *Trends Pharmacol Sci.* (2000) 21:149–54. doi: 10.1016/S0165-6147(00)01451-6

5. Stone TW. Kynurenic acid blocks nicotinic synaptic transmission to hippocampal interneurons in young rats. *Eur J Neurosci.* (2007) 25:2656–65. doi: 10.1111/j.1460-9568.2007.05540.x

6. Vécsei L, Miller J, MacGarvey U, Beal MF. Kynurenine and probenecid inhibit pentylenetetrazol- and NMDLA-induced seizures and increase kynurenic acid concentrations in the brain. *Brain Res Bull.* (1992) 28:233–8.

7. Vécsei L, Szalárdy L, Fülöp F, Toldi J. Kynurenines in the CNS: recent advances and new questions. *Nat Rev Drug Discov.* (2013) 12:64–82. doi: 10.1038/nrd3793

8. Robotka H, Toldi J, Vécsei L. L-kynurenine: metabolism and mechanism of neuroprotection. *Future Neurol.* (2008) 3:169–88. doi: 10.2217/14796708.3.2.169

9. Vamos E, Pardutz A, Klivenyi P, Toldi J, Vecsei L. The role of kynurenines in disorders of the central nervous system: possibilities for neuroprotection. *J Neurol Sci.* (2009) 283:21–27. doi: 10.1016/j.jns.2009.02.326

10. Schwarcz R, Bruno JP, Muchowski PJ, Wu H-Q. Kynurenines in the mammalian brain: when physiology meets pathology. *Nat Rev Neurosci.* (2012) 13:465–77. doi: 10.1038/nrn3257

11. Hilmas C, Pereira EF, Alkondon M, Rassoulpour A, Schwarcz R, Albuquerque EX. The brain metabolite kynurenic acid inhibits alpha7 nicotinic receptor activity and increases non-alpha7 nicotinic receptor expression: physiopathological implications. *J Neurosci Off J Soc Neurosci.* (2001) 21:7463–73. doi: 10.1523/JNEUROSCI.21-19-07463.2001

12. Wang J, Simonavicius N, Wu X, Swaminath G, Reagan J, Tian H, et al. Kynurenic acid as a ligand for orphan G protein-coupled receptor GPR35. *J Biol Chem.* (2006) 281:22021–8. doi: 10.1074/jbc.M603503200

13. Julliard W, Fechner JH, Mezrich JD. The aryl hydrocarbon receptor meets immunology: friend or foe? A little of both. *Front Immunol.* (2014) 5:458. doi: 10.3389/fimmu.2014.00458

14. Wirthgen E, Hoeflich A. Endotoxin-induced tryptophan degradation along the kynurenine pathway: the role of indolamine 2,3-dioxygenase and aryl hydrocarbon receptor-mediated immunosuppressive effects in endotoxin tolerance and cancer and its implications for immunoparalysis. *J Amino Acids.* (2015) 2015:973548. doi: 10.1155/2015/973548

15. Kiank C, Zeden J-P, Drude S, Domanska G, Fusch G, Otten W, et al. Psychological stress-induced, IDO1-dependent tryptophan catabolism: implications on immunosuppression in mice and humans. *PLoS ONE.* (2010) 5:e11825. doi: 10.1371/journal.pone.0011825

16. Małaczewska J, Siwicki AK, Wójcik RM, Turski WA, Kaczorek E. The effect of kynurenic acid on the synthesis of selected cytokines by murine splenocytes - in vitro and ex vivo studies. *Cent Eur J Immunol.* (2016) 41:39–46. doi: 10.5114/ceji.2016.58815

17. Tiszlavicz Z, Németh B, Fülöp F, Vécsei L, Tápai K, Ocsovszky I, et al. Different inhibitory effects of kynurenic acid and a novel kynurenic acid analogue on tumour necrosis factor-α (TNF-α) production by mononuclear cells, HMGB1 production by monocytes and HNP1-3 secretion by neutrophils. *Naunyn Schmiedebergs Arch Pharmacol.* (2011) 383:447–55. doi: 10.1007/s00210-011-0605-2

18. Lee TH, Wisniewski HG, Vilcek J. A novel secretory tumor necrosis factor-inducible protein (TSG-6) is a member of the family of hyaluronate binding proteins, closely related to the adhesion receptor CD44. *J Cell Biol.* (1992) 116:545–57.

19. Lesley J, Gál I, Mahoney DJ, Cordell MR, Rugg MS, Hyman R, et al. TSG-6 modulates the interaction between hyaluronan and cell surface CD44. *J Biol Chem.* (2004) 279:25745–54. doi: 10.1074/jbc.M313319200

20. Milner CM, Day AJ. TSG-6: a multifunctional protein associated with inflammation. *J Cell Sci.* (2003) 116:1863–73. doi: 10.1242/jcs.00407

21. Coulson-Thomas VJ, Lauer ME, Soleman S, Zhao C, Hascall VC, Day AJ, et al. Tumor necrosis factor-stimulated gene-6 (TSG-6) is constitutively expressed in adult central nervous system (CNS) and associated with astrocyte-mediated glial scar formation following spinal cord injury. *J Biol Chem.* (2016) 291:19939–52. doi: 10.1074/jbc.M115.710673

22. Lee RH, Pulin AA, Seo MJ, Kota DJ, Ylostalo J, Larson BL, et al. Intravenous hMSCs improve myocardial infarction in mice because cells embolized in lung are activated to secrete the anti-inflammatory protein TSG-6. *Cell Stem Cell.* (2009) 5:54–63. doi: 10.1016/j.stem.2009.05.003

23. Wisniewski HG, Maier R, Lotz M, Lee S, Klampfer L, Lee TH, et al. TSG-6: a TNF-, IL-1-, and LPS-inducible secreted glycoprotein associated with arthritis. *J Immunol Baltim Md.* (1993) 151:6593–01.

24. Oh JY, Roddy GW, Choi H, Lee RH, Ylöstalo JH, Rosa RH, et al. Anti-inflammatory protein TSG-6 reduces inflammatory damage to the cornea following chemical and mechanical injury. *Proc Natl Acad Sci USA.* (2010) 107:16875–80. doi: 10.1073/pnas.1012451107

25. Danchuk S, Ylostalo JH, Hossain F, Sorge R, Ramsey A, Bonvillain RW, et al. Human multipotent stromal cells attenuate lipopolysaccharide-induced acute lung injury in mice via secretion of tumor necrosis factor-α-induced protein 6. *Stem Cell Res Ther.* (2011) 2:27. doi: 10.1186/scrt68

26. Mittal M, Tiruppathi C, Nepal S, Zhao Y-Y, Grzych D, Soni D, et al. TNFα-stimulated gene-6 (TSG6) activates macrophage phenotype transition to prevent inflammatory lung injury. *Proc Natl Acad Sci USA.* (2016) 113:E8151–8. doi: 10.1073/pnas.1614935113

27. Day AJ, Milner CM. TSG-6: a multifunctional protein with anti-inflammatory and tissue-protective properties. *Matrix Biol.* (2019) 78–79:60–83. doi: 10.1016/j.matbio.2018.01.011

28. Choi H, Lee RH, Bazhanov N, Oh JY, Prockop DJ. Anti-inflammatory protein TSG-6 secreted by activated MSCs attenuates zymosan-induced mouse peritonitis by decreasing TLR2/NF-κB signaling in resident macrophages. *Blood.* (2011) 118:330–8. doi: 10.1182/blood-2010-12-327353

29. Megyeri K, Mándi Y, Degré M, Rosztóczy I. Induction of cytokine production by different Staphylococcal strains. *Cytokine.* (2002) 19:206–12. doi: 10.1006/cyto.2002.0876

30. Wang JE, Jørgensen PF, Almlöf M, Thiemermann C, Foster SJ, Aasen AO, et al. Peptidoglycan and lipoteichoic acid from Staphylococcus aureus induce tumor necrosis factor alpha, interleukin 6 (IL-6), and IL-10 production in both T cells and monocytes in a human whole blood model. *Infect Immun.* (2000) 68:3965–70. doi: 10.1128/iai.68.7.3965-3970.2000

31. Blasi F, Tarsia P, Aliberti S. Chlamydophila pneumoniae. *Clin Microbiol Infect Off Publ Eur Soc Clin Microbiol Infect Dis.* (2009) 15:29–35. doi: 10.1111/j.1469-0691.2008.02130.x

32. Virok D, Loboda A, Kari L, Nebozhyn M, Chang C, Nichols C, et al. Infection of U937 monocytic cells with Chlamydia pneumoniae induces extensive changes in host cell gene expression. *J Infect Dis.* (2003) 188:1310–21. doi: 10.1086/379047

33. Fülöp F, Szatmári I, Vámos E, Zádori D, Toldi J, Vécsei L. Syntheses, transformations and pharmaceutical applications of kynurenic acid derivatives. *Curr Med Chem.* (2009) 16:4828–42. doi: 10.2174/092986709789909602

34. Fülöp F, Szatmári I, Toldi J, Vécsei L. Modifications on the carboxylic function of kynurenic acid. *J Neural Transm Vienna Austr.* (2012) 119:109–14. doi: 10.1007/s00702-011-0721-7

35. Fülöp F, Szatmári I, Toldi J, Vécsei L. *Novel Types of c-3 Substituted Kinurenic Acid Derivatives With Improved Neuroprotective Activity.* (2017) Available online at: https://patents.google.com/patent/WO2017149333A1/en (accessed February 10, 2019).

36. Eszik I, Lantos I, Önder K, Somogyvári F, Burián K, Endrész V, et al. High dynamic range detection of Chlamydia trachomatis growth by direct quantitative PCR of the infected cells. *J Microbiol Methods.* (2016) 120:15–22. doi: 10.1016/j.mimet.2015.11.010

37. Wang G, Cao K, Liu K, Xue Y, Roberts AI, Li F, et al. Kynurenic acid, an IDO metabolite, controls TSG-6-mediated immunosuppression of human mesenchymal stem cells. *Cell Death Differ.* (2018) 25:1209–23. doi: 10.1038/s41418-017-0006-2

15

Inflammation-Induced Tryptophan Breakdown is Related with Anemia, Fatigue and Depression in Cancer

Lukas Lanser[1], Patricia Kink[1], Eva Maria Egger[1], Wolfgang Willenbacher[2,3], Dietmar Fuchs[4], Guenter Weiss[1] and Katharina Kurz[1]*

[1] *Department of Internal Medicine II, Medical University of Innsbruck, Innsbruck, Austria,* [2] *Department of Internal Medicine V, Medical University of Innsbruck, Innsbruck, Austria,* [3] *Oncotyrol Centre for Personalized Cancer Medicine, Medical University of Innsbruck, Innsbruck, Austria,* [4] *Division of Biological Chemistry, Biocenter, Medical University of Innsbruck, Innsbruck, Austria*

*Correspondence:
Katharina Kurz
katharina.kurz@i-med.ac.at

Many patients with cancer suffer from anemia, depression, and an impaired quality of life (QoL). These patients often also show decreased plasma tryptophan levels and increased kynurenine concentrations in parallel with elevated concentrations of Th1 type immune activation marker neopterin. In the course of anti-tumor immune response, the pro-inflammatory cytokine interferon gamma (IFN-γ) induces both, the enzyme indoleamine 2,3-dioxygenase (IDO) to degrade tryptophan and the enzyme GTP-cyclohydrolase I to form neopterin. High neopterin concentrations as well as an increased kynurenine to tryptophan ratio (Kyn/Trp) in the blood of cancer patients are predictive for a worse outcome. Inflammation-mediated tryptophan catabolism along the kynurenine pathway is related to fatigue and anemia as well as to depression and a decreased QoL in patients with solid tumors. In fact, enhanced tryptophan breakdown might greatly contribute to the development of anemia, fatigue, and depression in cancer patients. IDO activation and stimulation of the kynurenine pathway exert immune regulatory mechanisms, which may impair anti-tumor immune responses. In addition, tumor cells can degrade tryptophan to weaken immune responses directed against them. High IDO expression in the tumor tissue is associated with a poor prognosis of patients. The efficiency of IDO-inhibitors to inhibit cancer progression is currently tested in combination with established chemotherapies and with immune checkpoint inhibitors. Inflammation-mediated tryptophan catabolism and its possible influence on the development and persistence of anemia, fatigue, and depression in cancer patients are discussed.

Keywords: inflammation, tryptophan, kynurenine, cancer, anemia, fatigue, depression

INTRODUCTION

Cancer is a leading cause of death and disability worldwide with an increasing prevalence. Patients with malignant diseases often have sustained systemic immune activation, which is linked to tumor progression and a poor clinical outcome (1, 2). Initially, immune activation is an important mechanism to prevent carcinogenesis. However, this mechanism does not seem to work properly in patients with advanced cancer. Tumor cells are able to escape immune-mediated elimination by leukocytes due to loss of antigenicity and/or immunogenicity but also by creating an immunosuppressive microenvironment and by blocking anti-tumor immune response (3). Tryptophan (Trp) metabolism appears to play an important role within the tumor microenvironment (4).

In fact, enhanced Trp breakdown, reflected by decreased Trp and elevated kynurenine (Kyn) concentrations in the peripheral blood, is often observed in cancer patients and related to tumor progression, poor clinical outcome (**Table 1**) and an impaired quality of life (QoL) (58, 85). Trp breakdown in patients with malignancies is primarily mediated by increased tryptophan 2,3-dioxygenase (TDO) and indoleamine 2,3-dioxygenase 1 (IDO1) activities (86). The latter is primarily activated by pro-inflammatory cytokines of the T helper 1 (Th1) type immune response, particularly interferon gamma (IFN-γ) (87). IFN-γ also stimulates the formation of reactive oxygen species (ROS) as well as the expression of GTP-cyclohydrolase I (GCH-1) in target cells. In human monocytes/macrophages, this enzyme subsequently degrades GTP to form the pteridine neopterin, which has been established as a clinically useful marker for Th1 driven immune activation (88).

Higher neopterin concentrations mostly coincide with increased IDO-activation as reflected by a higher Kyn/Trp ratio (24, 46, 89, 90) and are related to tumor progression and an increased mortality rate (1, 91) in patients with malignant diseases.

Trp is essential for the growth and proliferation of all kinds of cells; therefore, local inflammation-induced Trp depletion is initially a defense mechanism of the immune system to limit growth of microbes but also of proliferating malignant cells (92). However, tumor cells seem to develop countermeasures via degradation of Trp, allowing them to escape this defense mechanism. Moreover, stimulation of IDO1 and Trp breakdown also impacts on Trp availability for immune cells over time and leads to the accumulation of Trp metabolites such as the kynurenines, which can directly modulate anti-tumor immune responses (93).

Apart from an activated immune system and enhanced Trp breakdown, patients with malignancies frequently suffer from anemia (94). Anemia is a main contributor to sustained fatigue (95), which is the most frequently reported symptom in cancer patients (96), affecting up to 78% (97). Actually, activities of daily living are mostly affected by cancer related fatigue (CRF) (98). Another common comorbidity is depression, affecting ~20% of cancer patients (99–101). All these comorbidities have been related to immune activation and the associated Trp breakdown.

This review discusses the current knowledge on and consequences of immune activation and Trp breakdown for the development and persistence of anemia, fatigue, and depression in cancer patients. Moreover, it gives an overview of possible therapeutic options for the treatment of comorbidities. At the beginning, a brief depiction of Trp metabolism and its relations to immune activation will be given.

TRYPTOPHAN METABOLISM

Trp is an essential amino acid that is required for protein biosynthesis. Therefore, it is essential for the growth and proliferation of cells. Trp must be supplied by diet or obtained from protein degradation, since it cannot be synthesized by human cells. The required daily amount for adults lies between 175 and 250 mg. Yet, the average daily intake for many individuals lies between 900 and 1,000 mg (102, 103). Thus, decreased Trp concentrations are suggested to be primarily caused by enhanced Trp breakdown.

Trp is also an important precursor for several bioactive metabolites including tryptamine, serotonin, melatonin, kynurenine (Kyn) and quinolinic acid (QUIN) and kynurenic acid (KYNA) as well as for the coenzyme NAD^+. These metabolites are mainly generated by two different biochemical pathways.

First, Trp can be catabolized by the enzyme tryptophan 5-hydroxylase (TPH) to 5-hydroxytryptophan (5-HTP) (**Figure 1**). 5-HTP is converted into 5-methoxytryptophan (5-MTP) by the hydroxyindole-O-methyltransferase (HIOMT) (104) and subsequently decarboxylated to 5-hydroxytryptamine (5-HT) by the vitamin B6 dependent aromatic-L-amino-acid decarboxylase (AADC) (105). 5-HT, better known as serotonin, is an important neurotransmitter that modulates numerous neuropsychological processes including mood, anxiety, anger, reward, and cognition (106). It is also involved in important processes outside the central nervous system (CNS), including regulatory functions in the gastrointestinal (GI) tract as well as cardiovascular and pulmonary system. Actually, over 90% of the total body serotonin is synthesized in the GI tract (107).

Although only 1% of the available Trp is converted by the Trp/5-HT pathway in healthy individuals, decreased Trp availability is associated with decreased serotonin concentrations and consequently with neuropsychologic disorders (105). In the pineal gland, aryl alkylamine N-acetyltransferase (AANAT) converts 5-HT into N-acetyl-5-hydroxytryptamine, which is further catabolyzed by the HIOMT to N-acetyl-5-methoxytryptamine (5-MT), better known as melatonin (108). Melatonin is primarily secreted at night and regulates the circadian rhythm under normal light/dark conditions (109). Finally, Trp can be directly decarboxylated by the AADC to tryptamine, which is an important neuromodulator of serotonin (110).

The second and quantitatively most important pathway is the decay to Kyn (**Figure 2**). Approximately 90% of the available Trp is oxidized to N-formylkynurenine by either tryptophan 2,3-dioxygenase (TDO; EC 1.13.11.11), indoleamine 2,3-dioxygenase 1 (IDO1; EC 1.13.11.52), or indoleamine 2,3-dioxygenase 2 (IDO2; 1.13.11.-). N-formylkynurenine is then subsequently hydrolyzed to Kyn by kynurenine formamidase. Kyn is further catalyzed by one of the four kynurenine aminotransferases (KATs) to KYNA. It can also be hydroxylated to 3-hydroxykynurenine (3-HK) by kynurenine 3-monooxygenase (KMO) and then converted to 3-hydroxyanthralinic acid (3-HAA) by the kynureninase (KYNU). Another important enzyme of the Kyn pathway, namely 3-hydroxyanthranilic acid dioxygenase (HAD), converts 3-HAA into 2-amino-3-carboxymuconate semialdehyde, which decays non-enzymatically into QUIN. Finally, phosphoribosyl transferase (QPRT) converts QUIN into nicotinamide, which is an important component of NAD^+ and $NADP^+$ being necessary for energy production (111).

TABLE 1 | Altered tryptophan metabolism in different cancer types and its relations to disease severity, progression, and survival.

Cancer type	Tryptophan metabolism within tumor tissues		Tryptophan metabolism in the peripheral blood	
	Findings	References	Findings	References
Acute myeloid leukemia	Up-regulation of IDO1 expression upon IFN-γ stimulation was related to an impaired overall survival	Folgiero et al. (5)	Increased Kyn levels were associated with a shorter overall survival	Mabuchi et al. (6)
	Increased IDO1 mRNA expression was correlated with an impaired overall survival	Fukuno et al. (7)	Kyn/Trp ratio was increased and associated with a shorter overall survival	Corm et al. (8)
	Increased IDO1 mRNA expression was related to an impaired overall survival and relapse-free survival	Chamuleau et al. (9)		
	Increased IDO1 expression inhibited T-cell proliferation	Tang et al. (10)		
Breast cancer	High IDO1 expression was associated with TNM stage, histological grade, lymph node metastasis, progression-free survival, and overall survival	Wei et al. (11)	Trp levels predict tumor progression and were associated with overall survival	Eniu et al. (12)
	Up-regulation of IDO1, TDO2, and KMO expression was found	Heng et al. (13)	Low Trp levels and an increased Kyn/Trp ratio were found	Lyon et al. (14)
	IDO1 expression increased with higher tumor stages	Isla Larrain et al. (15)	Increased Kyn/Trp ratio was associated with higher tumor grade and elevated neopterin levels	Girgin et al. (16)
	Increased IDO1 expression promotes tumor progression and is associated with an impaired overall survival	Chen et al. (17)		
	Higher IDO1 expression was associated with an impaired overall survival in estrogen receptor positive group	Soliman et al. (18)		
	Higher IDO1 expression was predictive for a better overall survival	Jacquemier et al. (19)		
	IDO1 expression was increased and correlated with tumor stages and lymph node metastasis	Yu et al. (20)		
Colorectal cancer	Increased IDO1 expression upon IFN-γ stimulation correlated with metastasis rate and an impaired overall survival	Ferdinande et al. (21)	Kyn/Trp ratio was increased and related to high neopterin levels and lymph node metastasis	Engin et al. (22)
	Increased IDO1 expression was associated with an impaired overall survival	Gao et al. (23)	Reduced Trp levels and an increased Kyn/Trp ratio was related to high neopterin levels and an impaired QoL	Huang et al. (24)
	Increased IDO1 expression upon IFN-γ stimulation correlated with reduced T-cell infiltration, higher metastasis rate and an impaired overall survival	Brandacher et al. (25)		
Gastrointestinal tumors	Increased IDO1 expression in esophageal cancer tissues was associated with differentiation grade, TNM stage, lymph node metastasis, and an impaired overall survival	Jia et al. (26)	Trp levels were decreased and associated with elevated neopterin levels	Iwagaki et al. (27)
	High IDO1 expression was a negative prognostic factor	Laimer et al. (28)		
	Increased IDO1 expression in esophageal cancer cells was related to disease progression and an impaired overall survival	Zhang et al. (29)		
Glioma	Up-regulation of IDO1, IDO2, and KMO expression upon IFN-γ stimulation was found	Adams et al. (30)	High Kyn/Trp ratio was correlated with an impaired overall survival	Zhai et al. (31)
	Increased IDO1 expression was correlated with an impaired overall survival	Mitsuka et al. (32)	Low Trp, KYNA and QUIN levels, and a high Kyn/Trp ratio were found	Adams et al. (30)
	Downregulation of IDO1 expression was associated with a better overall survival	Wainwright et al. (33)		
Gynecological cancer	Marginal IDO expression in patients in early stage cervical cancer predicted a favorable outcome	Heeren et al. (34)	Increased Kyn/Trp ratio correlated with advanced disease, poor response to therapy, and an impaired overall survival	Gostner et al. (35)

(Continued)

TABLE 1 | Continued

Cancer type	Tryptophan metabolism within tumor tissues		Tryptophan metabolism in the peripheral blood	
	Findings	References	Findings	References
	Increased IDO expression in endometrial carcinoma cells correlated with reduced T-cell infiltration and an impaired disease-specific survival	de Jong et al. (36)	Kyn/Trp ratio was increased and related to lymph node metastasis, FIGO stage, tumor size, parametrial invasion, and poor disease-specific survival in patients with cervical cancer	Ferns et al. (37)
	Increased IDO expression in cervical cancer cells was associated with higher tumor stage, lymph node metastasis, and an impaired overall survival	Inaba et al. (38)	Kyn/Trp ratio was increased in patients with ovarian cancer and associated with higher FIGO stages	Sperner-Unterweger et al. (39)
	High IDO1 expression in ovarian carcinoma cells correlated with reduced T-cell infiltration and an impaired overall survival	Inaba et al. (40)	Kyn/Trp ratio was increased	de Jong et al. (41)
	High IDO1 expression in endometrial cancer tissues was related to reduced T-cell infiltration, lymph node-metastasis, and poor progression-free survival	Ino et al. (42)	Increased QUIN levels and reduced KYNA levels were found in patients with primary ovarian cancer	Fotopoulou et al. (43)
	Increased IDO1 expression in ovarian cancer cells was correlated with impaired survival in patients with serous-type ovarian cancer	Okamoto et al. (44) and Takao et al. (45)	Elevated Trp levels and a decreased Kyn/Trp ratio was found and associated with elevated neopterin levels	Schroecksnadel et al. (46)
	High IDO1 expression in endometrial carcinoma cells was related to an impaired progression-free and overall survival	Ino et al. (47)		
Hepatocellular carcinoma	Increased IDO1 expression was associated with T-cell infiltration and an impaired overall survival	Li et al. (48)		
	Increased KMO expression was correlated with an impaired overall survival and an increased time to recurrence	Jin et al. (49)		
	Increased IDO1 expression upon IFN-γ stimulation correlates with metastasis rate and an impaired overall survival	Pan et al. (50)		
	Increased IDO1 expression in tumor infiltrating cells was associated with an increased progression-free survival	Ishio et al. (51)		
Kidney cancer	Up-regulation of IDO1 expression upon IFN-γ stimulation was found	Trott et al. (52)	Kyn/Trp ratio was increased and associated with a poorer progression-free survival	Lucarelli et al. (53)
	High IDO1 mRNA levels were associated with an increased overall survival	Riesenberg et al. (54) and Yuan et al. (55)		
Lung cancer	IDO1 expression was increased and correlated with TNM stage and lymph node-metastasis	Tang et al. (56)	Low Trp levels and a high Kyn/Trp ratio were associated with an increased lung cancer risk in the EPIC study;	Chuang et al. (57)
			In the International Lung cancer cohort consortium (5,364 smoking-matched case-control pairs) the highest quintiles of kynurenine, Kyn/Trp, quinolinic acid and neopterin were associated with a 20–30% higher risk and tryptophan with a 15% lower risk of lung cancer	Huang et al. (58)
	Enhanced Kyn production and increased TDO2 expression by cancer-associated fibroblasts was found	Hsu et al. (59)	Post-induction chemotherapy increased Kyn/Trp ratio was associated with an impaired progression-free and overall survival	Creelan et al. (60)
	No associations between IDO1 expression and clinicopathological parameters were found	Karanikas et al. (61)	Low Trp levels and a high Kyn/Trp ratio were found and associated with high neopterin levels, low hemoglobin levels, fatigue, and QoL	Kurz et al. (62)
	Increased IDO1 expression by infiltrating tumor cells was related to an impaired overall survival	Astigiano et al. (63)	Low Trp levels and a high Kyn/Trp ratio were found and associated with elevated neopterin levels	Engin et al. (64)

(Continued)

TABLE 1 | Continued

Cancer type	Tryptophan metabolism within tumor tissues		Tryptophan metabolism in the peripheral blood	
	Findings	References	Findings	References
			Low Trp levels and a higher Kyn/Trp ratio were found and related to tumor progression	Suzuki et al. (65)
Lymphoma	High IDO1 expression in tumor infiltrating immune cells was related to an increased overall survival	Nam et al. (66)	High Kyn levels and Kyn/Trp ratio were found and associated with tumor progression and a shorter overall survival in patients with adult T-cell leukemia/lymphoma	Masaki et al. (67)
	Up-regulation of IDO1 in non-Hodgkin lymphoma tissues was related to tumor progression, higher serum LDH and an impaired overall survival	Liu et al. (68)	High Kyn levels correlated with an impaired overall survival	Yoshikawa et al. (69)
	IDO1 expression was increased in stroma cells of Hodgkin lymphoma and correlated with an impaired overall survival	Choe et al. (70)	Low Trp levels and high Kyn levels were found and related to a shorter overall survival in patients with adult T-cell leukemia/lymphoma	Giusti et al. (71)
	High IDO1 expression in non-Hodgkin lymphoma tissues was related to a lower remission rates and an impaired overall survival	Ninomiya et al. (72)		
	IDO1 mRNA expression was increased in adult T-cell leukemia/lymphoma cells	Hoshi et al. (73)		
Melanoma	Increased IDO1 expression in nodal metastases was associated with an impaired overall survival	Pelak et al. (74)	Low Trp levels and a high Kyn/Trp ratio were found and associated with high neopterin levels and an impaired overall survival	Weinlich et al. (75)
	Increased IDO1 expression in nodal metastases was associated with clinical recurrence	Ryan et al. (76)	Patients who developed major depression during IFN-α therapy had a significantly higher Kyn/Trp ratio	Capuron et al. (77)
	Increased IDO1 expression in sentinel lymph nodes correlated with an impaired progression-free and overall survival	Speeckaert et al. (78)		
	Increased IDO1 expression in nodal metastases was associated with a poor survival	Brody et al. (79)		
Osteosarcoma	High IDO1 expression correlated with an impaired metastasis-free and overall survival	Urakawa et al. (80)		
Pancreatic cancer	Increased IDO1 expression upon IFN-γ stimulation correlated with lymph node metastasis and an impaired overall survival	Zhang et al. (81)	Higher HAA/HK ratio was associated with a reduced pancreatic cancer risk	Huang et al. (82)
Prostate cancer	IDO1 expression was increased and correlated with serum Kyn/Trp ratio	Feder-Mengus et al. (83)	High Kyn levels were associated with an impaired cancer-related survival	Pichler et al. (2)
Thyroid carcinoma	IDO1 expression was increased and associated with tumor aggressiveness	Moretti et al. (84)		

TDO, IDO1, and IDO2 are heme-containing enzymes and catalyze the first and rate-limiting step in Trp breakdown. TDO is mainly expressed in the liver and oxidizes excess Trp, thereby generating ATP and especially NAD$^+$. In mammals, NAD$^+$ is synthesized from Trp via the Preiss-Handler pathway in liver and kidney (112). Actually, the Trp concentration in the diet has been shown to influence the liver NAD$^+$ levels (113). TDO expression is stimulated by its substrate Trp (114) as well as by heme (115) and corticosteroids (116). NAD$^+$ inhibits TDO expression, thus forming a negative feedback loop (117). IDO1 can be expressed by many different cells, including antigen-presenting cells (APCs) like monocyte-derived macrophages, dendritic cells (DCs) and fibroblasts. Its expression is mainly induced by inflammatory stimuli such as IFN-γ, tumor necrosis factor alpha (TNF-α), IL-1, and IL-2 secreted by Th1 type cells,

inflammatory cytokines of innate immune cells as well as TGF-β, IL-10, and adenosine secreted by regulatory T cells (T$_{reg}$) (118). IDO1 expression is further stimulated by its own product Kyn via the aryl hydrocarbon receptor (AhR) (119–121) as well as by the cyclooxygenase-2 (COX-2) and prostaglandin E2 (PGE2) (122). Contrary to this, IDO1 expression is inhibited by the anti-inflammatory cytokines IL-4 and IL-13 (123, 124). Little is known about the physiological functions of the recently detected IDO2. It is primarily expressed in the liver, kidney, brain, placenta, and APCs including DCs and B cells; yet, IDO2 is significantly less active when compared to IDO1 (125). Similar to IDO1, IDO2 expression is stimulated by AhR activation (120). Interestingly, IDO2 negatively regulates IDO1 activity by competing for heme-binding (126). IFN-γ also stimulates KMO, KYNU and HAD activity (127).

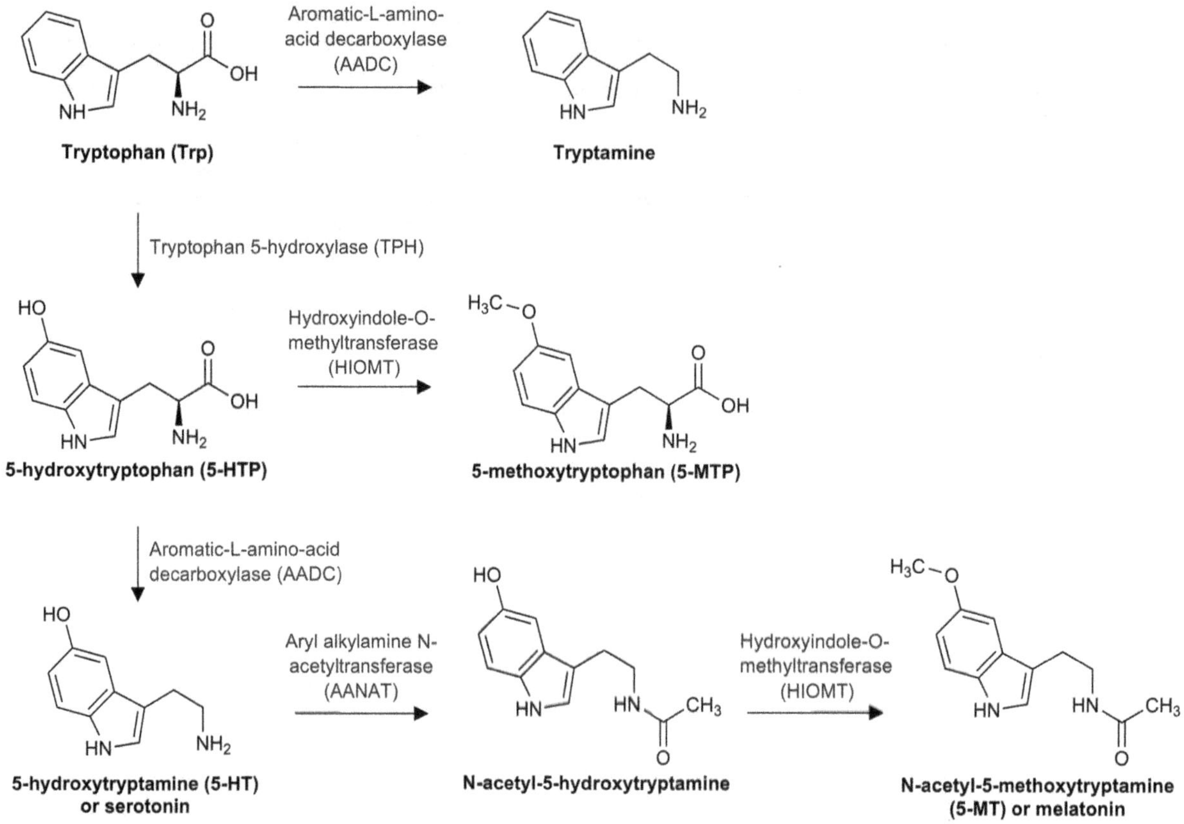

FIGURE 1 | Tryptophan pathway to serotonin and melatonin: This figure illustrates tryptophan breakdown to serotonin via the intermediate product 5-hydroxytryptophan (5-HTP) and the further conversion to melatonin via the intermediate product 5-acetyl-5-hydroxytryptamine.

TRYPTOPHAN BREAKDOWN VIA THE KYNURENINE PATHWAY MODULATES IMMUNE RESPONSE

An immunologicaly privileged milieu with a decreased reactivity to allogeneic (non-self) antigens is found in certain parts of the human body (e.g., brain, eye, testis, placenta). This immune tolerance prevents fetal rejection and immune responses against immunogenic sperms. An enhanced expression of TDO, IDO1, and IDO2, with a subsequent accumulation of Trp metabolites, is found in several parts of the human body including the placenta (128, 129), maternal and embryonic tissues in early conceptions (130, 131) as well as in the epididymis (132–134). Therefore, these enzymes are suggested to play an important role in immune tolerance. Immune tolerizing effects are also observed in the local tumor microenvironment. An enhanced Trp catabolism via Kyn pathway seems to be involved in immune paralysis against tumor cells. This may be primarily mediated by increased IDO1 expression and subsequent accumulation of Trp metabolites, since IDO1 is either expressed by many tumor cells themselves (see **Table 1**) or by tumor associated cells such as DCs or endothelial cells (ECs) (118).

Nearly all metabolites of the Kyn pathway affect immune activity via several mechanisms (**Figure 2**). Trp depletion slows down protein biosynthesis in immune cells and induces cell cycle arrest of T cells via eIF-2-alpha kinase GCN2, thus making them highly susceptible to Fas-ligand-mediated apoptosis (135, 136). Activation of GCN2 further promotes the generation of regulatory phenotypes (T_{reg}) in naive CD4$^+$ T cells (137). Activation of AhR by its endogenous ligand Kyn results in reduced T helper 17 (Th17) cell differentiation, while promoting the generation of T_{reg} cells (138, 139). T_{reg} cells, in turn, induce IDO1 expression in DCs, thus expanding their own population and forming a positive regulatory feedback loop (137). Th17 cells upregulate KMO expression, which reduces the availability of Kyn for AhR activation and consequently results in a reduced Th17 formation in the sense of a negative regulatory feedback loop (140). Finally, several metabolites of Trp breakdown such as Kyn, 3-HK, 3-HAA, QUIN, and picolinic acid were demonstrated to suppress the proliferation of CD4$^+$ lymphocytes, CD8$^+$ lymphocytes, and natural killer (NK) cells. Furthermore, they induce apoptosis of these cells probably mediated by oxygen free radicals (141–144), while 3-HAA induces apoptosis of monocytes/macrophages (145). However, apoptosis primarily occurs in Th1 cells and not in Th2 cells, thereby forming a negative feedback loop and preventing an excessive Th1 activation (141). In addition, the final product of the Kyn

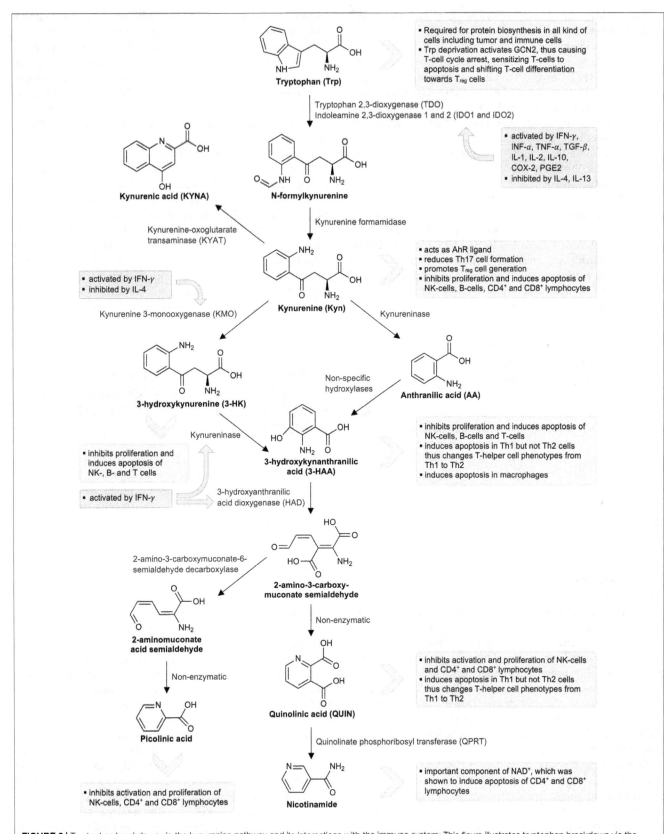

FIGURE 2 | Tryptophan breakdown via the kynurenine pathway and its interactions with the immune system: This figure illustrates tryptophan breakdown via the kynurenine pathway. The orange boxes indicate the effects of immune mediators on the kynurenine pathway and the yellow boxes indicate the effects of tryptophan metabolites on the immune system.

pathway NAD^+ also induces apoptosis in $CD4^+$ and $CD8^+$ lymphocytes (146).

Apart from immune modulating properties, Kyn metabolites may also help tumors to "optimize their microenvironment": Formation of QUIN by glioma cells was described to promote resistance to oxidative stress (147). Additionally, tumor cells might enhance their own IDO activity via an autocrine AhR-IL-6-STAT3 signaling loop (148), thereby suppressing T-cell proliferation. Upregulation of the tryptophanyl-tRNA synthetase WARS may protect Trp-degrading cancer cells from excessive intracellular Trp depletion via IFNγ and/or GCN2-signaling (149).

On the other hand, 5-MTP, which is produced by mesenchymal cells such as fibroblasts via 5-HTP, inhibits migration of cancer cells, tumor growth and cancer metastasis. This effect is probably mediated by 5-MTP derived inhibition of COX-2, which is constitutively overexpressed in cancer cells and promotes carcinogenesis (150). Therefore, reduced 5-MTP formation due to decreased Trp availability can contribute to tumor growth and cancer metastasis.

IMMUNE TOLERANCE RELATED TO INDOLEAMINE 2,3-DIOXYGENASE 1 ACTIVATION IN CANCER PATIENTS

IDO1 expression is a counter-regulatory mechanism to slow down potentially harmful over-activated immune responses. However, when the immune system attempts to fight a tumor, this counter-regulation is highly undesirable (151). In the majority of studies, an upregulation of IDO1 expression was associated with a poor clinical outcome (**Table 1**). Only in a small number of tumor entities, increased IDO1 activity was associated with a favorable prognosis (19, 54). The apparent inflammation-induced IDO1 expression in these patients probably indicates a stronger innate anti-tumor immune response.

It is suggested that IDO1 takes different positions in the three phases of cancer immunoediting: elimination, equilibrium, and escape (118). In the first phase (elimination), most tumor cells are recognized, and destroyed by the immune system. Low-level IDO1 production in the tumor microenvironment contributes to this tumor defense by inhibiting tumor proliferation (152). During the second phase (equilibrium), heterogeneity, and genetic instability progress in tumor cells that survived the elimination phase, thus enabling tumor cells to resist the immune response (153). In the last phase (escape), the tumor cells themselves as well as the tolerogenic immune cells produce large quantities of IDO1 (154), which results in immune tolerance described above (155, 156).

Due to these findings, inhibition of IDO1 as a therapeutic approach in cancer treatment has gained increasing attention in immuno-oncology. A recent study found that limitation of programmed cell death protein 1 (PD-1) inhibition might be due to an immunosuppressive tumor microenvironment based on IDO1 activation within macrophages (157). This suggests that IDO inhibition can be a potential therapeutic target in cancer patients, specifically in those who do not respond to immune checkpoint inhibitors. By now, clinical trials testing IDO1 inhibitors in combination with other chemotherapeutic or immunotherapeutic agents seem more promising than administration of IDO1 inhibitors alone. So far, five IDO1 inhibitors were studied as potential therapeutic options in cancer patients: indoximod [IDO pathway modulator; 1-methyl-D-tryptophan (1-MT)], epacadostat (selective IDO1 inhibitor; INCB024360), navoximod (GDC-0919), BMS-986205, and IDO1-targeting vaccines. All these IDO1 inhibitors were shown to be safe and well-tolerated (158–161). Epacadostat is the clinically most advanced IDO1 inhibitor and has been shown to inhibit tumor growth in mice models (162).

In human patients, epacadostat monotherapy was not effective (163, 164), while combined administration with PD-1 or cytotoxin T-lymphocyte-associated protein 4 (CTLA-4) inhibitors showed promising clinical activity in phase I/II studies (165–168). Unfortunately, a recent trial with combined administration of epacadostat with pembrolizumab found no superiority over pembrolizumab alone (169). Despite this setback, several ongoing trials investigate the effect of other (also structurally new) IDO1 inhibitors in combination with different immunotherapies (162).

INDOLEAMINE 2,3-DIOXYGENASE 2, TRYPTOPHAN 2,3-DIOXYGENASE, AND KYNURENINE 3-MONOOXYGENASE IN TUMOR IMMUNE TOLERANCE

Until now, IDO2 has been investigated far less than IDO1. Although IDO2 is expressed by cancer cells, it does not contribute to the accumulation of Trp metabolites to the same extent as IDO1 (170, 171). However, it was recently implicated that IDO2 affects B cell-mediated autoimmunity (172), and also contributes to carcinogenesis in models of pancreatic cancers (173). Interestingly, IDO2-deficiency was predictive for disease-free survival in patients receiving adjuvant radiotherapy (173).

Recent studies revealed that TDO may also be involved in tumor immune-escape. It was demonstrated that TDO is expressed in various tumors including glial tumors (174), breast cancers (175), lung cancers (59), colorectal carcinomas (176), melanomas, bladder carcinomas, and hepatocellular carcinomas (177). In glial tumors, TDO activity suppressed the anti-tumor immune responses via increased Kyn production (174). TDO was shown to be a promising therapeutic target to improve immune response to cancer cells (178). A recent study by Schramme et al. demonstrated that TDO inhibition increases the antitumor efficacy of immune checkpoint inhibitors (179).

Also, KMO activity may be involved in tumor immune tolerance. Recent studies have shown that its overexpression is related to rapid cancer progression and a poor prognosis (49, 180). Similar to inflammatory-induced IDO1 expression, KMO expression is induced by inflammatory stimuli (181, 182). Interestingly enough, the non-steroidal anti-inflammatory drug diclofenac is capable of binding human KMO, thereby inhibiting its activity (183). Since there is evidence that diclofenac also exerts anti-cancer effects (184), a possible explanation might be its interaction with Trp metabolism. Diclofenac inhibits COX-2 related IDO1 expression and KMO expression, thus reducing the accumulation of Trp catabolites.

FATIGUE AND DEPRESSION ARE RELATED TO IMMUNE ACTIVATION IN CANCER PATIENTS

Cancer related fatigue (CRF) is a complex multi-dimensional phenomenon that affects physical, cognitive and emotional activity, and behavior (185). It is associated with the cancer and its comorbidities themselves and often deteriorates during treatment (186). Actually, persisting fatigue limits the adherence of patients to cancer therapy (187). Chronic inflammation is proposed to be a leading cause of CRF. Higher inflammatory markers including IL-6, TNF-α, CRP, and neopterin were shown to correlate with fatigue in cancer patients prior to treatment, during treatment and also after treatment (62, 188–190).

Patients with lung cancer and moderate or severe fatigue are presented with lower Trp and hemoglobin concentrations, but with higher inflammatory markers (62). They furthermore assessed their QoL worse, and decreased QoL was associated with higher inflammatory markers and lower Trp concentrations. These results in 50 patients with lung cancer are well in line with earlier data showing significant correlations between fatigue/decreased QoL and immune-mediated Trp degradation in patients with different malignant diseases (85) as well as in patients with HIV-infection (191). Interestingly, correlations between inflammatory markers and decreased QoL were only seen in patients without antidepressant therapy in both HIV-infected and lung cancer patients. Also, in patients with colorectal cancer increased neopterin and decreased Trp levels correlated significantly with a decreased survival; QoL was worse in patients with low Trp (192).

A recent study in patients with solid tumors excluded patients with known depression or antidepressant treatment or established infection (90). Again, an association between immune activation and the QoL of patients as well as their depression susceptibility became evident. Fatigue was present in a high percentage of patients and was significantly associated with a decreased QoL, with decreased Trp and hemoglobin values (90). As low Trp or increased Kyn/Trp concentrations were associated with fatigue and decreased QoL, respectively, in several studies, this data indicates that immune activation and immune-mediated Trp degradation might contribute to the development of fatigue. Also, Kim and co-workers suggested a key role of inflammation-induced IDO-activation in CRF (193).

It is of importance that treatment with corticosteroids or anti-inflammatory drugs like celecoxib reduces fatigue in patients with advanced cancer (194, 195), suggesting that anti-inflammatory therapy improves fatigue by interfering with immune activation. A causal relationship between fatigue and immune activation has also been proposed in patients with other autoimmune diseases and infection (196) and treatment with TNF-α antagonists significantly reduces fatigue in patients with rheumatoid arthritis and psoriasis (197, 198).

Fatigue is one of the main symptoms of depression, which is another common comorbidity in subjects suffering from malignancies, affecting $\sim$20% of the patients (99–101). Depression is probably not only due to emotional distress but also due to immunological mechanisms, which might negatively affect the QoL and increase all-cause mortality (199–201). Enhanced Trp breakdown as a consequence of immune activation has been proposed to play a crucial role in the development of depression in cancer patients (202–204).

Recently, correlations between inflammation markers (neopterin and CRP) and depression scores in a population of patients with solid tumors were reported, and particularly in male patients, lower Trp levels were associated with higher depression scores and stronger fatigue (90).

This clinical data fit well with results from animal experiments: Depressive-like behavior related to immune activation was demonstrated to be associated with an upregulation of IDO1 (205–207) as well as KMO (208–210). Peripheral administration of lipopolysaccharide activated IDO, resulting in a distinct depressive-like behavioral syndrome (205). Interestingly, IDO inhibition prevented the development of depressive-like behavior (211), while Kyn administration dose dependently induced depressive-like behavior. Also the anti-inflammatory cytokine IL-10 was able to normalize IDO1 expression, thus relieving depressive-like behavior in mice (212).

Depression is also related to enhanced Trp breakdown and immune activation in patients with HIV-infection (191, 213), as well as in patients receiving immunotherapy [e.g., IL-2 or INF-α; (77, 214)].

Immune activation probably affects the development of CRF and depression also by other mechanisms: Pro-inflammatory cytokines, for one thing, directly affect basal ganglia and dopamine function and, for another, activate sensory nerves. This results in production of pro-inflammatory cytokines and prostaglandins by microglia in the CNS, which then affect the functionality of neurons, thereby contributing to fatigue (215). Immune activation furthermore influences the biosynthesis of the catecholamines dopamine, epinephrine and norepinephrine and the neurotransmitter serotonin (216).

INFLAMMATORY-INDUCED TRYPTOPHAN BREAKDOWN CONTRIBUTES TO THE DEVELOPMENT OF CANCER RELATED FATIGUE AND DEPRESSION

There are several pathophysiological mechanisms, which might explain how Trp metabolites cause CRF or neurobehavioral symptoms related to CRF such as depression.

Trp is a crucial amino acid in brain homeostasis and a precursor for serotonin and melatonin synthesis. It can cross the blood-brain barrier; therefore, reduced Trp availability may contribute to serotonin dysregulation and neurobehavioral manifestations (217, 218). However, also the accumulation of downstream metabolites of the Kyn pathway is suggested to trigger neurobehavioral symptoms (204, 205).

QUIN, which is primarily produced by monocytes/macrophages and microglia, generates free radicals, causes structural changes, and is a selective agonist at the glutamate receptor sensitive to N-methyl-D-aspartate (NMDA receptor) (219). Its accumulation results in excitotoxicity, neuronal cell death and disturbs glutamatergic transmission (220). QUIN cannot cross the blood brain barrier, which is why only QUIN synthesized by microglia or monocytes/macrophages migrated to the CNS influences neuroimmunology (221). On the contrary, KYNA is considered as a neuroprotective Trp metabolite, because it acts as antagonist at the NMDA and other glutamate receptors (222). Previous studies have demonstrated that KYNA can protect against QUIN related neuronal damage (223). This balance between neurotoxic and neuroprotective effects is expressed by the QUIN/KYNA ratio and related to the grade of pathway activity, but also immune activation (224). It was shown that depressed patients have a higher QUIN/KYNA ratio compared to healthy controls, thus moving the balance toward the neurodegenerative effects (225). The imbalance of neurotoxic and neuroprotective Trp metabolites is suggested to play a major role in the development of neuropsychiatric symptoms including CRF and depression (226). 3-HK also exerts neurotoxic effects by causing lipid peroxidation (227).

Although immune system activation frequently coincides with fatigue or depression in cancer patients, it has to be kept in mind, that fatigue or depression also can develop isolatedly in patients with other predisposing conditions (like anxiety or little social support). Probably the development of neuropsychiatric disturbances and depression is alleviated in the presence of an activated immune system and accelerated Trp breakdown, but it must not necessarily lead to depressed mood. Maybe the handling of bad news is impaired if Trp and thus serotonin availability is low.

Additionally, also other factors, like psychosocial aspects including demographical factors (age, gender, culture/ethnicity and social support), behavior/well-being (composed of stress/distress—including spiritual, anxiety, sleep disturbance, coping style, and pain) but also functional status (performance status, physical activity level, physical functioning, and productivity/work) contribute to the development, severity, and duration of CRF and depression. Moreover, an imbalance in the autonomic nervous system, disturbances in the hypothalamic-pituitary-adrenal axis and circadian rhythm as well as hypoxia or anemia are key players in the pathophysiology of CRF and depression (228, 229). These factors might in fact enforce vicious circles, such as e.g., psychosocial stress triggers oxidative stress and inflammation, and thus tumor progression (201).

INHIBITION OF TRYPTOPHAN BREAKDOWN FOR TREATMENT OF FATIGUE AND DEPRESSION

Experiments in mice demonstrated that the IDO pathway modulator indoximod inhibits depressive-like behavior (consecutive to bacterial infection) without altering the infectious immune response (211, 230). Moreover, the specific IDO1 inhibitor epacadostat was shown to reverse chronic

social defeat in mice (231). Another interesting compound, which might target IDO, is the antibiotic minocycline, which was demonstrated to reduce IDO activation and thus prevent depressive-like behavior in animal studies (232–234). Minocycline was also able to decrease IDO expression and the formation of pro-inflammatory cytokines in LPS-treated monocytic human microglial cells (235–237), suggesting that IDO inhibition might be responsible for the anti-depressive effects of minocycline. Also, in humans a large and statistically significant antidepressant effect of minocycline has been observed when comparing to placebo [see review and meta-analysis by Rosenblat and McIntyre (238)]. Due to the good tolerability, future larger RCTs investigating the potential of minocycline (238), but also of other anti-inflammatory treatments (239) are considered. Contrary to these findings, a recent study with mice showed no improvement of cancer-related behavioral symptoms when inhibiting IDO1 (either by an unspecific or a specific IDO inhibitor). Mice treated with 1-MT even had slightly more treatment-associated burrowing deficits. Genetic deletion of IDO on the other hand had no effect on the behavior of mice, but was associated with a worse tumor outcome (240). In consideration of these conflicting data, more studies investigating effects of IDO inhibition in cancer are needed. Clinical trials targeting TDO revealed antidepressant effects as well as amelioration of neurodegeneration following TDO inhibition, and seem to be a promising therapeutic target in cancer patients, especially with neurobehavioral symptoms (241, 242).

Inhibition of KMO also seems to be a possible therapeutic approach in the treatment of fatigue and depression by shifting Kyn metabolism toward the enhanced production of neuroprotective KYNA while decreasing production of neurotoxic QUIN. A recent mice trial revealed that KMO gene deletion substantially reduces 3-HK and QUIN concentrations while elevating KYNA concentrations (243). It was further shown to ameliorate neurodegeneration in patients with Alzheimer's and Parkinson's diseases (242). Therefore, KMO inhibition may be a promising therapeutic target in inflammation-related fatigue or depression by reducing generation of the neurotoxic Trp metabolites 3-HK and QUIN.

Another recent study showed decreased IDO1 and KMO expression in the murine brain as well as decreased IDO1 and IDO2 expression in human peripheral blood mononuclear cells as a consequence of antidepressant treatment (244, 245). This, in turn, demonstrates that reduction of psychosocial stress can also reduce inflammation-related factors.

NUTRITION, MICROBIOME, AND PHYSICAL ACTIVITY AND ITS ASSOCIATION WITH TRYPTOPHAN BREAKDOWN, FATIGUE, AND DEPRESSION

Monoaminergic antidepressants and also omega-3 fatty acids were demonstrated to reduce neurotoxic effects related to Trp breakdown (246). Omega-3 fatty acids contribute to the beneficial effects of the Mediterranean diet, which is regarded as anti-inflammatory diet (247). High adherence to this diet is linked to a lower risk of developing cancer and to a reduced cancer mortality in observational studies (248). A "Western" diet rich in refined sugars and long chain fatty acids and with low fiber content on the other hand enforces a type 1 pro-inflammatory state (249). Mouse experiments furthermore showed that Western diet exposure exacerbated hippocampal and hypothalamic proinflammatory cytokine expression and brain IDO activation after immune stimulation with LPS (250). Inflammation-induced Trp degradation in humans might then further intensify subdued psychosocial factors such as mood, negative thoughts and lack of energy or simply make patients more susceptible to them.

In fact, diet and the gut microbiome may influence inflammation and Trp metabolism by several ways (251): Microbiota metabolize phytochemicals (e.g., in vegetables) to indoles, which activate AhR as ligands, while other microbial-derived metabolites such as the short chain fatty acids butyrate, propionate, and acetate importantly mediate the crosstalk between host-microbiota and thereby have immune modulating effects (251). Actually Trp metabolic pathways are regarded as key biochemical pathways influencing the microbiota-neural-immune axis by translating information on the nutritional, inflammatory, microbial, and emotional state of the organism to the immune system (252–254) and by modulating intestinal immune response (251).

A recent review by Weber et al. proposed that preclinical and several clinical studies argued for the use of a ketogenic diet (KD) in combination with standard therapies in patients with cancer (255): KD had the potential to enhance the antitumor effects of classic chemo- and radiotherapy and to increase the QoL of patients (255). However, the heterogeneity between studies investigating these effects and low adherence to diet limit the current evidence (256). Interestingly, KD was shown to positively influence the Kyn pathway in rats (257). Increased β-hydroxybutyrate concentrations and an increased production of the neuroprotective KYNA were found in rat brain structures as a consequence of KD (258, 259). Also, a recent study in children revealed that Kyn levels significantly decreased and KYNA levels significantly increased 3 months after starting a KD (260).

Significant differences regarding Trp metabolism were reported between a low-glycemic load dietary pattern (characterized by whole grains, legumes, fruits, and vegetables) and a diet high in refined grains and added sugars on inflammation and energy metabolism pathways (261). In line with results of this study, a Mediterranean diet and other plant-based diets have been proposed to reduce fatigue in cancer survivors (262).

As cancer cells are very vulnerable to nutrient deprivation (especially glucose), fasting or fasting-mimicking diets (FMDs) might be another effective strategy to generate environments that can reduce the capability of cancer cells to adapt and survive and thus improve the effects of cancer therapies (263). Further studies investigating the effects of FMDs on Trp catabolism in the tumor microenvironment might therefore provide interesting new insights for future treatment approaches.

Besides, treatment with probiotics might be beneficial for cancer patients: In colorectal cancer survivors, probiotics (*Lactobacillus acidophilus* and *rhamnosus*) improved CRF, irritable bowel syndromes and QoL significantly in a double-blind placebo-controlled study (264); furthermore, probiotics and also melatonin supplementation appear to alleviate side effects of radiation therapy (265). Probiotic supplementation with *Lactobacillus plantarum* in combination with SSRI treatment improved cognitive performance and decreased Kyn concentrations in patients with major depression [compared to SSRI treatment alone, (266)]. Supplementation with a multispecies probiotic had a beneficial effect on Trp metabolism in trained athletes (267) and influenced Trp degradation and gut bacteria composition in patients with Alzheimer's disease (268). Additionally, highly adaptive lactobacilli where shown to produce the AhR ligand indole-3-aldehyde, which enabled IL-22 transcription for the fine tuning of host mucosal reactivity (269). Conclusively, these studies indicate that beneficial effects of probiotics on fatigue or depression might be due to alterations of Trp metabolism or anti-inflammatory effects [see review by (270)]. However, evidence is limited due to the heterogeneity of clinical trials. Therefore, further well-designed longitudinal placebo-controlled studies are desperately needed (271, 272).

Also, a recent review of clinical trials that assessed nutritional interventions for preventing and treating CRF suggests that supplementation with probiotics but also ginseng, or ginger may improve cancer survivors' energy levels and that nutritional interventions, alone or in combination with other interventions should be considered as therapy for fatigue in cancer survivors. Nevertheless, there is lacking evidence to determine the optimal diet to improve CRF in cancer patients (262, 273). Furthermore, also physical activity, psychosocial, mind-body, and pharmacological treatments have been proven to be effective (187).

Physical exercise also affects Trp metabolism and thereby might improve fatigue and depression. As this subject has been discussed elsewhere recently (274, 275), it will be discussed only briefly hereafter. Physical activity increases Trp availability in the brain, which results in an increased 5-HT synthesis and anti-depressant effects (276). Increased muscle use of branched-chain amino acids (BCAAs) favors the passing of Trp through the blood-brain barrier (277). In addition, endurance exercise increases concentrations of circulating free fatty acids, which displaces Trp from albumin, thus increasing free Trp concentrations (278). Additionally, physical activity increases the expression of kynurenine aminotransferases, which enhance the conversion of Kyn into KYNA (unable to cross the blood-brain barrier), thus protecting the brain from stress-induced changes (279). Interestingly, intense physical exercise induces the formation of several pro-inflammatory cytokines (280), which in turn activate IDO1 and Trp breakdown.

IMMUNE ACTIVATION CAUSING TRYPTOPHAN DEGRADATION AND (CONSEQUENTLY) ANEMIA

Another common comorbidity in cancer causing fatigue is anemia (95, 281). Anemic cancer patients have a worse QoL, an adverse outcome as well as a reduced rate of local tumor control compared to non-anemic cancer patients (282, 283).

Anemia is the most common "hematological complication," found in ~40–64% of patients with malignant diseases (94) and is mostly due to anemia of chronic disease (ACD) (284). ACD is caused by enhanced formation of pro-inflammatory cytokines, which can on the one hand directly inhibit erythropoiesis and on the other hand restrict the availability of iron for erythropoiesis. The latter is caused by an increased uptake and retention of iron within the cells of the reticuloendothelial system together with a suppression of iron absorption in the duodenum. The master regulator of iron homeostasis, hepcidin, has a decisive role in these processes. Similarly to Trp breakdown, this is initially a protective mechanism of the immune system to restrict available iron from microbes or tumor cells (285, 286).

IFN-γ, one of the main cytokines of Th1 type immune response, activates IDO and neopterin formation in hematopoietic stem cells and also exerts an influence on the proliferation of various stem cell populations (287). The intravenous injection of neopterin into mice resulted in a prolonged decrease in the number of erythroid progenitor cells and increased the number of myeloid progenitor cells (CFU-GMs) by activating stromal cells (288).

Trp metabolites like Kyn, on the other hand, increase hepcidin expression and inhibit erythropoietin (EPO) production by activating AhR (289). AhR competes with hypoxia-inducible factor 2α (HIF-2α), the key regulator of EPO production, for binding with HIF-1β (289, 290). Well in line with this finding, Kyn/Trp and neopterin were shown earlier to be associated inversely with hemoglobin concentrations and positively with hepcidin concentrations in patients with HIV-infection before antiretroviral therapy (287). Antiretroviral treatment slowed down immune-mediated Trp catabolism and improved iron metabolism and anemia (287).

Interestingly, in patients with different malignant diseases, increased Kyn/Trp and neopterin concentrations also coincided with lower hemoglobin values (85). Also, recent data confirms that anemic cancer patients present with higher inflammatory markers and a higher Kyn/Trp than non-anemic individuals (90). The same is also true for patients with anemia due to inflammation (291) and for HIV-infected patients (191).

Also, QUIN was shown to inhibit EPO production (292) by stimulating the production of nitric oxide (NO) (293) and inducing HIF-1α degradation (294).

In patients with myelodysplastic syndromes, a fundamental role for Trp metabolized along the serotonin pathway in normal erythropoiesis and in the physiopathology of MDS-related anemia was demonstrated recently: Decreased blood serotonin levels were related with impaired erythroid proliferating capacities, and treatment with fluoxetine, a common antidepressant, was effective in increasing serotonin levels and the number of erythroid progenitors (295).

Low serotonin concentrations are also associated with the development of depression. Vulser et al. actually showed a considerable association between anemia and depression in otherwise healthy adults (296). Increased Trp degradation might therefore be a connection between anemia and depression.

These findings show that impaired Trp availability but also accumulation of Trp metabolites, may affect erythropoiesis. In cancer patients, tumor cells produce TDO and IDO1, and both are equally capable of producing Kyn (174). However, they may only contribute to local Trp degradation and do not influence systemic Trp breakdown. On the other hand, IDO1 activity is also stimulated by the activated immune system and thereby contributes to systemic Trp catabolism. Therefore, inflammation-induced IDO1 activation and consecutive Trp breakdown might influence erythropoiesis. The most common symptom of anemia is fatigue, which is why both ACD and inflammation-induced Trp breakdown may be major contributors to overall-fatigue in patients with malignant diseases.

CONCLUSION

Inflammation-induced Trp breakdown in cancer patients is considered to play a key role in the pathophysiology of tumor immune tolerance. Accumulation of Trp metabolites as well as impaired Trp availability suppress the tumor immune response and may also greatly contribute to the development of comorbidities such as fatigue, depression, or anemia, which are all common in patients with malignancies. Although anemia is primarily caused by the enhanced immune response itself, inflammatory-induced Trp degradation may also be involved strongly. Studies have shown that inhibition of Trp breakdown might be a promising therapeutic option in cancer patients to counteract the immunosuppressive tumor microenvironment. Especially cancer patients with no response to immune checkpoint inhibitors might benefit from an additional IDO1 inhibition. Moreover, there is evidence that inhibition of IDO1, TDO, and KMO or other interventions targeting Trp metabolism (like diet or probiotics) may further improve neurobehavioral manifestations including CRF or depression. Further studies investigating the effects of IDO1, TDO, or KMO inhibition on tumor immune response should also take the impact on neurobehavioral manifestations into consideration.

AUTHOR CONTRIBUTIONS

LL and KK wrote the manuscript. PK, EE, WW, DF, and GW critically read and revised the paper. All authors listed approved the submitted version for publication.

FUNDING

This study received funding from Medizinische Universität Innsbruck.

ACKNOWLEDGMENTS

We hereby thank M.Sc. Simon Geisler and PD Johanna Gostner for technical support and interesting discussions.

REFERENCES

1. Rieder J, Lirk P, Hoffmann G. Neopterin as a potential modulator of tumor cell growth and proliferation. *Med Hypotheses.* (2003) 60:531–4. doi: 10.1016/S0306-9877(03)00002-1

2. Pichler R, Fritz J, Heidegger I, Steiner E, Culig Z, Klocker H, et al. Predictive and prognostic role of serum neopterin and tryptophan breakdown in prostate cancer. *Cancer Sci.* (2017) 108:663–70. doi: 10.1111/cas.13171

3. Beatty GL, Gladney WL. Immune escape mechanisms as a guide for cancer immunotherapy. *Clin Cancer Res.* (2015) 21:687–92. doi: 10.1158/1078-0432.CCR-14-1860

4. Opitz CA, Somarribas Patterson LF, Mohapatra SR, Dewi DL, Sadik A, Platten M, et al. The therapeutic potential of targeting tryptophan catabolism in cancer. *Br J Cancer.* (2020) 122:30–44. doi: 10.1038/s41416-019-0664-6

5. Folgiero V, Goffredo BM, Filippini P, Masetti R, Bonanno G, Caruso R, et al. Indoleamine 2,3-dioxygenase 1 (IDO1) activity in leukemia blasts correlates with poor outcome in childhood acute myeloid leukemia. *Oncotarget.* (2014) 5:2052–64. doi: 10.18632/oncotarget.1504

6. Mabuchi R, Hara T, Matsumoto T, Shibata Y, Nakamura N, Nakamura H, et al. High serum concentration of L-kynurenine predicts unfavorable outcomes in patients with acute myeloid leukemia. *Leuk Lymphoma.* (2016) 57:92–8. doi: 10.3109/10428194.2015.1041388

7. Fukuno K, Hara T, Tsurumi H, Shibata Y, Mabuchi R, Nakamura N, et al. Expression of indoleamine 2,3-dioxygenase in leukemic cells indicates an unfavorable prognosis in acute myeloid leukemia patients with intermediate-risk cytogenetics. *Leuk Lymphoma.* (2015) 56:1398–405. doi: 10.3109/10428194.2014.953150

8. Corm S, Berthon C, Imbenotte M, Biggio V, Lhermitte M, Dupont C, et al. Indoleamine 2,3-dioxygenase activity of acute myeloid leukemia cells can be measured from patients' sera by HPLC and is inducible by IFN-gamma. *Leuk Res.* (2009) 33:490–4. doi: 10.1016/j.leukres.2008.06.014

9. Chamuleau ME, van de Loosdrecht AA, Hess CJ, Janssen JJ, Zevenbergen A, Delwel R, et al. High INDO (indoleamine 2,3-dioxygenase) mRNA level in blasts of acute myeloid leukemic patients predicts poor clinical outcome. *Haematologica.* (2008) 93:1894–8. doi: 10.3324/haematol.13112

10. Tang XQ, Zhao ZG, Wang HX, Li QB, Lu J, Zou P. [Indoleamine 2, 3-dioxygenase activity in acute myeloid leukemia cells contributing to tumor immune escape]. *Zhongguo Shi Yan Xue Ye Xue Za Zhi.* (2006) 14:539–42.

11. Wei L, Zhu S, Li M, Li F, Wei F, Liu J, et al. High indoleamine 2,3-dioxygenase is correlated with microvessel density and worse prognosis in breast cancer. *Front Immunol.* (2018) 9:724. doi: 10.3389/fimmu.2018.00724

12. Eniu DT, Romanciuc F, Moraru C, Goidescu I, Eniu D, Staicu A, et al. The decrease of some serum free amino acids can predict breast cancer diagnosis and progression. *Scandinav J Clin Lab Investig.* (2019) 79:17–24. doi: 10.1080/00365513.2018.1542541

13. Heng B, Lim CK, Lovejoy DB, Bessede A, Gluch L, Guillemin GJ. Understanding the role of the kynurenine pathway in human breast cancer immunobiology. *Oncotarget.* (2016) 7:6506–20. doi: 10.18632/oncotarget.6467

14. Lyon DE, Walter JM, Starkweather AR, Schubert CM, McCain NL. Tryptophan degradation in women with breast cancer: a pilot study. *BMC Research Notes.* (2011) 4:156. doi: 10.1186/1756-0500-4-156

15. Isla Larrain MT, Rabassa ME, Lacunza E, Barbera A, Cretón A, Segal-Eiras A, et al. IDO is highly expressed in breast cancer and breast cancer-derived circulating microvesicles and associated to aggressive types of tumors by *in silico* analysis. *Tumor Biol.* (2014) 35:6511–9. doi: 10.1007/s13277-014-1859-3

16. Girgin G, Sahin TT, Fuchs D, Kasuya H, Yuksel O, Tekin E, et al. Immune system modulation in patients with malignant and benign breast disorders: tryptophan degradation and serum neopterin. *Int J Biol Markers.* (2009) 24:265–71. doi: 10.1177/172460080902400408

17. Chen JY, Li CF, Kuo CC, Tsai KK, Hou MF, Hung WC. Cancer/stroma interplay via cyclooxygenase-2 and indoleamine 2,3-dioxygenase promotes breast cancer progression. *Breast Cancer Res.* (2014) 16:410. doi: 10.1186/s13058-014-0410-1

18. Soliman H, Rawal B, Fulp J, Lee JH, Lopez A, Bui MM, et al. Analysis of indoleamine 2-3 dioxygenase (IDO1) expression in breast cancer tissue by immunohistochemistry. *Cancer Immunol Immunother.* (2013) 62:829–37. doi: 10.1007/s00262-013-1393-y

19. Jacquemier J, Bertucci F, Finetti P, Esterni B, Charafe-Jauffret E, Thibult ML, et al. High expression of indoleamine 2,3-dioxygenase in the tumour is associated with medullary features and favourable outcome in basal-like breast carcinoma. *Int J Cancer.* (2012) 130:96–104. doi: 10.1002/ijc.25979

20. Yu J, Sun J, Wang SE, Li H, Cao S, Cong Y, et al. Upregulated expression of indoleamine 2, 3-dioxygenase in primary breast cancer correlates with increase of infiltrated regulatory T cells in situ and lymph node metastasis. *Clin Dev Immunol.* (2011) 2011:469135. doi: 10.1155/2011/469135

21. Ferdinande L, Decaestecker C, Verset L, Mathieu A, Moles Lopez X, Negulescu AM, et al. Clinicopathological significance of indoleamine 2,3-dioxygenase 1 expression in colorectal cancer. *Br J Cancer.* (2012) 106:141–7. doi: 10.1038/bjc.2011.513

22. Engin A, Gonul II, Engin AB, Karamercan A, Sepici Dincel A, Dursun A. Relationship between indoleamine 2,3-dioxygenase activity and lymphatic invasion propensity of colorectal carcinoma. *World J Gastroenterol.* (2016) 22:3592–601. doi: 10.3748/wjg.v22.i13.3592

23. Gao YF, Peng RQ, Li J, Ding Y, Zhang X, Wu XJ, et al. The paradoxical patterns of expression of indoleamine 2,3-dioxygenase in colon cancer. *J Transl Med.* (2009) 7:71. doi: 10.1186/1479-5876-7-71

24. Huang A, Fuchs D, Widner B, Glover C, Henderson DC, Allen-Mersh TG. Serum tryptophan decrease correlates with immune activation and impaired quality of life in colorectal cancer. *Br J Cancer.* (2002) 86:1691–6. doi: 10.1038/sj.bjc.6600336

25. Brandacher G, Perathoner A, Ladurner R, Schneeberger S, Obrist P, Winkler C, et al. Prognostic value of indoleamine 2,3-dioxygenase expression in colorectal cancer: effect on tumor-infiltrating T cells. *Clin Cancer Res.* (2006) 12:1144–51. doi: 10.1158/1078-0432.CCR-05-1966

26. Jia Y, Wang H, Wang Y, Wang T, Wang M, Ma M, et al. Low expression of Bin1, along with high expression of IDO in tumor tissue and draining lymph nodes, are predictors of poor prognosis for esophageal squamous cell cancer patients. *Int J Cancer.* (2015) 137:1095–106. doi: 10.1002/ijc.29481

27. Iwagaki H, Hizuta A, Tanaka N, Orita K. Decreased serum tryptophan in patients with cancer cachexia correlates with increased serum neopterin. *Immunol Invest.* (1995) 24:467–78. doi: 10.3109/08820139509066843

28. Laimer K, Troester B, Kloss F, Schafer G, Obrist P, Perathoner A, et al. Expression and prognostic impact of indoleamine 2,3-dioxygenase in oral squamous cell carcinomas. *Oral Oncol.* (2011) 47:352–7. doi: 10.1016/j.oraloncology.2011.03.007

29. Zhang G, Liu WL, Zhang L, Wang JY, Kuang MH, Liu P, et al. Involvement of indoleamine 2,3-dioxygenase in impairing tumor-infiltrating CD8 T-cell functions in esophageal squamous cell carcinoma. *Clin Dev Immunol.* (2011) 2011:384726. doi: 10.1155/2011/384726

30. Adams S, Teo C, McDonald KL, Zinger A, Bustamante S, Lim CK, et al. Involvement of the kynurenine pathway in human glioma pathophysiology. *PLoS ONE.* (2014) 9:e112945. doi: 10.1371/journal.pone.0112945

31. Zhai L, Dey M, Lauing KL, Gritsina G, Kaur R, Lukas RV, et al. The kynurenine to tryptophan ratio as a prognostic tool for glioblastoma patients enrolling in immunotherapy. *J Clin Neurosci.* (2015) 22:1964–8. doi: 10.1016/j.jocn.2015.06.018

32. Mitsuka K, Kawataki T, Satoh E, Asahara T, Horikoshi T, Kinouchi H. Expression of indoleamine 2,3-dioxygenase and correlation with pathological malignancy in gliomas. *Neurosurgery.* (2013) 72:1031–8; discussion: 1038–9. doi: 10.1227/NEU.0b013e31828cf945

33. Wainwright DA, Balyasnikova IV, Chang AL, Ahmed AU, Moon KS, Auffinger B, et al. IDO expression in brain tumors increases the recruitment of regulatory T cells and negatively impacts survival. *Clin Cancer Res.* (2012) 18:6110–21. doi: 10.1158/1078-0432.CCR-12-2130

34. Heeren AM, van Dijk I, Berry D, Khelil M, Ferns D, Kole J, et al. Indoleamine 2,3-dioxygenase expression pattern in the tumor microenvironment predicts clinical outcome in early stage cervical cancer. *Front Immunol.* (2018) 9:1598. doi: 10.3389/fimmu.2018.01598

35. Gostner JM, Obermayr E, Braicu IE, Concin N, Mahner S, Vanderstichele A, et al. Immunobiochemical pathways of neopterin formation and tryptophan breakdown via indoleamine 2,3-dioxygenase correlate with circulating tumor cells in ovarian cancer patients- A study of the OVCAD consortium. *Gynecol Oncol.* (2018) 149:371–80. doi: 10.1016/j.ygyno.2018.02.020

36. de Jong RA, Kema IP, Boerma A, Boezen HM, van der Want JJ, Gooden MJ, et al. Prognostic role of indoleamine 2,3-dioxygenase in endometrial carcinoma. *Gynecol Oncol.* (2012) 126:474–80. doi: 10.1016/j.ygyno.2012.05.034

37. Ferns DM, Kema IP, Buist MR, Nijman HW, Kenter GG, Jordanova ES. Indoleamine-2,3-dioxygenase (IDO) metabolic activity is detrimental for cervical cancer patient survival. *Oncoimmunology.* (2015) 4:e981457. doi: 10.4161/2162402X.2014.981457

38. Inaba T, Ino K, Kajiyama H, Shibata K, Yamamoto E, Kondo S, et al. Indoleamine 2,3-dioxygenase expression predicts impaired survival of invasive cervical cancer patients treated with radical hysterectomy. *Gynecol Oncol.* (2010) 117:423–8. doi: 10.1016/j.ygyno.2010.02.028

39. Sperner-Unterweger B, Neurauter G, Klieber M, Kurz K, Meraner V, Zeimet A, et al. Enhanced tryptophan degradation in patients with ovarian carcinoma correlates with several serum soluble immune activation markers. *Immunobiology.* (2011) 216:296–301. doi: 10.1016/j.imbio.2010.07.010

40. Inaba T, Ino K, Kajiyama H, Yamamoto E, Shibata K, Nawa A, et al. Role of the immunosuppressive enzyme indoleamine 2,3-dioxygenase in the progression of ovarian carcinoma. *Gynecol Oncol.* (2009) 115:185–92. doi: 10.1016/j.ygyno.2009.07.015

41. de Jong RA, Nijman HW, Boezen HM, Volmer M, Ten Hoor KA, Krijnen J, et al. Serum tryptophan and kynurenine concentrations as parameters for indoleamine 2,3-dioxygenase activity in patients with endometrial, ovarian, and vulvar cancer. *Int J Gynecol Cancer.* (2011) 21:1320–7. doi: 10.1097/IGC.0b013e31822017fb

42. Ino K, Yamamoto E, Shibata K, Kajiyama H, Yoshida N, Terauchi M, et al. Inverse correlation between tumoral indoleamine 2,3-dioxygenase expression and tumor-infiltrating lymphocytes in endometrial cancer: its association with disease progression and survival. *Clin Cancer Res.* (2008) 14:2310–7. doi: 10.1158/1078-0432.CCR-07-4144

43. Fotopoulou C, Sehouli J, Pschowski R, VON Haehling S, Domanska G, Braicu EI, et al. Systemic changes of tryptophan catabolites via the indoleamine-2,3-dioxygenase pathway in primary cervical cancer. *Anticancer Res.* (2011) 31:2629–35.

44. Okamoto A, Nikaido T, Ochiai K, Takakura S, Saito M, Aoki Y, et al. Indoleamine 2,3-dioxygenase serves as a marker of poor prognosis in gene expression profiles of serous ovarian cancer cells. *Clin Cancer Res.* (2005) 11:6030–9. doi: 10.1158/1078-0432.CCR-04-2671

45. Takao M, Okamoto A, Nikaido T, Urashima M, Takakura S, Saito M, et al. Increased synthesis of indoleamine-2,3-dioxygenase protein is positively associated with impaired survival in patients with serous-type, but not with other types of, ovarian cancer. *Oncol Rep.* (2007) 17:1333–9. doi: 10.3892/or.17.6.1333

46. Schroecksnadel K, Winkler C, Fuith LC, Fuchs D. Tryptophan degradation in patients with gynecological cancer correlates with immune activation. *Cancer Lett.* (2005) 223:323–9. doi: 10.1016/j.canlet.2004.10.033

47. Ino K, Yoshida N, Kajiyama H, Shibata K, Yamamoto E, Kidokoro K, et al. Indoleamine 2,3-dioxygenase is a novel prognostic indicator for endometrial cancer. *Br J Cancer.* (2006) 95:1555–61. doi: 10.1038/sj.bjc.6603477

48. Li S, Han X, Lyu Q, Xie Q, Deng H, Mu L, et al. Mechanism and prognostic value of indoleamine 2,3-dioxygenase 1 expressed in hepatocellular carcinoma. *Cancer Sci.* (2018) 109:3726–36. doi: 10.1111/cas.13811

49. Jin H, Zhang Y, You H, Tao X, Wang C, Jin G, et al. Prognostic significance of kynurenine 3-monooxygenase and effects on proliferation, migration, and invasion of human hepatocellular carcinoma. *Sci Rep.* (2015) 5:10466. doi: 10.1038/srep10466

50. Pan K, Wang H, Chen MS, Zhang HK, Weng DS, Zhou J, et al. Expression and prognosis role of indoleamine 2,3-dioxygenase in hepatocellular carcinoma. *J Cancer Res Clin Oncol.* (2008) 134:1247–53. doi: 10.1007/s00432-008-0395-1

51. Ishio T, Goto S, Tahara K, Tone S, Kawano K, Kitano S. Immunoactivative role of indoleamine 2,3-dioxygenase in human hepatocellular carcinoma. *J Gastroenterol Hepatol.* (2004) 19:319–26. doi: 10.1111/j.1440-1746.2003.03259.x

52. Trott JF, Kim J, Abu Aboud O, Wettersten H, Stewart B, Berryhill G, et al. Inhibiting tryptophan metabolism enhances interferon therapy in kidney cancer. *Oncotarget.* (2016) 7:66540–57. doi: 10.18632/oncotarget.11658

53. Lucarelli G, Rutigliano M, Ferro M, Giglio A, Intini A, Triggiano F, et al. Activation of the kynurenine pathway predicts poor outcome in patients with clear cell renal cell carcinoma. *Urol Oncol.* (2017) 35:461.e15–461.e27. doi: 10.1016/j.urolonc.2017.02.011

54. Riesenberg R, Weiler C, Spring O, Eder M, Buchner A, Popp T, et al. Expression of indoleamine 2,3-dioxygenase in tumor endothelial cells correlates with long-term survival of patients with renal cell carcinoma. *Clin Cancer Res.* (2007) 13:6993–7002. doi: 10.1158/1078-0432.CCR-07-0942

55. Yuan F, Liu Y, Fu X, Chen J. Indoleamine-pyrrole 2,3-dioxygenase might be a prognostic biomarker for patients with renal cell carcinoma. *Zhong Nan Da Xue Xue Bao Yi Xue Ban.* (2012) 37:649–55. doi: 10.3969/j.issn.1672-7347.2012.07.001

56. Tang D, Yue L, Yao R, Zhou L, Yang Y, Lu L, et al. P53 prevent tumor invasion and metastasis by down-regulating IDO in lung cancer. *Oncotarget.* (2017) 8:54548–57. doi: 10.18632/oncotarget.17408

57. Chuang SC, Fanidi A, Ueland PM, Relton C, Midttun O, Vollset SE, et al. Circulating biomarkers of tryptophan and the kynurenine pathway and lung cancer risk. *Cancer Epidemiol Biomarkers Prev.* (2014) 23:461–8. doi: 10.1158/1055-9965.EPI-13-0770

58. Huang JY, Larose TL, Luu HN, Wang R, Fanidi A, Alcala K, et al. Circulating markers of cellular immune activation in prediagnostic blood sample and lung cancer risk in the Lung Cancer Cohort Consortium (LC3). *Int J Cancer.* (2019). doi: 10.1002/ijc.32555. [Epub ahead of print].

59. Hsu YL, Hung JY, Chiang SY, Jian SF, Wu CY, Lin YS, et al. Lung cancer-derived galectin-1 contributes to cancer associated fibroblast-mediated cancer progression and immune suppression through TDO2/kynurenine axis. *Oncotarget.* (2016) 7:27584–98. doi: 10.18632/oncotarget.8488

60. Creelan BC, Antonia S, Bepler G, Garrett TJ, Simon GR, Soliman HH. Indoleamine 2,3-dioxygenase activity and clinical outcome following induction chemotherapy and concurrent chemoradiation in Stage III non-small cell lung cancer. *Oncoimmunology.* (2013) 2:e23428. doi: 10.4161/onci.23428

61. Karanikas V, Zamanakou M, Kerenidi T, Dahabreh J, Hevas A, Nakou M, et al. Indoleamine 2,3-dioxygenase (IDO) expression in lung cancer. *Cancer Biol Ther.* (2007) 6:1258–62. doi: 10.4161/cbt.6.8.4446

62. Kurz K, Fiegl M, Holzner B, Giesinger J, Pircher M, Weiss G, et al. Fatigue in patients with lung cancer is related with accelerated tryptophan breakdown. *PLoS ONE.* (2012) 7:e36956. doi: 10.1371/journal.pone.0036956

63. Astigiano S, Morandi B, Costa R, Mastracci L, D'Agostino A, Ratto GB, et al. Eosinophil granulocytes account for indoleamine 2,3-dioxygenase-mediated immune escape in human non-small cell lung cancer. *Neoplasia.* (2005) 7:390–6. doi: 10.1593/neo.04658

64. Engin AB, Ozkan Y, Fuchs D, Yardim-Akaydin S. Increased tryptophan degradation in patients with bronchus carcinoma. *Eur J Cancer Care.* (2010) 19:803–8. doi: 10.1111/j.1365-2354.2009.01122.x

65. Suzuki Y, Suda T, Furuhashi K, Suzuki M, Fujie M, Hahimoto D, et al. Increased serum kynurenine/tryptophan ratio correlates with disease progression in lung cancer. *Lung Cancer.* (2010) 67:361–5. doi: 10.1016/j.lungcan.2009.05.001

66. Nam SJ, Kim S, Paik JH, Kim TM, Heo DS, Kim CW, et al. An increase in indoleamine 2,3-dioxygenase-positive cells in the tumor microenvironment predicts favorable prognosis in patients with diffuse large B-cell lymphoma treated with rituximab, cyclophosphamide, doxorubicin, vincristine, and prednisolone. *Leuk Lymphoma.* (2016) 57:1956–60. doi: 10.3109/10428194.2015.1117610

67. Masaki A, Ishida T, Maeda Y, Suzuki S, Ito A, Takino H, et al. Prognostic significance of tryptophan catabolism in adult T-cell leukemia/lymphoma. *Clin Cancer Res.* (2015) 21:2830–9. doi: 10.1158/1078-0432.CCR-14-2275

68. Liu XQ, Lu K, Feng LL, Ding M, Gao JM, Ge XL, et al. Up-regulated expression of indoleamine 2,3-dioxygenase 1 in non-Hodgkin lymphoma correlates with increased regulatory T-cell infiltration. *Leuk Lymphoma.* (2014) 55:405–14. doi: 10.3109/10428194.2013.804917

69. Yoshikawa T, Hara T, Tsurumi H, Goto N, Hoshi M, Kitagawa J, et al. Serum concentration of L-kynurenine predicts the clinical outcome of patients with diffuse large B-cell lymphoma treated with R-CHOP. *Eur J Haematol.* (2010) 84:304–9. doi: 10.1111/j.1600-0609.2009.01393.x

70. Choe JY, Yun JY, Jeon YK, Kim SH, Park G, Huh JR, et al. Indoleamine 2,3-dioxygenase (IDO) is frequently expressed in stromal cells of Hodgkin

lymphoma and is associated with adverse clinical features: a retrospective cohort study. *BMC Cancer.* (2014) 14:335. doi: 10.1186/1471-2407-14-335

71. Giusti RM, Maloney EM, Hanchard B, Morgan OS, Steinberg SM, Wachter H, et al. Differential patterns of serum biomarkers of immune activation in human T-cell lymphotropic virus type I-associated myelopathy/tropical spastic paraparesis, and adult T-cell leukemia/lymphoma. *Cancer Epidemiol Biomarkers Prev.* (1996) 5:699–704.

72. Ninomiya S, Hara T, Tsurumi H, Hoshi M, Kanemura N, Goto N, et al. Indoleamine 2,3-dioxygenase in tumor tissue indicates prognosis in patients with diffuse large B-cell lymphoma treated with R-CHOP. *Ann Hematol.* (2011) 90:409–16. doi: 10.1007/s00277-010-1093-z

73. Hoshi M, Ito H, Fujigaki H, Takemura M, Takahashi T, Tomita E, et al. Indoleamine 2,3-dioxygenase is highly expressed in human adult T-cell leukemia/lymphoma and chemotherapy changes tryptophan catabolism in serum and reduced activity. *Leuk Res.* (2009) 33:39–45. doi: 10.1016/j.leukres.2008.05.023

74. Pelak MJ, Snietura M, Lange D, Nikiel B, Pecka KM. The prognostic significance of indoleamine-2,3-dioxygenase and the receptors for transforming growth factor beta and interferon gamma in metastatic lymph nodes in malignant melanoma. *Pol J Pathol.* (2015) 66:376–82. doi: 10.5114/pjp.2015.57249

75. Weinlich G, Murr C, Richardsen L, Winkler C, Fuchs D. Decreased serum tryptophan concentration predicts poor prognosis in malignant melanoma patients. *Dermatology.* (2007) 214:8–14. doi: 10.1159/000096906

76. Ryan M, Crow J, Kahmke R, Fisher SR, Su Z, Lee WT. FoxP3 and indoleamine 2,3-dioxygenase immunoreactivity in sentinel nodes from melanoma patients. *Am J Otolaryngol.* (2014) 35:689–94. doi: 10.1016/j.amjoto.2014.08.009

77. Capuron L, Neurauter G, Musselman DL, Lawson DH, Nemeroff CB, Fuchs D, et al. Interferon-alpha-induced changes in tryptophan metabolism: *relationship to depression and paroxetine treatment. Biol Psychiatry.* (2003) 54:906–14. doi: 10.1016/S0006-3223(03)00173-2

78. Speeckaert R, Vermaelen K, van Geel N, Autier P, Lambert J, Haspeslagh M, et al. Indoleamine 2,3-dioxygenase, a new prognostic marker in sentinel lymph nodes of melanoma patients. *Eur J Cancer.* (2012) 48:2004–11. doi: 10.1016/j.ejca.2011.09.007

79. Brody JR, Costantino CL, Berger AC, Sato T, Lisanti MP, Yeo CJ, et al. Expression of indoleamine 2,3-dioxygenase in metastatic malignant melanoma recruits regulatory T cells to avoid immune detection and affects survival. *Cell Cycle.* (2009) 8:1930–4. doi: 10.4161/cc.8.12.8745

80. Urakawa H, Nishida Y, Nakashima H, Shimoyama Y, Nakamura S, Ishiguro N. Prognostic value of indoleamine 2,3-dioxygenase expression in high grade osteosarcoma. *Clin Exp Metast.* (2009) 26:1005–12. doi: 10.1007/s10585-009-9290-7

81. Zhang T, Tan XL, Xu Y, Wang ZZ, Xiao CH, Liu R. Expression and prognostic value of indoleamine 2,3-dioxygenase in pancreatic cancer. *Chin Med J.* (2017) 130:710–6. doi: 10.4103/0366-6999.201613

82. Huang JY, Butler LM, Midttun O, Ulvik A, Wang R, Jin A, et al. A prospective evaluation of serum kynurenine metabolites and risk of pancreatic cancer. *PLoS ONE.* (2018) 13:e0196465. doi: 10.1371/journal.pone.0196465

83. Feder-Mengus C, Wyler S, Hudolin T, Ruszat R, Bubendorf L, Chiarugi A, et al. High expression of indoleamine 2,3-dioxygenase gene in prostate cancer. *Eur J Cancer.* (2008) 44:2266–75. doi: 10.1016/j.ejca.2008.05.023

84. Moretti S, Menicali E, Voce P, Morelli S, Cantarelli S, Sponziello M, et al. Indoleamine 2,3-dioxygenase 1 (IDO1) is up-regulated in thyroid carcinoma and drives the development of an immunosuppressant tumor microenvironment. *J Clin Endocrinol Metab.* (2014) 99:E832–840. doi: 10.1210/jc.2013-3351

85. Schroecksnadel K, Fiegl M, Prassl K, Winkler C, Denz HA, Fuchs D. Diminished quality of life in patients with cancer correlates with tryptophan degradation. *J Cancer Res Clin Oncol.* (2007) 133:477–85. doi: 10.1007/s00432-007-0191-3

86. Platten M, Nollen EAA, Röhrig UF, Fallarino F, Opitz CA. Tryptophan metabolism as a common therapeutic target in cancer, neurodegeneration and beyond. *Nat Rev Drug Discov.* (2019) 18:379–401. doi: 10.1038/s41573-019-0016-5

87. Knutson KL, Disis ML. Tumor antigen-specific T helper cells in cancer immunity and immunotherapy. *Cancer Immunol Immunother.* (2005) 54:721–8. doi: 10.1007/s00262-004-0653-2

88. Murr C, Widner B, Wirleitner B, Fuchs D. Neopterin as a marker for immune system activation. *Curr Drug Metab.* (2002) 3:175–87. doi: 10.2174/1389200024605082

89. Denz H, Orth B, Weiss G, Herrmann R, Huber P, Wachter H, et al. Weight loss in patients with hematological neoplasias is associated with immune system stimulation. *Clin Investig.* (1993) 71:37–41. doi: 10.1007/BF00210961

90. Kink P, Egger E, Klaunzner M, Weiss G, Willenbacher W, Kasseroler M, et al. Tryptophan and phenylalanine metabolism and depression in patients with solid tumors. In: *Pteridines, 38th International Winter-Workshop Clinical, Chemical and Biochemical Aspects of Pteridines and Related Topics Innsbruck, February 26th–March 1st, 2019.* Innsbruck (2019).

91. Melichar B, Spisarova M, Bartouskova M, Krcmova LK, Javorska L, Studentova H. Neopterin as a biomarker of immune response in cancer patients. *Ann Transl Med.* (2017) 5:280. doi: 10.21037/atm.2017.06.29

92. Carlin JM, Ozaki Y, Byrne GI, Brown RR, Borden EC. Interferons and indoleamine 2,3-dioxygenase: role in antimicrobial and antitumor effects. *Experientia.* (1989) 45:535–41. doi: 10.1007/BF01990503

93. Timosenko E, Hadjinicolaou AV, Cerundolo V. Modulation of cancer-specific immune responses by amino acid degrading enzymes. *Immunotherapy.* (2017) 9:83–97. doi: 10.2217/imt-2016-0118

94. Gaspar BL, Sharma P, Das R. Anemia in malignancies: pathogenetic and diagnostic considerations. *Hematology.* (2015) 20:18–25. doi: 10.1179/1607845414Y.0000000161

95. Sobrero A, Puglisi F, Guglielmi A, Belvedere O, Aprile G, Ramello M, et al. Fatigue: a main component of anemia symptomatology. *Semin Oncol.* (2001) 28(2 Suppl. 8):15–8. doi: 10.1016/S0093-7754(01)90207-6

96. Stone P, Richards M, Hardy, J. Fatigue in patients with cancer. *Eur J Cancer.* (1998) 34:1670–76. doi: 10.1016/S0959-8049(98)00167-1

97. Narayanan V, Koshy C. Fatigue in cancer: a review of literature. *Indian J Palliat Care.* (2009) 15:19–25. doi: 10.4103/0973-1075.53507

98. LaVoy EC, Fagundes CP, Dantzer R. Exercise, inflammation, and fatigue in cancer survivors. *Exerc Immunol Rev.* (2016) 22:82–93.

99. Mitchell AJ, Chan M, Bhatti H, Halton M, Grassi L, Johansen C, et al. Prevalence of depression, anxiety, and adjustment disorder in oncological, haematological, and palliative-care settings: a meta-analysis of 94 interview-based studies. *Lancet Oncol.* (2011) 12:160–74. doi: 10.1016/S1470-2045(11)70002-X

100. Ng CG, Boks MP, Zainal NZ, de Wit NJ. The prevalence and pharmacotherapy of depression in cancer patients. *J Affect Disord.* (2011) 131:1–7. doi: 10.1016/j.jad.2010.07.034

101. Linden W, Vodermaier A, Mackenzie R, Greig D. Anxiety and depression after cancer diagnosis: prevalence rates by cancer type, gender, and age. *J Affect Disord.* (2012) 141:343–51. doi: 10.1016/j.jad.2012.03.025

102. Peters JC. Tryptophan nutrition and metabolism: an overview. *Adv Exp Med Biol.* (1991) 294:345–58. doi: 10.1007/978-1-4684-5952-4_32

103. Richard DM, Dawes MA, Mathias CW, Acheson A, Hill-Kapturczak N, Dougherty DM. L-Tryptophan: basic metabolic functions, behavioral research and therapeutic indications. *Int J Tryptophan Res.* (2009) 2:45–60. doi: 10.4137/IJTR.S2129

104. Cheng HH, Kuo CC, Yan JL, Chen HL, Lin WC, Wang KH, et al. Control of cyclooxygenase-2 expression and tumorigenesis by endogenous 5-methoxytryptophan. *Proc Natl Acad Sci USA.* (2012) 109:13231–6. doi: 10.1073/pnas.1209919109

105. Jacobsen JP, Medvedev IO, Caron MG. The 5-HT deficiency theory of depression: perspectives from a naturalistic 5-HT deficiency model, the tryptophan hydroxylase 2Arg439His knockin mouse. *Philos Trans R Soc Lond B Biol Sci.* (2012) 367:2444–59. doi: 10.1098/rstb.2012.0109

106. Canli T, Lesch KP. Long story short: the serotonin transporter in emotion regulation and social cognition. *Nat Neurosci.* (2007) 10:1103–9. doi: 10.1038/nn1964

107. Berger M, Gray JA, Roth BL. The expanded biology of serotonin. *Annu Rev Med.* (2009) 60:355–66. doi: 10.1146/annurev.med.60.042307.110802

108. Slominski A, Baker J, Rosano TG, Guisti LW, Ermak G, Grande M, et al. Metabolism of serotonin to N-acetylserotonin, melatonin, and 5-methoxytryptamine in hamster skin culture. *J Biol Chem.* (1996) 271:12281–6. doi: 10.1074/jbc.271.21.12281

109. Claustrat B, Leston J. Melatonin: physiological effects in humans. *Neurochirurgie.* (2015) 61:77–84. doi: 10.1016/j.neuchi.2015.03.002

110. Jones RS. Tryptamine: a neuromodulator or neurotransmitter in mammalian brain? *Prog Neurobiol.* (1982) 19:117–39. doi: 10.1016/0301-0082(82)90023-5

111. Nishizuka Y, Hayaishi O. Enzymic synthesis of niacin nucleotides from 3-hydroxyanthranilic acid in mammalian liver. *J Biol Chem.* (1963) 238:483–5.

112. Liu L, Su X, Quinn WJ III, Hui S, Krukenberg K, Frederick DW, et al. Quantitative analysis of NAD synthesis-breakdown fluxes. *Cell metabolism.* (2018) 27:1067–80.e5. doi: 10.1016/j.cmet.2018.03.018

113. Powanda MC, Wannemacher RW Jr. Evidence for a linear correlation between the level of dietary tryptophan and hepatic NAD concentration and for a systematic variation in tissue NAD concentration in the mouse and the rat. *J Nutr.* (1970) 100:1471–8. doi: 10.1093/jn/100.12.1471

114. Mehler AH, Knox WE. The conversion of tryptophan to kynurenine in liver. II. The enzymatic hydrolysis of formylkynurenine. *J Biol Chem.* (1950) 187:431–8.

115. Ren S, Correia MA. Heme: a regulator of rat hepatic tryptophan 2,3-dioxygenase? *Arch Biochem Biophys.* (2000) 377:195–203. doi: 10.1006/abbi.2000.1755

116. Danesch U, Gloss B, Schmid W, Schutz G, Schule R, Renkawitz R. Glucocorticoid induction of the rat tryptophan oxygenase gene is mediated by two widely separated glucocorticoid-responsive elements. *EMBO J.* (1987) 6:625–30. doi: 10.1002/j.1460-2075.1987.tb04800.x

117. Badawy AAB. Kynurenine pathway of tryptophan metabolism: regulatory and functional aspects. *Int J Tryptophan Res.* (2017) 10:1178646917691938. doi: 10.1177/1178646917691938

118. Hornyak L, Dobos N, Koncz G, Karanyi Z, Pall D, Szabo Z, et al. The role of indoleamine-2,3-dioxygenase in cancer development, diagnostics, and therapy. *Front Immunol.* (2018) 9:151. doi: 10.3389/fimmu.2018.00151

119. Pallotta MT, Fallarino F, Matino D, Macchiarulo A, Orabona C. AhR-mediated, non-genomic modulation of IDO1 function. *Front Immunol.* (2014) 5:497. doi: 10.3389/fimmu.2014.00497

120. Vogel CF, Goth SR, Dong B, Pessah IN, Matsumura F. Aryl hydrocarbon receptor signaling mediates expression of indoleamine 2,3-dioxygenase. *Biochem Biophys Res Commun.* (2008) 375:331–5. doi: 10.1016/j.bbrc.2008.07.156

121. Nguyen NT, Kimura A, Nakahama T, Chinen I, Masuda K, Nohara K, et al. Aryl hydrocarbon receptor negatively regulates dendritic cell immunogenicity via a kynurenine-dependent mechanism. *Proc Natl Acad Sci USA.* (2010) 107:19961–6. doi: 10.1073/pnas.1014465107

122. Hennequart M, Pilotte L, Cane S, Hoffmann D, Stroobant V, Plaen E, et al. Constitutive IDO1 expression in human tumors is driven by cyclooxygenase-2 and mediates intrinsic immune resistance. *Cancer Immunol Res.* (2017) 5:695–709. doi: 10.1158/2326-6066.CIR-16-0400

123. Musso T, Gusella GL, Brooks A, Longo DL, Varesio L. Interleukin-4 inhibits indoleamine 2,3-dioxygenase expression in human monocytes. *Blood.* (1994) 83:1408–11. doi: 10.1182/blood.V83.5.1408.1408

124. Chaves AC, Ceravolo IP, Gomes JA, Zani CL, Romanha AJ, Gazzinelli RT. IL-4 and IL-13 regulate the induction of indoleamine 2,3-dioxygenase activity and the control of Toxoplasma gondii replication in human fibroblasts activated with IFN-gamma. *Eur J Immunol.* (2001) 31:333–44. doi: 10.1002/1521-4141(200102)31:2<333::aid-immu333>3.0.co;2-x

125. Prendergast GC, Malachowski WJ, Mondal A, Scherle P, Muller AJ. Indoleamine 2,3-dioxygenase and its therapeutic inhibition in cancer. *Int Rev Cell Mol Biol.* (2018) 336:175–203. doi: 10.1016/bs.ircmb.2017.07.004

126. Lee YK, Lee HB, Shin DM, Kang MJ, Yi EC, Noh S, et al. Heme-binding-mediated negative regulation of the tryptophan metabolic enzyme indoleamine 2,3-dioxygenase 1 (IDO1) by IDO2. *Exp Mol Med.* (2014) 46:e121. doi: 10.1038/emm.2014.69

127. Mandi Y, Vecsei L. The kynurenine system and immunoregulation. *J Neural Transm.* (2012) 119:197–209. doi: 10.1007/s00702-011-0681-y

128. Minatogawa Y, Suzuki S, Ando Y, Tone S, Takikawa, O. Tryptophan pyrrole ring cleavage enzymes in placenta. *Adv Exp Med Biol.* (2003) 527:425–34. doi: 10.1007/978-1-4615-0135-0_50

129. Kudo Y, Boyd CA, Spyropoulou I, Redman CW, Takikawa O, Katsuki T, et al. Indoleamine 2,3-dioxygenase: distribution and function in the developing human placenta. *J Reprod Immunol.* (2004) 61:87–98. doi: 10.1016/j.jri.2003.11.004

130. Suzuki S, Tone S, Takikawa O, Kubo T, Kohno I, Minatogawa Y. Expression of indoleamine 2,3-dioxygenase and tryptophan 2,3-dioxygenase in early concepti. *Biochem J.* (2001) 355(Pt 2), 425–9. doi: 10.1042/bj3550425

131. Badawy AA. Tryptophan metabolism, disposition and utilization in pregnancy. *Biosci Rep.* (2015) 35:e00261. doi: 10.1042/BSR20150197

132. Britan A, Maffre V, Tone S, Drevet JR. Quantitative and spatial differences in the expression of tryptophan-metabolizing enzymes in mouse epididymis. *Cell Tissue Res.* (2006) 324:301–10. doi: 10.1007/s00441-005-0151-7

133. Fukunaga M, Yamamoto Y, Kawasoe M, Arioka Y, Murakami Y, Hoshi M, et al. Studies on tissue and cellular distribution of indoleamine 2,3-dioxygenase 2: the absence of IDO1 upregulates IDO2 expression in the epididymis. *J Histochem Cytochem.* (2012) 60:854–60. doi: 10.1369/0022155412458926

134. Jrad-Lamine A, Henry-Berger J, Damon-Soubeyrand C, Saez F, Kocer A, Janny L, et al. Indoleamine 2,3-dioxygenase 1 (ido1) is involved in the control of mouse caput epididymis immune environment. *PLoS ONE.* (2013) 8:e66494. doi: 10.1371/journal.pone.0066494

135. Lee GK, Park HJ, Macleod M, Chandler P, Munn DH, Mellor AL. Tryptophan deprivation sensitizes activated T cells to apoptosis prior to cell division. *Immunology.* (2002) 107:452–60. doi: 10.1046/j.1365-2567.2002.01526.x

136. Munn DH, Sharma MD, Baban B, Harding HP, Zhang Y, Ron D, et al. GCN2 kinase in T cells mediates proliferative arrest and anergy induction in response to indoleamine 2,3-dioxygenase. *Immunity.* (2005) 22:633–42. doi: 10.1016/j.immuni.2005.03.013

137. Fallarino F, Grohmann U, You S, McGrath BC, Cavener DR, Vacca C, et al. Tryptophan catabolism generates autoimmune-preventive regulatory T cells. *Transpl Immunol.* (2006) 17:58–60. doi: 10.1016/j.trim.2006.09.017

138. Mezrich JD, Fechner JH, Zhang X, Johnson BP, Burlingham WJ, Bradfield CA. An interaction between kynurenine and the aryl hydrocarbon receptor can generate regulatory T cells. *J Immunol.* (2010) 185:3190–8. doi: 10.4049/jimmunol.0903670

139. de Araujo EF, Feriotti C, Galdino NAL, Preite NW, Calich VLG, Loures FV. The IDO-AhR axis controls Th17/Treg immunity in a pulmonary model of fungal infection. *Front Immunol.* (2017) 8:880. doi: 10.3389/fimmu.2017.00880

140. Stephens GL, Wang Q, Swerdlow B, Bhat G, Kolbeck R, Fung M. Kynurenine 3-monooxygenase mediates inhibition of Th17 differentiation via catabolism of endogenous aryl hydrocarbon receptor ligands. *Eur J Immunol.* (2013) 43:1727–34. doi: 10.1002/eji.201242779

141. Fallarino F, Grohmann U, Vacca C, Bianchi R, Orabona C, Spreca A, et al. T cell apoptosis by tryptophan catabolism. *Cell Death Differ.* (2002) 9:1069–77. doi: 10.1038/sj.cdd.4401073

142. Frumento G, Rotondo R, Tonetti M, Damonte G, Benatti U, Ferrara GB. Tryptophan-derived catabolites are responsible for inhibition of T and natural killer cell proliferation induced by indoleamine 2,3-dioxygenase. *J Exp Med.* (2002) 196:459–68. doi: 10.1084/jem.20020121

143. Terness P, Bauer TM, Rose L, Dufter C, Watzlik A, Simon H, et al. Inhibition of allogeneic T cell proliferation by indoleamine 2,3-dioxygenase-expressing dendritic cells: mediation of suppression by tryptophan metabolites. *J Exp Med.* (2002) 196:447–57. doi: 10.1084/jem.20020052

144. Hayashi T, Mo JH, Gong X, Rossetto C, Jang A, Beck L, et al. 3-Hydroxyanthranilic acid inhibits PDK1 activation and suppresses experimental asthma by inducing T cell apoptosis. *Proc Natl Acad Sci USA.* (2007) 104:18619–24. doi: 10.1073/pnas.0709261104

145. Morita T, Saito K, Takemura M, Maekawa N, Fujigaki S, Fujii H, et al. L-tryptophan-kynurenine pathway metabolite 3-hydroxyanthranilic acid induces apoptosis in macrophage-derived cells under pathophysiological conditions. *Adv Exp Med Biol.* (1999) 467:559–63. doi: 10.1007/978-1-4615-4709-9_69

146. Seman M, Adriouch S, Scheuplein F, Krebs C, Freese D, Glowacki G, et al. NAD-induced T cell death: ADP-ribosylation of cell surface proteins by

ART2 activates the cytolytic P2X7 purinoceptor. *Immunity.* (2003) 19:571–82. doi: 10.1016/S1074-7613(03)00266-8

147. Sahm F, Oezen I, Opitz CA, Radlwimmer B, von Deimling A, Ahrendt T, et al. The endogenous tryptophan metabolite and NAD+ precursor quinolinic acid confers resistance of gliomas to oxidative stress. *Cancer Res.* (2013) 73:3225–34. doi: 10.1158/0008-5472.CAN-12-3831

148. Litzenburger UM, Opitz CA, Sahm F, Rauschenbach KJ, Trump S, Winter M, et al. Constitutive IDO expression in human cancer is sustained by an autocrine signaling loop involving IL-6, STAT3 and the AHR. *Oncotarget.* (2014) 5:1038–51. doi: 10.18632/oncotarget.1637

149. Adam I, Dewi DL, Mooiweer J, Sadik A, Mohapatra SR, Berdel B, et al. Upregulation of tryptophanyl-tRNA synthetase adapts human cancer cells to nutritional stress caused by tryptophan degradation. *Oncoimmunology.* (2018) 7:e1486353. doi: 10.1080/2162402X.2018.1486353

150. Wu KK, Cheng HH, Chang TC. 5-methoxyindole metabolites of L-tryptophan: control of COX-2 expression, inflammation and tumorigenesis. *J Biomed Sci.* (2014) 21:17. doi: 10.1186/1423-0127-21-17

151. Munn DH, Mellor AL. IDO in the tumor microenvironment: inflammation, counter-regulation, and tolerance. *Trends Immunol.* (2016) 37:193–207. doi: 10.1016/j.it.2016.01.002

152. Katz JB, Muller AJ, Prendergast GC. Indoleamine 2,3-dioxygenase in T-cell tolerance and tumoral immune escape. *Immunol Rev.* (2008) 222:206–21. doi: 10.1111/j.1600-065X.2008.00610.x

153. Dunn GP, Old LJ, Schreiber RD. The three Es of cancer immunoediting. *Annu Rev Immunol.* (2004) 22:329–60. doi: 10.1146/annurev.immunol.22.012703.104803

154. Shou D, Wen L, Song Z, Yin J, Sun Q, Gong W. Suppressive role of myeloid-derived suppressor cells (MDSCs) in the microenvironment of breast cancer and targeted immunotherapies. *Oncotarget.* (2016) 7:64505–11. doi: 10.18632/oncotarget.11352

155. Mellor AL, Keskin DB, Johnson T, Chandler P, Munn DH. Cells expressing indoleamine 2,3-dioxygenase inhibit T cell responses. *J Immunol.* (2002) 168:3771–6. doi: 10.4049/jimmunol.168.8.3771

156. Godin-Ethier J, Hanafi LA, Piccirillo CA, Lapointe R. Indoleamine 2,3-dioxygenase expression in human cancers: clinical and immunologic perspectives. *Clin Cancer Res.* (2011) 17:6985–91. doi: 10.1158/1078-0432.CCR-11-1331

157. Toulmonde M, Penel N, Adam J, Chevreau C, Blay JY, Le Cesne A, et al. Use of PD-1 targeting, macrophage infiltration, and IDO pathway activation in sarcomas: a phase 2 clinical trial. *JAMA Oncol.* (2018) 4:93–7. doi: 10.1001/jamaoncol.2017.1617

158. Iversen TZ, Engell-Noerregaard L, Ellebaek E, Andersen R, Larsen SK, Bjoern J, et al. Long-lasting disease stabilization in the absence of toxicity in metastatic lung cancer patients vaccinated with an epitope derived from indoleamine 2,3 dioxygenase. *Clin Cancer Res.* (2014) 20:221–32. doi: 10.1158/1078-0432.CCR-13-1560

159. Soliman HH, Jackson E, Neuger T, Dees EC, Harvey RD, Han H, et al. A first in man phase I trial of the oral immunomodulator, indoximod, combined with docetaxel in patients with metastatic solid tumors. *Oncotarget.* (2014) 5:8136–46. doi: 10.18632/oncotarget.2357

160. Perez RP, Riese MJ, Lewis KD, Saleh MN, Daud A, Berlin J, et al. Epacadostat plus nivolumab in patients with advanced solid tumors: preliminary phase I/II results of ECHO-204. *J Clin Oncol.* (2017) 35(Suppl. 15):3003. doi: 10.1200/JCO.2017.35.15_suppl.3003

161. Luke JJ, Tabernero J, Joshua A, Desai J, Varga AI, Moreno V, et al. BMS-986205, an indoleamine 2, 3-dioxygenase 1 inhibitor (IDO1i), in combination with nivolumab (nivo): Updated safety across all tumor cohorts and efficacy in advanced bladder cancer (advBC). *J Clin Oncol.* (2019) 37(Suppl. 7):358. doi: 10.1200/JCO.2019.37.7_suppl.358

162. Chen S, Song Z, Zhang A. Small-molecule immuno-oncology therapy: advances, challenges and new directions. *Curr Top Med Chem.* (2019) 19:180–5. doi: 10.2174/1568026619666190308131805

163. Michelagnoli M, Whelan J, Forsyth S, Otis Trial Management Group SI. A phase II study to determine the efficacy and safety of oral treosulfan in patients with advanced pre-treated Ewing sarcoma ISRCTN11631773. *Pediatr Blood Cancer.* (2015) 62:158–9. doi: 10.1002/pbc.25156

164. Kristeleit R, Davidenko I, Shirinkin V, El-Khouly F, Bondarenko I, Goodheart MJ, et al. A randomised, open-label, phase 2 study of the IDO1 inhibitor epacadostat (INCB024360) versus tamoxifen as therapy for biochemically recurrent (CA-125 relapse)-only epithelial ovarian cancer, primary peritoneal carcinoma, or fallopian tube cancer. *Gynecol Oncol.* (2017) 146:484–90. doi: 10.1016/j.ygyno.2017.07.005

165. Spira AI, Hamid O, Bauer TM, Borges VF, Wasser JS, Smith DC, et al. Efficacy/safety of epacadostat plus pembrolizumab in triple-negative breast cancer and ovarian cancer: Phase I/II ECHO-202 study. *J Clin Oncol.* (2017) 35:1103. doi: 10.1200/JCO.2017.35.15_suppl.1103

166. Mitchell TC, Hamid O, Smith DC, Bauer TM, Wasser JS, Olszanski AJ, et al. Epacadostat plus pembrolizumab in patients with advanced solid tumors: phase i results from a multicenter, open-label phase I/II Trial (ECHO-202/KEYNOTE-037). *J Clin Oncol.* (2018) 36:3223–30. doi: 10.1200/JCO.2018.78.9602

167. Gibney GT, Hamid O, Lutzky J, Olszanski AJ, Mitchell TC, Gajewski TF, et al. Phase 1/2 study of epacadostat in combination with ipilimumab in patients with unresectable or metastatic melanoma. *J Immunother Cancer.* (2019) 7:80. doi: 10.1186/s40425-019-0562-8

168. Jung KH, LoRusso P, Burris H, Gordon M, Bang YJ, Hellmann MD, et al. Phase I study of the indoleamine 2,3-dioxygenase 1 (IDO1) inhibitor navoximod (GDC-0919) administered with PD-L1 inhibitor (atezolizumab) in advanced solid tumors. *Clin Cancer Res.* (2019) 25:3220–8. doi: 10.1158/1078-0432.CCR-18-2740

169. Long GV, Dummer R, Hamid O, Gajewski TF, Caglevic C, Dalle S, et al. Epacadostat plus pembrolizumab versus placebo plus pembrolizumab in patients with unresectable or metastatic melanoma (ECHO-301/KEYNOTE-252): a phase 3, randomised, double-blind study. *Lancet Oncol.* (2019) 20:1083–97. doi: 10.1016/S1470-2045(19)30274-8

170. Lob S, Konigsrainer A, Zieker D, Brucher BL, Rammensee HG, Opelz G, et al. IDO1 and IDO2 are expressed in human tumors: levo- but not dextro-1-methyl tryptophan inhibits tryptophan catabolism. *Cancer Immunol Immunother.* (2009) 58:153–7. doi: 10.1007/s00262-008-0513-6

171. Hascitha J, Priya R, Jayavelu S, Dhandapani H, Selvaluxmy G, Sunder Singh S, et al. Analysis of Kynurenine/Tryptophan ratio and expression of IDO1 and 2 mRNA in tumour tissue of cervical cancer patients. *Clin Biochem.* (2016) 49:919–24. doi: 10.1016/j.clinbiochem.2016.04.008

172. Merlo LMF, Pigott E, DuHadaway JB, Grabler S, Metz R, Prendergast GC, et al. IDO2 is a critical mediator of autoantibody production and inflammatory pathogenesis in a mouse model of autoimmune arthritis. *J Immunol.* (2014) 192:2082–90. doi: 10.4049/jimmunol.1303012

173. Nevler A, Muller AJ, Sutanto-Ward E, DuHadaway JB, Nagatomo K, Londin E, et al. Host IDO2 gene status influences tumor progression and radiotherapy response in KRAS-driven sporadic pancreatic cancers. *Clin Cancer Res.* (2019) 25:724–34. doi: 10.1158/1078-0432.CCR-18-0814

174. Opitz CA, Litzenburger UM, Sahm F, Ott M, Tritschler I, Trump S, et al. An endogenous tumour-promoting ligand of the human aryl hydrocarbon receptor. *Nature.* (2011) 478:197–203. doi: 10.1038/nature10491

175. D'Amato NC, Rogers TJ, Gordon MA, Greene LI, Cochrane DR, Spoelstra NS, et al. A TDO2-AhR signaling axis facilitates anoikis resistance and metastasis in triple-negative breast cancer. *Cancer Res.* (2015) 75:4651–64. doi: 10.1158/0008-5472.CAN-15-2011

176. Chen IC, Lee KH, Hsu YH, Wang WR, Chen CM, Cheng YW. Expression pattern and clinicopathological relevance of the indoleamine 2,3-dioxygenase 1/tryptophan 2,3-dioxygenase protein in colorectal cancer. *Dis Markers.* (2016) 2016:8169724. doi: 10.1155/2016/8169724

177. Pilotte L, Larrieu P, Stroobant V, Colau D, Dolusic E, Frederick R, et al. Reversal of tumoral immune resistance by inhibition of tryptophan 2,3-dioxygenase. *Proc Natl Acad Sci USA.* (2012) 109:2497–502. doi: 10.1073/pnas.1113873109

178. Hua S, Chen F, Wang X, Wang Y, Gou S. Pt(IV) hybrids containing a TDO inhibitor serve as potential anticancer immunomodulators. *J Inorg Biochem.* (2019) 195:130–40. doi: 10.1016/j.jinorgbio.2019.02.004

179. Schramme F, Crosignani S, Frederix K, Hoffmann D, Pilotte L, Stroobant V, et al. Inhibition of tryptophan-dioxygenase activity increases the antitumor efficacy of immune checkpoint inhibitors. *Cancer Immunol Res.* (2020) 8:32–45. doi: 10.1158/2326-6066.CIR-19-0041

180. Chiu YH, Lei HJ, Huang KC, Chiang YL, Lin CS. Overexpression of kynurenine 3-monooxygenase correlates with cancer malignancy and

predicts poor prognosis in canine mammary gland tumors. *J Oncol.* (2019) 2019:6201764. doi: 10.1155/2019/6201764

181. Connor TJ, Starr N, O'Sullivan JB, Harkin A. Induction of indolamine 2,3-dioxygenase and kynurenine 3-monooxygenase in rat brain following a systemic inflammatory challenge: a role for IFN-gamma? *Neurosci Lett.* (2008) 441:29–34. doi: 10.1016/j.neulet.2008.06.007

182. Jones SP, Franco NF, Varney B, Sundaram G, Brown DA, de Bie J, et al. Expression of the kynurenine pathway in human peripheral blood mononuclear cells: implications for inflammatory and neurodegenerative disease. *PLoS ONE.* (2015) 10:e0131389. doi: 10.1371/journal.pone.0131389

183. Shave S, McGuire K, Pham NT, Mole DJ, Webster SP, Auer M. Diclofenac identified as a kynurenine 3-monooxygenase binder and inhibitor by molecular similarity techniques. *ACS Omega.* (2018) 3:2564–8. doi: 10.1021/acsomega.7b02091

184. Pantziarka P, Sukhatme V, Bouche G, Meheus L, Sukhatme VP. Repurposing Drugs in Oncology (ReDO)-diclofenac as an anti-cancer agent. *Ecancermedicalscience.* (2016) 10:610. doi: 10.3332/ecancer.2016.610

185. Radbruch L, Strasser F, Elsner F, Goncalves JF, Loge J, Kaasa S, et al. Fatigue in palliative care patients – an EAPC approach. *Palliat Med.* (2008) 22:13–32. doi: 10.1177/0269216307085183

186. Berger AM, Mooney K, Alvarez-Perez A, Breitbart WS, Carpenter KM, Cella D, et al. Cancer-related fatigue, version 2.2015. *J Natl Compr Canc Netw.* (2015) 13:1012–39. doi: 10.6004/jnccn.2015.0122

187. Bower JE. Cancer-related fatigue–mechanisms, risk factors, and treatments. *Nat Rev Clin Oncol.* (2014) 11:597–609. doi: 10.1038/nrclinonc.2014.127

188. Bower JE, Ganz PA, Aziz N, Fahey JL. Fatigue and proinflammatory cytokine activity in breast cancer survivors. *Psychosom Med.* (2002) 64:604–11. doi: 10.1097/00006842-200207000-00010

189. Saligan LN, Kim HS. A systematic review of the association between immunogenomic markers and cancer-related fatigue. *Brain Behav Immun.* (2012) 26:830–48. doi: 10.1016/j.bbi.2012.05.004

190. Bower JE, Lamkin DM. Inflammation and cancer-related fatigue: mechanisms, contributing factors, and treatment implications. *Brain Behav Immun.* (2013) 30(Suppl.): S48–57. doi: 10.1016/j.bbi.2012.06.011

191. Schroecksnadel K, Sarcletti M, Winkler C, Mumelter B, Weiss G, Fuchs D, et al. Quality of life and immune activation in patients with HIV-infection. *Brain Behav Immun.* (2008) 22:881–9. doi: 10.1016/j.bbi.2007.12.011

192. Huang A, Fuchst D, Widnert B, Glover C, Henderson DC, Allen-Mersh TG. Tryptophan and quality of life in colorectal cancer. In: Allegri G, Costa CVL, Ragazzi E, Steinhart H, Varesio L, editors. *Developments in Tryptophan and Serotonin Metabolism.* Boston, MA: Springer (2003). p. 353–8. doi: 10.1007/978-1-4615-0135-0_39

193. Kim S, Miller BJ, Stefanek ME, Miller AH. Inflammation-induced activation of the indoleamine 2,3-dioxygenase pathway: relevance to cancer-related fatigue. *Cancer.* (2015) 121:2129–36. doi: 10.1002/cncr.29302

194. Yennurajalingam S, Frisbee-Hume S, Palmer JL, Delgado-Guay MO, Bull J, Phan AT, et al. Reduction of cancer-related fatigue with dexamethasone: a double-blind, randomized, placebo-controlled trial in patients with advanced cancer. *J Clin Oncol.* (2013) 31:3076–82. doi: 10.1200/JCO.2012.44.4661

195. Guo Q, Li Q, Wang J, Liu M, Wang Y, Chen Z, et al. A comprehensive evaluation of clinical efficacy and safety of celecoxib in combination with chemotherapy in metastatic or postoperative recurrent gastric cancer patients: a preliminary, three-center, clinical trial study. *Medicine.* (2019) 98:e16234. doi: 10.1097/MD.0000000000016234

196. Dantzer R, Heijnen CJ, Kavelaars A, Laye S, Capuron L. The neuroimmune basis of fatigue. *Trends Neurosci.* (2014) 37:39–46. doi: 10.1016/j.tins.2013.10.003

197. Tyring S, Gottlieb A, Papp K, Gordon K, Leonardi C, Wang A, et al. Etanercept and clinical outcomes, fatigue, and depression in psoriasis: double-blind placebo-controlled randomised phase III trial. *Lancet.* (2006) 367:29–35. doi: 10.1016/S0140-6736(05)67763-X

198. Yount S, Sorensen MV, Cella D, Sengupta N, Grober J, Chartash EK. Adalimumab plus methotrexate or standard therapy is more effective than methotrexate or standard therapies alone in the treatment of fatigue in patients with active, inadequately treated rheumatoid arthritis. *Clin Exp Rheumatol.* (2007) 25:838–46.

199. Mystakidou K, Tsilika E, Parpa E, Katsouda E, Galanos A, Vlahos L. Assessment of anxiety and depression in advanced cancer patients and their relationship with quality of life. *Qual Life Res.* (2005) 14:1825–33. doi: 10.1007/s11136-005-4324-3

200. Mols F, Husson O, Roukema JA, van de Poll-Franse LV. Depressive symptoms are a risk factor for all-cause mortality: results from a prospective population-based study among 3,080 cancer survivors from the PROFILES registry. *J Cancer Surviv.* (2013) 7:484–92. doi: 10.1007/s11764-013-0286-6

201. Bortolato B, Hyphantis TN, Valpione S, Perini G, Maes M, Morris G, et al. Depression in cancer: The many biobehavioral pathways driving tumor progression. *Cancer Treat Rev.* (2017) 52:58–70. doi: 10.1016/j.ctrv.2016.11.004

202. Kurz K, Schroecksnadel S, Weiss G, Fuchs D. Association between increased tryptophan degradation and depression in cancer patients. *Curr Opin Clin Nutr Metab Care.* (2011) 14:49–56. doi: 10.1097/MCO.0b013e328340d849

203. Barreto FS, Chaves Filho AJ, de Araujo M, de Moraes MO, de Moraes ME, Maes M, et al. Tryptophan catabolites along the indoleamine 2,3-dioxygenase pathway as a biological link between depression and cancer. *Behav Pharmacol.* (2018) 29:165–80. doi: 10.1097/FBP.0000000000000384

204. Sforzini L, Nettis MA, Mondelli V, Pariante CM. Inflammation in cancer and depression: a starring role for the kynurenine pathway. *Psychopharmacology.* (2019) 236:2997–3011. doi: 10.1007/s00213-019-05200-8

205. O'Connor JC, Lawson MA, André C, Moreau M, Lestage J, Castanon N, et al. Lipopolysaccharide-induced depressive-like behavior is mediated by indoleamine 2,3-dioxygenase activation in mice. *Mol Psychiatry.* (2009) 14:511–22. doi: 10.1038/sj.mp.4002148

206. Norden DM, Devine R, Bicer S, Jing R, Reiser PJ, Wold LE, et al. Fluoxetine prevents the development of depressive-like behavior in a mouse model of cancer related fatigue. *Physiol Behav.* (2015) 140:230–5. doi: 10.1016/j.physbeh.2014.12.045

207. Doolin K, Allers KA, Pleiner S, Liesener A, Farrell C, Tozzi L, et al. Altered tryptophan catabolite concentrations in major depressive disorder and associated changes in hippocampal subfield volumes. *Psychoneuroendocrinology.* (2018) 95:8–17. doi: 10.1016/j.psyneuen.2018.05.019

208. Savitz J, Drevets WC, Wurfel BE, Ford BN, Bellgowan PS, Victor TA, et al. Reduction of kynurenic acid to quinolinic acid ratio in both the depressed and remitted phases of major depressive disorder. *Brain Behav Immun.* (2015) 46:55–9. doi: 10.1016/j.bbi.2015.02.007

209. Meier TB, Drevets WC, Wurfel BE, Ford BN, Morris HM, Victor TA, et al. Relationship between neurotoxic kynurenine metabolites and reductions in right medial prefrontal cortical thickness in major depressive disorder. *Brain Behav Immun.* (2016) 53:39–48. doi: 10.1016/j.bbi.2015.11.003

210. Parrott JM, Redus L, Santana-Coelho D, Morales J, Gao X, O'Connor JC. Neurotoxic kynurenine metabolism is increased in the dorsal hippocampus and drives distinct depressive behaviors during inflammation. *Transl Psychiatry.* (2016) 6:e918. doi: 10.1038/tp.2016.200

211. O'Connor JC, Lawson MA, Andre C, Briley EM, Szegedi SS, Lestage J, et al. Induction of IDO by bacille Calmette-Guerin is responsible for development of murine depressive-like behavior. *J Immunol.* (2009) 182:3202–12. doi: 10.4049/jimmunol.0802722

212. Laumet G, Edralin JD, Chiang AC, Dantzer R, Heijnen CJ, Kavelaars A. Resolution of inflammation-induced depression requires T lymphocytes and endogenous brain interleukin-10 signaling. *Neuropsychopharmacology.* (2018) 43:2597–605. doi: 10.1038/s41386-018-0154-1

213. Martinez P, Tsai AC, Muzoora C, Kembabazi A, Weiser SD, Huang Y, et al. Reversal of the Kynurenine pathway of tryptophan catabolism may improve depression in ART-treated HIV-infected Ugandans. *J Acquir Immune Defic Syndr.* (2014) 65:456–62. doi: 10.1097/QAI.0000000000000062

214. Maes M, Bonaccorso S, Marino V, Puzella A, Pasquini M, Biondi M, et al. Treatment with interferon-alpha (IFN alpha) of hepatitis C patients induces lower serum dipeptidyl peptidase IV activity, which is related to IFN alpha-induced depressive and anxiety symptoms and immune activation. *Mol Psychiatry.* (2001) 6:475–80. doi: 10.1038/sj.mp.4000872

215. Felger JC, Miller AH. Cytokine effects on the basal ganglia and dopamine function: the subcortical source of inflammatory malaise. *Front Neuroendocrinol.* (2012) 33:315–27. doi: 10.1016/j.yfrne.2012.09.003

216. Neurauter G, Schrocksnadel K, Scholl-Burgi S, Sperner-Unterweger B, Schubert C, Ledochowski M, et al. Chronic immune stimulation correlates with reduced phenylalanine turnover. *Curr Drug Metab.* (2008) 9:622–7. doi: 10.2174/138920008785821738

217. Fernstrom JD, Wurtman RJ. Brain serotonin content: physiological dependence on plasma tryptophan levels. *Science.* (1971) 173:149–52. doi: 10.1126/science.173.3992.149

218. Wichers MC, Koek GH, Robaeys G, Verkerk R, Scharpe S, Maes M. IDO and interferon-alpha-induced depressive symptoms: a shift in hypothesis from tryptophan depletion to neurotoxicity. *Mol Psychiatry.* (2005) 10:538–44. doi: 10.1038/sj.mp.4001600

219. Lugo-Huitron R, Ugalde Muniz P, Pineda B, Pedraza-Chaverri J, Rios C, Perez-de la Cruz V. Quinolinic acid: an endogenous neurotoxin with multiple targets. *Oxid Med Cell Longev.* (2013) 2013:104024. doi: 10.1155/2013/104024

220. Bender DA, McCreanor GM. Kynurenine hydroxylase: a potential rate-limiting enzyme in tryptophan metabolism. *Biochem Soc Trans.* (1985) 13:441–3. doi: 10.1042/bst0130441

221. Foster AC, Miller LP, Oldendorf WH, Schwarcz R. Studies on the disposition of quinolinic acid after intracerebral or systemic administration in the rat. *Exp Neurol.* (1984) 84:428–40. doi: 10.1016/0014-4886(84)90239-5

222. Perkins MN, Stone TW. An iontophoretic investigation of the actions of convulsant kynurenines and their interaction with the endogenous excitant quinolinic acid. *Brain Res.* (1982) 247:184–7. doi: 10.1016/0006-8993(82)91048-4

223. Foster AC, Vezzani A, French ED, Schwarcz R. Kynurenic acid blocks neurotoxicity and seizures induced in rats by the related brain metabolite quinolinic acid. *Neurosci Lett.* (1984) 48:273–8. doi: 10.1016/0304-3940(84)90050-8

224. Braidy N, Grant R. Kynurenine pathway metabolism and neuroinflammatory disease. *Neural Regen Res.* (2017) 12:39–42. doi: 10.4103/1673-5374.198971

225. Myint AM. Kynurenines: from the perspective of major psychiatric disorders. *FEBS J.* (2012) 279:1375–85. doi: 10.1111/j.1742-4658.2012.08551.x

226. Myint AM, Schwarz MJ, Steinbusch HW, Leonard BE. Neuropsychiatric disorders related to interferon and interleukins treatment. *Metab Brain Dis.* (2009) 24:55–68. doi: 10.1007/s11011-008-9114-5

227. Crozier-Reabe KR, Phillips RS, Moran GR. Kynurenine 3-monooxygenase from *Pseudomonas fluorescens*: substrate-like inhibitors both stimulate flavin reduction and stabilize the flavin-peroxo intermediate yet result in the production of hydrogen peroxide. *Biochemistry.* (2008) 47:12420–33. doi: 10.1021/bi8010434

228. Barsevick AM, Irwin MR, Hinds P, Miller A, Berger A, Jacobsen P, et al. Recommendations for high-priority research on cancer-related fatigue in children and adults. *J Natl Cancer Inst.* (2013) 105:1432–40. doi: 10.1093/jnci/djt242

229. Malhi GS, Mann JJ. Depression. *Lancet.* (2018) 392:2299–312. doi: 10.1016/S0140-6736(18)31948-2

230. Souza LC, Jesse CR, de Gomes MG, Del Fabbro L, Goes ATR, Donato F, et al. Activation of brain indoleamine-2,3-dioxygenase contributes to depressive-like behavior induced by an intracerebroventricular injection of streptozotocin in mice. *Neurochem Res.* (2017) 42:2982–95. doi: 10.1007/s11064-017-2329-2

231. Fuertig R, Azzinnari D, Bergamini G, Cathomas F, Sigrist H, Seifritz E, et al. Mouse chronic social stress increases blood and brain kynurenine pathway activity and fear behaviour: Both effects are reversed by inhibition of indoleamine 2,3-dioxygenase. *Brain Behav Immun.* (2016) 54:59–72. doi: 10.1016/j.bbi.2015.12.020

232. Xie W, Cai L, Yu Y, Gao L, Xiao L, He Q, et al. Activation of brain indoleamine 2,3-dioxygenase contributes to epilepsy-associated depressive-like behavior in rats with chronic temporal lobe epilepsy. *J Neuroinflamm.* (2014) 11:41. doi: 10.1186/1742-2094-11-41

233. Liu Y-N, Peng Y-L, Liu L, Wu T-Y, Zhang Y, Lian Y-J, et al. TNFα mediates stress-induced depression by upregulating indoleamine 2,3-dioxygenase in a mouse model of unpredictable chronic mild stress. *Eur Cytok Netw.* (2015) 26:15–25. doi: 10.1684/ecn.2015.0362

234. Reis DJ, Casteen EJ, Ilardi SS. The antidepressant impact of minocycline in rodents: a systematic review and meta-analysis. *Sci Rep.* (2019) 9:261–261. doi: 10.1038/s41598-018-36507-9

235. Henry CJ, Huang Y, Wynne A, Hanke M, Himler J, Bailey MT, et al. Minocycline attenuates lipopolysaccharide (LPS)-induced neuroinflammation, sickness behavior, and anhedonia. *J Neuroinflamm.* (2008) 5:15. doi: 10.1186/1742-2094-5-15

236. Bahrami Z, Firouzi M, Hashemi-Monfared A, Zahednasab H, Harirchian MH. The effect of minocycline on indolamine 2, 3 dioxygenase expression and the levels of kynurenic acid and quinolinic acid in LPS-activated primary rat microglia. *Cytokine.* (2018) 107:125–9. doi: 10.1016/j.cyto.2017.12.013

237. Clemens V, Regen F, Le Bret N, Heuser I, Hellmann-Regen J. Anti-inflammatory effects of minocycline are mediated by retinoid signaling. *BMC Neurosci.* (2018) 19:58. doi: 10.1186/s12868-018-0460-x

238. Rosenblat JD, McIntyre RS. Efficacy and tolerability of minocycline for depression: a systematic review and meta-analysis of clinical trials. *J Affect Disord.* (2018) 227:219–25. doi: 10.1016/j.jad.2017.10.042

239. Kohler O, Krogh J, Mors O, Benros ME. Inflammation in depression and the potential for anti-inflammatory treatment. *Curr Neuropharmacol.* (2016) 14:732–42. doi: 10.2174/1570159X14666151208113700

240. Vichaya EG, Vermeer DW, Budac D, Lee A, Grossberg A, Vermeer PD, et al. Inhibition of indoleamine 2,3 dioxygenase does not improve cancer-related symptoms in a murine model of human papilloma virus-related head and neck cancer. *Int J Tryptophan Res.* 12:1178646919872508. doi: 10.1177/1178646919872508

241. Salter M, Hazelwood R, Pogson CI, Iyer R, Madge DJ. The effects of a novel and selective inhibitor of tryptophan 2,3-dioxygenase on tryptophan and serotonin metabolism in the rat. *Biochem Pharmacol.* (1995) 49:1435–42. doi: 10.1016/0006-2952(95)00006-L

242. Breda C, Sathyasaikumar KV, Sograte Idrissi S, Notarangelo FM, Estranero JG, Moore GG, et al. Tryptophan-2,3-dioxygenase (TDO) inhibition ameliorates neurodegeneration by modulation of kynurenine pathway metabolites. *Proc Natl Acad Sci USA.* (2016) 113:5435–40. doi: 10.1073/pnas.1604453113

243. Giorgini F, Huang SY, Sathyasaikumar KV, Notarangelo FM, Thomas MA, Tararina M, et al. Targeted deletion of kynurenine 3-monooxygenase in mice: a new tool for studying kynurenine pathway metabolism in periphery and brain. *J Biol Chem.* (2013) 288:36554–66. doi: 10.1074/jbc.M113.503813

244. Brooks AK, Janda TM, Lawson MA, Rytych JL, Smith RA, Ocampo-Solis C, et al. Desipramine decreases expression of human and murine indoleamine-2,3-dioxygenases. *Brain Behav Immun.* (2017) 62:219–29. doi: 10.1016/j.bbi.2017.02.010

245. Duda W, Curzytek K, Kubera M, Connor TJ, Fagan EM, Basta-Kaim A, et al. Interaction of the immune-inflammatory and the kynurenine pathways in rats resistant to antidepressant treatment in model of depression. *Int Immunopharmacol.* (2019) 73:527–38. doi: 10.1016/j.intimp.2019.05.039

246. Borsini A, Alboni S, Horowitz MA, Tojo LM, Cannazza G, Su KP, et al. Rescue of IL-1beta-induced reduction of human neurogenesis by omega-3 fatty acids and antidepressants. *Brain Behav Immun.* (2017) 65:230–8. doi: 10.1016/j.bbi.2017.05.006

247. Román GC, Jackson RE, Gadhia R, Román AN, Reis J. Mediterranean diet: the role of long-chain ω-3 fatty acids in fish; polyphenols in fruits, vegetables, cereals, coffee, tea, cacao and wine; probiotics and vitamins in prevention of stroke, age-related cognitive decline, and Alzheimer disease. *Rev Neurol.* (2019) 175:724–41. doi: 10.1016/j.neurol.2019.08.005

248. Schwingshackl L, Schwedhelm C, Galbete C, Hoffmann G. Adherence to mediterranean diet and risk of cancer: an updated systematic review and meta-analysis. *Nutrients.* (2017) 9:E1063. doi: 10.3390/nu9101063

249. Myles IA. Fast food fever: reviewing the impacts of the Western diet on immunity. *Nutr J.* (2014) 13:61. doi: 10.1186/1475-2891-13-61

250. André C, Dinel AL, Ferreira G, Layé S, Castanon N. Diet-induced obesity progressively alters cognition, anxiety-like behavior and lipopolysaccharide-induced depressive-like behavior: focus on brain indoleamine 2,3-dioxygenase activation. *Brain Behav Immun.* (2014) 41:10–21. doi: 10.1016/j.bbi.2014.03.012

251. Agus A, Planchais J, Sokol H. Gut microbiota regulation of tryptophan metabolism in health and disease. *Cell Host Microbe.* (2018) 23:716–24. doi: 10.1016/j.chom.2018.05.003

252. Martin CR, Osadchiy V, Kalani A, Mayer EA. The brain-gut-microbiome axis. *Cell Mol Gastroenterol Hepatol.* (2018) 6:133–48. doi: 10.1016/j.jcmgh.2018.04.003

253. Rankin LC, Artis D. Beyond host defense: emerging functions of the immune system in regulating complex tissue physiology. *Cell.* (2018) 173:554–67. doi: 10.1016/j.cell.2018.03.013

254. Wang G, Huang S, Wang Y, Cai S, Yu H, Liu H, et al. Bridging intestinal immunity and gut microbiota by metabolites. *Cell Mol Life Sci.* (2019) 76:3917–37. doi: 10.1007/s00018-019-03190-6

255. Weber DD, Aminzadeh-Gohari S, Tulipan J, Catalano L, Feichtinger RG, Kofler B. Ketogenic diet in the treatment of cancer - where do we stand? *Mol Metab.* (2019). doi: 10.1016/j.molmet.2019.06.026. [Epub ahead of print].

256. Sremanakova J, Sowerbutts AM, Burden S. A systematic review of the use of ketogenic diets in adult patients with cancer. *J Hum Nutr Diet.* (2018) 31:793–802. doi: 10.1111/jhn.12587

257. Heischmann S, Gano LB, Quinn K, Liang LP, Klepacki J, Christians U, et al. Regulation of kynurenine metabolism by a ketogenic diet. *J Lipid Res.* (2018) 59:958–66. doi: 10.1194/jlr.M079251

258. Zarnowski T, Choragiewicz T, Tulidowicz-Bielak M, Thaler S, Rejdak R, Zarnowski I, et al. Ketogenic diet increases concentrations of kynurenic acid in discrete brain structures of young and adult rats. *J Neural Transm.* (2012) 119:679–84. doi: 10.1007/s00702-011-0750-2

259. Zarnowski T, Tulidowicz-Bielak M, Zarnowska I, Mitosek-Szewczyk K, Wnorowski A, Jozwiak K, et al. Kynurenic acid and neuroprotective activity of the ketogenic diet in the eye. *Curr Med Chem.* (2017) 24:3547–58. doi: 10.2174/0929867324666170509120257

260. Zarnowska I, Wróbel-Dudzinska D, Tulidowicz-Bielak M, Kocki T, and Mitosek-Szewczyk K, Gasior M, et al. Changes in tryptophan and kynurenine pathway metabolites in the blood of children treated with ketogenic diet for refractory epilepsy. *Seizure.* (2019) 69:265–72. doi: 10.1016/j.seizure.2019.05.006

261. Navarro SL, Tarkhan A, Shojaie A, Randolph TW, Gu H, Djukovic D, et al. Plasma metabolomics profiles suggest beneficial effects of a low-glycemic load dietary pattern on inflammation and energy metabolism. *Am J Clin Nutr.* (2019) 110:984–92. doi: 10.1093/ajcn/nqz169

262. Inglis JE, Lin PJ, Kerns SL, Kleckner IR, Kleckner AS, Castillo DA, et al. Nutritional interventions for treating cancer-related fatigue: a qualitative review. *Nutr Cancer.* (2019) 71:21–40. doi: 10.1080/01635581.2018.1513046

263. Nencioni A, Caffa I, Cortellino S, Longo VD. Fasting and cancer: molecular mechanisms and clinical application. *Nat Rev Cancer.* (2018) 18:707–19. doi: 10.1038/s41568-018-0061-0

264. Lee JY, Chu SH, Jeon JY, Lee MK, Park JH, Lee DC, et al. Effects of 12 weeks of probiotic supplementation on quality of life in colorectal cancer survivors: a double-blind, randomized, placebo-controlled trial. *Dig Liver Dis.* (2014) 46:1126–32. doi: 10.1016/j.dld.2014.09.004

265. Stubbe CE, Valero M. Complementary strategies for the management of radiation therapy side effects. *J Adv Pract Oncol.* (2013) 4:219–31. doi: 10.6004/jadpro.2013.4.4.3

266. Rudzki L, Ostrowska L, Pawlak D, Malus A, Pawlak K, Waszkiewicz N, et al. Probiotic *Lactobacillus plantarum* 299v decreases kynurenine concentration and improves cognitive functions in patients with major depression: a double-blind, randomized, placebo controlled study. *Psychoneuroendocrinology.* (2019) 100:213–22. doi: 10.1016/j.psyneuen.2018.10.010

267. Strasser B, Geiger D, Schauer M, Gostner JM, Gatterer H, Burtscher M, et al. Probiotic supplements beneficially affect tryptophan-kynurenine metabolism and reduce the incidence of upper respiratory tract infections in trained athletes: a randomized, double-blinded, placebo-controlled trial. *Nutrients.* (2016) 8:E752. doi: 10.3390/nu8110752

268. Leblhuber F, Steiner K, Schuetz B, Fuchs D, Gostner JM. Probiotic supplementation in patients with Alzheimer's dementia - an explorative intervention study. *Curr Alzheimer Res.* (2018) 15:1106–13. doi: 10.2174/1389200219666180813144834

269. Zelante T, Iannitti RG, Cunha C, De Luca A, Giovannini G, Pieraccini G, et al. Tryptophan catabolites from microbiota engage aryl hydrocarbon receptor and balance mucosal reactivity via interleukin-22. *Immunity.* (2013) 39:372–85. doi: 10.1016/j.immuni.2013.08.003

270. Park C, Brietzke E, Rosenblat JD, Musial N, Zuckerman H, Ragguett RM, et al. Probiotics for the treatment of depressive symptoms: an anti-inflammatory mechanism? *Brain Behav Immun.* (2018) 73:115–24. doi: 10.1016/j.bbi.2018.07.006

271. Wallace CJK, Milev R. The effects of probiotics on depressive symptoms in humans: a systematic review. *Ann Gen Psychiatry.* (2017) 16:14. doi: 10.1186/s12991-017-0138-2

272. Nikolova V, Zaidi SY, Young AH, Cleare AJ, Stone JM. Gut feeling: randomized controlled trials of probiotics for the treatment of clinical depression: systematic review and meta-analysis. *Ther Adv Psychopharmacol.* (2019) 9:2045125319859963. doi: 10.1177/2045125319859963

273. Baguley BJ, Skinner TL, Wright ORL. Nutrition therapy for the management of cancer-related fatigue and quality of life: a systematic review and meta-analysis. *Br J Nutr.* (2019) 122:527–41. doi: 10.1017/S000711451800363X

274. Metcalfe AJ, Koliamitra C, Javelle F, Bloch W, Zimmer P. Acute and chronic effects of exercise on the kynurenine pathway in humans - a brief review and future perspectives. *Physiol Behav.* (2018) 194:583–7. doi: 10.1016/j.physbeh.2018.07.015

275. Gostner JM, Geisler S, Stonig M, Mair L, Sperner-Unterweger B, Fuchs D. Tryptophan metabolism and related pathways in psychoneuroimmunology: the impact of nutrition and lifestyle. *Neuropsychobiology.* 79:89–99. doi: 10.1159/000496293

276. Wegner M, Helmich I, Machado S, Nardi AE, Arias-Carrion O, Budde H. Effects of exercise on anxiety and depression disorders: review of meta-analyses and neurobiological mechanisms. *CNS Neurol Dis Drug Targets.* (2014) 13:1002–14. doi: 10.2174/1871527313666140612102841

277. Meeusen R. Exercise, nutrition and the brain. *Sports Med.* (2014) 44(Suppl. 1):S47–56. doi: 10.1007/s40279-014-0150-5

278. Valente-Silva P, Ruas JL. Tryptophan-kynurenine metabolites in exercise and mental health. In: Spiegelman B, editor. *Hormones, Metabolism and the Benefits of Exercise.* Cham: Springer (2017). p. 83–91. doi: 10.1007/978-3-319-72790-5_7

279. Agudelo LZ, Femenía T, Orhan F, Porsmyr-Palmertz M, Goiny M, Martinez-Redondo V, et al. Skeletal muscle PGC-1α1 modulates kynurenine metabolism and mediates resilience to stress-induced depression. *Cell.* (2014) 159:33–45. doi: 10.1016/j.cell.2014.07.051

280. Sprenger H, Jacobs C, Nain M, Gressner AM, Prinz H, Wesemann W, et al. Enhanced release of cytokines, interleukin-2 receptors, and neopterin after long-distance running. *Clin Immunol Immunopathol.* (1992) 63:188–95. doi: 10.1016/0090-1229(92)90012-D

281. Kallich JD, Tchekmedyian NS, Damiano AM, Shi J, Black JT, Erder MH. Psychological outcomes associated with anemia-related fatigue in cancer patients. *Oncology.* (2002) 16:117–24.

282. Sabbatini P. The relationship between anemia and quality of life in cancer patients. *Oncologist.* (2000) 5(Suppl. 2):19–23. doi: 10.1634/theoncologist.5-suppl_2-19

283. Knight K, Wade S, Balducci L. Prevalence and outcomes of anemia in cancer: a systematic review of the literature. *Am J Med.* (2004) 116(Suppl. 7A):11–26S. doi: 10.1016/j.amjmed.2003.12.008

284. Weiss G, Goodnough LT. Anemia of chronic disease. *N Engl J Med.* (2005) 352:1011–23. doi: 10.1056/NEJMra041809

285. Ganz T. Anemia of Inflammation. *N Engl J Med.* (2019) 381:1148–57. doi: 10.1056/NEJMra1804281

286. Weiss G, Ganz T, Goodnough LT. Anemia of inflammation. *Blood.* (2019) 133:40–50. doi: 10.1182/blood-2018-06-856500

287. Kurz K, Schroecksnadel S, Seifert M, Sarcletti M, Fuchs D, Weiss G, et al. Iron metabolic changes and immune activation in patients with HIV-1 infection before and after ART. *Pteridines.* (2010) 21:47. doi: 10.1515/pteridines.2010.21.1.29

288. Tsuboi I, Harada T, Hirabayashi Y, Kanno J, Inoue T, Aizawa S. Inflammatory biomarker, neopterin, predominantly enhances myelopoiesis, which suppresses erythropoiesis via activated stromal cells. *Immunobiology.* (2010) 215:348–55. doi: 10.1016/j.imbio.2009.05.004

289. Eleftheriadis T, Pissas G, Antoniadi G, Liakopoulos V, Stefanidis I. Kynurenine, by activating aryl hydrocarbon receptor, decreases erythropoietin and increases hepcidin production in HepG2 cells: a new

mechanism for anemia of inflammation. *Exp Hematol.* (2016) 44:60–7.e1. doi: 10.1016/j.exphem.2015.08.010

290. Platten M, Wick W, Van den Eynde BJ. Tryptophan catabolism in cancer: beyond IDO and tryptophan depletion. *Cancer Res.* (2012) 72:5435–40. doi: 10.1158/0008-5472.CAN-12-0569

291. Weiss G, Schroecksnadel K, Mattle V, Winkler C, Konwalinka G, Fuchs D. Possible role of cytokine-induced tryptophan degradation in anaemia of inflammation. *Eur J Haematol.* (2004) 72:130–4. doi: 10.1046/j.0902-4441.2003.00197.x

292. Pawlak D, Koda M, Pawlak S, Wolczynski S, Buczko W. Contribution of quinolinic acid in the development of anemia in renal insufficiency. *Am J Physiol Renal Physiol.* (2003) 284:F693–700. doi: 10.1152/ajprenal.00327.2002

293. Braidy N, Grant R, Adams S, Brew BJ, Guillemin GJ. Mechanism for quinolinic acid cytotoxicity in human astrocytes and neurons. *Neurotox Res.* (2009) 16:77–86. doi: 10.1007/s12640-009-9051-z

294. Huang LE, Willmore WG, Gu J, Goldberg MA, Bunn HF. Inhibition of hypoxia-inducible factor 1 activation by carbon monoxide and nitric oxide. Implications for oxygen sensing and signaling. *J Biol Chem.* (1999) 274:9038–44. doi: 10.1074/jbc.274.13.9038

295. Sibon D, Coman T, Rossignol J, Lamarque M, Kosmider O, Bayard E, et al. Enhanced renewal of erythroid progenitors in myelodysplastic anemia by peripheral serotonin. *Cell Rep.* (2019) 26:3246–56.e4. doi: 10.1016/j.celrep.2019.02.071

296. Vulser H, Wiernik E, Hoertel N, Thomas F, Pannier B, Czernichow S, et al. Association between depression and anemia in otherwise healthy adults. *Acta Psychiatr Scand.* (2016) 134:150–60. doi: 10.1111/acps.12595

16

The Immunomodulator 1-Methyltryptophan Drives Tryptophan Catabolism Toward the Kynurenic Acid Branch

Elisa Wirthgen[1], Anne K. Leonard[2], Christian Scharf[3] and Grazyna Domanska[4*]

[1] Department of Pediatrics, Rostock University Medical Center, Rostock, Germany, [2] Institute of Biochemistry, University Medicine Greifswald, Greifswald, Germany, [3] Department of Otorhinolaryngology, Head and Neck Surgery, University Medicine Greifswald, Greifswald, Germany, [4] Institute of Immunology and Transfusion Medicine, University Medicine Greifswald, Greifswald, Germany

*Correspondence:
Grazyna Domanska
grazyna.domanska@
med.uni-greifswald.de

Background: Animal model studies revealed that the application of 1-methyltryptophan (1-MT), a tryptophan (TRP) analog, surprisingly increased plasma levels of the TRP metabolite, kynurenic acid (KYNA). Under inflammatory conditions, KYNA has been shown to mediate various immunomodulatory effects. Therefore, the present study aims to confirm and clarify the effects of 1-MT on TRP metabolism in mice as well as in humans.

Methods: Splenocytes from Balb/C or indoleamine 2,3-dioxygenase knockout ($IDO1^{-/-}$) mice or whole human blood were stimulated with 1-MT for 6, 24, or 36 h. C57BL/6 mice received 1-MT in drinking water for 5 days. Cell-free supernatants and plasma were analyzed for TRP and its metabolites by tandem mass spectrometry (MS/MS).

Results: 1-MT treatment induced an increase in TRP and its metabolite, KYNA in Balb/C, $IDO^{-/-}$ mice, and in human blood. Concurrently, the intermediate metabolite kynurenine (KYN), as well as the KYN/TRP ratio, were reduced after 1-MT treatment. The effects of 1-MT on TRP metabolites were similar after the *in vivo* application of 1-MT to C57BL/6 mice.

Conclusions: The data indicate that 1-MT induced an increase of KYNA *ex vivo* and *in vivo* confirming previously described results. Furthermore, the results of $IDO^{-/-}$ mice indicate that this effect seems not to be mediated by IDO1. Due to the proven immunomodulatory properties of KYNA, a shift toward this branch of the kynurenine pathway (KP) may be one potential mode of action by 1-MT and should be considered for further applications.

Keywords: 1-MT, IDO, KYNA, kynurenine pathway, tryptophan

INTRODUCTION

1-methyltryptophan (1-MT) is a TRP analog described first in 1991 (1) as a potential competitive inhibitor of the enzyme indoleamine 2,3-dioxygenase (IDO1). IDO1 is one rate-limiting enzyme of the kynurenine pathway (KP) (**Figure 1**), which plays a crucial role in the regulation of the immune response, notably as a counter-regulatory mechanism in the context of inflammation (2, 3). In

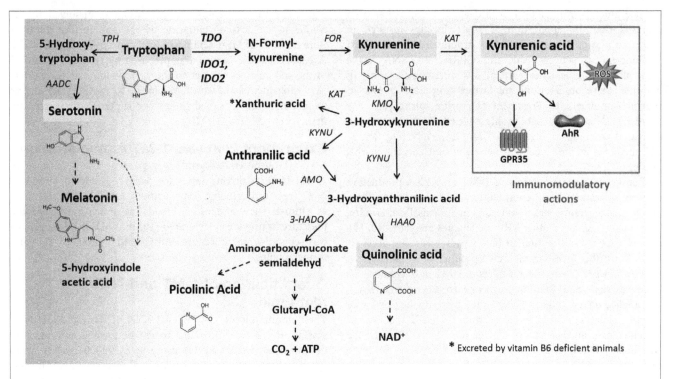

FIGURE 1 | Main pathways of TRP degradation, including relevant enzymes [modified after (2, 3)]. Black arrows mark enzymatic reactions and dashed arrows include more than one catalytic reaction step. Metabolites analyzed in this study are shaded gray. The catabolism of TRP by the enzymes TDO, IDO1/IDO2 represents the rate-limiting step of the kynurenine pathway in which 95% of dietary TRP is oxidized. One percentage of dietary tryptophan for the synthesis of serotonin. Apart from neuromodulatory properties (not shown), KYNA is an agonist of the broadly expressed receptors GPR35 and AhR. Furthermore, KYNA functions as an ROS scavenger. KYNA production. In addition to the presented canonical pathway of KYNA formation, alternative routes of KYNA production, promoted by the presence of ROS, are described (4). AADC, aromatic L-amino acid decarboxylase; AANAT, N-acetyltransferase; AhR, hydrocarbon receptor; AMO, anthranilate 3-monooxygenase; FOR, formamidase; GPR35: G-protein-coupled receptor 35; HAAO, 3-hydroxyanthranilic acid oxidase; HADO, 3-hydroxyanthranilic acid 3,4-dioxygenase; IDO, indolamine 2,3-dioxygenase; KAT, kynurenine aminotransferase; KMO, kynurenine 3-monooxygenase; KYNU, kynureninase; TDO, tryptophan 2,3-dioxygenase; TPH, tryptophan hydroxylase; ROS, reactive oxygen species.

cell free assays, it has been shown that 1-MT binds to the ferrous IDO complex but cannot be catalytically converted to kynurenine due to the additional methyl group (1). 1-MT is known for its low toxicity and great pharmacokinetic properties such as good intestinal absorption, low clearance, and low binding to plasmatic proteins (5, 6). Two stereoisomers of 1-MT, 1-methyl-D-tryptophan (D-1-MT also known as Indoximod) and 1-methyl-L-tryptophan (L-1-MT) are well studied and potential inhibitors of IDO. Indoximod is under investigation in several clinical trials (7–9) while L-1-MT or the combination of both isoforms DL-1-MT is used as IDO inhibitors in preclinical studies *in vivo* and *in vitro* (10–12). According to the reported IC_{50} values of L-1-MT (120 μM) and D-1-MT (2.5 mM) in HeLa cells (13), it is currently assumed that both L- and D-1-MT are weak IDO inhibitors *in vivo* (14, 15). Indeed, the D-isomer completely fails to inhibit the enzyme activity in inflammatory stimulated HeLa cells (9). The lack of IDO inhibition might be due to a low affinity of the inhibitor to the enzyme concurrent with a physiologically limited accumulation of the inhibitor to serum levels similar to those of TRP (16). Nevertheless, significant effects of these drugs on immune response were reported *in vivo* and *in vitro* (2, 16) revealing modes of actions other than IDO1 inhibition. Unexpectedly,

the oral or subcutaneous applications of 1-MT in Balb/C mice (10) and pigs (11), resulted in increased plasma levels of the TRP metabolite kynurenic acid (KYNA), a stable end product of KP, rather than KYN, which is an intermediate metabolite of KP. Due to the proven immunomodulatory properties of KYNA (3), a shift of KP toward the KYNA branch may be one potential mode of action by 1-MT, which may also be relevant for the application in humans. As previously described in detail (3), under inflammatory conditions, KYNA mediates mainly immunosuppressive effects, notably by targeting the G-protein-coupled receptor 35 (GPR35)- or aryl hydrocarbon receptor (AhR)-associated signaling pathways (2, 17, 18). For instance, KYNA reduces the expression and secretion of TNFα (10, 19–21) and diminishes the secretion of high-mobility group box 1 in monocytes (20, 22). Furthermore, there is evidence that KYNA induces downregulation of IL23/IL17 axis (23), which is assumed to have beneficial effects as an anti-inflammatory treatment in many immune-mediated diseases (24). The anti-inflammatory effects of KYNA, as frequently observed in *in vitro* models, are also confirmed *in vivo* in mice. It has been shown that, in a mouse model of LPS-induced septic shock, KYNA treatment attenuated LPS induced pro-inflammatory mediators such as TNF-α and nitric oxide (NO) and significantly rescued animals from LPS-induced death (22, 25). It has been reported that the application of 1-MT in pigs resulted in increased plasma levels of KYNA of around $5\,\mu M$ (11) which is sufficient to activate AhR and GPR35 as KYNA has a great affinity to the latter even at low micromolar range. In addition, these observations are further supported *ex vivo* in murine immune cells. Treatment of murine splenocytes with $5\,\mu M$ KYNA exerted a slight proliferative effect concurrent with increased secretion of IL-1β and IL-6 (26), suggesting that 1-MT mediates its biological and yet significant effects via AhR and/or GPR35.

Taking the observed effects of 1-MT on KYNA production into consideration, the present study aimed at verifying these effects in other mouse strains as well as in humans. Furthermore, additional insights on other TRP metabolites are provided. We treated animals and/or human blood with 1-MT for different times. To further investigate if KYNA production is related to the activity of the IDO enzyme, the effect of 1-MT in IDO knockout mice was examined. In addition to *ex vivo* experiments, 1-MT was applied *in vivo* in the C57BL/6 mice to verify the previously described effects of 1-MT in Balb/C mice (10). TRP metabolism in cell culture supernatants or plasma was characterized by the metabolites of TRP and its downstream metabolites kynurenine (KYN), quinolinic acid (QUIN), KYNA, and serotonin (5-HT). As a marker for increased IDO1 activity, the ratio of KYN to TRP was calculated.

MATERIALS AND METHODS

Animals

Female Balb/C ($n = 6$), $IDO1^{-/-}$, and C57BL/6 mice ($n = 41$) were maintained in the breeding facility at the University of Greifswald, Germany. $IDO1^{-/-}$ mice with a Balb/C background ($n = 6$) were provided by M. Moser (Brussels, Belgium) with the permission of A. Mellor (Augusta, Georgia, U.S.A.). As described in detail (27), the $IDO1^{-/-}$ mice were generated using a DNA construct that targets the murine IDO gene in embryonic stem cells. The defective gene expression was verified in tissues with a high level of constitutive IDO1 expression by PCR and Western Blot. All mice were kept in groups (6–9 mice/cage) under controlled conditions with 12/12 light/dark cycle and access to food and water *ad libitum*. All animal experiments were approved by the Animal Protection Committee of Mecklenburg-Vorpommern, Germany (AZ 7221.3-1.1-083/12).

Experiment 1: Stimulation of Murine Splenocytes and Human Whole Blood With 1-MT

Mice were euthanized as previously described (10). Spleens were aseptically removed into sterile, cold RPMI 1640 medium (Biochrom KG Berlin, Germany), and cell suspensions were prepared within 1 h after harvesting the organ. For *ex vivo* stimulation of whole blood cell cultures, human blood from six individual healthy donors was obtained from the Institute of Immunology and Transfusion Medicine, Greifswald after a written consent for scientific use. 1-MT (L-isomer, purity 95%;

Sigma-Aldrich, Deisenhofen, Germany) was dissolved in 1 N NaOH to a stock concentration of 1M, and further dilutions were made in RPMI medium to a final concentration of $600\,\mu M$. A NaOH solvent control was prepared by adding 1 N NaOH to the cell culture medium to the same volume as used for 1-MT. After incubation with 1-MT for 6, 24, or 36 h. TRP and its metabolites were analyzed in cell-free supernatants by tandem mass spectrometry (MS/MS).

Experiment 2: *in vivo* 1-MT Administration

1-MT (DL-isomer, 2 mg/ml) was given to C57BL/6 mice ($n = 24$) in the drinking water for 5 days. A control group ($n = 17$) received drinking water without 1-MT. After treatment, all animals were euthanized, blood was drawn by retroorbital puncture as previously described (10) into EDTA-tubes, plasma was separated and stored at $-80°C$ until analysis of TRP and its metabolites.

Quantification of 1-MT and TRP Metabolites

The determination of 1-MT, TRP, KYN, KYNA, and QUIN in plasma or cell-free supernatants was performed as previously described in detail (28, 29) using an API2000 tandem mass spectrometer equipped with an electrospray ion source (ABSciex, Darmstadt, Germany). As an indicator of IDO1 activation, the ratio of KYN and TRP (KYN × 100/TRP) was calculated (30).

Statistics

Statistical analyses of experiment 1 was performed using SAS software, version 9.4 (SAS Institute Inc., Cary, NC, USA). The continuous response variables (TRP, KYN, KYNA, QUIN, 5-HT) were analyzed by Analysis of Variance (ANOVA) comprising the fixed effects treatment (1-MT, Control), and sampling time (6, 24, 36 h) and their interaction (treatment × time). In order to compare the six sets of measurements, the data were analyzed by fitting and testing generalized linear models applying the GLIMMIX procedure. The repeated statement in the GLIMMIX procedure was used with respect to repeated measurements on the same subject. Tukey–Kramer procedure was used for pair-wise multiple comparisons of TRP metabolites within one species. For the presentation of the results, the least square means (LS-means) and their standard errors (SE) were calculated and tested for each fixed effect in the model using the Tukey–Kramer procedure for all pair-wise comparisons. Data of experiment 2 were analyzed using the SigmaPlot 14.0 software. Differences between the treatment and the control group were compared with Welch's *t*-test or Mann-Whitney U test according to unequal variances of the treatment and the control group or failure of the normality test, respectively. The effects and differences were considered significant at $p < 0.05$.

RESULTS

1-MT Modifies TRP Metabolism and Increases KYNA *ex vivo*

To investigate whether 1-MT induces the production of KYNA *ex vivo*, murine splenocytes and human blood were stimulated with 1-MT for either 6, 24, or 36 h according to the experimental design 1. Due to the weak inhibitory potential of L-1-MT (IC_{50} = 120 μM) (13), a relatively high concentration i.e., 600 μM L-1-MT was chosen to achieve effective inhibition of IDO. To further investigate if KYNA production is dependent on a functional IDO enzyme, the effect of 1-MT in IDO knockout mice was examined. TRP and its metabolites were measured in supernatants of cell culture.

Pair-wise comparisons between 1-MT treatment and controls (main effect: Treatment) are presented in **Table 1**. Thereby, the concentrations of TRP were increased by 1-MT in Balb/C and $IDO1^{-/-}$ mice as well as in human blood. That does not seem surprising since the applied L-1-MT contains 5% L-TRP, which corresponds to a concentration of 30 μM. In both murine and human cell culture supernatants, the increased level of TRP concentration corresponded to decreased levels of KYN, and 5-HT indicating downregulation of TRP breakdown. The downstream TRP metabolite QUIN was reduced by 1-MT in mice but not in human blood, suggesting species-specific differences. The observation of a diminished degradation of TRP

TABLE 1 | Pairwise comparisons of the treatment effect (1-MT vs. control) using Tukey-Kramer test.

	1-MT	Control	SE	P-value
	LSM	LSM		
TRP (μM)				
Balb/C	250.94	227.44	3.24	**0.003**
IDO1$^{-/-}$	221.61	202.00	4.43	**0.030**
Human	220.78	197.00	5.08	**0.002**
KYN (μM)				
Balb/C	1.72	2.26	0.11	**0.001**
IDO1$^{-/-}$	1.45	1.90	0.07	**0.001**
Human	1.62	2.34	0.18	**0.001**
KYNA (μM)				
Balb/C	4.95	4.06	1.05	**0.047**
IDO1$^{-/-}$	2.56	1.20	0.16	**<0.001**
Human	4.09	1.37	0.29	**<0.001**
QUIN (μM)				
Balb/C	0.42	0.52	0.02	**0.002**
IDO1$^{-/-}$	0.38	0.45	0.01	**<0.001**
Human	0.33	0.32	0.01	0.64
5-HT (μM)				
Balb/C	1.20	1.37	0.03	**<0.001**
IDO1$^{-/-}$	1.12	1.28	0.02	**<0.001**
Human	1.01	1.08	0.01	**0.002**
KYN/TRP ratio				
Balb/C	0.69	1.00	0.06	**0.001**
IDO1$^{-/-}$	0.66	0.94	0.03	**<0.001**
Human	0.73	1.22	0.12	**0.002**

Concentrations of the metabolites TRP, KYN, KYNA, QUIN, 5-HT were measured in cell culture supernatants of isolated splencocytes (Balb/C, IDO1$^{-/-}$) and human whole blood cell culture. As marker for IDO activity KYN/TRP ratio was calculated. Results are presented as LS-means (LSM) ± SE averaged over three incubation times (6, 24, 36 h) per subject. 1-MT: n = 18 (six per species); Control: n = 18 (six per species). P-values < 0.05 are marked in bold.

via KP was further supported by the results of KYN to TRP ratio, often used as a marker for IDO activity (28). This ratio was decreased by 1-MT at all time points both in mice and human cell cultures, indicating that 1-MT inhibited the activity of IDO. Despite the presumed IDO inhibition by the high concentrations of 1-MT, the synthesis of kynurenine was not reduced completely, indicating a lack of effective IDO inhibition. The treatment effect on TRP and its metabolites KYN, 5-HT, and QUIN were comparable between different times of incubation with 1-MT (treatment × time, $p > 0.05$) (**Figures 2A–C**).

1-MT induced an increase of KYNA in cell culture supernatants of murine splenocytes as well as in human blood, confirming studies in pigs and mice (10, 11). Interestingly, this effect was also detected in $IDO1^{-/-}$ mice, revealing that KYNA production was not related to a functional IDO enzyme. In splenocytes of $IDO1^{-/-}$ mice and human blood, increased levels of KYNA were detected after 6, 24, and 36 h of stimulation with 1-MT, indicating a TRP breakdown toward the KYNA branch. Interestingly, in Balb/C mice, KYNA levels were lower in the treatment group compared to controls after 6 h of stimulation with 1-MT (treatment × time, $p < 0.05$). However, this effect might not reflect a reduced KYNA production but is rather the consequence of an increased KYNA concentration in the control group.

1-MT Modifies TRP Metabolism and Increases KYNA *in vivo*

We next investigated whether 1-MT induces the production of KYNA after *in vivo* application. According to the design of experiment 2, 1-MT was given to C57BL/6 in drinking water over a period of 5 days. Afterward, TRP and its metabolites were measured in plasma. The results are presented in **Figure 3**. After 5 days, 1-MT concentration in plasma was reached to ~25.5 μM, whereas in control animals the concentration was below the detection range (LLOQ: <2.3 μM) (data are not shown). The ratio of KYN to TRP was decreased after 1-MT treatment indicating a diminished TRP breakdown. However, it is assumed that the plasma concentrations achieved *in vivo* do not effectively block IDO activity, indicating that this effect is not related to the activity of the IDO enzyme. Similar to *ex vivo* findings, the pairwise comparisons reveal that the 1-MT treatment increased plasma levels of TRP and KYNA. In contrast, the concentrations of QUIN and 5-HT were not significantly affected by 1-MT treatment.

Together with the previously published findings from mice and pigs, the present study reveals that 1-MT induces an increase of KYNA concentrations in different species, including humans. Furthermore, these effects seem to be independent of IDO activity.

DISCUSSION

In this study, effects of 1-MT on TRP metabolism were investigated in mice and humans to provide additional insights into potential modes of action of 1-MT as previously described in mice and pigs (10, 11). The results of experiment 1 show

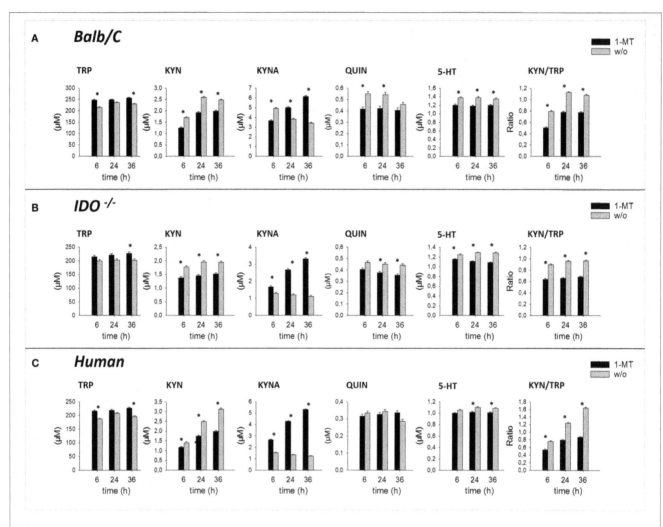

FIGURE 2 | Effect of 1-MT on TRP metabolism in cultured splenocytes isolated from Balb/C mice **(A)**, $IDO^{-/-}$ mice **(B)**, and in human whole blood cell culture **(C)**. TRP and its metabolites KYN, KYNA, QUIN were measured in cell culture supernatants after 6, 24, or 36 h incubation with 1-MT (600 μM) by MS/MS. KYN/TRP ratio was calculated as a marker for IDO1 activity. The results are presented as LS-means + SE. Significant differences between the 1-MT and the control group were calculated using the Tukey-Kramer test and are shown for each incubation time. $n = 6$ per species, $^*P < 0.05$.

that 1-MT increased the concentrations of TRP in supernatants of cultured murine splenocytes, human blood cell culture, and murine plasma. These results confirm the data from pigs where plasma concentrations of TRP are increased after 24 h of treatment with 1-MT subcutaneously (11). The effect of increased TRP concentrations may be a result of indirect supplementation of TRP contained in commercially available 1-MT, though the applied 1-MT has a purity of at least 95%. As confirmed by previous studies, 1-MT contains ≤5% TRP (11, 31), which may affect the results of *in vitro* or *ex vivo* studies, independently of IDO activity. However, the indirect TRP supplementation does not sufficiently explain the results *in vivo* because the amount of TRP contained in 1-MT is negligible compared to the dietary derived TRP amounts, which are positively regulated by tryptophan 2,3-dioxygenase (TDO) (mainly expressed in the liver) to maintain the homeostasis of TRP (32). It has been further described that both isomers of 1-MT mimic TRP (14, 33),

which may feign an amino acid oversupply and, therefore, may reduce the uptake of endogenous TRP to somatic cells resulting in increased TRP levels. Although it could not be clarified conclusively whether TRP contamination of 1-MT and/or other effects such as TRP mimetics caused the increase of TRP, the summary of results from previous studies, including the present study, indicate that it seems to be a general effect. Since higher TRP concentrations lead to an activation of TDO, one can assume that TRP supplementation may result in an accelerated TRP degradation concurrent with increased production of TRP downstream metabolites. For instance, in human glioblastoma cells, the TRP contamination of 1-MT (L-isomer) resulted in an increased production of KYN, indicating an accelerated degradation of TRP via KP (31). This was supported by studies in pigs where TRP supplementation resulted in an overall activation of the KP as well as the 5-HT system (34). In contrast, the results of our present study show that the 1-MT-induced elevation of

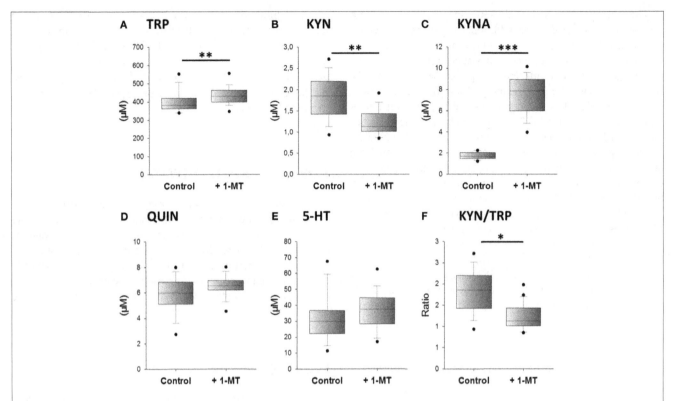

FIGURE 3 | Effects of 1-MT application on plasma concentrations of TRP **(A)**, KYN **(B)**, KYNA **(C)**, QUIN **(D)**, 5-HT **(E)**, and the calculated KYN/TRP ratio **(F)**. 1-MT was applied via drinking water for 5 days. Control animals received drinking water without 1-MT. TRP and its metabolites were measured using MS/MS. The KYN/TRP ratio was used as a marker for IDO1 activity. The results are presented as boxplot including the median, the interquartile range, and the min and max values. Significant differences between the 1-MT- and control groups were calculated using the Welsh's test **(B–F)** or the Mann-Whitney U test **(A)**. 1-MT: $n = 24$; MYR: $n = 17$; ***$P < 0.001$, **$P < 0.01$, *$P < 0.05$.

TRP, which was associated with increased production of KYNA with a decrease of other TRP metabolites such as KYN or 5-HT in mice as well as in human blood. Also, the ratio of KYN to TRP, often used as a marker for IDO activity, was decreased in all investigated species after both *ex vivo* and *in vivo* application of 1-MT. In the present study, these results reveal an enhanced degradation of TRP directed to one specific branch of the KP (see also **Figure 1**) which not only seems to be a consequence of increased TRP levels but is also related to 1-MT. Although in the present study, the effect of 1-MT on KYN to TRP ratio seems to be uniform between *ex vivo* and *in vivo* studies, the *in vivo* treatment of healthy Balb/C mice (10) or pigs (11) did not significantly affect the KYN to TRP ratio indicating species/strain-specific responses to 1-MT or effects of the experimental design. Nevertheless, the results from mice and pigs (10, 11) showed independently from each other that 1-MT induced an increase of KYNA indicating that this effect is not restricted to a specific animal model. Furthermore, the findings in human blood indicate that this effect may be even relevant for the application of 1-MT in humans.

The finding that 1-MT induced an elevation of KYNA, but not the intermediate metabolite KYN, raises the question of whether TRP is metabolized directly to KYNA rather than through IDO activity. Computational modeling of data evaluated from a previously reported study in pigs (11) reveals that it is more likely that increased levels of TRP are directly degraded to KYNA (35). It is assumed that the major production of KYNA is attributed to kynurenine aminotransferases (KATs), enzymes with a broad spectrum of substrates besides KYN. *In vitro* analysis show that TRP is a substrate for the enzyme KAT II with a similar *Km*-value as the substrate KYN (36). Interestingly, in the present study, KYNA was also increased in IDO knockout mice, supporting the hypothesis that this effect is not related to a functional IDO enzyme. This is supported by the finding that increased KYNA levels were also measured after *in vivo* application of 1-MT, although the plasma concentrations of 1-MT ($\sim$25 μM) were too low to inhibit IDO effectively.

The finding that other TRP metabolites of KP or serotonin pathway are decreased, or unaffected indicates that the KYNA production is not mediated by one of the rate-limiting enzymes of KP (canonical pathway) but might be mediated by other TRP degrading enzymes or non-enzymatically. According to this hypothesis, alternative mechanisms of KYNA production (4) might be involved. For instance, it was described that enzymes such as the aromatic amino acid transaminase are able to catalyze TRP to intermediate metabolites which serve as KYNA precursors in the presence of reactive oxygen radicals (ROS) (4).

The theory that increased TRP may promote KYNA production was tested in an additional experiment. Thereby, the application of 5% TRP (contained in L-1-MT) induced an increase of KYNA production 3 h after application but not after longer incubation time, indicating that the additional TRP is metabolized via the kynurenine pathway (data not shown). However, the KYNA production by L- and D-1-MT was 2 to 3-fold higher compared to L-TRP alone, which leads one to assume that the TRP contamination is not an exclusive explanation for the increased KYNA values. According to this, it is suggested that other mechanisms might be involved in the increased production of KYNA. Although there is currently a lack of data, it cannot be ruled out that 1-MT itself is metabolized or transformed to TRP or other TRP related metabolites by a yet unknown pathway. These questions remain to be clarified in further studies.

In the present study, it seems surprising that the loss of functional IDO1 in the IDO KO mice has no effect on the 1-MT-induced changes of TRP metabolites. These data implicate that other tryptophan-catabolizing enzymes like IDO2 and tryptophan 2,3-dioxygenase (TDO) might compensate for the lack of IDO1. This theory is supported by other studies demonstrating that IDO1 deficiency does not affect the inflammation in murine models of arthritis, pregnancy, or bacterial infection (27, 37, 38).

CONCLUSIONS

The results from the present study indicate that the administration of 1-MT induces a shift of KP toward the branch of KYNA. This effect was shown independently in two mice strains as well as in human blood. Furthermore, the results from IDO knockout mice, as well as the decreased levels of KYN *in vivo*, indicate that the 1-MT-induced increase of KYNA seems not to be dependent on IDO1 activity. This was confirmed by the *in vivo* results where 1-MT levels were too low for an effective IDO1 inhibition; nevertheless, KYNA was increased in plasma. The increase of KYNA may be one potential mode of action by 1-MT and should be considered for preclinical studies and therapeutic applications in humans. Furthermore, the application of 1-MT might have therapeutic implications as it may provide a method to increase KYNA while preserving IDO1 activity. Due to its immunoregulatory role, the inhibition of IDO1 may not be appropriate for different therapeutic approaches.

AUTHOR CONTRIBUTIONS

GD conceived the project, designed and performed the experiments, and analyzed MS data. GD and EW wrote the manuscript. EW analyzed the data, created the figures, and wrote the first draft of the manuscript. AL and CS assisted with performing of the MS analysis and critically revised the manuscript for important intellectual content. All authors critically reviewed the manuscript and approved the final version.

FUNDING

EW was supported by the Rostock University Medical Center (UMR, FORUN 889021).

ACKNOWLEDGMENTS

The authors are grateful to Christian Manteuffel from the Leibniz Institute for Farm Animal Biology (FBN) for statistical consulting and technical support with SAS software. The authors are also thankful to Murthy N. Darisipudi from the Department of Immunology of University Medicine Greifswald for supporting the linguistic editing of the manuscript.

REFERENCES

1. Cady SG, Sono M. 1-Methyl-dl-tryptophan, β-(3-benzofuranyl)-dl-alanine (the oxygen analog of tryptophan), and β-[3-benzo (b) thienyl]-dl-alanine (the sulfur analog of tryptophan) are competitive inhibitors for indoleamine 2, 3-dioxygenase. *Arch Biochem Biophys*. (1991) 291:326–33. doi: 10.1016/0003-9861(91)90142-6

2. Wirthgen E, Hoeflich A. Endotoxin-induced tryptophan degradation along the kynurenine pathway: the role of indolamine 2, 3-dioxygenase and aryl hydrocarbon receptor-mediated immunosuppressive effects in endotoxin tolerance and cancer and its implications for immunoparalysis. *J Amino Acids*. (2015) 2015:973548. doi: 10.1155/2015/973548

3. Wirthgen E, Hoeflich A, Rebl A, Günther J. Kynurenic acid: the janus-faced role of an immunomodulatory tryptophan metabolite and its link to pathological conditions. *Front Immunol*. (2018) 8:1957. doi: 10.3389/fimmu.2017.01957

4. Ramos-Chávez LA, Lugo Huitrón R, González Esquivel D, Pineda B, Ríos C, Silva-Adaya D, et al. Relevance of alternative routes of kynurenic acid production in the brain. *Oxid Med Cell Longev*. (2018) 2018:5272741. doi: 10.1155/2018/5272741

5. Jia L, Schweikart K, Tomaszewski J, Page JG, Noker PE, Buhrow SA, et al. Toxicology and pharmacokinetics of 1-methyl-d-tryptophan: absence of toxicity due to saturating absorption. *Food Chem Toxicol*. (2008) 46:203–11. doi: 10.1016/j.fct.2007.07.017

6. Liu X, Newton RC, Friedman SM, Scherle PA. Indoleamine 2, 3-dioxygenase, an emerging target for anti-cancer therapy. *Curr*

Cancer Drug Targets. (2009) 9:938–52. doi: 10.2174/1568009097901 92374

7. Uyttenhove C, Pilotte L, Théate I, Stroobant V, Colau D, Parmentier N, et al. Evidence for a tumoral immune resistance mechanism based on tryptophan degradation by indoleamine 2, 3-dioxygenase. *Nat Med.* (2003) 9:1269–74. doi: 10.1038/nm934

8. Muller AJ, DuHadaway JB, Donover PS, Sutanto-Ward E, Prendergast GC. Inhibition of indoleamine 2, 3-dioxygenase, an immunoregulatory target of the cancer suppression gene Bin1, potentiates cancer chemotherapy. *Nat Med.* (2005) 11:312–9. doi: 10.1038/nm1196

9. Hou DY, Muller AJ, Sharma MD, DuHadaway J, Banerjee T, Johnson M, et al. Inhibition of indoleamine 2,3-dioxygenase in dendritic cells by stereoisomers of 1-methyl-tryptophan correlates with antitumor responses. *Cancer Res.* (2007) 67:792–801. doi: 10.1158/0008-5472.CAN-06-2925

10. Kiank C, Zeden J-P, Drude S, Domanska G, Fusch G, Otten W, et al. Psychological stress-induced, IDO1-dependent tryptophan catabolism: implications on immunosuppression in mice and humans. *PLoS ONE.* (2010) 5:e11825. doi: 10.1371/journal.pone.0011825

11. Wirthgen E, Otten W, Tuchscherer M, Tuchscherer A, Domanska G, Brenmoehl J, et al. Effects of 1-methyltryptophan on immune responses and the kynurenine pathway after lipopolysaccharide challenge in pigs. *Int J Mol Sci.* (2018) 19:3009. doi: 10.3390/ijms19103009

12. Löb S, Königsrainer A, Zieker D, Brücher BL, Rammensee H-G, Opelz G, et al. IDO1 and IDO2 are expressed in human tumors: levo-but not dextro-1-methyl tryptophan inhibits tryptophan catabolism. *Cancer Immunol Immunother.* (2009) 58:153–7. doi: 10.1007/s00262-008-0513-6

13. Liu X, Shin N, Koblish HK, Yang G, Wang Q, Wang K, et al. Selective inhibition of IDO1 effectively regulates mediators of antitumor immunity. (2010) 115:3520–30. doi: 10.1182/blood-2009-09-246124

14. Fox E, Oliver T, Rowe M, Thomas S, Zakharia Y, Gilman PB, et al. Indoximod: an immunometabolic adjuvant that empowers T cell activity in cancer. *Front Oncol.* (2018) 8:370. doi: 10.3389/fonc.2018.00370

15. Prendergast GC, Smith C, Thomas S, Mandik-Nayak L, Laury-Kleintop L, Metz R, et al. Indoleamine 2,3-dioxygenase pathways of pathogenic inflammation and immune escape in cancer. *Cancer Immunol Immunother CII.* (2014) 63:721–35. doi: 10.1007/s00262-014-1549-4

16. Günther J, Däbritz J, Wirthgen E. Limitations and off-target effects of tryptophan-related IDO inhibitors in cancer treatment. *Front Immunol.* (2019) 10:1801. doi: 10.3389/fimmu.2019.01801

17. Wang J, Simonavicius N, Wu X, Swaminath G, Reagan J, Tian H, et al. Kynurenic acid as a ligand for orphan G protein-coupled receptor GPR35. *J Biol Chem.* (2006) 281:22021–8. doi: 10.1074/jbc.M603503200

18. DiNatale BC, Murray IA, Schroeder JC, Flaveny CA, Lahoti TS, Laurenzana EM, et al. Kynurenic acid is a potent endogenous aryl hydrocarbon receptor ligand that synergistically induces interleukin-6 in the presence of inflammatory signaling. *Toxicol Sci.* (2010) 115:89–97. doi: 10.1093/toxsci/kfq024

19. Steiner L, Gold M, Mengel D, Dodel R, Bach J-P. The endogenous α7 nicotinic acetylcholine receptor antagonist kynurenic acid modulates amyloid-β-induced inflammation in BV-2 microglial cells. *J Neurol Sci.* (2014) 344:94–9. doi: 10.1016/j.jns.2014.06.032

20. Tiszlavicz Z, Németh B, Fülöp F, Vécsei L, Tápai K, Ocsovszky I, et al. Different inhibitory effects of kynurenic acid and a novel kynurenic acid analogue on tumour necrosis factor-α (TNF-α) production by mononuclear cells, HMGB1 production by monocytes and HNP1-3 secretion by neutrophils. *Naunyn Schmiedeberg's Arch Pharmacol.* (2011) 383:447–55. doi: 10.1007/s00210-011-0605-2

21. Mándi Y, Endrész V, Mosolygó T, Burián K, Lantos I, Fülöp F, et al. The opposite effects of kynurenic acid and different kynurenic acid analogs on tumor necrosis factor-α (TNF-α) production and tumor necrosis factor-stimulated gene-6 (TSG-6) expression. *Front Immunol.* (2019) 10:1406. doi: 10.3389/fimmu.2019.01406

22. Moroni F, Cozzi A, Sili M, Mannaioni G. Kynurenic acid: a metabolite with multiple actions and multiple targets in brain and periphery. *J Neural Transm.* (2012) 119:133–9. doi: 10.1007/s00702-011-0763-x

23. Elizei SS, Poormasjedi-Meibod M-S, Wang X, Kheirandish M, Ghahary A. Kynurenic acid downregulates IL-17/1L-23 axis *in vitro. Mol Cell Biochem.* (2017) 431:55–65. doi: 10.1007/s11010-017-2975-3

24. Gaffen SL, Jain R, Garg AV, Cua DJ. The IL-23-IL-17 immune axis: from mechanisms to therapeutic testing. *Nat Rev Immunol.* (2014) 14:585. doi: 10.1038/nri3707

25. Moroni F, Fossati S, Chiarugi A, Cozzi A (editors). Kynurenic acid actions in brain and periphery. In: *International Congress Series.* Elsevier (2007).

26. Małaczewska J, Siwicki AK, Wójcik RM, Turski WA, Kaczorek E. The effect of kynurenic acid on the synthesis of selected cytokines by murine splenocytes - *in vitro* and *ex vivo* studies. *Cent Eur J Immunol.* (2016) 41:39–46. doi: 10.5114/ceji.2016.58815

27. Baban B, Chandler P, McCool D, Marshall B, Munn DH, Mellor AL. Indoleamine 2,3-dioxygenase expression is restricted to fetal trophoblast giant cells during murine gestation and is maternal genome specific. *J Reprod Immunol.* (2004) 61:67–77. doi: 10.1016/j.jri.2003.11.003

28. Wirthgen E, Tuchscherer M, Otten W, Domanska G, Wollenhaupt K, Tuchscherer A, et al. Activation of indoleamine 2, 3-dioxygenase by LPS in a porcine model. *Innate Immun.* (2014) 20:30–9. doi: 10.1177/1753425913481252

29. Wirthgen E, Kanitz E, Tuchscherer M, Tuchscherer A, Domanska G, Weitschies W, et al. Pharmacokinetics of 1-methyl-L-tryptophan after single and repeated subcutaneous application in a porcine model. *Exp Anim.* (2016) 65:147–55. doi: 10.1538/expanim.15-0096

30. Suzuki Y, Suda T, Asada K, Miwa S, Suzuki M, Fujie M, et al. Serum indoleamine 2,3-dioxygenase activity predicts prognosis of pulmonary tuberculosis. *Clin Vaccine Immunol CVI.* (2012) 19:436–42. doi: 10.1128/CVI.05402-11

31. Schmidt SK, Siepmann S, Kuhlmann K, Meyer HE, Metzger S, Pudelko S, et al. Influence of tryptophan contained in 1-Methyl-Tryptophan on antimicrobial and immunoregulatory functions of indoleamine 2,3-dioxygenase. *PLoS ONE.* (2012) 7:e44797. doi: 10.1371/journal.pone.00 44797

32. Kanai M, Nakamura T, Funakoshi H. Identification and characterization of novel variants of the tryptophan 2, 3-dioxygenase gene: differential regulation in the mouse nervous system during development. *Neurosci Res.* (2009) 64:111–7. doi: 10.1016/j.neures.2009.02.004

33. Metz R, Rust S, DuHadaway JB, Mautino MR, Munn DH, Vahanian NN, et al. IDO inhibits a tryptophan sufficiency signal that stimulates mTOR: a novel IDO effector pathway targeted by D-1-methyl-tryptophan. *Oncoimmunology.* (2012) 1:1460–8. doi: 10.4161/onci.21716

34. Stracke J, Otten W, Tuchscherer A, Witthahn M, Metges CC, Puppe B, et al. Dietary tryptophan supplementation and affective state in pigs. *J Vet Behav.* (2017) 20:82–90. doi: 10.1016/j.jveb.2017.03.009

35. Kleimeier D, Domanska G, Kanitz E, Otten W, Wirthgen E, Bröker BM, et al. Effects of 1-Methyltryptophan on the kynurenine pathway in pigs. In: *5th International Symposium Systems Biology of Microbial Infection.* Jena (2019).

36. Han Q, Cai T, Tagle DA, Robinson H, Li J. Substrate specificity and structure of human aminoadipate aminotransferase/kynurenine aminotransferase II. *Biosci Rep.* (2008) 28:205–15. doi: 10.1042/BSR200 80085

37. Put K, Brisse E, Avau A, Imbrechts M, Mitera T, Janssens R, et al. IDO1 deficiency does not affect disease in mouse models of systemic juvenile idiopathic arthritis and secondary hemophagocytic lymphohistiocytosis. *PLoS ONE.* (2016) 11:e0150075. doi: 10.1371/journal.pone.0150075

38. Divanovic S, Sawtell NM, Trompette A, Warning JI, Dias A, Cooper AM, et al. Opposing biological functions of tryptophan catabolizing enzymes during intracellular infection. *J Infect Dis.* (2012) 205:152–61. doi: 10.1093/infdis/jir621

17

IDO Targeting in Sarcoma: Biological and Clinical Implications

Imane Nafia[1], Maud Toulmonde[2], Doriane Bortolotto[1], Assia Chaibi[1], Dominique Bodet[1], Christophe Rey[1], Valerie Velasco[2], Claire B. Larmonier[2], Loïc Cerf[1], Julien Adam[3], François Le Loarer[2], Ariel Savina[4], Alban Bessede[1*†] and Antoine Italiano[2,5*†]

[1] Explicyte Immuno-Oncology, Bordeaux, France, [2] Department of Medical Oncology, Institut Bergonié, Bordeaux, France, [3] Department of Pathology, Gustave Roussy, Villejuif, France, [4] Institut Roche, Paris, France, [5] Inserm U1218, Bordeaux, France

*Correspondence:
Alban Bessede
a.bessede@explicyte.com
Antoine Italiano
a.italiano@bordeaux.unicancer.fr

† These authors share
senior authorship

Sarcomas are heterogeneous malignant mesenchymal neoplasms with limited sensitivity to immunotherapy. We recently demonstrated an increase in Kynurenine Pathway (KP) activity in the plasma of sarcoma patients treated with pembrolizumab. While the KP has already been described to favor immune escape through the degradation of L-Tryptophan and production of metabolites including L-Kynurenine, Indoleamine 2,3 dioxygenase (IDO1), a first rate-limiting enzyme of the KP, still represents an attractive therapeutic target, and its blockade had not yet been investigated in sarcomas. Using immunohistochemistry, IDO1 and CD8, expression profiles were addressed within 203 cases of human sarcomas. At a preclinical level, we investigated the modulation of the KP upon PDL1 blockade in a syngeneic model of sarcoma through mRNA quantification of key KP enzymes within the tumor. Furthermore, in order to evaluate the possible anti-tumor effect of IDO blockade in combination with PDL1 blockade, an innovative IDO inhibitor (GDC-0919) was used. Its effect was first assessed on Kynurenine to Tryptophan ratio at plasmatic level and also within the tumor. Following GDC-0919 treatment, alone or in combination with anti-PDL1 antibody, tumor growth, immune cell infiltration, and gene expression profiling were measured. IDO1 expression was observed in 39.1% of human sarcoma cases and was significantly higher in tumors with high CD8 infiltration. In the pre-clinical setting, blockade of PDL1 led to a strong anti-tumor effect and was associated with an intratumoral inflammatory cytokines signature driven by Ifng but also with a modulation of the KP enzymes including Ido1 and Ido2. IDO1 inhibition using GDC-0919 resulted in (i) a significant decrease of plasmatic Kynurenine to Tryptophan ratio and in (ii) a decrease of tumoral Kynurenine. However, GDC-0919 used alone or combined with anti-PDL1, did not show anti-tumoral activity and did not affect the tumor immune cell infiltrate. In order to elucidate the mechanism(s) underlying the lack of effect of GDC-0919, we analyzed the gene expression profile of intratumoral biopsies. Interestingly, we have found that GDC-0919 induced a downregulation of the expression of pvr and granzymes, and an upregulation of inhba and Dtx4 suggesting a potential role of the IDO pathway in the control of NK function.

Keywords: sarcomas, immunotherapy, indoleamine, kynurenine, PDL1

INTRODUCTION

Soft-tissue sarcomas (STS) represent a heterogeneous group of rare tumors including more than 70 different histological subtypes (1). The identification of new therapies for STS patients is of crucial importance. Indeed, 40 to 50% STS patients will develop metastatic disease. Once metastases are detected, the treatment is mainly based on palliative chemotherapy and median survival of patients in this setting is about 12 to 20 months (2).

Historically, sarcomas represent the first tumor model for which immunotherapy has been suggested as a relevant therapeutic strategy (3). The PD1-PDL1 interaction is a major pathway hijacked by tumors to suppress immune control. The normal function of PD1, expressed on the surface of activated T cells under healthy conditions, is to down-modulate unwanted or excessive immune responses, including autoimmune reactions. Recent studies have shown that PDL1 was expressed in 58% of cases of STS, osteosarcomas and GIST (4–7) and that this overexpression has been associated with poor prognosis (6, 7). Targeting the PD1/PDL1 interaction was associated with impressive anti-tumor activity in a pre-clinical model of osteosarcoma (8).

We and others have shown that PD1 targeting has only modest efficacy in patients with advanced STS (9–12). By analyzing tumor samples from patients treated with the PD1 antagonist Pembrolizumab, we observed a high level of IDO1 expression (12). IDO1 is a major regulator of the Tryptophan (Trp) catabolism pathway that has been linked to impairment of anti-tumor immunity and tumor growth in several models (13, 14). Kynurenine, which is notably produced by IDO1, is a key metabolite of this pathway that can promote selective expansion of regulatory T cells (Tregs) (15). Strikingly, we found a statistically significant increase in the kynurenine/tryptophan ratio, a robust pharmacodynamic marker of the IDO1/Kynurenine pathway (KP), between pre-treatment and on-treatment plasma samples of sarcoma patients treated with Pembrolizumab. Notably, this upregulation of the kynurenine/tryptophan ratio was also correlated with a higher density of IDO1 expression in pre-treated tumor samples (11).

IDO1/2 are major regulators of the KP, which is involved in immune homeostasis and tolerance—including fetomaternal tolerance—and avoiding acute and chronic hyperinflammatory reactions and autoimmunity. These enzymes induce biostatic tryptophan starvation, which limits lymphocyte expansion, and produce a series of catabolites, collectively known as kynurenines. L-kynurenine—the first, stable tryptophan catabolite in this pathway—induces T helper type-1 cell apoptosis and acts as an endogenous activator of the ligand-operated transcription factor aryl hydrocarbon receptor (AhR), thus promoting Treg cell generation and expansion. A novel oncotherapeutic approach, based on the inhibition of IDO1/2 by 1-methyl-tryptophan (1-MT) has demonstrated a synergistic efficacy when used in combination with conventional chemotherapy (16). Recent preclinical data have also evidenced that IDO1 deficient mice (Ido1−/−) were more sensitive to immune checkpoint inhibitors, including anti-CTLA4, anti-PD1, and anti-PDL1,

thus highlighting the crucial role of IDO1 in resistance to those treatments. The same authors have shown that the prototypical IDO1 inhibitor, 1-MT, can synergize with the same immunotherapies (17).

Altogether, such data led us to hypothesize that the IDO1/KP pathway could preferentially contribute to the immune-suppressive phenotype of STS cells and be an important mechanism of the primary resistance to PD1 inhibition observed in sarcoma patients (8), and that targeting this pathway with an innovative compound would improve anti-PD1/PDL1 efficacy in this setting.

Currently, several investigational agents inhibiting the IDO-Kyn-Trp pathway such as IDO1, combination IDO1/TDO inhibitors, AhR inhibitors as well as a recombinant kynureninase are in clinical development or late preclinical testing (18). We investigated the pre-clinical activity of a specific IDO inhibitor—GDC-0919—and its capacity to synergize with PD1 inhibition in a preclinical model of STS.

RESULTS

Histological Profiling Identifies Expression of IDO1 in Human STS

In order to investigate IDO1 expression in human STS, we performed an immunohistochemistry-based analysis for IDO1, PDL1, and CD8 markers of 203 cases of sarcomas with genomic complex (**Figure 1A**). Their characteristics are described in **Table 1**. The median density of CD8+ was 32.5 cells/mm^2 (range 0–2663). Neither metastases-free survival nor overall survival was significantly different between patients with level of CD8 TL tumor density below or above the median (**Supplementary Figure 1**). IDO expression was observed in 79 cases (39.1%). The proportion of tumors with positive IDO1 staining was significantly higher in the group with higher levels of CD8+ TL tumor density than in the group with lower levels (65.3% vs. 12.9%, $p < 0.001$) (**Figure 1B**). Moreover, PDL1 expression was positive on tumor cells and on immune cells in 46 cases (22.7%), and almost exclusively in tumors with higher levels of CD8 TL tumor density (*data not shown*).

The KP Is Active in Human Sarcoma Cell Lines and Is Reversed by GDC-0919

In order to evaluate the capacity of human sarcoma cells to produce Kynurenine as an immunosuppressive mechanism, we exposed two sarcoma cell lines—namely IB115 (dedifferentiated liposarcoma) and IB136 (leiomyosarcoma)—to increasing concentrations of human interferon gamma (hIFNg) for 48 h before cell supernatant collection for Kynurenine measurement by mean of an immuno-assay (ImmuSmol). We observed a hIFNg dose-dependent increase of Kynurenine, which was more pronounced for IB115 than for IB136 cell lines (**Figure 2A**). We then evaluated the capacity of the IDO1 inhibitor GDC-0919 to prevent from hIFNg-induced Kynurenine production. To this end, IB115 and IB136 cells were exposed to 1×10^3 UI/mL and 1×10^4 UI/mL hIFNg, respectively, in co-treatment with increasing concentrations of GDC-0919 (**Figure 2B**). As

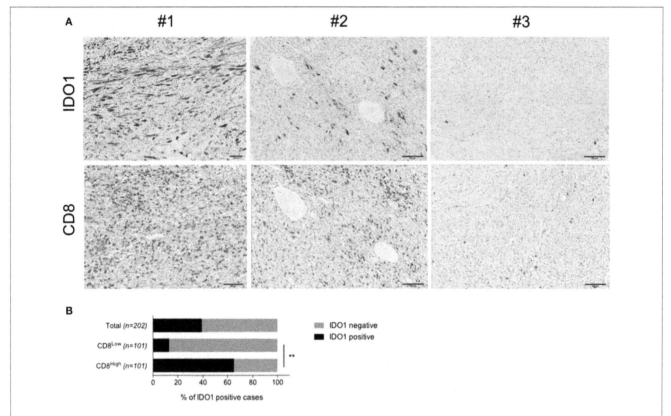

FIGURE 1 | IDO1 is expressed in human sarcoma and its tumor microenvironment. **(A)** Immunohistochemical staining for IDO1 in a cases with positive tumor cells (#1), immune cells (#2) or no positivity (#3). Stainings for CD8 in sequential sections are shown. **(B)** Quantification of IDO1 positivity within the total cohort ($n = 203$), patients harboring either high (CD8^{High}, $n = 101$) or low (CD8^{Low}, $n = 101$) CD8 infiltration. Data are represented as percentage. **$p < 0.01$.

expected, treatment with GDC-0919 significantly inhibited the production of Kynurenine with IC_{50} values at $5.1\ 10^{-7}$M and $2.4\ 10^{-7}$M for IB115 and IB136 cell lines, respectively.

MCA205 Sarcoma Preclinical Model Harbors KP Activity

In order to characterize the respective levels of activity of the IDO-Kyn-Trp pathway in different syngeneic mouse tumor models, we quantified Kynurenine and Tryptophan levels in the extracellular space of the tumor using intratumoral microdialysis in each of the following models: CT26 colon cancer, A20 lymphoma, EMT6 breast cancer, and MC205 sarcoma models. Microdialysis in a "non-tumor bearing" area was performed on the opposite flank and served as a control. As depicted in **Figure 3**, MCA205 mouse model displayed the highest level of Kynurenine to Tryptophan ratio with a significant difference between tumor and non-tumor regions thus suggesting the expression and activity of Tryptophan-degrading enzymes.

Modulation of the KP Upon Anti-PDL1 Treatment in the MCA205 Mouse Model

We then investigated the gene expression profiles of KP and immune-related genes in MCA205 tumor biopsies collected on vehicle and anti-PDL1 treated mice 13 days post tumor inoculation. Interestingly, we observed an increase in Tryptophan-degrading enzymes upon PDL1 blockade—*Ido1* and *Ido2*—while no change was observed for *Tdo2* (**Figure 4**). Correlation studies between genes encoding for KP enzymes and immune markers pointed that *Ido1* level was correlated to Il6 ($R^2 = 0.69$) and to a lesser extent to Ifng ($R^2 = 0.36$) (**Supplementary Figure 2**). Besides *Ido1* and *Ido2*, we also observed an induction of genes encoding downstream enzymes in the IDO-KYN-TRP pathway such as Kynureninase (*Kynu*) or kynurenine monooxygenase (*Kmo*) which converts Kynurenine to Anthranilic acid or to 3-hydroxyKynurenine, respectively. Hydroxyanthranilate oxygenase (*Haao*) favoring the degradation of the immunosuppressive metabolite Hydroxyanthranilic acid was also significantly upregulated (**Figure 4**) thus highlighting a global effect of PDL1 blockade on the pathway. As expected, anti-PDL1 favored the induction of an immune response within the tumor as highlighted by *Tnfa, Il6, Ifng, Il2*, and *Tgfb* induction—Ifng expression levels being significantly correlated with survival (*Data not shown*). Tumor-draining lymph nodes (TDLNs) are a critical compartment for the control of the anti-tumor immune response. We thus investigated the expression level of the same genes in this compartment, which only revealed a non-significant induction of Ido1. The other enzymes of the pathway were not affected (**Supplementary Figure 3**).

TABLE 1 | Patient characteristics.

	Nb of patients	%
Median age (min-max) 62 years (18-95)		
GENDER		
Male	111	54.6
Female	92	45.4
LOCATION		
Limb	155	76.4
Trunk wall	21	10.4
Head and neck	2	1
Internal trunk	25	12.3
Median tumor size (min-max) 97 mm (10-)		
HISTOLOGY		
LPS	20	9.8
US/MFH	56	27.6
LMS	74	36.4
MYXOFIBROSARCOMA	30	14.8
Others	23	12.3
GRADE		
1	10	4.9
2	53	26.1
3	140	69.0
DEPTH		
Deep	145	71.5
Both superficial & deep	36	17.7
Superficial	22	10.8

Treatment With IDO Inhibitor Limits Kynurenine Production

Before investigating the benefit of IDO inhibition in the preclinical sarcoma model, we evaluated the impact of GDC-0919—a novel IDO1 inhibitor—on Kynurenine and Tryptophan levels both at peripheral and tumoral levels. Two doses of GDC-0919—100 and 200mg/kg, po, bid—were explored in a LPS model known to promote Kynurenine production. As expected, Kyn/Trp ratio increase was induced upon LPS administration and was reversed in a same extent with 100 and 200mg/kg of GDC-0919 (**Supplementary Figure 4**). Treatment of MCA205 tumor bearing mice with GDC-0919 either as a single agent (100mg/kg, po, bid) or in combination with an anti-PDL1 antibody yielded a significant decrease in plasmatic Kynurenine to Tryptophan ratio. However, this event was only transient as no significant difference was observed at the latest time-points (ie., Day 13 post tumor inoculation) (**Figure 5**). By using intratumoral microdialysis, we evaluated the effect of GDC-0919 on the tumoral extracellular contents of kynurenine pathway metabolites 13 days after tumor cell inoculation. As expected, GDC-0919 induced a substantial decrease in Kynurenine, Kynurenine to Tryptophan ratio, and Kynurenic acid. Interestingly, combining an anti-PDL1 antibody to GDC-0919 favored the decrease of upstream metabolites (Kynurenine and Kynurenic acid) while partially preventing the decrease in 3HAA, a downstream metabolite of the pathway (**Figure 5**).

IDO Inhibition Does Not Optimize Anti-PDL1 Mediated Anti-tumor Response

As depicted by tumor growth assessment, anti-PDL1 administration triggered a significant anti-tumor response resulting in 1 out of 15 tumor rejection. IDO1 blockade using GDC-0919 did not confer significant benefit either alone or in combination with anti-PDL1—even if a trend of optimization was observed with a tumor rejection observed on 3 out of 15 mice tested (**Figure 6**). In order to investigate the *in vivo* mechanism of action of the different treatment regimens, tumor infiltrating leukocytes (TILs) were assessed through extensive flow cytometry analysis (**Figure 7**). As expected, PDL1 blockade favored tumor infiltration by CD45+ leukocytes, mainly composed of a higher fraction of CD4+ and CD8+ T cells also harboring a more pronounced activated state as depicted by intracellular IFNgamma staining. Combination of anti-PDL1 with GDC-0919 did not change the observed features. Administration of GDC-0919 alone limited the tumor proportions of CD3+ lymphocytes and CD4+ T cells, which were also shown to be less activated based on the IFNgamma staining. As to the myeloid cell subsets, anti-PDL1 limited macrophages infiltration (CD11b+/F4/80+ cells) and concomitantly i) favored a M1 state – defined as CD38+/Egr2- and ii) limited the M2 immunosuppressive cell subset (CD38-/Egr2+). Unlike anti-PDL1, GDC-0919 used as a single agent favored macrophages infiltration of the tumor. Combining GDC-0919 to the anti-PDL1 antibody did not result in significant changes in comparison to anti-PDL1 used as a single agent. Analysis of Myeloid Derived Suppressor Cells (MDSCs) by mean of CD11b and Gr1 staining revealed that anti-PDL1 limited their infiltration within the tumor – especially $CD11b+/Gr1^{Low}$ and $CD11b+/Gr1^{Int}$ populations. No changes in $CD11b+/Gr1^{High}$ were observed. GDC-0919 had no impact on these cell populations, neither alone nor in combination with anti-PDL1.

Gene Expression Modulation Upon GDC-0919 Treatment

In order to characterize the molecular response induced by IDO1 blockade, intratumoral biopsies—collected 13 days post tumor inoculation—were subjected to a gene expression analysis using Nanostring technology and the PanIO360 panel. As expected, PDL1 blockade was shown to strongly modulate different genes belonging to several pathways including interferon signaling (**Supplementary Figure 5**). GDC-0919 applied alone favored the modulation of several genes including the downregulation of Gzma and Gzme (encoding for Granzyme A and E, respectively) but also Prf1 (encoding for Perforin) (**Figure 8A**). When combined with anti-PDL1, GDC-0919 triggered several gene expression changes, including the upregulation of the inhibitory molecule Tigit that could participate in the lack of synergistic effect of GDC-0919 and anti-PDL1. As to identify genes specifically modulated upon GDC-0919—either alone or combined with anti-PDL1—we assessed genes for which a significant difference has been observed in GDC-0919 vs. Vehicle and anti-PDL1 vs. anti-PDL1 + GDC-0919. Interestingly, only a few genes were found significantly modulated in both

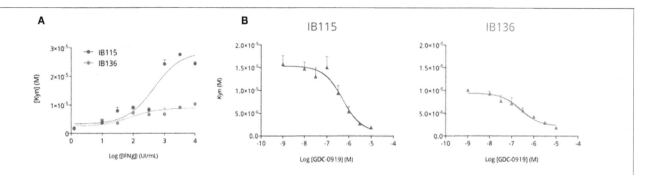

FIGURE 2 | Primary human sarcoma cell lines display an inducible Tryptophan-degrading activity. **(A)** Two primary human sarcoma cell lines, IB115 and IB136, were treated with increasing concentrations of recombinant human Interferon gamma and cell culture supernatants were collected 48 h after treatment initiation for Kynurenine level assessment by mean of ELISA. **(B)** Both IB115 and IB136 were treated with a fixed concentration of Interferon gamma—10^3 U/mL and 10^4 U/mL respectively—and concomitantly treated with an increasing concentration of GDC-0919 (IDO inhibitor) for 48 h. Cell culture supernatants were processed for Kynurenine content measurement (ELISA). Means ± SEM are represented.

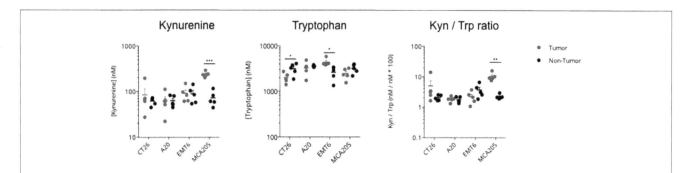

FIGURE 3 | Intratumoral activity of the KP in several syngeneic mouse models. Four different syngeneic mouse models—CT26 colon cancer, A20 lymphoma, EMT6 breast cancer, and MCA205 sarcoma—were processed at an average tumor volume of 200 mm³, for non-tumor (contralateral) and intratumoral microdialysis. Collected microdialysates were then processed for simultaneous measurement of Kynurenine and Tryptophan content by LC/MS; Kynurenine to Tryptophan ratio was then calculated. For statistical analysis, student t-test was used. $^*p < 0.05$, $^{**}p < 0.01$, $^{***}p < 0.001$. Means ± SEM are represented.

situations (**Figure 8B**) including a downregulation of Granzyme a, Pvr (encoding for the poliovirus receptor, CD155), and Spp1 (encoding for the Osteopontin) and an upregulation of inhba, encoding for the inhibin—a member of the Tgfbeta signaling, and the E3 Ubiquitin ligase Dtx4.

DISCUSSION

Despite the revolution of cancer immunotherapy revealed by the use of immune checkpoint blockers, it still remains a challenge to optimize clinical response through combination therapies targeting resistance mechanisms. Considering preclinical and clinical evidence, blockade of IDO-driven tryptophan catabolism represents an exciting therapeutic avenue to potentiate cancer immunotherapy for which several candidates have been developed and tested in different clinical settings (19). We have recently demonstrated a modulation of the KP at the peripheral level in the PEMBROSARC trial assessing the efficacy of Pembrolizumab in STS patients, thus highlighting this pathway as a possible and relevant resistance mechanism to PD1 inhibition in STS (12).

We investigated here a large cohort of human STS for several immune markers (CD8, IDO1, PDL1). High CD8+ TL infiltration has been associated with favorable prognosis in different malignancies (20). In our series, neither metastases-free survival nor overall survival was significantly different between patients with level of CD8 TL tumor density below or above the median, or IDO1 positive or negative tumors. However, the proportion of tumors with positive IDO1 staining was significantly higher in the group with higher levels of CD8+ TL tumor density than in the group with lower levels. Moreover, PDL1 expression was positive in tumor cells in seven (12%) and in immune cells in 26 (44%) of the 59 samples analyzed, and almost exclusively in tumors with higher levels of CD8 TL tumor density. These findings are in line with our previous work showing IDO1 expression as a frequent hallmark of STS (12). Altogether, these data suggest a peculiar role of the IDO pathway in sarcoma progression and thus therapeutic potential of IDO inhibitors in a subset of sarcomas.

Here, by using a preclinical model of fibrosarcoma, we evaluated the benefit on *in vitro* and *in vivo* anti-tumor response of IDO1 blockade through a pharmacological approach using GDC-0919 alone or in combination with an immune

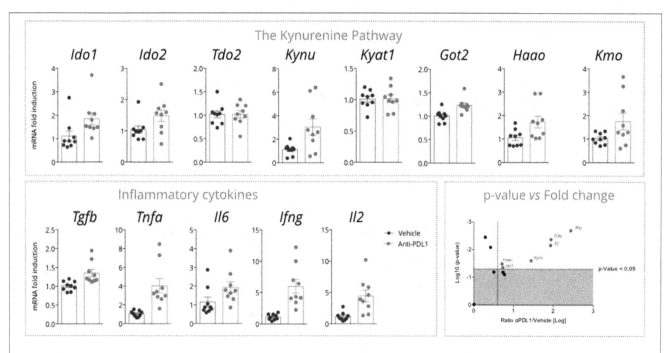

FIGURE 4 | Gene expression assessment in tumor samples collected from a MCA205 tumor-bearing model treated or not with anti-PDL1. Tumor samples were retrieved 13 days post tumor inoculation, and subjected to RT-qPCR for expression analysis of genes encoding for the different enzymes of the KP and key inflammatory cytokines. On the right bottom, display of the p-values vs. the log transformed ratio of tumor mRNA level between PDL1 and Vehicle. Means ± SEM are represented. *Ido1*, Indoleamine 2,3 dioxygenase 1; *Ido2*, Indoleamine 2,3 dioxygenase 2; *Tdo2*, Tryptophan dioxygenase; *Kynu*, Kynureninase; *Kyat1*; Kynurenine Aminotransferase 1; *Got2*, Kynurenine Aminotransferase 4; *Haao*, Hydroxyananthranilate oxygenase; *Kmo*, Kynurenine Monooxygenase.

checkpoint blocker. This IDO1 inhibitor demonstrated (i) a good pharmacological activity *in vitro* on human cell lines and (ii) the expected *in vivo* pharmacodynamic profile with peripheral and intratumoral decrease of Kynurenine. These results are consistent with those reported from the phase I study investigating GDC-0919 as a single agent and in combination with Atezolizumab in patients with advanced solid tumors (21). Indeed, GDC-0919 significantly reduced plasma Kynurenine in comparison to pre-dose levels. However, we observed that GDC-0919 alone or combined with anti-PDL1, only yielded to a transient decrease in plasmatic Kynurenine level thus suggesting a delayed compensatory mechanism restoring in turn Kynurenine production. As to investigate whether this feature is also observable within the tumor compartment, a longitudinal intratumoral microdialysis could be performed. Also, in future pre-clinical and/or clinical studies investigating the impact of IDO1 blockade, expression assessment of the other tryptophan degrading enzymes (IDO2, TDO2) could be evaluated. Nevertheless, whether alone or combined with anti-PDL1, GDC-0919 did not show anti-tumoral activity and did not significantly affect the tumor immune cell infiltrate, thereby corroborating the data obtained in patients. Indeed, the overall response rates observed in a cohort of 75 patients treated with GDC-0919 and Atezolizumab were not significantly different from those expected with Atezolizumab alone (21). Moreover, serial tumor biopsies did not show any significant intratumoral increase in CD8 or tumor infiltrating leukocytes (21).

In order to elucidate the mechanism(s) underlying the lack of effect of GDC-0919, intratumoral biopsies were performed and subjected to gene expression profiling and analysis under GDC-0919 alone and in combination with anti-PDL1. Interestingly, we have shown that the IDO1 inhibitor either as single agent or combined with anti-PDL1 significantly induced a downregulation of the expression of pvr and granzymes, and an upregulation of inhba and Dtx4. Inhba is a ligand in the transforming growth factor β (TGF-β) superfamily, which has been shown to regulate Ido1 via the Smad signaling pathway (22). A recent study has demonstrated that inhba plays a crucial role in inhibiting NK cell proliferation and production of granzyme B thereby leading to impairment of tumor susceptibility to NK cell-mediated killing (23). Finally, the Dtx4 E3-Ubiquitin ligase—known to promote TBK1 degradation and Type 1 interferon response (24)—was found to be upregulated. Evidences from the literature support the implication of NK cells in the anti-tumor activity of PD1/PDL1 blockers (25). Altogether, our data suggest a potential role for inhibitors of the IDO pathway in the down-regulation of NK function, which could explain why IDO inhibition did not result in a synergistic effect when combined with PD1/PDL1 blockers. These new evidences thus warrants further investigation to delineate the mechanism of action underlying the impact of GDC-0919 on NK cell activity toward tumor cells and calls the interest to analyze NK cell features/biology in cancer patients undergoing treatment regimen combining immune checkpoint blockers (ICB) with

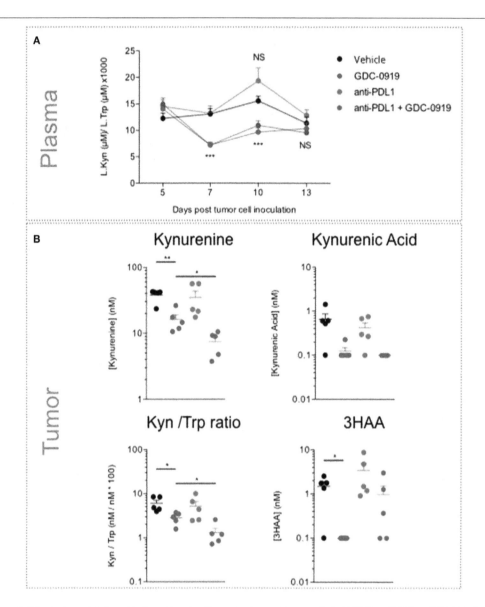

FIGURE 5 | Assessment of Tryptophan catabolism at both peripheral and tumor levels upon pharmacological inhibition of IDO1 and PDL1 blockade. MCA205 tumor-bearing mice were treated with either GDC-0919, anti-PDL1, or combination of both. **(A)** Mice were bled at different time-points following tumor inoculation, and Kynurenine to Tryptophan ratio was analyzed by mean of ELISA. **(B)** Thirteen days post tumor inoculation, animals from all the experimental groups were processed for intratumoral microdialysis and several metabolites of the KP—Kynurenine, Tryptophan, Kynurenine to Tryptophan ratio, Kynurenic Acid, and 3-OH Anthranilic acid—were quantified in the collected dialysates by LC/MS. For statistical analysis, student t-test was used. *$p < 0.05$, **$p < 0.01$, ***$p < 0.001$, NS, not significant. Means ± SEM are represented. In A, experimental groups are compared to Vehicle-treated animals.

IDO inhibitors—all of these to give insights in order to design novel therapeutic strategies improving ICB efficacy.

MATERIALS AND METHODS

Human Tumor Samples

All Formalin Fixed Paraffin Embedded (FFPE) tumors used in this work were collected at the Institut Bergonié (Bordeaux, France). For each case, tumor histology was confirmed by an experienced pathologist before staining processing.

Study Approval

The study was approved by the Institutional Review Board of the Institut Bergonié (Bordeaux, France), and the methods were carried out in accordance with the approved guidelines and with written informed consent from all patients. All animal experiments were performed with the approval of the Institutional Animal Use and Care Committee.

Immunohistochemistry

FFPE specimens were processed for immunohistochemistry with respective antibodies specific for IDO1 (clone UMAB126,

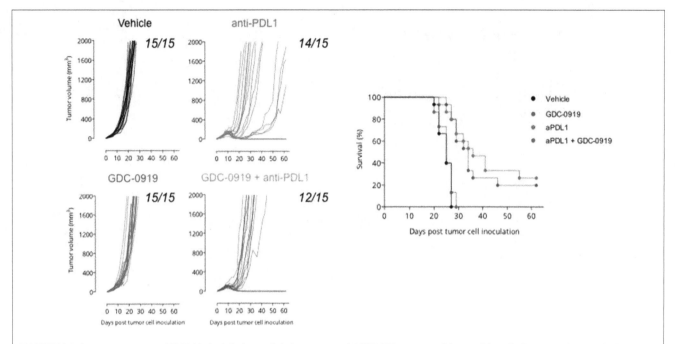

FIGURE 6 | Anti-tumor assessment of IDO1 blockade in the preclinical sarcoma model. MCA205 sarcoma cell line was injected subcutaneously and animals were then treated or not (Vehicle) with either (i) anti-PDL1 starting from day 6 post tumor inoculation and then repeated every 3 days for a total of 4 injections or (ii) GDC-0919 starting from day 6 post tumor inoculation and then treated orally twice daily or combination of both (as described in Material and Methods). Tumor growth kinetics (left panel), and survival curves (right panel) are depicted. Each graph represents 1 experiment with 15 animals per group.

Origen), CD8 (clone SP16, Spring Bioscience), and anti-PDL1 (clone SP263, Ventana) according to conventional protocols using a Ventana Benchmark Ultra automated platform Briefly, tissue sections were deparaffinized, and processed for epitope retrieval in CC1 buffer. After primary antibody incubation, amplification and detection steps used either an UltraView or an OptiView kit, DAB was used as a chromogen and counterstaining was performed with haematoxylin. Brightfield images were acquired using a VS120 virtual slides platform (Olympus). CD8+ cells density was evaluated using a dedicated image analysis algorithm as previously described (26). IDO1 staining was scored semi-quantitatively in tumor cells taking into account both the percentage of positive cells and their intensity from 0 to 3). Expression of PD-L1 in tumor cells (percentage of tumor cells stained) and immune cells (percentage of tumor area occupied by PD-L1 positive immune cells) was evaluated by a trained pathologist (JA). Positivity was defined as ≥1% either in tumor cells or immune cells.

Cell Culture

The human cell lines used in this study were derived from human surgical STS specimens collected at the Institut Bergonié (Bordeaux, France) after obtaining patient consent [16]. All cell lines were cultured in RPMI 1640 medium containing GlutaMAX™ supplement (Life Technologies), 10% (v/v) fetal bovine serum (FBS), 1% penicillin/streptomycin and 0.2% Normocin (InvivoGen) at 37°C with 5% CO2. Murine cell lines—A20, 4T1, CT26, and MCA205—used for syngeneic mouse models were cultured in their appropriate media according

to ATCC specifications. Cell lines were checked for their mycoplasma-free status before use.

Animal Models

All mice were housed in A2 animal facility. All animal studies were carried out under protocols approved by the Institutional Animal Care and Use Committee at University of Bordeaux. Colon CT26, Lymphoma A20, Breast EMT6, and Sarcoma MCA205 cancer cell lines were cultured in vitro according to ATCC specifications, and were checked for their mycoplasma-free status before use. A cell suspension was prepared according to the viable cell count and was inoculated in either Balb/c (CT26, A20, and EMT6) or C57BL/6J (MCA205) mice purchased from Charles River (L'Abresle, France). Anti-PD-L1 monoclonal antibody (a-PDL1, clone 10F9-G2; purchased from BioXCell) was applied intraperitoneally at 5mg/kg and treatment was repeated 4 times, on days 6, 9, 12, and 15. GDC-0919 was freshly prepared every day in 1% Carboxymethylcellulose prepared in order to administer 100mg/kg twice daily. Treatment was applied from day 6 to day 26 post tumor inoculation (21-days treatment duration). Starting from day 6 post MCA205 tumor cell inoculation, all experimental animal groups were monitored 3 times a week for tumor volume measured by physical examination and according to the formula "V = Length * Width2/2." In order to perform kynurenine and Tryptophan level assessment in plasma, animals were bled on days 5, 7, 10, and 13 post tumor inoculation, ~2h after the morning treatments. Blood was collected by retroorbital venipuncture using EDTA tubes (Microvette, Sarstedt), and samples were then

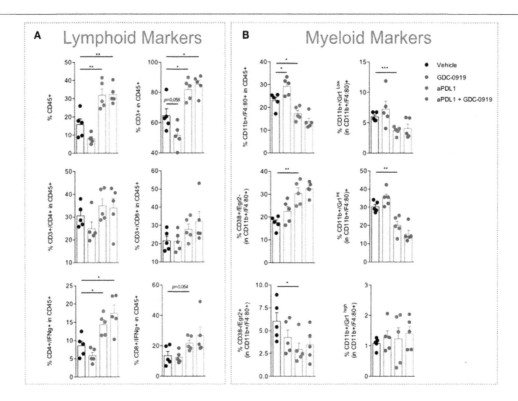

FIGURE 7 | Characterization of tumor-infiltrating leukocytes upon KP blockade. MCA205 sarcoma cell line was subcutaneously inoculated and animals were then treated or not (Vehicle) with either (i) anti-PDL1 or (ii) GDC-0919 or combination of both (as described in Material and Methods). Thirteen days after tumor inoculation, tumors were retrieved and processed for cell suspension preparation and then analyzed by flow cytometry for **(A)** lymphoid or **(B)** myeloid markers. Student t-test was used. *$p < 0.05$, **$p < 0.01$, ***$p < 0.001$, n.s.: not significant. Means ± SEM are represented.

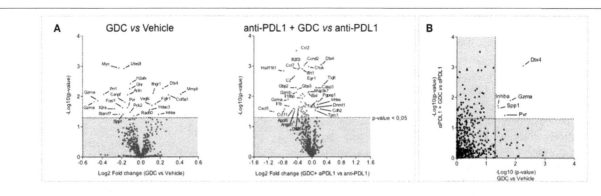

FIGURE 8 | Highlight of possible resistance mechanisms to IDO1 blockade through tumor gene expression profiling. **(A)** Volcano plot of NanoString gene expression analysis in tumor samples comparing GDC-0919 vs. Vehicle groups (left panel) and GDC-0919 + anti-PDL1 vs. anti-PDL1 (right panel). **(B)** Plot representation of p-value comparing GDC-0919 vs. Vehicle groups (X axis) and GDC-0919 + anti-PDL1 vs. anti-PDL1 (Y axis). Green dots indicate downregulations; Red dots indicate upregulations. Dashed line depicts a 0,05 significativity.

processed for Kynurenine and Tryptophan dosage by ELISA (ImmuSmol, #ISE-2227).

Intratumoral Microdialysis

Thirteen days post tumor cell inoculation, mice from satellite group were anesthetized by isoflurane inhalation (Compact Anesthesia module, MINERVE) and connected to the microdialysis platform (CMA microdialysis, Sweden). A microdialysis probe (CMA) was inserted within the tumor and, unless indicated in the controlateral non-tumor region, and flushed continuously with a microperfusion buffer prior to the collection of the dialysates. After this stabilization period, dialysate collection was performed over 60 min. Tubes were stored at −80°C until metabolite dosage by LC/MS including L-Tryptophan, L-Kynurenine, Kynurenic acid, 3-Hydroxyanthranilic acid.

KP Metabolites Quantification by Liquid Chromatography Coupled To Mass Spectrometry (LC/MS)

Five microliter of microdialysate samples were diluted in 45μL of acetonitrile. Diluted samples were vortexed and analyzed by LC/MS system consisting of a Waters ACQUITY UPLC® equipped with an UPLC CSH column and coupled to a Waters XEVO™ TQ-XS Mass Spectrometer (Waters Corporation, Milford, MA, USA) operating in the positive ion electrospray multiple reaction monitoring mode. Quantification was performed using standard calibration curves and internal labeled standards.

Digital Multiplexed Gene Expression Analysis

Tumor biopsy samples were collected from syngeneic sarcoma MCA205 tumor-bearing mice 13 days after tumor cell inoculation, further homogenized in Trizol (Fermentas, Fisher Scientific SAS; Illkirch, France) and RNA was isolated using a standard chloroform/isopropanol protocol (27). After RNA extraction, DNAse digestion step and RNA control quality, extracted RNAs were dosed using microvolume spectrophotometry by Nanodrop 8000 platform (ThermoFisher, Waltham, MA, USA). RNA samples were subsequently diluted in RNase-free water to a concentration of 20 ng/μL. A Reporter CodeSet MasterMix was created by adding 70 μL hybridization buffer to the PanCancer IO 360™ Gene Expression Panel [Probeset XT_Mm_IO360 (NanoString Technologies, Seattle, WA, USA)]. Hybridization reactions of 100 ng RNA were incubated for 24 h at 65°C and ramped down to 4°C followed by digital barcode counting using NanoString nCounter Digital Analyzer (NanoString Technologies, Seattle, WA, USA). Background thresholding was fixed to count value of 20. The geometric mean of positive controls was used to compute positive control normalization parameters. Samples with normalization factors outside 0.3–3.0 were excluded. The geometric mean of housekeeping genes was used to compute the reference normalization factor. Samples with reference factors outside the 0.10–10.0 range were also excluded. Analysis of gene expression was done using the Advanced Analysis module on the nSolver software (NanoString Technologies, Seattle, WA, USA).

RTqPCR Gene Expression Analysis

Cryopreserved tumor biopsies were subjected to tissue preparation procedure by tissue lysis and stainless steel beads prior to RNA extraction according to a Trizol protocol. After RNA extraction, samples followed a DNAse digestion step, RNA control quality on Bioanalyzer 2100 (Agilent, Santa Clara, CA, USA) and quantification on Nanodrop 1000 spectrophotometer (ThermoFisher, Waltham, MA, USA). cDNAs were prepared using PowerAid Premium reverse Transcriptase enzyme (ThermoFisher, Waltham, MA, USA). qPCR procedure was performed using LightCycler 480 (Roche Diagnostics, Mannheim, Germany) in Sybr green (Life Technologies Corp., Carlsbad, CA, USA), primers were designed and validated. Reference genes were selected with GeNorm algorithm.

Flow Cytometry for Immune Cell Infiltrate Analysis

At day 13 post tumor cell inoculation, satellite animals from each experimental groups were sacrificed, and tumors were collected. Tumors were processed for organ dissociation using the GentleMACS system (Miltenyi Biotec). Tumor homogenates were then processed for immunostaining and profiling analysis by flow cytometry for the (i) lymphoïd panel—Viability marker/CD45/CD3/CD4/CD8/IFNg, and (ii) myeloid panel—Viability marker/CD45/CD11b/F4:80/CD38/Egr2/Gr1. For the lymphoid panel analysis and in particular for IFNgamma, cells were first stimulated with a cocktail of PMA, Ionomycin and Brefeldin A.

Statistical Analysis

Two tailed Student's t-test was utilized to derive statistical significance. The minimal level of significance was $p < 0.05$ (Graph PadPRISM version 6, La Jolla, California, USA).

AUTHOR CONTRIBUTIONS

IN, AI, and AS, designed and supervised the study as a whole. MT, JA, and FL designed and supervised the histological part. CR and VV performed the immunohistochemistry. AC performed the TILs analysis. DBor performed the majority of in-vivo experiments. DBod performed the Kynurenine and Tryptophan dosage by ELISA. LC and CL performed analyses of gene expression data. AB and AI wrote the manuscript.

REFERENCES

1. Jo VY, Fletcher CD. WHO classification of soft tissue tumours: an update based on the 2013 (4th) edition. *Pathology.* (2014) 46:95–104. doi: 10.1097/PAT.0000000000000050

2. Italiano A, Mathoulin-Pelissier S, Cesne AL, Terrier P, Bonvalot S, Collin F, et al. Trends in survival for patients with metastatic soft-tissue sarcoma. *Cancer.* (2011) 117:1049–54. doi: 10.1002/cncr.25538

3. Coley WB. II Contribution to the knowledge of sarcoma. *Ann Surg.* (1891) 14:199–220. doi: 10.1097/00000658-189112000-00015

4. Kim JR, Moon YJ, Kwon KS, Bae JS, Wagle S, Kim KM, et al. Tumor infiltrating PD1-positive lymphocytes and the expression of PD-L1 predict poor prognosis of soft tissue sarcomas. *PLoS ONE.* (2013) 8:e82870. doi: 10.1371/journal.pone.0082870

5. D'Angelo SP, Shoushtari AN, Agaram NP, Kuk D, Qin LX, Carvajal RD, et al. Prevalence of tumor-infiltrating lymphocytes and PD-L1 expression in the soft tissue sarcoma microenvironment. *Hum Pathol.* (2015) 46:357–65. doi: 10.1016/j.humpath.2014.11.001

6. Shen JK, Cote GM, Choy E, Yang P, Harmon D, Schwab J, et al. Programmed cell death ligand 1 expression in osteosarcoma. *Cancer Immunol Res.* (2014) 2:690–8. doi: 10.1158/2326-6066.CIR-13-0224

7. Bertucci F, Finetti P, Mamessier E, Pantaleo MA, Astolfi A, Ostrowski J, et al. PDL1 expression is an independent prognostic factor in localized GIST. *Oncoimmunology.* (2015) 4:e1002729. doi: 10.1080/2162402X.2014.1002729

8. Lussier DM, O'Neill L, Nieves LM, McAfee MS, Holechek SA, Collins AW, et al. Enhanced T-cell immunity to osteosarcoma through antibody blockade of PD-1/PD-L1 interactions. *J Immunother.* (2015) 38:96–106. doi: 10.1097/CJI.0000000000000065

9. Tawbi HA, Burgess M, Bolejack V, Van Tine BA, Schuetze SM, Hu J, et al. Pembrolizumab in advanced soft-tissue sarcoma and bone sarcoma (SARC028): a multicentre, two-cohort, single-arm, open-label, phase 2 trial. *Lancet Oncol.* (2017) 18:1493–501. doi: 10.1016/S1470-2045(17)30624-1

10. D'Angelo SP, Mahoney MR, Van Tine BA, Atkins J, Milhem MM, Jahagirdar BN, et al. Nivolumab with or without ipilimumab treatment for metastatic sarcoma (Alliance A091401): two open-label, non-comparative, randomised, phase 2 trials. *Lancet Oncol.* (2018) 19:416–26. doi: 10.1016/S1470-2045(18)30006-8

11. Toulmonde M, Italiano A. PD-1 inhibition in sarcoma still needs investigation. *Lancet Oncol.* (2018) 19:e6. doi: 10.1016/S1470-2045(17)30921-X

12. Toulmonde M, Penel N, Adam J, Chevreau C, Blay JY, Le Cesne A, et al. Use of PD-1 targeting, macrophage infiltration, and IDO pathway activation in sarcomas: a phase 2 clinical trial. *JAMA Oncol.* (2018) 4:93–7. doi: 10.1001/jamaoncol.2017.1617

13. Munn DH, Sharma MD, Hou D, Baban B, Lee JR, Antonia SJ, et al. Expression of indoleamine 2,3-dioxygenase by plasmacytoid dendritic cells in tumor-draining lymph nodes. *J Clin Invest.* (2004) 114:280–90. doi: 10.1172/JCI21583

14. Brandacher G, Perathoner A, Ladurner R, Schneeberger S, Obrist P, Winkler C, et al. Prognostic value of indoleamine 2,3-dioxygenase expression in colorectal cancer: effect on tumor-infiltrating T cells. *Clin Cancer Res.* (2006) 12:1144–51. doi: 10.1158/1078-0432.CCR-05-1966

15. Acovic A, Simovic Markovic B, Gazdic M, Arsenijevic A, Jovicic N, Gajovic N, et al. Indoleamine 2,3-dioxygenase-dependent expansion of T-regulatory cells maintains mucosal healing in ulcerative colitis. *Therap Adv Gastroenterol.* (2018) 11:1756284818793558. doi: 10.1177/1756284818793558

16. Muller AJ, DuHadaway JB, Donover PS, Sutanto-Ward E, Prendergast GC. Inhibition of indoleamine 2,3-dioxygenase, an immunoregulatory target of the cancer suppression gene Bin1, potentiates cancer chemotherapy. *Nat Med.* (2005) 11:312–9. doi: 10.1038/nm1196

17. Holmgaard RB, Zamarin D, Munn DH, Wolchok JD, Allison JP. Indoleamine 2,3-dioxygenase is a critical resistance mechanism in antitumor Tcell immunotherapy targeting CTLA-4. *J Exp Med.* (2013) 210:1389–402. doi: 10.1084/jem.20130066

18. Labadie BW, Bao R, Luke JJ. Reimagining IDO pathway inhibition in cancer immunotherapy via downstream focus on the tryptophan-kynurenine-aryl hydrocarbon axis. *Clin Cancer Res.* (2019) 25:1462–71. doi: 10.1158/1078-0432.CCR-18-2882

19. Ricciuti B, Leonardi GC, Puccetti P, Fallarino F, Bianconi V, Sahebkar A, et al. Targeting indoleamine-2,3-dioxygenase in cancer: scientific rationale and clinical evidence. *Pharmacol Ther.* (2019) 196:105–16. doi: 10.1016/j.pharmthera.2018.12.004

20. Gentles AJ, Newman AM, Liu CL, Bratman SV, Feng W, Kim D, et al. The prognostic landscape of genes and infiltrating immune cells across human cancers. *Nat Med.* (2015) 21:938–45. doi: 10.1038/nm.3909

21. Jung KH, LoRusso P, Burris H, Gordon M, Bang YJ, Hellmann MD, et al. Phase I study of the indoleamine 2,3-Dioxygenase 1 (IDO1) inhibitor navoximod (GDC-0919) administered with PD-L1 inhibitor (Atezolizumab) in advanced solid tumors. *Clin Cancer Res.* (2019) 25:3220–8. doi: 10.1158/1078-0432.CCR-18-2740

22. Guiton R, Henry-Berger J, Drevet JR. The immunobiology of the mammalian epididymis: the black box is now open! *Basic Clin Androl.* (2013) 23:8. doi: 10.1186/2051-4190-23-8

23. Rautela J, Dagley LF, de Oliveira CC, Schuster IS, Hediyeh-Zadeh S, Delconte RB, et al. Therapeutic blockade of activin-A improves NK cell function and antitumor immunity. *Sci Signal.* (2019) 12:eaat7527. doi: 10.1126/scisignal.aat7527

24. Cui J, Li Y, Zhu L, Liu D, Songyang Z, Wang HY, et al. NLRP4 negatively regulates type I interferon signaling by targeting the kinase TBK1 for degradation via the ubiquitin ligase DTX4. *Nat Immunol.* (2012) 13:387–95. doi: 10.1038/ni.2239

25. Hsu J, Hodgins JJ, Marathe M, Nicolai CJ, Bourgeois-Daigneault MC, Trevino TN, et al. Contribution of NK cells to immunotherapy mediated by PD-1/PD-L1 blockade. *J Clin Invest.* (2018) 128:4654–68. doi: 10.1172/JCI99317

26. Ou D, Adam J, Garberis I, Blanchard P, Nguyen F, Levy A, et al. Clinical relevance of tumor infiltrating lymphocytes, PD-L1 expression and correlation with HPV/p16 in head and neck cancer treated with bio- or chemo-radiotherapy. *Oncoimmunology.* (2017) 6:e1341030. doi: 10.1080/2162402X.2017.1341030

27. Chomczynski P, Sacchi N. Single-step method of RNA isolation by acid guanidinium thiocyanate-phenol-chloroform extraction. *Anal Biochem.* (1987) 162:156–9. doi: 10.1016/0003-2697(87)90021-2

18

Tryptophan Catabolism and Response to Therapy in Locally Advanced Rectal Cancer (LARC) Patients

Sara Crotti[1]*, Alessandra Fraccaro[2], Chiara Bedin[1], Antonella Bertazzo[3],
Valerio Di Marco[2], Salvatore Pucciarelli[4] and Marco Agostini[1,4]*

[1] Nano-Inspired Biomedicine Laboratory, Institute of Paediatric Research—Città della Speranza, Padua, Italy, [2] Department of Chemical Sciences, University of Padua, Padua, Italy, [3] Department of Pharmaceutical and Pharmacological Sciences, University of Padua, Padua, Italy, [4] First Surgical Clinic Section, Department of Surgical, Oncological and Gastroenterological Sciences, University of Padua, Padua, Italy

*Correspondence:
Sara Crotti
s.crotti@irpcds.org
Marco Agostini
m.agostini@unipd.it

In locally advanced rectal cancer patients (LARC), preoperative chemoradiation improves local control and sphincter preservation. The response rate to treatment varies substantially between 20 and 30%, and it is an important prognostic factor. Indeed, nonresponsive patients are subjected to higher rates of local and distant metastases, and worse survival compared to patients with complete response. In the search of predictive biomarkers for response prediction to therapy in LARC patients, we found increased plasma tryptophan levels in nonresponsive patients. On the basis of plasma levels of 5-hydroxy-tryptophan and kynurenine, the activities of tryptophan 5-hydroxylase 1 (TPH1) and indoleamine-2,3-dioxygenases 1 (IDO1)/tryptophan-2,3-dioxygenase (TDO2) have been obtained and data have been correlated with gene expression profiles. We demonstrated that TDO2 overexpression in nonresponsive patients correlates with kynurenine plasma levels. Finally, through the gene expression and targeted metabolomic analysis in paired healthy mucosa-rectal cancer tumor samples, we evaluated the impact of tryptophan catabolism at tissue level in responsive and nonresponsive patients.

Keywords: tryptophan, rectal cancer, IDO1, TDO2, TPH1, kynurenine pathway, serotonin pathway

INTRODUCTION

Cancer is a major cause of death in industrialized countries, and colorectal cancer (CRC) is one of the most common tumors in both male and female (1). About 30% of CRC cases concern the rectal tract of the large intestine, approximately the last 15 cm of the intestinal tract. In the most advanced stages of the disease, the tumor delocalizes and begins its proliferation in areas of the body different from the one in which it arose. Due to the different blood and lymph node ducts to which they are connected, colon cancer mainly develops liver metastases while rectal cancer develops, in addition to the liver ones, also thoracic metastases. Prevention and diagnosis strategies for rectal and colon cancer are mostly the same; the planned therapy, however, is shared only for some traits.

Preoperative chemoradiotherapy (pCRT) is worldwide accepted as a standard treatment for locally advanced rectal cancer (LARC) with stage II and III aiming at improving local tumor control, and inducing tumor downsizing and downstaging (2). Standard treatment includes administration of ionizing radiation for 45–50.4 Gy associated with 5-fluorouracil administration during radiation therapy and few modifications (e.g., adding Oxaliplatin) are introduced to ameliorate primary tumor response and, consequently, patients' outcome. Typically, complete pathologic response rate to pCRT is between 20 and 30% (3). It follows that patients with *a priori* resistant tumor should not be included in the treatment, which is associated with substantial adverse effects and higher rates of local and distant metastases. The search of predictive biomarkers for response prediction to therapy in rectal cancer would improve the patients' management. In this frame, in adjunction to clinical features (4, 5), the potentiality of liquid biopsy has been extensively employed to identify circulating predictive biomarkers (6, 7). Indeed, a number of putative biomarkers including proteins (8, 9), circulating peptides (10),

and circulating tumor cells or nucleic acids (11–13) have been proposed. However, recently an increased focus on the tumor microenvironment offered further opportunities to understand the tumor response biology and the relations between pCRT and the radiation-induced response (14, 15), together with tumor-specific immune response (16).

Physiologically, several pro-inflammatory mediators and T cells cytotoxic activity are modulated by tryptophan (TRP) and its metabolites, as an adaptation mechanism to restrict excessive acute immune response in tissues (17). Tryptophan is the precursor of several active compounds, collectively named TRYCATs (**Figure 1**). At the tumor microenvironment, TRP catabolism is promoted by indoleamine 2,3-dioxygenase (IDO1) overexpression under pro-inflammatory conditions, and it plays an important role in modulating antitumor immune response

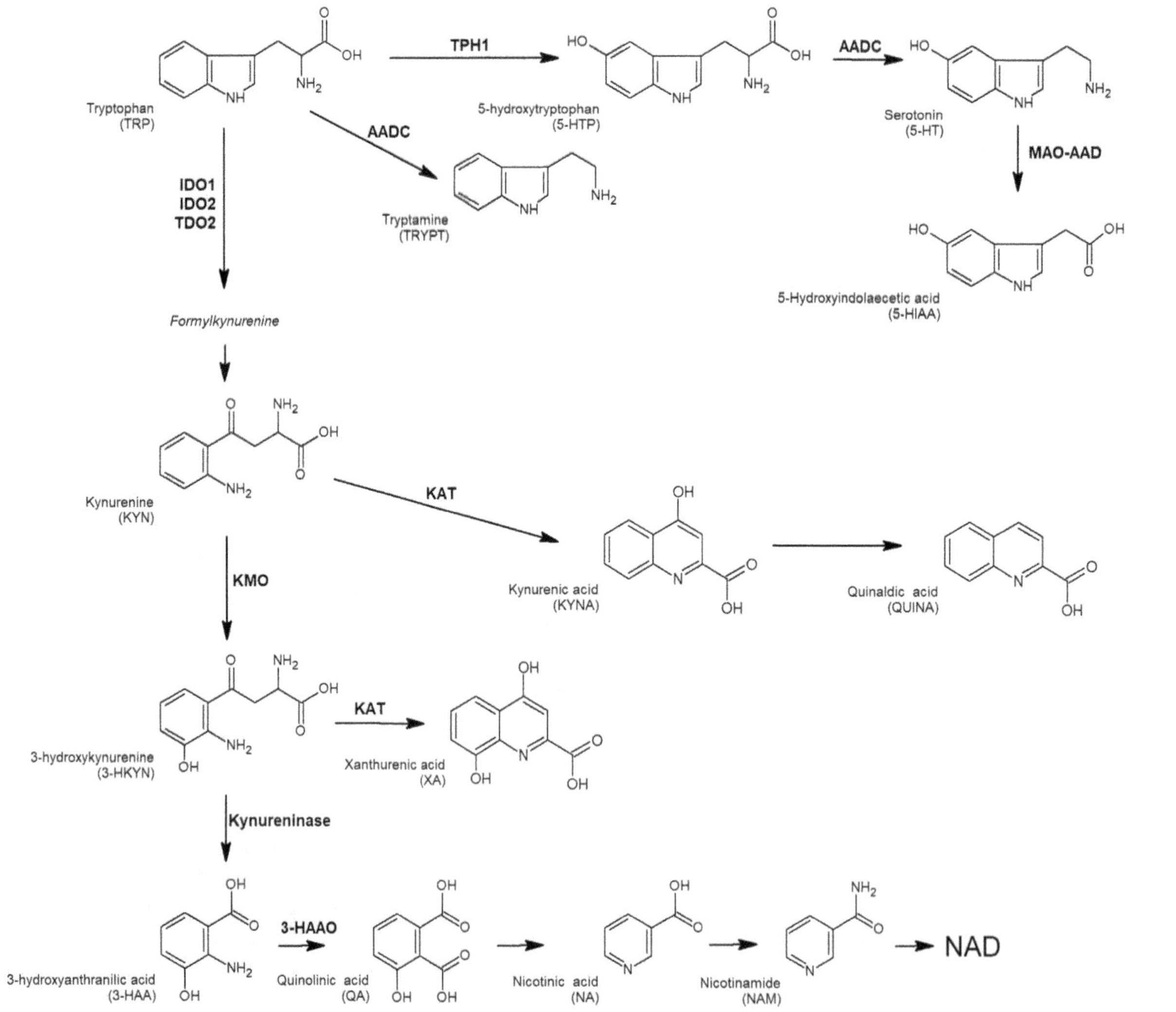

FIGURE 1 | TRP and its key catabolites (TRYCATs) produced via three biochemical pathways: the kynurenine pathway, tryptamine pathway, and serotonin pathway. Enzymes involved: AADC, aromatic L-amino acid decarboxylase; AD, aldehyde dehydrogenase; 3-HAAO, 3-hydroxyanthranilate 3,4-dioxygenase; IDO1, indoleamine-2,3-dioxygenases 1; IDO2, indoleamine-2,3-dioxygenases 2; KAT, L-kynurenine aminotransferase; KMO, kynurenine monooxygenase; MAO-A, monoamine oxidase A; TDO, tryptophan-2,3-dioxygenase; TPH1, tryptophan hydroxylase 1.

(18–20). In CRC, IDO1 expression at the tumor invasion front correlates with disease progression and worse clinical outcome (21) and is associated with the frequency of liver metastases (22). As observed in other tumors, local TRP depletion in CRC plays an important role in either antitumor immune response suppression or cancer cell proliferation/survival support (23–25). Beside IDO1, a second enzyme involved in TRP metabolism, tryptophan-2,3-dioxygenase (TDO2) is expressed in a significant proportion of human tumors and is involved in proliferation, migration, invasion, and immunoresistance (26–28). A valuable way to measure local catabolism is represented by plasma or blood quantification of TRP and its main metabolites, i.e., 5-hydroxy-tryptophan (5-HTP), kynurenine (KYN), and serotonin (5-HT). Consequently, circulating levels of TRP can be used as a "proxy" for tumor microenvironment metabolism.

In this frame, we highlighted that CRC-associated inflammation is capable of modulating circulating levels of TRP and its metabolites along the adenoma–carcinoma sequence. Indeed, decreased TRP concentration and increased IDO1 and tryptophan hydroxylase 1 (TPH1) enzymatic activities were detectable in plasma samples concomitant to precancerous lesion (high grade-adenomas) or in association to risk factors (inflammatory bowel diseases) (29). Moreover, we defined the TRP catabolism as a possible source of prognostic marker for familial adenomatous polyposis patients, based on IDO1 and TPH1 activity with high sensitivities and specificities (up to 92%) (30). Agostini et al. have firstly suggested the link between IDO1 and chemoresistance of rectal cancer patients in a de novo meta-analysis on rectal tumor tissues (31). IDO1 and other two genes involved in the immune system pathway (AKR1C3 and CXCL10) have been identified as a gene set associated with pCRT response and survival. Consistently with these results, we focused our attention on TRP metabolism as a hallmark of immune host response modulation in LARC. In this study, both at circulating and at tissue level, we investigated metabolic and genetic markers of the TRP catabolism before pCRT in LARC patients in order to find out new predictive biomarkers measuring the response to therapy.

MATERIALS AND METHODS
Chemicals
Isotopically labeled internal standards d$_5$-tryptophan (TRPd, 98.8%), d$_4$-serotonin (5HTd, 98.7%), and d$_5$-kynurenic acid (KINAd, 99.2%) were purchased from CDN isotopes (Quebec, Canada) while $^{13}C_6$-nicotinamide (NAmC, 99.4%) was purchased from Sigma Aldrich (Milan, Italy). Analytical standards for tryptophan (TRP), kynurenine (KYN), 5-hydroxy-tryptophan (5-HTP), serotonin (5-HT), tryptamine (Tryp), kynurenic acid (KYNA), quinaldic acid (QA), xanthurenic acid (XA), 3-hydroxyanthranilic acid (3-HAA), 5-hydroxyindoleacetic acid (5-HIAA), nicotinic acid (NA), quinolinic acid (QuiA), and nicotinamide (NAm) have been purchased from Sigma Aldrich (Milan, Italy). LC-MS-grade solvents (acetonitrile, methanol, chloroform, isopropanol), and suprapure trifluoroacetic acid (TFA) were purchased

TABLE 1 | Clinical and demographic characteristics of all LARC patients.

Characteristic		N	%
Age	Median (range yrs.)	66 (31–79)	
Sex	Male	52	63%
	Female	30	37%
Tumor distance from anal verge	≤7 cm	26	32%
	>7 cm	39	48%
	Not available	17	20%
TRG	1–2	37	45%
	3–5	45	55%
Specimens	Plasma	45	
	Tissues	69	
Paired samples	Plasma–tumor samples	32	
	Healthy mucosa–tumor samples	13	

Tumor regression grade (TRG) is calculated according to Mandard et al. (32). TRG 1–2, responders; TRG 3–5, nonresponders.

from Romil. TRIzol™ reagent was obtained from Thermo Fisher Scientific.

LC-MS/MS and LC-UV/FLD Analyses
Mass spectrometry measurements were performed by using an API 4000 triple quadrupole mass spectrometer (AB SCIEX, MA, USA) coupled to an Ultimate 3000 UPLC system (Thermo Fisher). Analyzed metabolites were TRP, KYN, 5-HTP, 5-HT, Tryp, KYNA, QA, XA, 3-HAA, 5-HIAA, NA, QuiA, and NAm. Scheduled MRM transitions, instrumental parameters, and chromatographic conditions were reported in **Supplementary Material S1**.

HPLC-UV/FLD analyses of plasma samples to detect and quantify TRP, KYN, 5-HTP, and 5-HT were performed as previously reported (29).

Sample Collection
This study was conducted according to the principles expressed in the Declaration of Helsinki. Biological specimens (de-personalized plasma and tissue biopsies) were obtained from the Tissue Biobank of the First Surgical Clinic of Padua Hospital (Italy). The protocol was approved by the ethics committee of the institution (Comitato Etico del Centro Oncologico Regionale, Approved Protocol Number: P448). Selected samples were obtained from rectal cancer patients before preoperative chemoradiotherapy (pCRT) which consisted of external-beam radiotherapy (>6 MV) using a conventional fractionation (>50 Gy in 28 fractions, 1.8 Gy per day, 5 sessions per week) and 5-fluorouracil administered as neoadjuvant chemotherapy drug by bolus or continuous venous infusion. Elective surgery was performed after 7 weeks (median value) to completion of preoperative chemoradiotherapy (interquartile range 6–8 weeks), and patients' response to pCRT was evaluated after histological evaluation of surgical resection as the tumor regression grade (TRG) according to Mandard et al. (32). All demographic and clinical data are presented in **Table 1**.

TABLE 2 | Tryptophan (TRP), kynurenine (KYN), 5-hydroxy-tryptophan (5-HTP), serotonin (5-HT) plasma levels and tumor tissue expression of enzymes involved in TRP metabolism.

	Plasma metabolite levels				
	TRG 1–2 (*n* = 17)		TRG 3–5 (*n* = 28)		*p*-value
	Median	Q1, Q3	Median	Q1, Q3	
TRP µg/mL	8.43	7.06, 10.71	10.24	8.37, 11.93	<0.05
KYN µg/mL	0.31	0.24, 0.46	0.41	0.30, 0.53	
5HTP µg/mL	0.06	0.05, 0.07	0.05	0.04, 0.06	
5HT µg/mL	0.01	0.005, 0.01	0.01	0.001, 0.02	

	Gene expression of involved enzymes				
	TRG 1–2 (*n* = 25)		TRG 3–5 (*n* = 27)		*p*-value
	Median	Q1, Q3	Median	Q1, Q3	
IDO1 (RQ)	66.87	23.08, 138.6	57.46	25.73, 98.07	
TDO2 (RQ)	67.21	40.12, 148.7	185.8	57.74, 250.0	<0.05
TPH1 (RQ)	1.68	0.66, 6.44	2.97	0.82, 12.0	

RQ, relative quantitation.

Sample Preparation

Healthy rectum mucosa and tumor pre-therapy biopsies were processed to isolate total RNA by TRIzol™ reagent following the manufacturer's protocol. After chloroform addition, the aqueous upper layer was transferred for the subsequent gene expression analysis while the lower organic phase containing the interphase layer was stored at −20°C for metabolite quantification. RNA concentration and purity were estimated as the ratio 260/280 nm by the NanoDrop 2000 spectrophotometer (Thermo Scientific, USA). Only samples with a ratio between 1.7 and 2.1 were considered suitable for downstream analysis. Reverse transcription and quantitative real-time PCR (qPCR) were performed as described in **Supplementary Material S2**.

TRP and its metabolites were extracted from the lower organic phase obtained during the RNA isolation by adding an equal volume of acidified cold water (0.05% TFA) containing known amounts of the following internal standards: TRPd, 5HTd, KINAd, and NAmC. The mixture was centrifuged at 4°C for 5 min (12,000 rpm) using a Heraeus Fresco 21 centrifuge (Thermo Electron Corp.). Extracted analytes were transferred into a new tube and dried under vacuum. The residual organic layer, containing the interphase, was treated with ethanol (300 µL) to eliminate DNA, and residual protein pellet was extracted according to TRIzol™ manufacturer's instructions. Total protein amount was finally quantified by the Pierce BCA Protein Assay Kit (Thermo Fisher).

Statistical Analysis

Statistical analysis was performed with GraphPad Prism, version 5.00, 2007 (La Jolla, CA, USA). Normality of data was evaluated using the D'Agostino-Pearson omnibus normality test, and parametric (or nonparametric) statistical analyses were completed accordingly. Spearman rank test was used to determine the strength and direction of the relationship between variables.

RESULTS AND DISCUSSION

Circulating TRP Metabolite Levels and Response to Therapy

TRP catabolism in 45 LARC patients was assessed through plasma level quantification of TRP and its major metabolites (KYN, 5-HTP, and 5-HT) by means of HPLC-UV-VIS/FLD analysis. Usually, TRP plasma levels are physiologically regulated by the hepatic TDO2 enzyme. However, under non-physiological conditions (e.g., in presence of inflammation or cancer), overexpression of IDO1/TDO2 enzymes can actively contribute to TRP catabolism. The median TRP concentration was 9.01 µg/mL (8.68–10.01, 95% CI) which is—as expected—very close to the TRP concentration we observed in our previous investigation for control (i.e., healthy subjects) plasma samples (29). Indeed, we already demonstrated that TRP catabolism increases more in people affected by colon cancer than those affected by rectal cancer. Differently, in the present study, the cohort of rectal cancer patients was collected to check for differences between TRG 1–2 and TRG 3–5 patients and not for diagnostic evaluation (i.e., comparison with healthy subjects). Data reported in **Table 2** suggest that a statistically significant increase of TRP in TRG 3–5 patients is present, together with an increasing trend of KYN levels. No difference is present between 5-HTP and 5-HT plasma levels. When IDO1/TDO2 and TPH1 enzymatic activities are estimated from these data, following the usual approach (29), a lower TPH1 enzymatic activity ($p < 0.01$) resulted for TRG 3–5 patients (**Figure 2A**, box-plots). This decrease underlines a possible involvement of serotonin pathway in tumor response, while the IDO1/TDO2 activity, which is an

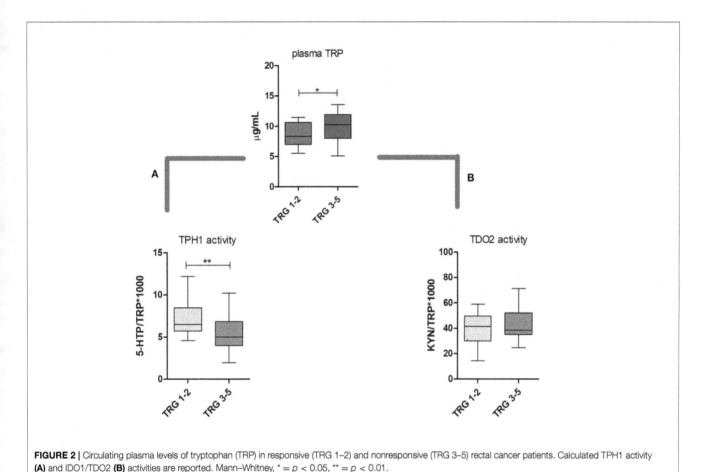

FIGURE 2 | Circulating plasma levels of tryptophan (TRP) in responsive (TRG 1–2) and nonresponsive (TRG 3–5) rectal cancer patients. Calculated TPH1 activity **(A)** and IDO1/TDO2 **(B)** activities are reported. Mann–Whitney, $* = p < 0.05$, $** = p < 0.01$.

estimation of kynurenine pathway, shows only a nonstatistically significant increasing trend (**Figure 2B**, box-plots).

To evaluate this hypothesis, we decided to perform a gene expression analysis of IDO1, TDO2, and TPH1 in order to clarify whether in TRG 3–5 patients the decrease in TPH1 systemic activity actually means a downregulation of TPH1 gene expression. However, as underlined by gene expression data reported in **Table 2**, there is no difference for TPH1 and IDO1 between TRG 1–2 and TRG 3–5 patients. On the contrary, TDO2 shows instead a statistically significant increase in TRG 3–5 patients ($p < 0.05$). Even after data normalization to healthy rectal mucosa ($n = 17$ samples, not paired), TDO2 was still overexpressed in TRG 3–5 patients only (tumor/healthy mucosa average ratio: 1.035 for TRG 1–2 and 2.230 for TRG 3–5), while TPH1 was equally downregulated in both patients' groups (tumor/healthy mucosa average ratio: 0.015 for TRG 1–2 and 0.022 for TRG 3–5). To further verify whether these metabolic and gene expression alterations may be consistent, Spearman's rank correlation test was employed to analyze the results from only the paired plasma-tumor samples ($n = 32$). Plasma levels of detected metabolites (both precursors TRP and its products KYN, 5-HTP, and 5-HT) and the calculated enzymatic activities of IDO1, TDO2, and TPH1 have been compared against their quantified genes expression. Obtained results indicated that in rectal cancer patients, KYN plasma levels

are strongly correlated with TDO2 gene expression ($r = 0.6026$, $p < 0.001$, $n = 32$) and, after patients' stratification according to their response to therapy, only those having TRG 3–5 still showed a positive correlation between KYN and TDO2 ($r = 0.556$, $p < 0.05$, $n = 17$).

Following the same procedure, we found that neither IDO1 nor TPH1 gene expressions were correlated with their metabolites or calculated activities in rectal cancer patients. Other authors previously showed this discrepancy for IDO1 (33). To explain this behavior, it should be noted that that enzymatic process coordination depends upon temporal regulation of both substrates and enzymes. Moreover, changes in mRNA levels of IDO1 and TPH1 just indicate cell metabolic changes and may moderately correlate with changes in enzymes activity. Consequently, as for most of proteins, disparity between mRNA levels and protein abundance make it difficult to predict real activity for these enzymes (34).

Local Quantification of TRP Metabolites Better Reflects Gene Expression

To clarify whether it is possible to correlate the amount of TRP and its metabolites to enzyme activity and their gene expression in LARC patients, we developed and validated an analytical method for the simultaneous evaluation of TRP catabolism at both metabolic and genetic levels. By this method, metabolite

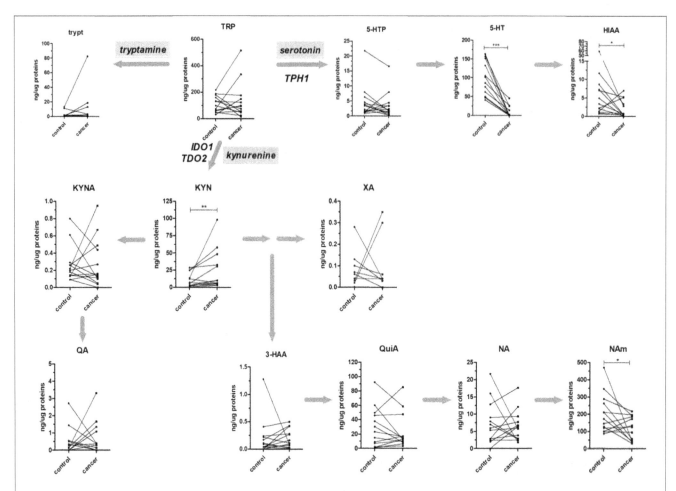

FIGURE 3 | Absolute amounts (presented as ng of metabolite per μg of total proteins) of TRP along the kynurenine and serotonin pathways in 13 healthy mucosa (control) and rectal cancer (cancer) paired samples. The tryptamine metabolic pathway is presented for completeness. Matched samples are connected together. Results from Wilcoxon signed rank test are reported ($*p < 0.05$; $**p < 0.01$; $***p < 0.001$).

quantification and gene expression analysis were obtained in the same tissue samples, by means of a sequential extraction procedure. In brief, paired biopsies (healthy mucosa and rectal cancer counterpart) have been extracted with TRIzol™ following the manufacturers' protocol. The resultant upper aqueous phase was used for quantitative real-time PCR of IDO1, TDO2, and TPH1 genes, while the lower organic phase was added by the four internal standards (TRPd, 5HTd, KINAd, and NAmC) before metabolite extraction (see Sample Preparation section for details).

A total of 13 metabolites have been quantified by a single scheduled LC-MRM analysis. These metabolites were tryptophan (TRP), kynurenine (KYN), 5-hydroxy-tryptophan (5-HTP), serotonin (5-HT), tryptamine (Tryp), kynurenic acid (KYNA), quinaldic acid (QA), xanthurenic acid (XA), 3-hydroxyanthranilic acid (3-HAA), 5-hydroxyindoleacetic acid (5-HIAA), nicotinic acid (NA), quinolinic acid (QuiA), and nicotinamide (NAm). Instrumental parameters and scheduled transitions employed to quantify and qualify metabolites are resumed in **Supplementary Material S3**. Good performances in terms of LLOQ, LOD, CV %, and accuracy

% for all metabolites have been obtained, with exception to Tryp and 3-HAA (**Supplementary Material S3**). For these two metabolites, the present method was not able to provide enough reproducibility and then quantitative results should be considered as approximate.

The method was applied to the analysis of 13 paired healthy mucosa/rectal cancer samples, and obtained results are reported in **Figure 3**. All the major metabolites along the kynurenine and serotonin pathways have been quantified; in addition, Tryp has been included in the present study for completeness, even if tryptamine pathway accounts only for the <1% of TRP catabolism (35). For both types of samples, no difference was present in the TRP tissue level (average values: 97.98 and 95.06 ng/μg of proteins, for healthy mucosa and rectal cancer, respectively). However, in cancer tissues a trend of decrease along the serotonin pathway was observable for 5-HTP and further confirmed by the statistically significant decrease of 5-HT ($p < 0.001$, Wilcoxon signed-rank test) and its final catabolite 5-HIAA ($p < 0.05$, Wilcoxon signed-rank test). This strong decrease in serotonin level is reasonably due to the lack of enterochromaffin cells, which are normally present in

TABLE 3 | Normalized (tumor/healthy mucosa) gene expression (nRQ) for all paired samples.

	All samples (n = 13 pairs)				
	Mean	Min, Max	Trend in tumor	Correlation with metabolites	p-value
IDO1 (nRQ)	0.71	0.10, 2.41	=	NAm (r = 0.424)	<0.05
TDO2 (nRQ)	1.56	0.09, 10.04	↑		
Calculated activity	230 (111)	8.6, 636 (2.19, 441)	↑	KYN (r = 0.803) TRP (r = −0.461)	<0.0001 <0.05
TPH1 (nRQ)	0.43	0.001, 3.65	↓	5-HT (r = 0.810)	<0.0001
Calculated activity	36.3 (40.7)	1.2, 148 (8.6, 115.7)	=	5-HTP (r = 0.680)	<0.0001

Data are presented as mean fold change and minimum and maximum (Min, Max) values. Enzymatic activity is reported as calculated mean value for rectal cancer samples (healthy mucosa) and relative minimum, maximum. "Trend in tumor" column highlights fold changes at least >1.5 (or <0.67). Correlation between gene expression and TRP metabolites was evaluated using Spearman's rank test and only significant results are reported.

healthy rectal mucosa but not in cancer tissue. These cells are a specialized subset of enteroendocrine cells and the largest producer of 5-HT in the body (~95%), which is critical to gastrointestinal motility (36). On the contrary, KYN increased significantly in rectal cancer tissues ($p < 0.01$, Wilcoxon signed-rank test). This increase could be the result of a diminished TRP consumption along the serotonin pathway and could explain, at least theoretically, the unaltered total TRP levels in rectal cancer tissues. Increased KYN levels in colon cancer tissues and human colon cancer cells have been recently correlated with the tumor proliferation through the activation of the aryl hydrocarbon receptor (AHR) (37). KYN exerts also immuno-modulating effects at the tumor microenvironment (38) and is the precursor of quinaldic acid (QA), xanthurenic acid (XA), and nicotinamide (NAm) (**Figure 3**). QA and XA levels were comparable between healthy mucosa and rectal cancer samples. On the contrary, NAm, which is the precursor for redox cofactor NAD^+, was decreased in rectal cancer samples ($p < 0.05$, Wilcoxon signed-rank test). NAm decrease may be a hallmark of increased energetic demand in tumor; indeed, cancer cells are able to reprogram their metabolism (nutrient uptake, intracellular metabolism, and gene expression) for sustaining survival, growth, and metastasis. In particular, to satisfy their NAD^+ demand, tumors can overcome the limitation of a *de novo* synthesis from TRP and adopt a salvage pathway, which "recycles" existing NA and NAm (39).

The gene expression of rate-limiting step enzymes IDO1, TDO2, and TPH1 and their calculated activity were finally obtained for each sample (**Table 3**). For all the three enzymes, the mean of normalized RQ (cancer/healthy mucosa) was calculated and presented as fold change (F.C.). Obtained data revealed that in rectal cancer samples the kynurenine pathway was characterized by TDO2 overexpression, while IDO1 expression remained practically unchanged (using a 1.5-fold ratio criterion). These data are consistent with others reported in literature, in which TDO2 expression in several human tumor cell lines and tissues has been demonstrated (26, 28, 40–42). Similarly, a rise in the calculated enzymatic activity (KYN/TRP*1,000) in rectal cancer tissues compared to mucosa was detected (mean activity: 111 and 230 for healthy mucosa and rectal cancer, respectively; $p < 0.05$, Wilcoxon signed-rank test). This increase positively correlated with KYN produced and negatively correlated with the

enzyme substrate TRP (**Table 3**) suggesting that, in rectal cancer, TDO2 may be responsible for increased KYN levels.

Most importantly, the THP1 downregulation observed for this group of rectal cancer is consistent with that previously observed in the plasma–tissue correlation (actual fold change: 0.43). Differently to the previous observation, however, actual 5-HT tissue levels strongly correlated with THP1 expression and the calculated THP1 activity positively correlated with 5-HTP production (**Table 3**). Collectively, these results indicated that local quantification of TRP metabolites better reflects gene expression and enzymatic activity.

Preliminary Correlation Between TRP Metabolism and Response Prediction

In our first analysis on paired plasma–tissue samples, we suggested that a decreased THP1 activity together with TDO2 overexpression was a common hallmark of lack of response to therapy in rectal cancer patients (**Figure 2** and **Table 2**). In our second analysis on 13 paired control/cancer samples, we aimed at verifying these results and at correlating them to metabolite production at the tissue level. Again, we found that, after stratification of gene expression data, IDO1 was substantially unchanged in TRG 1–2 and TRG 3–5 patients, while TDO2 overexpression was peculiar of nonresponsive patients only (**Table 4**). Consistently to TDO2 overexpression, an increase in the calculated enzymatic activity along the kynurenine pathway has been detected in these patients (136 vs. 311, for TRG 1–2 and TRG 3–5, respectively). TPH1-normalized gene expression decreased in both TRG 1–2 patients (nRQ = 0.19) and TRG 3–5 patients (nRQ = 0.66), even if in the latter the decrease was less consistent. Conversely, calculated THP1 activity showed an opposite trend (43 vs. 29, for TRG 1–2 and TRG 3–5, respectively).

Metabolic data have been finally stratified according to patients' TRG, and obtained results are reported in **Figure 4**. For both kynurenine and serotonin pathways, no statistical differences have been observed, probably due to the low sample size ($n = 6$ and $n = 7$ for TRG 1–2 and TRG 3–5, respectively). Even if a trend of decrease in 5-HT and HIAA tissue levels of TRG 3–5 patients can be inferred from the data, this trend is not supported by gene expression data (**Table 4**).

TABLE 4 | Normalized (tumor/healthy mucosa) gene expression (*nRQ*) after patients' stratification according to their TRG (responders: TRG 1–2; nonresponders: TRG 3–5).

	TRG 1–2 (n = 6 pairs)		TRG 3–5 (n = 7 pairs)		
	Mean	Min, max	Mean	Min, max	Trend in TRG 3–5
IDO1 (nRQ)	0.66	0.13, 2.00	0.789	0.10, 2.41	=
TDO2 (nRQ)	0.88	0.40, 1.99	2.13	0.09, 10.04	↑
Calculated activity	136	8.6, 292.5	311	11.6, 636.6	↑
TPH1 (nRQ)	0.19	0.002, 0.44	0.66	0.001, 3.65	↑
Calculated activity	43	1.2, 149	29	2.6, 94.7	=

Data are presented as mean fold change and minimum and maximum (Min, Max) values. "Trend in tumor" column highlights fold changes at least >1.5 (or <0.67). Enzymatic activity is reported as calculated mean value for rectal cancer samples (healthy mucosa) and relative minimum and maximum.

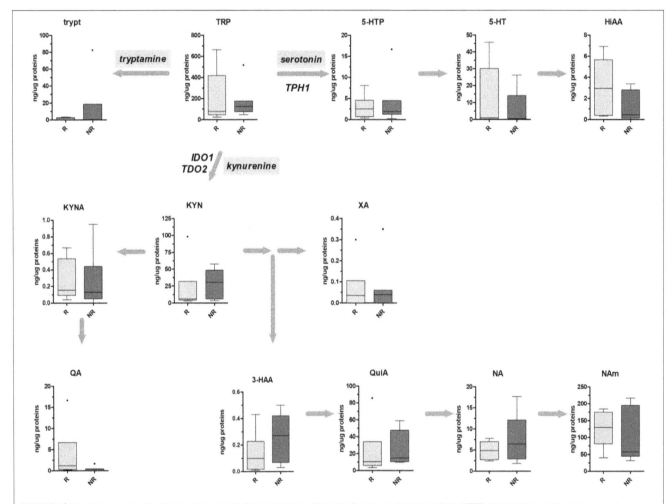

FIGURE 4 | Box-plots representing the absolute amounts (presented as ng of metabolite per μg of total proteins) of TRP along the kynurenine and serotonin pathways in six TRG 1–2 (responders, R) and seven TRG 3–5 (nonresponders, NR) rectal cancer patients. Outliers are also reported.

CONCLUSION

In this work, metabolic and genetic markers of the TRP catabolism before pCRT in LARC patients have been investigated in plasma and tissue samples. In plasma, changes in TRP levels firstly evidenced the difference between responsive (TRG 1–2) and nonresponsive (TRG 3–5) patients. Moreover, TRG 3–5 patients revealed an increased activity along the kynurenine pathway, which correlates with TDO2 overexpression. However, discordant results were obtained from the analysis of the serotonin pathway. Indeed, the decrease in THP1 activity calculated both in plasma and in tissues showed opposite results with respect to the tissue expression. This probably suggests the presence of a posttranscriptional regulation in THP1 protein abundance, which in turn affects its activity in TRG 3–5 patients. Of note, the THP1 posttranscriptional regulation and the diurnal variation of TPH1 activity in the central nervous system have been demonstrated (43–45), but none seems to be reported about cancer. Collectively, these results indicate that mechanisms regulating TRP catabolism may be different between responsive and nonresponsive LARC patients. To confirm these data, further analyses should be performed to increase the sample size and to better investigate the mechanisms involved in tumor response to therapy.

AUTHOR CONTRIBUTIONS

SC: conceptualization and writing - original draft. AF:

investigation. CB and AB: investigation and writing - review and editing. VM: writing - review and editing. SP: clinical data management. MA: project supervision. All authors contributed to the article and approved the submitted version.

FUNDING

The research leading to these results has received funding from AIRC under IG 2016 - ID. 19104 project – P.I. Agostini Marco.

REFERENCES

1. Rawla P, Sunkara T, Barsouk A. Epidemiology of colorectal cancer: incidence, mortality, survival, and risk factors. *Przeglad Gastroenterol.* (2019) 14:89–103. doi: 10.5114/pg.2018.81072

2. Bosset JF, Collette L, Calais G, Mineur L, Maingon P, Radosevic-Jelic L, et al. Chemotherapy with preoperative radiotherapy in rectal cancer. *N Engl J Med.* (2006) 355:1114–23. doi: 10.1056/NEJMoa060829

3. Brown CL, Ternent CA, Thorson AG, Christensen MA, Blatchford GJ, Shashidharan M, et al. Response to preoperative chemoradiation in stage II and III rectal cancer. *Dis Colon Rectum.* (2003) 46:1189–93. doi: 10.1007/s10350-004-6714-y

4. Pucciarelli S, Toppan P, Friso ML, Russo V, Pasetto L, Urso E, et al. Complete pathologic response following preoperative chemoradiation therapy for middle to lower rectal cancer is not a prognostic factor for a better outcome. *Dis Colon Rectum.* (2004) 47:1798–807. doi: 10.1007/s10350-004-0681-1

5. Das P, Skibber JM, Rodriguez-Bigas MA, Feig BW, Chang GJ, Wolff RA, et al. Predictors of tumor response and downstaging in patients who receive preoperative chemoradiation for rectal cancer. *Cancer.* (2007) 109:1750–5. doi: 10.1002/cncr.22625

6. Agostini M, Crotti S, Bedin C, Cecchin E, Maretto I, D'Angelo E, et al. Predictive response biomarkers in rectal cancer neoadjuvant treatment. *Front Biosci.* (2014) 6:110–9. doi: 10.2741/S418

7. Bedin C, Crotti S, D'Angelo E, D'Aronco S, Pucciarelli S, Agostin M. Circulating biomarkers for response prediction of rectal cancer to neoadjuvant chemoradiotherapy. *Curr Med Chem.* (2019) 27:1–21. doi: 10.2174/0929867326666190507084839

8. Helgason HH, Engwegen JYMN, Zapatka M, Vincent A, Cats A, Boot H, et al. Identification of serum proteins as prognostic and predictive markers of colorectal cancer using surface enhanced laser desorption ionization-time of flight mass spectrometry. *Oncol Rep.* (2010) 24:57–64. doi: 10.3892/or_00000828

9. Repetto O, De Re V, De Paoli A, Belluco C, Alessandrini L, Canzonieri V, et al. Identification of protein clusters predictive of tumor response in rectal cancer patients receiving neoadjuvant chemo-radiotherapy. *Oncotarget.* (2017) 8:28328–41. doi: 10.18632/oncotarget.16053

10. Crotti S, Enzo MV, Bedin C, Pucciarelli S, Maretto I, Del Bianco P, et al. Clinical predictive circulating peptides in rectal cancer patients treated

with neoadjuvant chemoradiotherapy. *J Cell Physiol.* (2015) 230:1822–8. doi: 10.1002/jcp.24894

11. Magni E, Botteri E, Ravenda PS, Cassatella MC, Bertani E, Chiappa A, et al. Detection of circulating tumor cells in patients with locally advanced rectal cancer undergoing neoadjuvant therapy followed by curative surgery. *Int J Colorectal Dis.* (2014) 29:1053–9. doi: 10.1007/s00384-014-1958-z

12. Azizian A, Kramer F, Jo P, Wolff HA, Beissbarth T, Skarupke R, et al. Preoperative prediction of lymph node status by circulating Mir-18b and Mir-20a during chemoradiotherapy in patients with rectal cancer. *World J Surg.* (2015) 39:2329–35. doi: 10.1007/s00268-015-3083-8

13. D'Angelo E, Fassan M, Maretto I, Pucciarelli S, Zanon C, Digito M, et al. Serum miR-125b is a non-invasive predictive biomarker of the pre-operative chemoradiotherapy responsiveness in patients with rectal adenocarcinoma. *Oncotarget.* (2016) 7:28647–57. doi: 10.18632/oncotarget.8725

14. Park JH, Richards CH, McMillan DC, Horgan PG, Roxburgh CSD. The relationship between tumour stroma percentage, the tumour microenvironment and survival in patients with primary operable colorectal cancer. *Ann Oncol.* (2014) 25:644–51. doi: 10.1093/annonc/mdt593

15. Trumpi K, Ubink I, Trinh A, Djafarihamedani M, Jongen JM, Govaert KM, et al. Neoadjuvant chemotherapy affects molecular classification of colorectal tumors. *Oncogenesis.* (2017) 6:e357. doi: 10.1038/oncsis.2017.48

16. Matsutani S, Shibutani M, Maeda K, Nagahara H, Fukuoka T, Nakao S, et al. Significance of tumor-infiltrating lymphocytes before and after neoadjuvant therapy for rectal cancer. *Cancer Sci.* (2018) 109:966–79. doi: 10.1111/cas.13542

17. Comai S, Bertazzo A, Brughera M, Crotti S. Tryptophan in health and disease. *Adv Clin Chem.* (2020) 95:165–218. doi: 10.1016/bs.acc.2019.08.005

18. Theate I, van Baren N, Pilotte L, Moulin P, Larrieu P, Renauld JC, et al. Extensive profiling of the expression of the indoleamine 2,3-dioxygenase 1 protein in normal and tumoral human tissues. *Cancer Immunol Res.* (2015) 3:161–72. doi: 10.1158/2326-6066.CIR-14-0137

19. Amobi A, Qian F, Lugade AA, Odunsi K. Tryptophan catabolism and cancer immunotherapy targeting IDO mediated immune suppression. *Adv Exp Med Biol.* (2017) 1036:129–44. doi: 10.1007/978-3-319-67577-0_9

20. Schramme F, Crosignani S, Frederix K, Hoffmann D, Pilotte L, Stroobant V, et al. Inhibition of tryptophan-dioxygenase activity increases the antitumor efficacy of immune checkpoint inhibitors. *Cancer Immunol Res.* (2020) 8:32–45. doi: 10.1158/2326-6066.CIR-19-0041

21. Ferdinande L, Decaestecker C, Verset L, Mathieu A, Moles Lopez X, Negulescu AM, et al. Clinicopathological significance of indoleamine 2,3-dioxygenase 1 expression in colorectal cancer. *Br J Cancer*. (2012) 106:141–7. doi: 10.1038/bjc.2011.513

22. Brandacher G, Perathoner A, Ladurner R, Schneeberger S, Obrist P, Winkler C, et al. Prognostic value of indoleamine 2,3-dioxygenase expression in colorectal cancer: effect on tumor-infiltrating T cells. *Clin Cancer Res*. (2006) 12:1144–51. doi: 10.1158/1078-0432.CCR-05-1966

23. Fallarino F, Grohmann U, You S, McGrath BC, Cavener DR, Vacca C, et al. The combined effects of tryptophan starvation and tryptophan catabolites down-regulate T cell receptor zeta-chain and induce a regulatory phenotype in naive T cells. *J Immunol*. (2006) 176:6752–61. doi: 10.4049/jimmunol.176.11.6752

24. Thaker AI, Rao MS, Bishnupuri KS, Kerr TA, Foster L, Marinshaw JM, et al. IDO1 metabolites activate beta-catenin signaling to promote cancer cell proliferation and colon tumorigenesis in mice. *Gastroenterology*. (2013) 145:416–25 e411–4. doi: 10.1053/j.gastro.2013.05.002

25. Pflugler S, Svinka J, Scharf I, Crncec I, Filipits M, Charoentong P, et al. IDO1(+) Paneth cells promote immune escape of colorectal cancer. *Commun Biol*. (2020) 3:252. doi: 10.1038/s42003-020-0989-y

26. D'Amato NC, Rogers TJ, Gordon MA, Greene LI, Cochrane DR, Spoelstra NS, et al. A TDO2-AhR signaling axis facilitates anoikis resistance and metastasis in triple-negative breast cancer. *Cancer Res*. (2015) 75:4651–64. doi: 10.1158/0008-5472.CAN-15-2011

27. van Baren N, Van den Eynde BJ. Tryptophan-degrading enzymes in tumoral immune resistance. *Front Immunol*. (2015) 6:34. doi: 10.3389/fimmu.2015.00034

28. Pham QT, Oue N, Sekino Y, Yamamoto Y, Shigematsu Y, Sakamoto N, et al. TDO2 overexpression is associated with cancer stem cells and poor prognosis in esophageal squamous cell carcinoma. *Oncology*. (2018) 95:297–308. doi: 10.1159/000490725

29. Crotti S, D'Angelo E, Bedin C, Fassan M, Pucciarelli S, Nitti D, et al. Tryptophan metabolism along the kynurenine and serotonin pathways reveals substantial differences in colon and rectal cancer. *Metabolomics*. (2017) 13:148. doi: 10.1007/s11306-017-1288-6

30. Crotti S, Bedin C, Bertazzo A, Digito M, Zuin M, Urso ED, et al. Tryptophan metabolism as source of new prognostic biomarkers for FAP patients. *Int J Tryptophan Res*. (2019) 12:1178646919890293. doi: 10.1177/1178646919890293

31. Agostini M, Janssen KP, Kim IJ, D'Angelo E, Pizzini S, Zangrando A, et al. An integrative approach for the identification of prognostic and predictive biomarkers in rectal cancer. *Oncotarget*. (2015) 6:32561–74. doi: 10.18632/oncotarget.4935

32. Mandard AM, Dalibard F, Mandard JC, Marnay J, Henry-Amar M, Petiot JF, et al. Pathologic assessment of tumor regression after preoperative chemoradiotherapy of esophageal carcinoma. Clinicopathologic correlations. *Cancer*. (1994) 73:2680–6. doi: 10.1002/1097-0142(19940601)73:11<2680::AID-CNCR2820731105>3.0.CO;2-C

33. Puccetti P, Fallarino F, Italiano A, Soubeyran I, MacGrogan G, Debled M, et al. Accumulation of an endogenous tryptophan-derived metabolite in colorectal and breast cancers. *PLoS ONE*. (2015) 10:e0122046. doi: 10.1371/journal.pone.0122046

34. Tian Q, Stepaniants SB, Mao M, Weng L, Feetham MC, Doyle MJ, et al. Integrated genomic and proteomic analyses of gene expression in Mammalian cells. *Mol Cell Proteomics*. (2004) 3:960–9. doi: 10.1074/mcp.M400055-MCP200

35. Stavrum AK, Heiland I, Schuster S, Puntervoll P, Ziegler M. Model of tryptophan metabolism, readily scalable using tissue-specific gene expression data. *J Biol Chem*. (2013) 288:34555–66. doi: 10.1074/jbc.M113.474908

36. Terry N, Margolis KG. Serotonergic mechanisms regulating the GI tract: experimental evidence and therapeutic relevance. *Handb Exp Pharmacol*. (2017) 239:319–42. doi: 10.1007/164_2016_103

37. Venkateswaran N, Lafita-Navarro MC, Hao YH, Kilgore JA, Perez-Castro L, Braverman J, et al. MYC promotes tryptophan uptake and metabolism by the kynurenine pathway in colon cancer. *Genes Dev*. (2019) 33:1236–51. doi: 10.1101/gad.327056.119

38. Opitz CA, Litzenburger UM, Sahm F, Ott M, Tritschler I, Trump S, et al. An endogenous tumour-promoting ligand of the human aryl hydrocarbon receptor. *Nature*. (2011) 478:197–203. doi: 10.1038/nature10491

39. Houtkooper RH, Canto C, Wanders RJ, Auwerx J. The secret life of NAD+: an old metabolite controlling new metabolic signaling pathways. *Endocr Rev*. (2010) 31:194–223. doi: 10.1210/er.2009-0026

40. Pilotte L, Larrieu P, Stroobant V, Colau D, Dolusic E, Frederick R, et al. Reversal of tumoral immune resistance by inhibition of tryptophan 2,3-dioxygenase. *Proc Natl Acad Sci USA*. (2012) 109:2497–502. doi: 10.1073/pnas.1113873109

41. Hsu YL, Hung JY, Chiang SY, Jian SF, Wu CY, Lin YS, et al. Lung cancer-derived galectin-1 contributes to cancer associated fibroblast-mediated cancer progression and immune suppression through TDO2/kynurenine axis. *Oncotarget*. (2016) 7:27584–98. doi: 10.18632/oncotarget.8488

42. Tina E, Prosen S, Lennholm S, Gasparyan G, Lindberg M, Gothlin Eremo A. Expression profile of the amino acid transporters SLC7A5, SLC7A7, SLC7A8 and the enzyme TDO2 in basal cell carcinoma. *Br J Dermatol*. (2019) 180:130–40. doi: 10.1111/bjd.16905

43. Sitaram BR, Lees GJ. Diurnal rhythm and turnover of tryptophan hydroxylase in the pineal gland of the rat. *J Neurochem*. (1978) 31:1021–6. doi: 10.1111/j.1471-4159.1978.tb00142.x

44. Sugden D, Grady R Jr, Mefford IN. Measurement of tryptophan hydroxylase activity in rat pineal glands and pinealocytes using an HPLC assay with electrochemical detection. *J Pineal Res*. (1989) 6:285–92. doi: 10.1111/j.1600-079X.1989.tb00424.x

45. Huang Z, Liu T, Chattoraj A, Ahmed S, Wang MM, Deng J, et al. Posttranslational regulation of TPH1 is responsible for the nightly surge of 5-HT output in the rat pineal gland. *J Pineal Res*. (2008) 45:506–14. doi: 10.1111/j.1600-079X.2008.00627.x

19

Tryptophan and its Metabolites in Lung Cancer: Basic Functions and Clinical Significance

Chenwei Li[1] and Hui Zhao[2]*

[1] Department of Respiratory Medicine, The Second Affiliated Hospital of Dalian Medical University, Dalian, China,
[2] Department of Health Examination Center, The Second Affiliated Hospital of Dalian Medical University, Dalian, China

*Correspondence:
Hui Zhao
zhaohui@dmu.edu.cn

Lung cancer is the most lethal malignancy worldwide. Recently, it has been recognized that metabolic reprogramming is a complex and multifaceted factor, contributing to the process of lung cancer. Tryptophan (Try) is an essential amino acid, and Try and its metabolites can regulate the progression of lung cancer. Here, we review the pleiotropic functions of the Try metabolic pathway, its metabolites, and key enzymes in the pathogenic process of lung cancer, including modulating the tumor environment, promoting immune suppression, and drug resistance. We summarize the recent advance in therapeutic drugs targeting the Try metabolism and kynurenine pathway and their clinical trials.

Keywords: tryptophan, lung cancer, kynurenine pathway, IDO, TDO

INTRODUCTION

Lung cancer (LC) is one of the most common malignancies worldwide and has a high mortality rate (1). Previous studies have shown that lung carcinogenesis is attributed to the gain-functional mutation of several cancer-associated genes, including the epidermal growth factor receptor (EGFR), Kirsten rat sarcoma viral oncogene homolog (KRAS), and v-raf murine sarcoma viral oncogene homolog B1 (BRAF) (2–4). Actually, therapeutic drugs targeting these molecules have been demonstrated to prolong the survival of LC patients, particularly for non-small cell lung cancer (NSCLC) patients. However, therapeutic efficacy of these drugs is limited due to rapid development of drug resistance in LC patients (4–6). Therefore, other effective treatments are urgently needed. Currently, cancer has been thought not to be a genetic disease, rather than a metabolic disease, which is associated with tumor immune escape (7, 8). It is well known that tumor cells usually undergo aerobic glycolysis for their glucose metabolism, known as the Warburg effect (9). Moreover, extensive studies have revealed that alternations in metabolisms are not only for glucose, but also for amino acid, lipid, nucleotide, and others in cancer (10). Notably, tryptophan (Try) metabolism is a particularly compelling physiological context in LC because of its complex and multifaceted effect on LC cells and cancer-associated cells in immune escape (11).

Try cannot be synthesized directly by the human body and has the lowest levels in the human body among 20 essential amino acids such that it depends on food protein. Similar to other essential amino acids, Try is essential for biosynthesizing cellular protein and formatting cytoskeleton (12). In the circulation, most Try binds to albumin for transportation and only 10%–20% of it remain free amino acid (13, 14). The free Try is mainly degraded through the kynurenine (KYN) pathway and is metabolized to form serotonin or other metabolites (15). Try plays a significantly physiological role in synthesizing proteins. However, the metabolic formation of serotonin and the KYN pathway-mediated metabolism, together with the lack of its endogenous production, may make Try shortage that can impair the protein synthesis. In the KYN pathway, Try is firstly converted to formyl-kynurenine, which is rapidly degraded to KYN by key enzymes of indoleamine-pyrrole 2,3-dioxygenase (IDO)1, IDO2, and tryptophan 2,3-dioxygenase (TDO), particularly by IDO1 (14, 16). Next, KYN is catalyzed into a series of metabolites, including anthranilic acid (AA), kynurenic acid (KA), xanthurenic acid (XA), 3-hydroxyanthranilic (3-HAA), quinolinic acid (QA), and NAD+ (17). In the lung, Try degradation is mainly catalyzed by IDO1 because IDO1 is constitutively expressed in many organs while TDO is predominantly expressed in the liver (18). Previous studies have shown that most Try metabolites in the KYN pathway are associated with the development of many diseases, including cancer. Actually, the IDO1-related Try metabolites are associated with lung cancer development (19, 20). This review aims to summarize the research advance in how Try and its metabolites contribute to the development and progression of LC.

THE EXPRESSION AND BIOLOGICAL FUNCTIONS OF Try METABOLITES IN LC

Try and Its Metabolites in LC

A previous study has indicated that circulating Try levels decrease in patients with lung, gastric, colorectal, breast, and prostate cancer (21). Recent studies using liquid chromatography mass spectrometry (LC-MS) have found that plasma Try and XA levels decrease and 3-HAA increases in 19 NSCLC patients, relative to 10 non-tumor healthy controls (22, 23). Similarly, high-performance liquid chromatography-fluorescence detection (HPLC-FD) or gas chromatography mass spectrometry (GC-MS) analyses reveal that the concentrations of serum Try in LC patients are significantly lower than that in the controls (24, 25). Moreover, patients with lung adenocarcinoma (LADC) tend to have lower serum Try concentrations than those with lung squamous carcinoma (LSCC), which may be related to its regulatory function in the proliferation and metastasis of different types of cancers (24). However, there is no significant difference in the levels of serum Try during the progression of lung cancer. Accordingly, the levels of serum or plasma Try may be useful for the diagnosis of LC with a specificity of >92% (24). Interestingly, a study reveals that cisplatin-resistant LC cells consume more Try than non-resistant cells (26), suggesting that Try levels may be associated with the development of drug resistance in LC cells. However, how the levels of circulating Try are associated with levels of Try in the tumor microenvironment remains to be investigated.

The decrease in circulating Try may be attributed to several reasons. First, the enhanced expression and activity of Try-metabolizing enzymes in LC patients can promote Try metabolism, decreasing the levels of Try in the circulation and

tumor (27). Second, LC patients may have malnutrition and poor digestion/absorption so that they may intake less Try from foods (24). Last, over-consumption of Try-contained foods may disorder Try metabolism, especially in advanced stage of lung cancer (24, 28) because Try is an essential component for cytoskeleton and protein synthesis in LC.

Decreased circulating Try is a crucial metabolic feature in LC patients. Accordingly, Try levels may combine with other metabolic molecules for diagnosis of LC. Actually, the levels of serum Try, alanine, valine, isoleucine, histidine, and ornithine have a diagnostic value for NSCLC with an area under the receiver-operator characteristic (ROC) of >0.80, and effectively discriminate neoplastic patients from healthy subjects (29, 30). LC patients display decreased levels of serum Try, threonine, citrulline, and histidine and increased proline, isoleucine, phenylalanine, and ornithine, leading to an area under curve (AUC) of 0.80, but the Try metabolite profile does not distinguish different pathological types of LC (29, 31). Consistently, HPLC-FD analysis indicates that a combination of six metabolites [L-tryptophan, hypoxanthine, inosine, indoleacrylic acid, acylcarnitine C10:1, and lysoPC (18:2)] effectively separates NSCLC patients from non-tumor subjects with an AUC of 0.99 (32).

IDO1, IDO2, and TDO in LC
IDO1

The IDO1 is a key enzyme in the KYN pathway, particularly in the lung. Previous studies have detected IDO expression in tumor cells, blood vessels, stromal cells of NSCLC patients, as well as in dendritic cells (DCs) in the tumor environment and tumor-related lymph nodes in patients with LC (33). However, the function of IDO1 in endothelial cells has yet been understood (34). The expression of IDO promotes KYN accumulation, which may dilate blood vessels (35). Accordingly, it is possible that IDO1 deficiency may reduce vascular-related adverse reaction of some therapeutic drugs pharmacologically (35). Besides, IDO1 mRNA transcripts are upregulated in lung tissues (36) and the serum KYN : Try ratio (KTR), an indicative of IDO activity, is greater in LC patients than healthy subjects (37), supporting the notion that higher KTR is associated with increased risk for LC (38), especially for LSCC in heavy smokers, because AhR (aryl hydrocarbon receptor) activates the carcinogenesis pathway of benzo(a)pyrene (BaP), a strong lung carcinogen derived from tobacco smoking (39). High levels of IDO1 expression can enhance LC cell invasion in vitro and distant metastasis into the brain, liver, and bone in vivo, while IDO1 inhibition attenuates their invasion and distant metastasis in rodents (40). Similarly, IDO1 inhibition also inhibits the lung metastasis of breast cancer and improves the survival of tumor-bearing animals (41, 42). Furthermore, IDO1-deficient mice are partially resistant to cancer growth in a Lewis rat model of lung carcinoma (43).

The activity and expression of IDO1 are associated with diagnosis, prognosis, and therapeutic responses in LC (44–48). IDO1 activity may be a valuable biomarker for evaluating the response to immunotherapy, and its levels may help in choosing therapy for LC patients, who are sensitive to immunotherapy (49).

Similarly, increased IDO1 activity is detected in LC patients, who initially respond to immune checkpoint inhibitors (ICIs) and later exhibit cancer progression, leading to a worse prognosis (44). Furthermore, increased IDO1 activity is closely associated with worse survival of NSCLC patients receiving explicit radiotherapy (48, 50). However, these studies were performed in small groups of patients. Therefore, further prospective studies with a larger population are necessary to validate the prognostic value of IDO1 activity in LC patients following radiotherapy. Interestingly, elevated IDO1 expression is associated with better outcome in lung adenosquamous carcinoma patients, especially for those after surgical resection of the tumor (51). The discrepancy may stem from different studying populations. While previous studies mainly focus on patients with unresectable LC and patients receiving chemotherapy or chemoradiation, this study centers on LC patients after radical surgery (51). It is possible that IDO1 activity may have different values in prognosis of different stages of LC following varying therapeutic strategies.

IDO2 and TDO

IDO2 and TDO are other key enzymes for Try degradation (52–55). Although the IDO1 and IDO2 genes are highly homologous at human chromosome 8 and tightly connected (56, 57), the IDO2 catalytic activity is much weaker than that of IDO1 *in vitro* and *in vivo* (58). Actually, there is no significant difference in the concentrations of plasma Try and KYN between wild-type and IDO2-deficient mice (59). Human TDO gene sequence has a low homology (16%) with the IDO1, but their protein catalytic domains have a high similarity (60) and TDO is predominantly expressed in the liver (61). Similar to IDO1, upregulated IDO2 and TDO may be associated with immune escape in some types of tumors (53, 55, 62, 63). Previous studies have reported that TDO enhances the migration and invasion of glioblastoma and breast cancer cells *in vitro* and treatment with a TDO inhibitor significantly inhibits distant metastasis in mice (64–66). Furthermore, IDO2$^{-/-}$ mice display a decreased tumor size compared with wild-type mice (67). Pharmacological inhibition of TDO reduces the number of lung tumor nodules in mice (68). Apparently, enhanced IDO2 and TDO expression and activity may promote the progression and metastasis of LC and their activity is indistinguishable (49). Similar to the function of IDO1, upregulated IDO2 expression is linked to worse prognosis in NSCLC (53). Therefore, IDO2 inhibitors may be valuable for targeting LC and IDO2 may be a biomarker for immunotherapy (69). Moreover, there is little information on whether IDO2 expression is associated with resistance to cisplatin in LC patients and what the value of IDO2 is in diagnosis and prognosis of LC (26, 63). Therefore, further studies are warranted to address these questions.

Try METABOLITES AND IMMUNE ESCAPE IN LC

The immune escape is a "hallmark of cancer" (70, 71). Tumor immune escape refers to the phenomenon, in which tumor cells can grow and metastasize by avoiding recognition and attack by the immune system through various mechanisms (72). Currently, IDO1 has been suggested to be important for immune escape of LC. First, upregulated IDO1 expression promotes the degradation of Try and the accumulation of its metabolites (such as KYN, 3-HAA and others) in LC. These metabolites act on various immune cells, including T cells (naïve CD4+ T cells, Th17, and Treg), antigen-presenting cells (APC, DCs, and macrophages), and NK cells, and lead to immune escape. The promising mechanisms by which Try metabolites induce cancer immune tolerance and immunosuppression are summarized in **Figure 1**.

First, Try is an essential amino acid for immune cell proliferation, and Try depletion results in T-cell apoptosis, which is one major reason for cancer immunosuppression (73). The decreased Try levels can inhibit T-cell proliferation by activating general control over nonderepressible 2 (GCN2) kinase and suppressing the mTOR signaling, a target of rapamycin (74–76). The GCN2 is a serine/threonine kinase and can phosphorylate eukaryotic initiation factor 2a kinase (eIF2a) in the presence of low concentration of Try, inhibiting protein synthesis and T cell proliferation (74). Activated GCN2 can also promote the differentiation of naïve CD4+ T cells into Tregs (16, 74, 77). Furthermore, GCN2 can alter the phenotype of DCs and macrophages (75, 76, 78), making them prone to immunosuppression to promote tumorigenesis. In contrast, other studies argue that GCN2 is a sensor of amino acid starvation and its activation is not dependent on a low Try level, rather than deficiency in many amino acids (79, 80). Actually, T cells with GCN2 deficiency have similar activity to wild-type T cells in B16 melanoma-bearing mice (79), which contradicts the tumor promotion of GCN2. Apparently, there may be another mechanism that senses Try-deprived condition to regulate T cell immunity against tumor. The mTOR signaling appears to be a possible candidate (81, 82) because inhibition of mTOR complex 1 (mTORC1) can induce T-cell autophagy and anergy in the tumor microenvironment (83). Moreover, mTORC1 inhibition can also induce Treg cells to suppress anti-tumor immune responses (82).

Second, increased KYN can lead to immune tolerance by inhibiting T cell proliferation and inducing T cell apoptosis to promote tumor growth (38). The KYN is a ligand of AhR, and its activation promotes Treg cell differentiation that can directly inhibit anti-tumor immune responses, contributing to cancer immune escape (77, 84). The AhR activation can also direct DCs and macrophages toward an immune-suppressive phenotype (85–87). The AhR activation enhances IL-10 synthesis and secretion, and inhibits the IFN-β signaling in DCs, but induces IL-10 and IFN-α production in NK cells, respectively. Consistently, higher frequency of Tregs is detected in mice bearing cisplatin-resistant tumors than those bearing cisplatin-sensitive tumors (26).

Third, the downstream metabolites (such as 3-HAA and QA) of KYN can also induce T-cell apoptosis (88), contributing to immune tolerance. Recent studies have shown that QA can inhibit the proliferation of cancer-specific CD8+ cytotoxic T

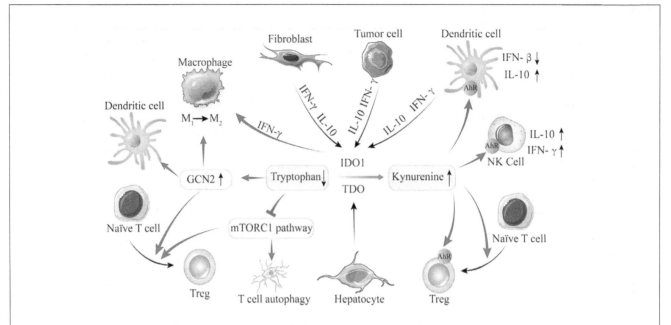

FIGURE 1 | The Try-IDO1/TDO-KYN pathway and immune escape. IDO1 is constitutively expressed in fibroblast, tumor cells, and DCs, and can be upregulated by IL-10 and IFN-γ, whereas TDO is only expressed in hepatocytes. When IDO1 and TDO are activated, they promote Try degradation and KYN accumulation. Try depletion can activate GCN2 and inhibit the mTORC1 signaling. The KYN can bind to AhR in NK cells, Tregs, and DCs. Therefore, the Try-IDO1/TDO-KYN pathway cooperatively modulates immune cells (e.g., DCs, macrophage, Treg, and T cells) to regulate anti-inflammatory cytokine production, leading to enhanced immunosuppression in the tumor microenvironment.

and NK cells to promote tumor growth (89). Furthermore, LC patients with lower plasma 3-HAA, the precursor of QA, benefit more from ICI treatment, suggesting that plasma 3-HAA levels may be a biomarker for predicting the response of LC patients to ICIs (23). The lower plasma 3-HAA may reflect less immunosuppression in patients because 3-HAA can promote Treg responses to produce high levels of TGF-β that decrease effector T-cell function, leading to immunosuppression (90). However, its precise mechanism in tumor immunity is not clear.

Next, IDO1 expression can be regulated by cytokines, such as IL-10 and IFN-γ (91, 92) while IDO1 inhibition can enhance T-cell proliferation and infiltration in the tumor environment and IL-2 production (93). Furthermore, IDO1 or IDO2 deficiency can modulate the tumor microenvironment by reducing KTR, enhancing immune cell infiltration and IFN-γ production (67). TDO and IDO2 act as the Try-metabolizing enzymes and can also promote Try degradation, resulting in immune regulation similar to IDO1. However, there are few reports and further studies are needed.

Last, IDO1 and TDO catalyze the production of several downstream Try metabolites, such as KYN (64, 84), KA (94), and XA (66), which can activate the AhR and may contribute to the immune modulation of IDO1 and TDO. Interestingly, KYN can directly bind and activate the AhR, with a high affinity at low picomolar levels (95). However, whether similar mechanisms also apply to other polar metabolites that activate the AhR, such as KA, remains to be investigated. In addition, AhR can regulate IDO-related regulatory phenotype in DCs (96). Here, an autocrine IDO–KYN/AhR–IDO feedback loop may contribute to the immune modulation (97, 98).

THE CLINICAL APPLICATIONS OF Try METABOLITES IN LC

Enhanced IDO1 expression and activity can evade immunosurveillance and are associated with poor prognosis of LC. Therefore, inhibition of IDO1 may be an ideal strategy for intervention of LC. There are several direct IDO1 inhibitors available, including epacadostat and navoximod that neither directly kill tumor cells, nor spontaneously initiate an immune response (99). Unlike epacadostat, the Try mimetic indoximod (D-1MT, 1-methyl-D-tryptophan) is the first non-enzyme inhibitory drug that targets the IDO1 pathway and can inhibit lung tumor growth *in vivo* (100–102). Indoximod can directly act on immune cells by creating an artificially Try-related signal, relieving the IDO1-mediated immunosuppression (99). There are ongoing clinical trials that investigate anti-IDO1 agents as monotherapy or adjuvant therapies with other drugs for various solid tumors. The clinical trials of anti-IDO1 agents for different combination strategies, such as combination with ICIs, other immunomodulators, and chemotherapy, are summarized in **Table 1**.

Epacadostat, a small-molecule IDO1 inhibitor, was developed by Incyte and is being tested for its therapeutic efficacy and safety in an advanced stage of clinical trial (103). The phase I/II KeyNote 037/ECHO 301 trial to test the safety and efficacy of different doses of epacadostat combined with 200 mg pembrolizumab (i.e., an anti-PD1 agent) every 3 weeks (Q3W) in 62 patients with different types of cancers has achieved promising results (104). There were 24% of patients experiencing high-grade toxicities but no treatment-related

TABLE 1 | Clinical trials for the potential drugs targeting the IDO1/TDO-KYN pathway.

Indication	Tumor type	Combination	Status	ClinicalTrials.gov	Phase
IDO inhibitor: Epacadostat	Metastatic NSCLC	Pembrolizumab	Complete	NCT03322540	II
	Metastatic NSCLC	Pembrolizumab and Platinum-based Chemotherapy	Completed	NCT03322566	II
	NSCLC	Nivolumab	Terminated	NCT03348904	III
	Extensive Stage Small Cell Lung Cancer	Pembrolizumab	Withdrawn	NCT03402880	II
	NSCLC, UC	Atezolizumab	Terminated	NCT02298153	I
	Advanced Solid Tumor, NSCLC	Sirolimus	Recruiting	NCT03217669	I
	Solid Tumor, Advanced Malignancies, Metastatic Cancer	Azacitidine and Pembrolizumab	Completed	NCT02959437	I/II
	Solid Tumor, Head and Neck Cancer, Lung Cancer, UC	Durvalumab (MEDI4736)	Completed	NCT02318277	I/II
	B-cell Malignancies, CRC, Head and Neck Cancer, LC, Lymphoma, Melanoma, Ovarian Cancer, Glioblastoma	Nivolumab	Completed	NCT02327078	I/II
	Microsatellite-instability High CRC, Endometrial Cancer, Head and Neck Cancer, HCC, GC, Lung Cancer, Lymphoma, RCC, Ovarian Cancer, Solid Tumor, UC, Melanoma, Bladder Cancer, TNBC	Pembrolizumab	Active, not recruiting	NCT02178722	I/II
	NSCLC	Pembrolizumab and chemotherapy	Completed	NCT02862457	I
	Solid Tumor	INCB001158 and Pembrolizumab	Terminated	NCT03361228	I/II
	Advanced Malignancies, Metastatic Cancer	INCAGN01876 and Immune Therapies	Completed	NCT03277352	I/II
	Solid Tumor	Pembrolizumab and Chemotherapy	Completed	NCT03085914	I/II
	Solid Tumor	Nivolumab and Immune Therapies	Active, not recruiting	NCT03347123	I/II
IDO inhibitor: Navoximod	Advanced solid tumor	–	Completed	NCT02048709	I
IDO inhibitor: BMS-986205	NSCLC	Nivolumab and Chemotherapy	Withdrawn	NCT03417037	III
	Advanced Cancer, Melanoma, NSCLC	Nivolumab and Ipilimumab	Recruiting	NCT02658890	I/II
IDO inhibitor: MK-7162	Advanced solid tumor	Pembrolizumab	Recruiting	NCT03364049	I
IDO inhibitor: LY3381916	LY3381916 alone or in combination with LY3300054 in solid tumors	LY3300054	Recruiting	NCT03343613	I
IDO inhibitor: KHK2455	Locally advanced or metastatic solid tumors	Mogamulizumab	Recruiting	NCT02867007	I
IDO pathway modulator: Indoximod (D-1-MT)	NSCLC, Progression of NSCLC, NSCLC Recurrent	Tergenpumatucel-L and docetaxel	Active, not recruiting	NCT02460367	I
	Metastatic or refractory solid tumors	N/A	Completed	NCT00567931	I
	Relapsed or Refractory Solid Tumors	–	Terminated	NCT00739609	I
IDO pathway modulator: NLG-802	Advanced solid tumors	N/A	Recruiting	NCT03164603	I
Dual IDO1/TDO inhibitor: HTI1090/ SHR9146	Advanced solid tumors	SHR-1210 and apatinib	Not yet recruiting	NCT03491631	I
	Advanced solid tumors	N/A	Recruiting	NCT03208959	I
IDO Peptide Vaccination	NSCLC	–	Completed	NCT01219348	I

Data accessed from https://www.clinicaltrials.gov/ on January 15, 2021. UC, urothelial cancer; CRC, colorectal cancer; HCC, hepatocellular carcinoma; RCC, renal carcinoma; N/A, not applicable.

death and 12 out of 22 patients obtained objective responses. Unfortunately, a further phase III clinical trial with epacadostat 100 mg twice a day (BID) and pembrolizumab 200 mg (Q3W) failed to improve progression-free survival (PFS) in patients with metastatic melanoma (105). Because of the limitations of this trial, further clinical trials are necessary to test its therapeutic efficacy and safety.

The phase I ECHO-110 study was designed to test epacadostat at different doses combined with atezolizumab (i.e., an anti-PD-L1 agent) 1,200 mg Q3W in 29 patients with stage IIIB/IV NSCLC, who had previously been treated with ≥1 prior line of platinum-based chemotherapy (≥2 cycles), but not with checkpoint/IDO inhibitors. Similarly, 7 out of 29 patients displayed high-grade toxicities but no treatment-related death. Epacadostat at a dose up to 300 mg BID combined with atezolizumab 1,200 mg Q3W was well-tolerated in patients with previously treated NSCLC (103). However, only one patient achieved objective response. The low therapeutic efficacy may stem from the fact of almost all patients with negative PD-L1 expression. Similarly, the single-arm combination of the ECHO-301 trial also failed, lining with the results from other Phase II and III trials conducted in different settings (17) and was converted into the randomized phase II trials of epacadostat combined with pembrolizumab in LC patients. In addition, the KEYNOTE-715-06/ECHO-306-06 trials with the combination of epacadostat, pembrolizumab, and platinum-based chemotherapy did not obtain promising benefit in overall response rate in NSCLC patients (Clinicaltrial.gov.). These observations suggest that the combination of Epacadostat and a PD-1/PD-L1 blockade may not be valuable for patients with PD-L1 negative LC. However, whether this treatment strategy can achieve positive responses in PD-L1 expressing NSCLC or whether combination with platinum-based chemotherapy can achieve a better outcome in NSCLC patients has not been clarified. The ongoing, randomized, phase 2 ECHO-305 (NCT03322540) and ECHO-306 (NCT03322566) trials may give promising results.

New IDO inhibitors, such as navoximod (NLG-919/GDC-0919) and BMS-986205, are also being tested in clinical trials (106). In a phase I study of the IDO1 inhibitor, combination of navoximod and atezolizumab displayed acceptable safety, tolerability, and pharmacokinetics, but not clear beneficial evidence of navoximod in patients with advanced solid tumors (107).

There are questions on whether epacadostat doses used in the ECHO-301 trial could effectively inhibit IDO1 activity in the tumor microenvironment and whether targeting multiple enzymes in the KYN pathway to control Try metabolism would benefit to these patients (58).

There are also ongoing trials testing IDO1 and TDO dual inhibitors such as HTI-1090 (SHR9146) as a monotherapy for solid tumors (NCT03208959). The dual inhibitor of DN1406131 is being tested for its safety in healthy subjects (NCT03641794) while RG70099 from Curadev/Roche is still in preclinical development (108).

In a word, most researchers have focused on IDO/TDO inhibitors for the treatment of LC, and some of them have already been tested in clinical trials. However, the current therapeutic efficacy appears limited. Thus, further studies are necessary to understand the biological functions of Try and its metabolites in the development and progression of LC. Given that the KYN downstream metabolites have profound functions in regulating T cell immunity against LC, these metabolites and their catalyzing enzymes may be explored for development of therapies for LC. Similarly, combination of IDO/TDO inhibitors and other therapies (chemotherapy, radiotherapy, targeted therapy, and immunotherapy) should be pursued to determine the safety and therapeutic efficacy in LC. Previous studies have demonstrated that patient's metabolism (BMI variation and hypercholesterolemia)

has a significant impact on the outcome of PD1 inhibitor treatment in LC patients (109, 110). Some drugs can regulate body metabolism and are significantly related to clinical outcomes of ICI treatment in LC patients (111, 112). Metformin, an effective agent for the management of type 2 diabetes mellitus, in combination with ICI treatment can improve the anticancer effects of ICIs (113, 114). Statins can inhibit cholesterol production (115) and is associated with better clinical outcome of anti-PD1 treatment in advanced NSCLC patients in an intensity-dependent manner (111). However, IDO1 as an immune checkpoint is not as well studied as PD1, and the role of patient metabolism and drugs involved in its regulation on the outcome of patients treated with IDO/TDO inhibitors needs to be further confirmed. If demonstrated, IDO/TDO inhibitors may benefit many patients with LC.

CONCLUSION

Currently, modulation of Try metabolism has been used for diagnosis, prognosis, and therapies for LC. The levels of circulating IDO activity and downstream metabolites (3-HAA, QA, KA, etc.) can be used to predict the efficacy of different treatments in LC (116, 117). However, the results are inconsistent, which may be caused by limitations, such as small sample size, inconsistent measurement methods, influence of the gender, tumor stage, and tumor heterogeneity. Hence, further studies are needed in multi-centers with a larger population, standardized measurement methods, paired samples, and detailed analysis for different stages and pathological types of LC. Currently, some metabolites, enzyme inhibitors targeting immune checkpoints, and modulators have been developed for the diagnosis and treatment of LC. Because the change in metabolomics is one of the factors for the development of cancer, it will be wise to integrate the role of metabolomic changes in the pathogenesis of LC and consider other factors together for the development of therapeutic strategies for LC. Therefore, further studies are necessary to understand the process of complicated Try metabolism and its regulation in different types and stages of LC.

AUTHOR CONTRIBUTIONS

CL performed the literature search and drafted the manuscript and figures. HZ edited and revised the manuscript. All authors contributed to the article and approved the submitted version.

FUNDING

This work was supported by grants from the National Natural Science Foundation of China 81703087, the United Fund of the Second Hospital of Dalian Medical University and Dalian Institute of Chemical Physics, Chinese Academy of Sciences (UF-ZD-202011), and the Project of Education Department of Liaoning Province (LZ2020009).

REFERENCES

1. Siegel RL, Miller KD, Fuchs HE, Jemal A. Cancer Statistics, 2021. *CA: A Cancer J Clin* (2021) 71(1):7–33. doi: 10.3322/caac.21654

2. Tan DS, Yom SS, Tsao MS, Pass HI, Kelly K, Peled N, et al. The International Association for the Study of Lung Cancer Consensus Statement on Optimizing Management of EGFR Mutation-Positive Non-Small Cell Lung Cancer: Status in 2016. *J Thorac Oncol* (2016) 11:946–63. doi: 10.1016/j.jtho.2016.05.008

3. Antonio M, Lara F, Sara M, Maria GS, Luigi G, Antonio C, et al. Clinical Features and Outcome of Patients With Non-Small-Cell Lung Cancer Harboring BRAF Mutations. *J Clin Oncol* (2011) 29(26):3574–9. doi: 10.1200/JCO.2011.35.9638

4. Jänne PA, Shaw AT, Pereira JR, Jeannin G, Vansteenkiste J, Barrios C, et al. Selumetinib Plus Docetaxel for KRAS -Mutant Advanced Non-Small-Cell Lung Cancer: A Randomised, Multicentre, Placebo-Controlled, Phase 2 Study. *Lancet Oncol* (2013) 14(1):38–47. doi: 10.1016/S1470-2045(12) 70489-8

5. Rosell R, Carcereny E, Gervais R, Vergnenegre A, Massuti B, Felip E, et al. Erlotinib Versus Standard Chemotherapy as First-Line Treatment for European Patients With Advanced EGFR Mutation-Positive Non-Small-Cell Lung Cancer (EURTAC): A Multicentre, Open-Label, Randomised Phase 3 Trial. *Lancet Oncol* (2012) 13(3):239–46. doi: 10.1016/S1470-2045 (11)70393-X

6. A JP, Chih-Hsin YJ, Dong-Wan K, David P, Yuichiro O, S RS, et al. AZD9291 in EGFR Inhibitor-Resistant Non-Small-Cell Lung Cancer. *N Engl J Med* (2015) 372(18):1689–99. doi: 10.1056/NEJMoa1411817

7. Wishart DS. Is Cancer a Genetic Disease or a Metabolic Disease? *EBioMedicine* (2015) 2(6):478–9. doi: 10.1016/j.ebiom.2015.05.022

8. Hanahan D, Weinberg RA. Hallmarks of Cancer: The Next Generation. *Cell* (2011) 144:646–74. doi: 10.1016/j.cell.2011.02.013

9. Burk D, Schade AL. On Respiratory Impairment in Cancer Cells. *Science* (1956) 124:270–2. doi: 10.1126/science.124.3215.267

10. Fahrmann JF, Vykoukal JV, Ostrin EJ. Amino Acid Oncometabolism and Immunomodulation of the Tumor Microenvironment in Lung Cancer. *Front Oncol* (2020) 10:276. doi: 10.3389/fonc.2020.00276

11. Godin-Ethier J, Hanafi LA, Piccirillo CA, Lapointe R. Indoleamine 2,3-Dioxygenase Expression in Human Cancers: Clinical and Immunologic Perspectives. *Clin Cancer Res* (2011) 17:6985–91. doi: 10.1158/1078-0432.CCR-11-1331

12. Weljie AM, Jirik FR. Hypoxia-Induced Metabolic Shifts in Cancer Cells: Moving Beyond the Warburg Effect. *Int J Biochem Cell Biol* (2011) 43:981–9. doi: 10.1016/j.biocel.2010.08.009

13. Pardridge WM. Tryptophan Transport Through the Blood-Brain Barrier: *In Vivo* Measurement of Free and Albumin-Bound Amino Acid. *Life Sci* (1979) 25(17):1519–28. doi: 10.1016/0024-3205(79)90378-3

14. Cervenka I, Agudelo LZ, Ruas JL. Kynurenines: Tryptophan's Metabolites in Exercise, Inflammation, and Mental Health. *Science* (2017) 357(6349): eaaf9794. doi: 10.1126/science.aaf9794

15. Schwarcz R, Stone TW. The Kynurenine Pathway and the Brain: Challenges, Controversies and Promises. *Neuropharmacology* (2017) 112:237–47. doi: 10.1016/j.neuropharm.2016.08.003

16. Munn DH, Mellor AL. IDO in the Tumor Microenvironment: Inflammation, Counter-Regulation, and Tolerance. *Trends Immunol* (2016) 37:193–207. doi: 10.1016/j.it.2016.01.002

17. Platten M, Nollen EAA, Röhrig UF, Fallarino F, Opitz CA. Tryptophan Metabolism as a Common Therapeutic Target in Cancer, Neurodegeneration and Beyond. *Nat Rev Drug Discov* (2019) 18(5):379–401. doi: 10.1038/s41573-019-0016-5

18. Dai X, Zhu BT. Indoleamine 2,3-Dioxygenase Tissue Distribution and Cellular Localization in Mice: Implications for Its Biological Functions. *J Histochem Cytochem* (2010) 58:17–28. doi: 10.1369/jhc.2009.953604

19. Yoshida R, Imanishi J, Oku T, Kishida T, Hayaishi O. Induction of Pulmonary Indoleamine 2,3-Dioxygenase by Interferon. *Proc Natl Acad Sci USA* (1981) 78:129–32. doi: 10.1073/pnas.78.1.129

20. Yoshida R, Urade Y, Tokuda M, Hayaishi O. Induction of Indoleamine 2,3-Dioxygenase in Mouse Lung During Virus Infection. *Proc Natl Acad Sci USA* (1979) 76:4084–6. doi: 10.1073/pnas.76.8.4084

21. Miyagi Y, Higashiyama M, Gochi A, Akaike M, Ishikawa T, Miura T, et al. Plasma Free Amino Acid Profiling of Five Types of Cancer Patients and Its Application for Early Detection. *PLoS One* (2011) 6:e24143. doi: 10.1371/journal.pone.0024143

22. Weckwerth W, Morgenthal K. Metabolomics: From Pattern Recognition to Biological Interpretation. *Drug Discov Today* (2005) 10:1551–8. doi: 10.1016/S1359-6446(05)03609-3

23. Karayama M, Masuda J, Mori K, Yasui H, Hozumi H, Suzuki Y, et al. Comprehensive Assessment of Multiple Tryptophan Metabolites as Potential Biomarkers for Immune Checkpoint Inhibitors in Patients With Non-Small Cell Lung Cancer. *Clin Transl Oncol* (2021) 23(2):418–23. doi: 10.1007/s12094-020-02421-8

24. Ren YP, Tang AG, Zhou QX, Xiang ZY. Clinical Significance of Simultaneous Determination of Serum Tryptophan and Tyrosine in Patients With Lung Cancer. *J Clin Lab Anal* (2011) 25:246–50. doi: 10.1002/jcla.20467

25. Miyamoto S, Taylor SL, Barupal DK, Taguchi A, Wohlgemuth G, Wikoff WR, et al. Systemic Metabolomic Changes in Blood Samples of Lung Cancer Patients Identified by Gas Chromatography Time-of-Flight Mass Spectrometry. *Metabolites* (2015) 5:192–210. doi: 10.3390/metabo5020192

26. Nguyen DJM, Theodoropoulos G, Li YY, Wu C, Sha W, Feun LG, et al. Targeting the Kynurenine Pathway for the Treatment of Cisplatin-Resistant Lung Cancer. *Mol Cancer Res* (2020) 18:105–17. doi: 10.1158/1541-7786.MCR-19-0239

27. Munn DH, Mellor AL. Indoleamine 2,3-Dioxygenase and Tumor-Induced Tolerance. *J Clin Invest* (2007) 117:1147–54. doi: 10.1172/JCI31178

28. Pisters PW, Pearlstone DB. Protein and Amino Acid Metabolism in Cancer Cachexia: Investigative Techniques and Therapeutic Interventions. *Crit Rev Clin Lab Sci* (1993) 30:223–72. doi: 10.3109/10408369309084669

29. Shingyoji M, Iizasa T, Higashiyama M, Imamura F, Saruki N, Imaizumi A, et al. The Significance and Robustness of a Plasma Free Amino Acid (PFAA) Profile-Based Multiplex Function for Detecting Lung Cancer. *BMC Cancer* (2013) 13:77. doi: 10.1186/1471-2407-13-77

30. Jun M, Masahiko H, Akira I, Tomio N, Hiroshi Y, Takashi D, et al. Possibility of Multivariate Function Composed of Plasma Amino Acid Profiles as a Novel Screening Index for Non-Small Cell Lung Cancer: A Case Control Study. *BMC Cancer* (2010) 10:690. doi: 10.1186/1471-2407-10-690

31. Kim HJ, Jang SH, Ryu JS, Lee JE, Kim YC, Lee MK, et al. The Performance of a Novel Amino Acid Multivariate Index for Detecting Lung Cancer: A Case Control Study in Korea. *Lung Cancer* (2015) 90:522–7. doi: 10.1016/j.lungcan.2015.10.006

32. Ruiying C, Zeyun L, Yongliang Y, Zijia Z, Ji Z, Xin T, et al. A Comprehensive Analysis of Metabolomics and Transcriptomics in Non-Small Cell Lung Cancer. *PLoS One* (2020) 15:e0232272. doi: 10.1371/journal.pone.0232272

33. Munn DH, Sharma MD, Lee JR, Jhaver KG, Johnson TS, Keskin DB, et al. Potential Regulatory Function of Human Dendritic Cells Expressing Indoleamine 2,3-Dioxygenase. *Science* (2002) 297:1867–70. doi: 10.1126/science.1073514

34. Theate I, van Baren N, Pilotte L, Moulin P, Larrieu P, Renauld JC, et al. Extensive Profiling of the Expression of the Indoleamine 2,3-Dioxygenase 1 Protein in Normal and Tumoral Human Tissues. *Cancer Immunol Res* (2015) 3:161–72. doi: 10.1158/2326-6066.CIR-14-0137

35. Wang Y, Liu H, McKenzie G, Witting PK, Stasch JP, Hahn M, et al. Kynurenine Is an Endothelium-Derived Relaxing Factor Produced During Inflammation. *Nat Med* (2010) 16:279–85. doi: 10.1038/nm.2092

36. Karanikas V, Zamanakou M, Kerenidi T, Dahabreh J, Hevas A, Nakou M, et al. Indoleamine 2,3-Dioxygenase (IDO) Expression in Lung Cancer. *Cancer Biol Ther* (2007) 6:1258–62. doi: 10.4161/cbt.6.8.4446

37. Suzuki Y, Suda T, Furuhashi K, Suzuki M, Fujie M, Hahimoto D, et al. Increased Serum Kynurenine/Tryptophan Ratio Correlates With Disease Progression in Lung Cancer. *Lung Cancer* (2010) 67:361–5. doi: 10.1016/j.lungcan.2009.05.001

38. Chuang SC, Fanidi A, Ueland PM, Relton C, Midttun O, Vollset SE, et al. Circulating Biomarkers of Tryptophan and the Kynurenine Pathway and Lung Cancer Risk. *Cancer Epidemiol Biomarkers Prev* (2014) 23:461–8. doi: 10.1158/1055-9965.EPI-13-0770

39. Huang JY, Larose TL, Luu HN, Wang R, Fanidi A, Alcala K, et al. Circulating Markers of Cellular Immune Activation in Prediagnostic Blood Sample and

Lung Cancer Risk in the Lung Cancer Cohort Consortium (Lc3). *Int J Cancer* (2020) 146:2394–405. doi: 10.1002/ijc.32555

40. Tang D, Yue L, Yao R, Zhou L, Yang Y, Lu L, et al. P53 Prevent Tumor Invasion and Metastasis by Down-Regulating IDO in Lung Cancer. *Oncotarget* (2017) 8:54548–57. doi: 10.18632/oncotarget.17408

41. Levina V, Su Y, Gorelik E. Immunological and Nonimmunological Effects of Indoleamine 2,3-Dioxygenase on Breast Tumor Growth and Spontaneous Metastasis Formation. *Clin Dev Immunol* (2012) 2012:173029. doi: 10.1155/2012/173029

42. Smith C, Chang MY, Parker KH, Beury DW, DuHadaway JB, Flick HE, et al. IDO Is a Nodal Pathogenic Driver of Lung Cancer and Metastasis Development. *Cancer Discov* (2012) 2(8):722–35. doi: 10.1158/2159-8290.CD-12-0014

43. Schafer CC, Wang Y, Hough KP, Sawant A, Grant SC, Thannickal VJ, et al. Indoleamine 2,3-Dioxygenase Regulates Anti-Tumor Immunity in Lung Cancer by Metabolic Reprogramming of Immune Cells in the Tumor Microenvironment. *Oncotarget* (2016) 7:75407–24. doi: 10.18632/oncotarget.12249

44. Agullo-Ortuno MT, Gomez-Martin O, Ponce S, Iglesias L, Ojeda L, Ferrer I, et al. Blood Predictive Biomarkers for Patients With Non-Small-Cell Lung Cancer Associated With Clinical Response to Nivolumab. *Clin Lung Cancer* (2020) 21:75–85. doi: 10.1016/j.cllc.2019.08.006

45. Uyttenhove C, Pilotte L, Theate I, Stroobant V, Colau D, Parmentier N, et al. Evidence for a Tumoral Immune Resistance Mechanism Based on Tryptophan Degradation by Indoleamine 2,3-Dioxygenase. *Nat Med* (2003) 9:1269–74. doi: 10.1038/nm934

46. Zamanakou M, Germenis AE, Karanikas V. Tumor Immune Escape Mediated by Indoleamine 2,3-Dioxygenase. *Immunol Lett* (2007) 111:69–75. doi: 10.1016/j.imlet.2007.06.001

47. Wang Y, Hu GF, Wang ZH. The Status of Immunosuppression in Patients With Stage IIIB or IV Non-Small-Cell Lung Cancer Correlates With the Clinical Characteristics and Response to Chemotherapy. *Onco Targets Ther* (2017) 10:3557–66. doi: 10.2147/OTT.S136259

48. Wang W, Huang L, Jin JY, Pi W, Ellsworth SG, Jolly S, et al. A Validation Study on IDO Immune Biomarkers for Survival Prediction in Non-Small Cell Lung Cancer: Radiation Dose Fractionation Effect in Early-Stage Disease. *Clin Cancer Res* (2020) 26:282–9. doi: 10.1158/1078-0432.CCR-19-1202

49. Botticelli A, Mezi S, Pomati G, Cerbelli B, Cerbelli E, Roberto M, et al. Tryptophan Catabolism as Immune Mechanism of Primary Resistance to Anti-PD-1. *Front Immunol* (2020) 11:1243. doi: 10.3389/fimmu.2020.01243

50. Wang W, Huang L, Jin JY, Jolly S, Zang Y, Wu H, et al. IDO Immune Status After Chemoradiation May Predict Survival in Lung Cancer Patients. *Cancer Res* (2018) 78:809–16. doi: 10.1158/0008-5472.CAN-17-2995

51. Ma W, Duan H, Zhang R, Wang X, Xu H, Zhou Q, et al. High Expression of Indoleamine 2, 3-Dioxygenase in Adenosquamous Lung Carcinoma Correlates With Favorable Patient Outcome. *J Cancer* (2019) 10:267–76. doi: 10.7150/jca.27507

52. Löb S, Königsrainer A, Zieker D, Brücher BLDM, Rammensee H-G, Opelz G, et al. IDO1 and IDO2 Are Expressed in Human Tumors: Levo- But Not Dextro-1-Methyl Tryptophan Inhibits Tryptophan Catabolism. *Cancer Immunol Immunother* (2009) 58:153–7. doi: 10.1007/s00262-008-0513-6

53. Mandarano M, Bellezza G, Belladonna ML, Vannucci J, Gili A, Ferri I, et al. Indoleamine 2,3-Dioxygenase 2 Immunohistochemical Expression in Resected Human Non-Small Cell Lung Cancer: A Potential New Prognostic Tool. *Front Immunol* (2020) 11:839. doi: 10.3389/fimmu.2020.00839

54. Witkiewicz AK, Costantino CL, Metz R, Muller AJ, Prendergast GC, Yeo CJ, et al. Genotyping and Expression Analysis of IDO2 in Human Pancreatic Cancer: A Novel, Active Target. *J Am Coll Surg* (2009) 208(5):781–7. doi: 10.1016/j.jamcollsurg.2008.12.018

55. Michael P, Nikolaus VKD, Iris O, Wolfgang W, Katharina O. Cancer Immunotherapy by Targeting IDO1/TDO and Their Downstream Effectors. *Front Immunol* (2015) 5:673. doi: 10.3389/fimmu.2014.00673

56. Yuasa HJ, Mizuno K, Ball HJ. Low Efficiency IDO2 Enzymes Are Conserved in Lower Vertebrates, Whereas Higher Efficiency IDO1 Enzymes Are Dispensable. *FEBS J* (2015) 282:2735–45. doi: 10.1111/febs.13316

57. Fatokun AA, Hunt NH, Ball HJ. Indoleamine 2,3-Dioxygenase 2 (IDO2) and the Kynurenine Pathway: Characteristics and Potential Roles in Health and Disease. *Amino Acids* (2013) 45:1319–29. doi: 10.1007/s00726-013-1602-1

58. Yuasa HJ, Ball HJ, Ho YF, Austin CJ, Whittington CM, Belov K, et al. Characterization and Evolution of Vertebrate Indoleamine 2, 3-Dioxygenases IDOs From Monotremes and Marsupials. *Comp Biochem Physiol B Biochem Mol Biol* (2009) 153:137–44. doi: 10.1016/j.cbpb.2009.02.002

59. Jusof FF, Bakmiwewa SM, Weiser S, Too LK, Metz R, Prendergast GC, et al. Investigation of the Tissue Distribution and Physiological Roles of Indoleamine 2,3-Dioxygenase-2. *Int J Tryptophan Res* (2017) 10:1178646917735098. doi: 10.1177/1178646917735098

60. Cheong JE, Sun L. Targeting the IDO1/TDO2-KYN-AhR Pathway for Cancer Immunotherapy - Challenges and Opportunities. *Trends Pharmacol Sci* (2018) 39:307–25. doi: 10.1016/j.tips.2017.11.007

61. Moon PK, Tran S, Minhas PS. Revisiting IDO and Its Value As a Predictive Marker for Anti-PD-1 Resistance. *J Transl Med* (2019) 17:31. doi: 10.1186/s12967-019-1784-8

62. Platten M, Wick W, Van den Eynde BJ. Tryptophan Catabolism in Cancer: Beyond IDO and Tryptophan Depletion. *Cancer Res* (2012) 72:5435–40. doi: 10.1158/0008-5472.CAN-12-0569

63. Nicolas VB, Van den Eynde BJ. Tumoral Immune Resistance Mediated by Enzymes That Degrade Tryptophan. *Cancer Immunol Res* (2015) 3(9):978–85. doi: 10.1158/2326-6066.CIR-15-0095

64. Opitz CA, Litzenburger UM, Sahm F, Ott M, Tritschler I, Trump S, et al. An Endogenous Tumour-Promoting Ligand of the Human Aryl Hydrocarbon Receptor. *Nature* (2011) 478:197–203. doi: 10.1038/nature10491

65. Wikoff WR, Grapov D, Fahrmann JF, DeFelice B, Rom WN, Pass HI, et al. Metabolomic Markers of Altered Nucleotide Metabolism in Early Stage Adenocarcinoma. *Cancer Prev Res (Phila)* (2015) 8:410–8. doi: 10.1158/1940-6207.CAPR-14-0329

66. Novikov O, Wang Z, Stanford EA, Parks AJ, Ramirez-Cardenas A, Landesman E, et al. An Aryl Hydrocarbon Receptor-Mediated Amplification Loop That Enforces Cell Migration in ER-/PR-/Her2- Human Breast Cancer Cells. *Mol Pharmacol* (2016) 90:674–88. doi: 10.1124/mol.116.105361

67. Yamasuge W, Yamamoto Y, Fujigaki H, Hoshi M, Nakamoto K, Kunisawa K, et al. Indoleamine 2,3-Dioxygenase 2 Depletion Suppresses Tumor Growth in a Mouse Model of Lewis Lung Carcinoma. *Cancer Sci* (2019) 110:3061–7. doi: 10.1111/cas.14179

68. Hsu YL, Hung JY, Chiang SY, Jian SF, Wu CY, Lin YS, et al. Lung Cancer-Derived Galectin-1 Contributes to Cancer Associated Fibroblast-Mediated Cancer Progression and Immune Suppression Through TDO2/kynurenine Axis. *Oncotarget* (2016) 7:27584–98. doi: 10.18632/oncotarget.8488

69. Liu Y, Xu P, Liu H, Fang C, Guo H, Chen X, et al. Silencing IDO2 in Dendritic Cells: A Novel Strategy to Strengthen Cancer Immunotherapy in a Murine Lung Cancer Model. *Int J Oncol* (2020) 57:587–97. doi: 10.3892/ijo.2020.5073

70. Luo J, Solimini NL, Elledge SJ. Principles of Cancer Therapy: Oncogene and Non-Oncogene Addiction. *Cell* (2009) 136:823–37. doi: 10.1016/j.cell.2009.02.024

71. Prendergast GC. Immune Escape as a Fundamental Trait of Cancer: Focus on IDO. *Oncogene* (2008) 27(28):3889–900. doi: 10.1038/onc.2008.35

72. Jiang X, Wang J, Deng X, Xiong F, Ge J, Xiang B, et al. Role of the Tumor Microenvironment in PD-L1/PD-1-Mediated Tumor Immune Escape. *Mol Cancer* (2019) 18:10. doi: 10.1186/s12943-018-0928-4

73. Mellor AL, Munn DH. IDO Expression by Dendritic Cells: Tolerance and Tryptophan Catabolism. *Nat Rev Immunol* (2004) 4:762–74. doi: 10.1038/nri1457

74. Munn DH, Sharma MD, Baban B, Harding HP, Zhang Y, Ron D, et al. GCN2 Kinase in T Cells Mediates Proliferative Arrest and Anergy Induction in Response to Indoleamine 2,3-Dioxygenase. *Immunity* (2005) 22:633–42. doi: 10.1016/j.immuni.2005.03.013

75. Rodriguez PC, Quiceno DG, Ochoa AC. L-Arginine Availability Regulates T-Lymphocyte Cell-Cycle Progression. *Blood* (2007) 109:1568–73. doi: 10.1182/blood-2006-06-031856

76. Ravishankar B, Liu H, Shinde R, Chaudhary K, Xiao W, Bradley J, et al. The Amino Acid Sensor GCN2 Inhibits Inflammatory Responses to Apoptotic Cells Promoting Tolerance and Suppressing Systemic Autoimmunity. *Proc Natl Acad Sci USA* (2015) 112:10774–9. doi: 10.1073/pnas.1504276112

77. Fallarino F, Grohmann U, You S, McGrath BC, Cavener DR, Vacca C, et al. The Combined Effects of Tryptophan Starvation and Tryptophan

Catabolites Down-Regulate T Cell Receptor Zeta-Chain and Induce a Regulatory Phenotype in Naive T Cells. *J Immunol* (2006) 176:6752–61. doi: 10.4049/jimmunol.176.11.6752

78. Liu H, Huang L, Bradley J, Liu K, Bardhan K, Ron D, et al. GCN2-Dependent Metabolic Stress Is Essential for Endotoxemic Cytokine Induction and Pathology. *Mol Cell Biol* (2014) 34(3):428–38. doi: 10.1128/MCB.00946-13

79. Sonner JK, Deumelandt K, Ott M, Thomé CM, Rauschenbach KJ, Schulz S, et al. The Stress Kinase GCN2 Does Not Mediate Suppression of Antitumor T Cell Responses by Tryptophan Catabolism in Experimental Melanomas. *OncoImmunology* (2016) 5(12):e1240858. doi: 10.1080/2162402X.2016.1240858

80. Castilho BA, Shanmugam R, Silva RC, Ramesh R, Himme BM, Sattlegger E. Keeping the Eif2 Alpha Kinase Gcn2 in Check. *BBA - Mol Cell Res* (2014) 1843(9):1948–68. doi: 10.1016/j.bbamcr.2014.04.006

81. Metz R, Rust S, DuHadaway JB, Mautino MR, Munn DH, Vahanian NN, et al. IDO Inhibits a Tryptophan Sufficiency Signal That Stimulates mTOR: A Novel IDO Effector Pathway Targeted by D-1-Methyl-Tryptophan. *OncoImmunology* (2012) 1(9):1460–8. doi: 10.4161/onci.21716

82. Cobbold SP, Adams E, Farquhar CA, Nolan KF, Howie D, Lui KO, et al. Infectious Tolerance *via* the Consumption of Essential Amino Acids and mTOR Signaling. *Proc Natl Acad Sci USA* (2009) 106:12055–60. doi: 10.1073/pnas.0903919106

83. Johnson TS, Munn DH. Host Indoleamine 2,3-Dioxygenase: Contribution to Systemic Acquired Tumor Tolerance. *Immunol Invest* (2012) 41:765–97. doi: 10.3109/08820139.2012.689405

84. Mezrich JD, Fechner JH, Zhang X, Johnson BP, Burlingham WJ, Bradfield CA. An Interaction Between Kynurenine and the Aryl Hydrocarbon Receptor can Generate Regulatory T Cells. *J Immunol (Baltimore Md.: 1950)* (2010) 185(6):3190–8. doi: 10.4049/jimmunol.0903670

85. Quintana FJ, Murugaiyan G, Farez MF, Mitsdoerffer M, Tukpah AM, Burns EJ, et al. An Endogenous Aryl Hydrocarbon Receptor Ligand Acts on Dendritic Cells and T Cells to Suppress Experimental Autoimmune Encephalomyelitis. *Proc Natl Acad Sci USA* (2010) 107:20768–73. doi: 10.1073/pnas.1009201107

86. Jaronen M, Quintana FJ. Immunological Relevance of the Coevolution of IDO1 and AHR. *Front Immunol* (2014) 5:521. doi: 10.3389/fimmu.2014.00521

87. Manlapat AK, Kahler DJ, Chandler PR, Munn DH, Mellor AL. Cell-Autonomous Control of Interferon Type I Expression by Indoleamine 2,3-Dioxygenase in Regulatory CD19+ Dendritic Cells. *Eur J Immunol* (2007) 37:1064–71. doi: 10.1002/eji.200636690

88. Fallarino F, Grohmann U, Vacca C, Bianchi R, Orabona C, Spreca A, et al. T Cell Apoptosis by Tryptophan Catabolism. *Cell Death Differ* (2002) 9:1069–77. doi: 10.1038/sj.cdd.4401073

89. Frumento G, Rotondo R, Tonetti M, Damonte G, Benatti U, Ferrara GB. Tryptophan-Derived Catabolites Are Responsible for Inhibition of T and Natural Killer Cell Proliferation Induced by Indoleamine 2,3-Dioxygenase. *J Exp Med* (2002) 196:459–68. doi: 10.1084/jem.20020121

90. Gargaro M, Vacca C, Massari S, Scalisi G, Manni G, Mondanelli G, et al. Engagement of Nuclear Coactivator 7 by 3-Hydroxyanthranilic Acid Enhances Activation of Aryl Hydrocarbon Receptor in Immunoregulatory Dendritic Cells. *Front Immunol* (2019) 10:1973. doi: 10.3389/fimmu.2019.01973

91. Dubinett S, Sharma S. Towards Effective Immunotherapy for Lung Cancer: Simultaneous Targeting of Tumor-Initiating Cells and Immune Pathways in the Tumor Microenvironment. *Immunotherapy* (2009) 1:721–5. doi: 10.2217/imt.09.56

92. Halak BK, Maguire HCJr, Lattime EC. Tumor-Induced Interleukin-10 Inhibits Type 1 Immune Responses Directed at a Tumor Antigen as Well as a Non-Tumor Antigen Present at the Tumor Site. *Cancer Res* (1999) 59(4):911–7.

93. Labadie BW, Bao R, Luke JJ. Reimagining IDO Pathway Inhibition in Cancer Immunotherapy *via* Downstream Focus on the Tryptophan-Kynurenine-Aryl Hydrocarbon Axis. *Clin Cancer Res* (2019) 25:1462–71. doi: 10.1158/1078-0432.CCR-18-2882

94. DiNatale BC, Murray IA, Schroeder JC, Flaveny CA, Lahoti TS, Laurenzana EM, et al. Kynurenic Acid Is a Potent Endogenous Aryl Hydrocarbon Receptor Ligand That Synergistically Induces Interleukin-6 in the Presence of Inflammatory Signaling. *Toxicol Sci* (2010) 115:89–97. doi: 10.1093/toxsci/kfq024

95. Seok SH, Ma ZX, Feltenberger JB, Chen H, Chen H, Scarlett C, et al. Trace Derivatives of Kynurenine Potently Activate the Aryl Hydrocarbon Receptor (AHR). *J Biol Chem* (2018) 293:1994–2005. doi: 10.1074/jbc.RA117.000631

96. Takenaka MC, Quintana FJ. Tolerogenic Dendritic Cells. *Semin Immunopathol* (2017) 39:113–20. doi: 10.1007/s00281-016-0587-8

97. Li Q, Harden JL, Anderson CD, Egilmez NK. Tolerogenic Phenotype of IFN-γ-Induced IDO+ Dendritic Cells Is Maintained *via* an Autocrine IDO-Kynurenine/AhR-IDO Loop. *J Immunol* (2016) 197:962–70. doi: 10.4049/jimmunol.1502615

98. Nguyen NT, Kimura A, Nakahama T, Chinen I, Masuda K, Nohara K, et al. Aryl Hydrocarbon Receptor Negatively Regulates Dendritic Cell Immunogenicity *via* a Kynurenine-Dependent Mechanism. *Proc Natl Acad Sci USA* (2010) 107:19961–6. doi: 10.1073/pnas.1014465107

99. Prendergast GC, Malachowski WP, DuHadaway JB, Muller AJ. Discovery of IDO1 Inhibitors: From Bench to Bedside. *Cancer Res* (2017) 77:6795–811. doi: 10.1158/0008-5472.CAN-17-2285

100. Liu KT, Liu YH, Liu HL, Chong IW, Yen MC, Kuo PL. Neutrophils Are Essential in Short Hairpin RNA of Indoleamine 2,3- Dioxygenase Mediated-Antitumor Efficiency. *Mol Ther Nucleic Acids* (2016) 5:e397. doi: 10.1038/mtna.2016.105

101. Munn DH, Mellor AL. IDO and Tolerance to Tumors. *Trends Mol Med* (2004) 10:15–8. doi: 10.1016/j.molmed.2003.11.003

102. Hou DY, Muller AJ, Sharma MD, DuHadaway J, Banerjee T, Johnson M, et al. Inhibition of Indoleamine 2,3-Dioxygenase in Dendritic Cells by Stereoisomers of 1-Methyl-Tryptophan Correlates With Antitumor Responses. *Cancer Res* (2007) 67:792–801. doi: 10.1158/0008-5472.CAN-06-2925

103. Hellmann MD, Gettinger S, Chow LQM, Gordon M, Awad MM, Cha E, et al. Phase 1 Study of Epacadostat in Combination With Atezolizumab for Patients With Previously Treated Advanced Nonsmall Cell Lung Cancer. *Int J Cancer* (2020) 147:1963–9. doi: 10.1002/ijc.32951

104. Mitchell TC, Hamid O, Smith DC, Bauer TM, Wasser JS, Olszanski AJ, et al. Epacadostat Plus Pembrolizumab in Patients With Advanced Solid Tumors: Phase I Results From a Multicenter, Open-Label Phase I/II Trial (ECHO-202/KEYNOTE-037). *J Clin Oncol* (2018) 36:3223–30. doi: 10.1200/JCO.2018.78.9602

105. Muller AJ, Manfredi MG, Zakharia Y, Prendergast GC. Inhibiting IDO Pathways to Treat Cancer: Lessons From the ECHO-301 Trial and Beyond. *Semin Immunopathol* (2019) 41:41–8. doi: 10.1007/s00281-018-0702-0

106. Liu M, Wang X, Wang L, Ma X, Gong Z, Zhang S, et al. Targeting the IDO1 Pathway in Cancer: From Bench to Bedside. *J Hematol Oncol* (2018) 11:100. doi: 10.1186/s13045-018-0644-y

107. Jung KH, LoRusso P, Burris H, Gordon M, Bang YJ, Hellmann MD, et al. Phase I Study of the Indoleamine 2,3-Dioxygenase 1 (IDO1) Inhibitor Navoximod (GDC-0919) Administered With PD-L1 Inhibitor (Atezolizumab) in Advanced Solid Tumors. *Clin Cancer Res* (2019) 25:3220–8. doi: 10.1158/1078-0432.CCR-18-2740

108. Gyulveszi G, Fischer C, Mirolo M, Stern M, Green L, Ceppi M, et al. Abstract LB-085: RG70099: A Novel, Highly Potent Dual IDO1/TDO Inhibitor to Reverse Metabolic Suppression of Immune Cells in the Tumor Micro-Environment. *Cancer Res* (2016) 76(14_Supplement):LB-085. doi: 10.1158/1538-7445.AM2016-LB-085

109. Cortellini A, Ricciuti B, Tiseo M, Bria E, Banna GL, Aerts JG, et al. Baseline BMI and BMI Variation During First Line Pembrolizumab in NSCLC Patients With a PD-L1 Expression >/= 50%: A Multicenter Study With External Validation. *J Immunother Cancer* (2020) 8(2):e001403. doi: 10.1136/jitc-2020-001403

110. Perrone F, Minari R, Bersanelli M, Bordi P, Tiseo M, Favari E, et al. The Prognostic Role of High Blood Cholesterol in Advanced Cancer Patients Treated With Immune Checkpoint Inhibitors. *J Immunother* (2020) 43:196–203. doi: 10.1097/cji.0000000000000321

111. Cantini L, Pecci F, Hurkmans DP, Belderbos RA, Lanese A, Copparoni C, et al. High-Intensity Statins Are Associated With Improved Clinical Activity of PD-1 Inhibitors in Malignant Pleural Mesothelioma and Advanced Non-Small Cell Lung Cancer Patients. *Eur J Cancer* (2021) 144:41–8. doi: 10.1016/j.ejca.2020.10.031

112. Liu W, Wang Y, Luo J, Liu M, Luo Z. Pleiotropic Effects of Metformin on the Antitumor Efficiency of Immune Checkpoint Inhibitors. *Front Immunol* (2020) 11:586760. doi: 10.3389/fimmu.2020.586760

113. Afzal MZ, Dragnev K, Sarwar T, Shirai K. Clinical Outcomes in non-Small-Cell Lung Cancer Patients Receiving Concurrent Metformin and Immune Checkpoint Inhibitors. *Lung Cancer Manag* (2019) 8:LMT11. doi: 10.2217/lmt-2018-0016

114. Scharping NE, Menk AV, Whetstone RD, Zeng X, Delgoffe GM. Efficacy of PD-1 Blockade Is Potentiated by Metformin-Induced Reduction of Tumor Hypoxia. *Cancer Immunol Res* (2017) 5:9–16. doi: 10.1158/2326-6066.Cir-16-0103

115. Fatehi Hassanabad A. Current Perspectives on Statins as Potential Anti-Cancer Therapeutics: Clinical Outcomes and Underlying Molecular Mechanisms. *Transl Lung Cancer Res* (2019) 8:692–9. doi: 10.21037/tlcr.2019.09.08

116. Prodinger J, Loacker LJ, Schmidt RL, Ratzinger F, Greiner G, Witzeneder N, et al. The Tryptophan Metabolite Picolinic Acid Suppresses Proliferation and Metabolic Activity of CD4+ T Cells and Inhibits C-Myc Activation. *J Leukoc Biol* (2016) 99:583–94. doi: 10.1189/jlb.3A0315-135R

117. Wirthgen E, Hoeflich A, Rebl A, Gunther J. Kynurenic Acid: The Janus-Faced Role of an Immunomodulatory Tryptophan Metabolite and Its Link to Pathological Conditions. *Front Immunol* (2017) 8:1957. doi: 10.3389/fimmu.2017.01957

Permissions

The contributors of this book come from diverse backgrounds, making this book a truly international effort. This book will bring forth new frontiers with its revolutionizing research information and detailed analysis of the nascent developments around the world.

We would like to thank all the contributing authors for lending their expertise to make the book truly unique. They have played a crucial role in the development of this book. Without their invaluable contributions this book wouldn't have been possible. They have made vital efforts to compile up to date information on the varied aspects of this subject to make this book a valuable addition to the collection of many professionals and students.

This book was conceptualized with the vision of imparting up-to-date information and advanced data in this field. To ensure the same, a matchless editorial board was set up. Every individual on the board went through rigorous rounds of assessment to prove their worth. After which they invested a large part of their time researching and compiling the most relevant data for our readers.

The editorial board has been involved in producing this book since its inception. They have spent rigorous hours researching and exploring the diverse topics which have resulted in the successful publishing of this book. They have passed on their knowledge of decades through this book. To expedite this challenging task, the publisher supported the team at every step. A small team of assistant editors was also appointed to further simplify the editing procedure and attain best results for the readers.

Apart from the editorial board, the designing team has also invested a significant amount of their time in understanding the subject and creating the most relevant covers. They scrutinized every image to scout for the most suitable representation of the subject and create an appropriate cover for the book.

The publishing team has been an ardent support to the editorial, designing and production team. Their endless efforts to recruit the best for this project, has resulted in the accomplishment of this book. They are a veteran in the field of academics and their pool of knowledge is as vast as their experience in printing. Their expertise and guidance has proved useful at every step. Their uncompromising quality standards have made this book an exceptional effort. Their encouragement from time to time has been an inspiration for everyone.

The publisher and the editorial board hope that this book will prove to be a valuable piece of knowledge for researchers, students, practitioners and scholars across the globe.

List of Contributors

Freek J. H. Sorgdrager
European Research Institute for the Biology of Ageing, University Medical Center Groningen, University of Groningen, Groningen, Netherlands
Laboratory of Neurochemistry and Behavior, Department of Biomedical Sciences, Institute Born-Bunge, University of Antwerp, Antwerp, Belgium
Department of Neurology and Alzheimer Center, University Medical Center Groningen, University of Groningen, Groningen, Netherlands
Department of Laboratory Medicine, University Medical Center Groningen, University of Groningen, Groningen, Netherlands

Petrus J. W. Naudé
Department of Neurology and Alzheimer Center, University Medical Center Groningen, University of Groningen, Groningen, Netherlands
Department of Molecular Neurobiology, Groningen Institute for Evolutionary Life Sciences (GELIFES), University of Groningen, Groningen, Netherlands

Ido P. Kema
Department of Laboratory Medicine, University Medical Center Groningen, University of Groningen, Groningen, Netherlands

Ellen A. Nollen
European Research Institute for the Biology of Ageing, University Medical Center Groningen, University of Groningen, Groningen, Netherlands

Peter P. De Deyn
Laboratory of Neurochemistry and Behavior, Department of Biomedical Sciences, Institute Born-Bunge, University of Antwerp, Antwerp, Belgium
Department of Neurology and Alzheimer Center, University Medical Center Groningen, University of Groningen, Groningen, Netherlands
Department of Neurology, Memory Clinic of Hospital Network Antwerp (ZNA) Middelheim and Hoge Beuken, Antwerp, Belgium

Soumya R. Mohapatra
DKTK Brain Cancer Metabolism Group, German Cancer Research Center (DKFZ), Heidelberg, Germany

Ahmed Sadik
DKTK Brain Cancer Metabolism Group, German Cancer Research Center (DKFZ), Heidelberg, Germany
Faculty of Bioscience, Heidelberg University, Heidelberg, Germany

Lars-Oliver Tykocinski
Division of Rheumatology, Department of Medicine V, University Hospital of Heidelberg, Heidelberg, Germany

Jørn Dietze and Ines Heiland
Department of Arctic and Marine Biology, UiT The Arctic University of Norway, Tromsø, Norway

Gernot Poschet
Centre for Organismal Studies (COS), University of Heidelberg, Heidelberg, Germany

Christiane A. Opitz
DKTK Brain Cancer Metabolism Group, German Cancer Research Center (DKFZ), Heidelberg, Germany
Neurology Clinic and National Center for Tumor Diseases, University Hospital of Heidelberg, Heidelberg, Germany

Claudio Costantini, Marina M. Bellet, Giorgia Renga, Claudia Stincardini, Monica Borghi, Marilena Pariano, Barbara Cellini, Luigina Romani and Teresa Zelante
Department of Experimental Medicine, University of Perugia, Perugia, Italy

Nancy Keller
Department of Medical Microbiology and Immunology, Department of Bacteriology, University of Wisconsin-Madison, Madison, WI, United States

Lorenzo Gaetani and Massimiliano Di Filippo
Section of Neurology, Department of Medicine, University of Perugia, Perugia, Italy

Francesca Boscaro and Giuseppe Pieraccini
Mass Spectrometry Centre (CISM), Department of Health Sciences, University of Florence, Florence, Italy

Paolo Calabresi
Section of Neurology, Department of Neuroscience, Agostino Gemelli Hospital, Catholic University of the Sacred Heart, Rome, Italy

John R. Moffett, Peethambaran Arun, Narayanan Puthillathu, Ranjini Vengilote and Aryan M. Namboodiri
Departments of Anatomy, Physiology and Genetics and Neuroscience Program, Uniformed Services University Medical School, Bethesda, MD, United States

Luigina Romani and Teresa Zelante
Department of Experimental Medicine, University of Perugia, Perugia, Italy

John A. Ives
The Center for Brain, Mind, and Healing, Samueli Institute, Alexandria, VA, United States

Abdulla A-B Badawy
Independent Consultant, Cardiff, United Kingdom

Giorgia Manni, Giada Mondanelli, Giulia Scalisi, Maria Teresa Pallotta, Dario Nardi, Eleonora Padiglioni, Rita Romani, Vincenzo Nicola Talesa, Paolo Puccetti, Francesca Fallarino and Marco Gargaro
Department of Experimental Medicine, University of Perugia, Perugia, Italy

Livia De Picker, Violette Coppens, Bernard Sabbe and Manuel Morrens
Faculty of Medicine and Health Sciences, Collaborative Antwerp Psychiatric Research Institute, University of Antwerp, Antwerp, Belgium
University Department of Psychiatry, Campus Duffel, Antwerp, Belgium

Erik Fransen
StatUa Center for Statistics, University of Antwerp, Antwerp, Belgium

Maarten Timmers
Janssen Research and Development, Janssen Pharmaceutica N.V., Beerse, Belgium
Reference Center for Biological Markers of Dementia (BIODEM), Institute Born-Bunge, University of Antwerp, Antwerp, Belgium

Peter de Boer
Janssen Research and Development, Janssen Pharmaceutica N.V., Beerse, Belgium

Herbert Oberacher
Core Facility Metabolomics, Institute of Legal Medicine, Medical University of Innsbruck, Innsbruck, Austria

Dietmar Fuchs
Biocenter, Division of Biological Chemistry, Medical University of Innsbruck, Innsbruck, Austria

Robert Verkerk
Department of Pharmaceutical Sciences, University of Antwerp, Antwerp, Belgium

Hanna Kehnscherper, Julia Gesche, Nina Irmscher, Christian Junghanss and Claudia Maletzki
Medical Clinic III - Hematology, Oncology, Palliative Care, Department of Internal Medicine, Rostock University Medical Center, Rostock, Germany

Christin Riess
University Children's Hospital, Rostock University Medical Centre, Rostock, Germany
Institute for Medical Microbiology, Virology, and Hygiene, Rostock University Medical Centre, Rostock, Germany
Medical Clinic III - Hematology, Oncology, Palliative Care, Department of Internal Medicine, Rostock University Medical Center, Rostock, Germany

Björn Schneider and Annette Zimpfer
Institute of Pathology, Rostock University Medical Center, University of Rostock, Rostock, Germany

Fatemeh Shokraie, Carl Friedrich Classen and Elisa Wirthgen
University Children's Hospital, Rostock University Medical Centre, Rostock, Germany

Grazyna Domanska
Institute of Immunology and Transfusion Medicine, University of Greifswald, Greifswald, Germany

Daniel Strüder
Department of Otorhinolaryngology, Head and Neck Surgery "Otto Koerner", Rostock University Medical Center, Rostock, Germany

Takumi Kudo
DKTK CCU Neuroimmunology and Brain Tumor Immunology, German Cancer Research Center (DKFZ), Heidelberg, Germany
Department of Neurology, Medical Faculty Mannheim, Heidelberg University, Mannheim, Germany
Department of Neurosurgery, Tokyo Medical and Dental University, Tokyo, Japan

Mirja T. Prentzell and Soumya R. Mohapatra
DKTK Brain Cancer Metabolism Group, German Cancer Research Center (DKFZ), Heidelberg, Germany

Felix Sahm
DKTK CCU Neuroimmunology and Brain Tumor Immunology, German Cancer Research Center (DKFZ), Heidelberg, Germany
Department of Neuropathology, Institute of Pathology, University Hospital Heidelberg, Heidelberg, Germany

Zhongliang Zhao and Ingrid Grummt
DKTK Division Molecular Biology of the Cell, German Cancer Research Center (DKFZ), Heidelberg, Germany

Wolfgang Wick
DKTK CCU Neurooncology, German Cancer Research Center (DKFZ), Heidelberg, Germany
Neurology Clinic and National Center for Tumor Diseases, University Hospital of Heidelberg, Heidelberg, Germany

Christiane A. Opitz
DKTK Brain Cancer Metabolism Group, German Cancer Research Center (DKFZ), Heidelberg, Germany
Neurology Clinic and National Center for Tumor Diseases, University Hospital of Heidelberg, Heidelberg, Germany

Michael Platten and Edward W. Green
DKTK CCU Neuroimmunology and Brain Tumor Immunology, German Cancer Research Center (DKFZ), Heidelberg, Germany
Department of Neurology, Medical Faculty Mannheim, Heidelberg University, Mannheim, Germany

Sofia Cussotto, Inês Delgado, Sandra Dexpert, Agnès Aubert and Lucile Capuron
University of Bordeaux, INRAE, Bordeaux INP, NutriNeuro, UMR 1286, Bordeaux, France

Andrea Anesi
Department of Food Quality and Nutrition, Research and Innovation Centre, Fondazione Edmund Mach (FEM), San Michele all'Adige, Italy

Cédric Beau, Damien Forestier, Patrick Ledaguenel and Eric Magne
Service de Chirurgie Digestive et Parietale, Clinique Tivoli, Bordeaux, and Clinique Jean Villar, Bruges, France

Fulvio Mattivi
Department of Food Quality and Nutrition, Research and Innovation Centre, Fondazione Edmund Mach (FEM), San Michele all'Adige, Italy
Department of Cellular, Computational and Integrative Biology (CIBIO), University of Trento, Trento, Italy

Fanni A. Boros
Department of Neurology, Faculty of Medicine, Albert Szent-Györgyi Clinical Center, University of Szeged, Szeged, Hungary

László Vécsei
Department of Neurology, Faculty of Medicine, Albert Szent-Györgyi Clinical Center, University of Szeged, Szeged, Hungary
MTA-SZTE Neuroscience Research Group of the Hungarian Academy of Sciences, University of Szeged, Szeged, Hungary
Department of Neurology, Interdisciplinary Excellence Centre, University of Szeged, Szeged, Hungary

Juliane Günther
Research Group Epigenetics, Metabolism and Longevity, Leibniz Institute for Farm Animal Biology, Dummerstorf, Germany

Jan Däbritz and Elisa Wirthgen
Department of Pediatrics, Rostock University Medical Center, Rostock, Germany

Yi-Shu Huang, Joy Ogbechi, Felix I. Clanchy, Richard O. Williams and Trevor W. Stone
The Kennedy Institute of Rheumatology, NDORMS, University of Oxford, Oxford, United Kingdom

Yvette Mándi, Valéria Endrész, Timea Mosolygó, Katalin Burián and Ildikó Lantos
Department of Medical Microbiology and Immunobiology, University of Szeged, Szeged, Hungary

Ferenc Fülöp, István Szatmári and Bálint Lőrinczi
Institute of Pharmaceutical Chemistry and Research Group for Stereochemistry, Hungarian Academy of Sciences, University of Szeged, Szeged, Hungary

Attila Balog
Department of Rheumatology and Immunology, University of Szeged, Szeged, Hungary

Lukas Lanser, Patricia Kink, Eva Maria Egger, Guenter Weiss and Katharina Kurz
Department of Internal Medicine II, Medical University of Innsbruck, Innsbruck, Austria

Wolfgang Willenbacher
Department of Internal Medicine V, Medical University of Innsbruck, Innsbruck, Austria
Oncotyrol Centre for Personalized Cancer Medicine, Medical University of Innsbruck, Innsbruck, Austria

Dietmar Fuchs
Division of Biological Chemistry, Biocenter, Medical University of Innsbruck, Innsbruck, Austria

Elisa Wirthgen
Department of Pediatrics, Rostock University Medical Center, Rostock, Germany

Anne K. Leonard
Institute of Biochemistry, University Medicine Greifswald, Greifswald, Germany

Christian Scharf
Department of Otorhinolaryngology, Head and Neck Surgery, University Medicine Greifswald, Greifswald, Germany

Grazyna Domanska
Institute of Immunology and Transfusion Medicine, University Medicine Greifswald, Greifswald, Germany

Imane Nafia, Doriane Bortolotto, Assia Chaibi, Dominique Bodet, Christophe Rey, Loïc Cerf and Alban Bessede
Explicyte Immuno-Oncology, Bordeaux, France

Maud Toulmonde, Valerie Velasco, Claire B. Larmonier and François Le Loarer
Department of Medical Oncology, Institut Bergonié, Bordeaux, France

Julien Adam
Department of Pathology, Gustave Roussy, Villejuif, France

Ariel Savina
Institut Roche, Paris, France

Antoine Italiano
Department of Medical Oncology, Institut Bergonié, Bordeaux, France
Inserm U1218, Bordeaux, France

Sara Crotti and Chiara Bedin
Nano-Inspired Biomedicine Laboratory, Institute of Paediatric Research—Città della Speranza, Padua, Italy

Alessandra Fraccaro and Valerio Di Marco
Department of Chemical Sciences, University of Padua, Padua, Italy

Antonella Bertazzo
Department of Pharmaceutical and Pharmacological Sciences, University of Padua, Padua, Italy

Salvatore Pucciarelli
First Surgical Clinic Section, Department of Surgical, Oncological and Gastroenterological Sciences, University of Padua, Padua, Italy

Marco Agostini
Nano-Inspired Biomedicine Laboratory, Institute of Paediatric Research—Città della Speranza, Padua, Italy
First Surgical Clinic Section, Department of Surgical, Oncological and Gastroenterological Sciences, University of Padua, Padua, Italy

Chenwei Li
Department of Respiratory Medicine, The Second Affiliated Hospital of Dalian Medical University, Dalian, China

Hui Zhao
Department of Health Examination Center, The Second Affiliated Hospital of Dalian Medical University, Dalian, China

Index

Printed in the USA
CPSIA information can be obtained
at www.ICGtesting.com
JSHW051623061123
51533JS00005B/85